D1558651

Also by Herbert Weinstock

TCHAIKOVSKY
(1943)

CHOPIN: THE MAN AND HIS MUSIC
(1949)

DONIZETTI AND THE WORLD OF OPERA IN ITALY, PARIS, AND
VIENNA IN THE FIRST HALF OF THE NINETEENTH CENTURY
(1963)

VINCENZO BELLINI: HIS LIFE AND HIS OPERAS
(1971)

Collaborations with Wallace Brockway:

MEN OF MUSIC: THEIR LIVES, TIMES, AND ACHIEVEMENTS
(1939; second edition, revised, 1950)

THE WORLD OF OPERA
(1962; a second edition, revise, of *The Opera,* 1941)

ROSSINI:
A Biography

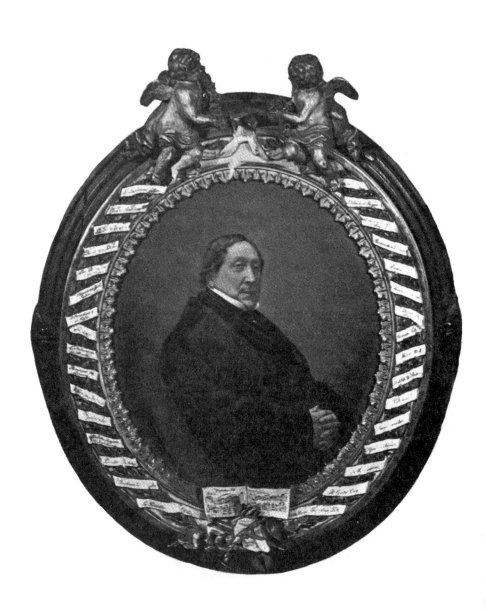

ROSSINI

A BIOGRAPHY

by

Herbert Weinstock

LIMELIGHT EDITIONS
NEW YORK
1987

First Limelight Edition April 1987

Copyright © 1968 by Herbert Weinstock
Reprinted by arrangement with Alfred A. Knopf, Inc.

Library of Congress Cataloging-in-Publication Data

Weinstock, Herbert, 1905–
Rossini, a biography.

Reprint. Originally published:
New York: Knopf, 1968.
Bibliography: p.
Includes index.
1. Rossini, Gioacchino, 1792–1868.   2. Composers—
Biography.   I. Title.
ML410.R8W35   1987   780'.92'4 [B]   87-2588
ISBN 0-87910-071-0
ISBN 0-87910-102-4 (pbk.)

For Ben Meiselman

Acknowledgments

FOR MANY INVALUABLE ACTS of kindness and for essential assistance in assembling the materials for this book, and then in writing it, I am consciously indebted to a very large number of people. I want especially to thank Mr. William Ashbrook, Terre Haute, Indiana; Dr. Guglielmo Barblan, Milan; Mr. Harold M. Barnes, Paris; Professore Francesco Bossarelli, Naples; Dr. and Mrs. Alfredo Bonaccorsi, Florence; Mlle Hélène Boschot, Paris; Mr. Wallace Brockway, New York; Mr. Giorgio Camici, Paris; Mr. Harry Cardello, New Hyde Park, New York; Mme Marthe Cudell, Brussels; Dr. Victor de Sabata, Jr., Milan; Mme Monique de Smet, Louvain; Mr. Vincent de Sola, New York; Dr. Luigi Elleni, Forlì; Dr. Napoleone Fanti, Bologna; Dr. Richard J. Fauliso, Hartford, Connecticut; M. V. Fédorov, Paris; Mr. Richard Franko Goldman, New York; Mr. Patrick Gregory, New York; Mr. Cecil Hopkinson, London; Mr. Charles Jahant, Landover Hills, Maryland; Mr. Alfred A. Knopf, New York; Mr. Terry McEwen, New York; Dr. Leslie A. Marchand, New Brunswick, New Jersey; Mrs. Elinore J. Marvel, New York; Professore Giovanni Masiello and Professoressa Dina Zanetti Masiello, Rome; Mr. Ben Meiselman, New York; Mrs. Esther Mendelsohn, New York; Mr. Richard Miller, New York; Dr. and Mrs. Hans Moldenhauer, Spokane, Washington; Professoressa Anna Mondolfi, Naples; Mr. Sam Morgenstern, New York; Mr. Andrew Porter, London; Dr. Dante Raiteri, Florence; Mr. Paul C. Richards, Brookline, Massachusetts; Mr. Irving Schwerké, Appleton, Wisconsin; Mr. Walter Talevi, Rome; Mr. Virgil Thomson, New York; Mr. Floriano Vecchi, New York; Signorina Renata Vercesi, Milan; Dr. Walter Vichi, Forlì; Mr. Edward N. Waters. Washington, D.C.; and Mr. William Weaver, Monte San Savino. To many others—friends, correspondents, people met casually—I express gratitude that is no less sincere because necesarily expressed without the publication of their very numerous names.

In addition to the unpurchasable assistance received from librarians mentioned above, I received invaluable help from generous individuals in the following libraries: Bologna (the Conservatorio G. B. Martini); Brussels (the Conservatoire Royal de Musique); Forlì (the Raccolta Piancastelli in the Biblioteca Comunale); Florence (the Biblioteca Nazionale and the Conservatorio Luigi Cherubini); Milan (the Conservatorio Giuseppe Verdi); Naples (the Conservatorio San Pietro a Maiella); New York (the New York Public Library); Paris (the Bibliothèque Nationale, the Bibliothèque de l'Opéra, and the library of the Conservatoire de Musique); Rome (the Biblioteca Nazionale and the Conservatorio di Santa Cecilia); and Washington, D.C. (the Library of Congress).

—HERBERT WEINSTOCK

Contents

Illustrations

The Teatro alla Scala, Milan, about 1812 (photograph from the Museo Teatrale alla Scala, Milan)

Domenico Donzelli, portrait in the Museo Donizettiano, Bergamo (photograph by Lucchetti, Bergamo)

Giuditta Pasta in the title role of *Tancredi*, portrait in the Rossini birthplace, Pesaro

Geltrude Righetti-Giorgi, the first Rosina (from Giuseppe Radiciotti's *Gioacchino Rossini*)

Gilbert-Louis Duprez as Arnold in *Guillaume Tell*, portrait in the Rossini birthplace, Pesaro

An original stage-set painting for *Aureliano in Palmira*, La Scala, 1813 (photograph from the Museo Teatrale alla Scala, Milan)

An original stage-set design for *La Gazza ladra*, 1817 (photograph from the Museo Teatrale alla Scala, Milan)

Domenico Barbaja, portrait in the Museo Teatrale alla Scala, Milan (photograph from there)

Olympe Pélissier (from Giuseppe Radiciotti's *Gioacchino Rossini*)

FOLLOWING PAGE 280

Rossini, sketch by Guglielmo De Sanctis, 1862 (from Giuseppe Radiciotti's *Gioacchino Rossini*)

Rossini, portrait by Ary Scheffer, 1843 (from Giuseppe Radiciotti's *Gioacchino Rossini*)

Rossini about 1858, photograph by Nadar in the Conservatoire Royal de Musique, Brussels (photograph by W. Broes, Brussels)

Wall of memorial room in the Conservatorio Rossini, Pesaro, with original deathbed sketch of Rossini by Gustave Doré (from a postcard)

Rossini about 1860 (photograph by Numa Blanc in the author's collection)

Rossini in 1864, marble medallion by H. Chevalier (from Alexis-Jacob Azevedo's *G. Rossini*)

Introduction

"To the best of my belief there is no demand whatever for a life of Rossini in English"—thus the late Francis Toye. When Toye's *Rossini: A Study in Tragi-Comedy* was first published in London in 1934, Rossini was regarded outside Italy as the psychologically puzzling composer of one comic opera and some bouncing, melodious overtures. *Il Barbiere di Siviglia*, an aging if not senile opera, was kept in the repertoire of opera houses chiefly to provide pretty, agile sopranos (who should not have been singing its Rosina at all) with another pretext for enjoyable, reprehensible *fioriture*, tenors with an opportunity to display heart-twanging tones in cantilena, and assorted other singers with established license to overplay roles debased from Beaumarchais. The only Rossini opera then being heard at all, *Il Barbiere* was seldom heard as Rossini had composed it.

The operatic scene has changed since 1934. After the Second World War, pre-Verdi Italian operas of the early nineteenth century, most notably the works of Rossini, Donizetti, and Bellini, began to emerge from the sound-deadening mists in which they had remained hidden. Increasingly, Rossini was heard. Now he has begun to be viewed not merely as the concocter of one *opera buffa* and a sheaf of overtures, but, somewhat less fragmentarily, also as the begetter of several whole *opere buffe* and even, on occasion, of noncomic music in addition to the *Stabat Mater*. As against Mr. Toye's wry confession of 1934, my own belief is that some "demand" may now exist for a life of Rossini in English.

Mr. Toye's was the only appreciable biography of the "Swan of Pesaro" to be written and published in English in this century.* Blessedly well written, it was based largely upon the standard biography in Italian, Giuseppe Radiciotti's three-volume *Gioacchino Rossini: Vita documentata, opere ed influenze su l'arte* (Tivoli, 1927–9). Any later writer on Rossini must contract a very large debt to the patient, scrupulous Radiciotti. But that debt must be contracted cautiously. Mr. Toye con-

sulted those three imposing volumes (1,431 large pages) too unques-
tioningly and appears not to have gone outside them to primary sources.
His book seldom can be faulted for its presentation of the more traditionally received aspects of Rossini's life, character, and art. But count-
less details that he accepted have been proved incorrect by the published
results of later research by many writers, both Italian (headed by Alfredo
Bonaccorsi) and non-Italian. Today we have numerous possibilities for
understanding Rossini's life and works which were unknown to both
Radiciotti and Toye.

In 1934, for example, Carlo Piancastelli had four years more to live;
his huge collection of autographs, Roman coins, incunabula, manuscripts,
books, pamphlets, paintings, and drawings—he owned some eight hundred Rossini autograph letters and very numerous related documents—
had not yet been deposited in the Biblioteca Comunale at Forlì, some
forty miles southeast of Bologna. The Rossini materials in the Raccolta
Piancastelli approximately triple the number of Rossini's letters available
to scholars before 1934. Rossini does not belong among the great letter
writers. Guido Biagi described his epistolary style at its best when he
said: "He wrote unpretentiously, in a language and orthography all
his own, with short phrases borrowed from his librettos, and in the
joking tone of *recitativo semiserio,* lacking only the usual doublebass
accompaniment."[n] For a biographer, nonetheless, the letters and other
documents at Forlì are of nearly first importance.

Unhappily, even the Piancastelli Collection adds comparatively
little to the sparse sources on the personal life of Rossini during the
years when he was composing operas. As the late Frank Walker wrote
in 1960[n]: "A great difficulty for any biographer of Rossini is that the
active part of his life is very inadequately documented. He was thirty-
seven when 'William Tell,' his last opera, was produced, and we have
only about thirty letters to cover the whole of this period. The floods
of correspondence date from the years when he had practically abandoned composition. New light on the Neapolitan period, 1815–1822,
and his early relations with [Domenico] Barbaja and Isabella Colbran
would be particularly welcome."

I have been able to consult nearly ninety of Rossini's letters written
from 1815 through 1829,[n] about three times Mr. Walker's number, but
not nearly enough to invalidate his point. If, as seems certain, Mr. Walker
intended to write a biography of Rossini, his death in 1962 was an even
greater loss to musical history than has been recognized. After his death,

I bought a small part of his library from his brother, Mr. A. G. Walker, and his marginal notations in books and pamphlets that I thus acquired have led me to many fresh sources of information and interpretation.

Books about Rossini's life and music naturally abounded in Italian during and after his lifetime; they were also numerous in French. The most renowned of them, and disastrously the most often quoted, is Stendhal's *Vie de Rossini*, first published in 1824, when its subject was only thirty-two years old and had not yet composed any of his operas to French texts, the *Stabat Mater*, or the *Petite Messe solennelle*. Stendhal's book has been available in English translation since 1957.[n] In English, as in French, it is more interesting now as a psychological self-portrait of its author, a parade of enthusiasms and detestations, than as a biography of the young Rossini. At least once in each three pages, it is magnificently, romantically—in a sense creatively—wrong. Under the date of January 24, 1824, Eugène Delacroix recorded in his *Journal* one of the earliest reactions to the *Vie de Rossini*: "After leaving [Georges] Rouget's, after dinner, laziness propelled me to the library, where I skimmed through the life of Rossini; I surfeited myself with it, and made a mistake by doing so. As a matter of fact, that Stendhal is rude, arrogant when he is right, and often nonsensical." Delacroix's summary judgment was just. Unhappily, Stendhal's inventions have infested almost every book on Rossini written since 1824.

I began the present book in the hope of writing a "life and works" that would both tell the story of Rossini's life and critically analyze his achievement. But I have had to abandon all description and analysis of scores not essential to the biography itself. Rossini lived seventy-six years and composed thirty-nine operas, two large nonoperatic works, and hundreds of small pieces. To have combined exegesis of the music with narration of his life story would have been to produce a book of monstrous size. The present volume is therefore, rather, a "life and times."

I have tried to express borrowed opinions only in direct or clearly identified indirect quotation. This book presents Rossini (need it be said?) as I see him: as a very copious and original musical creator, a maker of delicious and moving operas, and an influence upon many other composers, particularly Donizetti, Bellini, and Verdi. But it does not try to picture him as a "great" composer or even as a "great" operatic creator. The exclusive adoration of Olympians and monumental masterpieces stultifies both a just view of musical history and essential variety in listening. I love Rossini no less because I cannot regard him as creatively the peer of twenty other composers whom we all can name. As a human being, he was—and remains—as complex and fascinating as any of them, and as rewarding.

—HERBERT WEINSTOCK

A NOTE ON THE SPELLING OF ROSSINI'S FIRST NAME

ROSSINI'S first name is spelled "Gioacchino" in nearly all modern references to him. It is, of course, the Italian equivalent of the German "Joachim"; its classic Italian form was "Giovacchino." But Rossini himself, in a very large majority of the hundreds of surviving autographs, spelled it "Gioachino," as did many of the writers contemporary with him. I have therefore decided to give the name as he himself bore it; in quoted material, I have spelled it as printed or written.

—H. W.

A NOTE ON NOTES

DESPITE A STRONG CONVICTION that a footnote should be just that—that is, should appear at the bottom of the page on which the indication for it occurs—I reluctantly decided against that sensible system for the present book because of the large number of notes and the amount of space they required. A superior italic *n* (*ⁿ*) herein means that a relevant note is to be found in the section beginning on page 389. In that section— for ease of reference—each such note is preceded (in quotation marks) by the two words that lead up to the related indication (*ⁿ*) in the text.

—H. W.

ROSSINI

"Non ebbe infanzia artistica
e fu subito lui"

—GUIDO PANNAIN

"*What an artist's biographer looks for are the cracks in the mask, the rents in the veil. A man, a biographer stubbornly feels, is always more precious than any art he may produce, even the greatest, and rightly or wrongly he believes that the discovery of the man intensifies perception of the art.*"

—Francis Steegmuller

"*Quelques-uns diront: 'Que nous importe la vie de Balzac? Seule compte son œuvre.' Cette querrelle, très ancienne, m'a toujours paru vaine. Nous savons qu'il serait impossible d'expliquer l'œuvre par la vie; nous savons que les grands événements, dans la vie d'un créateur, sont ses œuvres. Mais l'existence d'un grand homme est, en soi, un prodigieux sujet d'intérêt.*"

—André Maurois

"*The splendour of the dresses, the blaze of the candles, the perfumes, all those rounded arms, and fine shoulders; bouquets, the sound of Rossini's music, pictures by Ciceri! I am beside myself!*"

—Stendhal
(Scott-Moncrieff translation)

CHAPTER I

1792-1810

G IOACHINO ANTONIO ROSSINI was born on February 29, 1792, five months and a few days after the marriage of his parents. His birthplace was Pesaro, an Adriatic port of the Marches, then part of the States of the Church, under the rule of Rome. He was the only child of Giuseppe Antonio and Anna Guidarini Rossini.

Giuseppe Antonio Rossini came of a family whose history long was said to have been starred with minor distinctions. These undocumented traditions pictured the Rossinis (or Russinis) as patricians at Cotignola (Lugo) in the sixteenth century. And certainly a Fabrizio Rossini served as governor of Ravenna—fifteen miles east of Lugo—and died in 1570 while the town's emissary to Alfonso d'Este, duca di Ferrara. But the composer never took seriously his relatives' attempts to claim descent from Fabrizio and other real or imagined Rossinis of local prominence. In 1739 an earlier Giuseppe Antonio Rossini, born at Lugo in 1703, had had a son called Gioachino Sante Rossini, who later married a girl called Antonia Olivieri. Their son, still another Giuseppe Antonio, born at Lugo on March 10, 1758, was to become the composer's father. Two centuries after Fabrizio Rossini's death, the family that produced Gioachino Antonio Rossini was poor and undistinguished.

Little is known about the ancestry of Rossini's mother, Anna Guidarini. Her maternal grandfather, Paolo Romagnoli of Urbino, had had a daughter named Lucia. Lucia Romagnoli had married a Pesaro baker, Domenico Guidarini, by whom she had had four children: Anna, born on July 26, 1771; Annunziata, who later married one Andrea Ricci; Francesco Maria; and Maria, who married a Bolognese named Mazzotti. Pesaro police records of 1798–9 reveal that Annunziata

Guidarini was accused of practicing prostitution; some of her reputation for sexual insouciance was shared, justly or unjustly, by her older sister, Anna. Both Maria Guidarini Mazzotti and Francesco Maria Guidarini were to be mentioned in Rossini's will.

Nothing musical is recorded of any of Rossini's forebears earlier than his parents. Both of them, however, were for a time practicing musicians. Giuseppe played the trumpet and the horn, and during the Carnival opera season of 1788–9 at the Teatro del Sole (in use from 1637 to 1816) in Pesaro, he was a member of the orchestra. He also served as town trumpeter—a sort of herald—in both Lugo and Pesaro and played briefly in the band of the Ferrara garrison.

Anna Rossini, who was beautiful when young, had a good natural soprano voice. Although untrained musically, she acquired roles by ear well enough to obtain employment for some years in provincial opera houses. She made her debut at the Teatro Civico in Bologna when Giuseppe Rossini was a member of its orchestra. Their son was to tell the German conductor-composer Ferdinand Hiller[n] that his mother had "had a beautiful voice, which she used out of necessity. Poor mama!" he added. "She wasn't really unintelligent, but she didn't know a note of music. She sang by ear." To his Belgian friend Edmond Michotte he said of her: "She sang all the time, even when doing household chores. In fact, she was ignorant about music, but she had a prodigious memory ... and for that reason easily learned the roles assigned to her. Her naturally expressive voice was beautiful and full of grace—sweet, like her appearance."[n]

On March 14, 1789, the *gonfaloniere* of Pesaro read out to the town council a letter in which Giuseppe Rossini begged to be considered for the first town-trumpetership that might fall vacant. He described himself in it as "Trumpet of the Community of Lugo, the same man who played to applause at the past Carnival's opera." The councilors granted his plea by a vote of twenty-one in favor, four opposed. On March 25, Giuseppe wrote to thank them for having voted him a one-year *sopravvivenza*, or right of succession. On April 28, 1790, the council, having discharged Luigi Ricci, one of the town's two trumpeters, notified him that the trumpetership was his for one year.

Giuseppe had entered into negotiations with Ricci late in 1789, while still earning a thin living at Lugo. He finally had agreed to pay Ricci a lifelong annuity of twenty scudi[n] (Ricci had demanded twenty-four) in return for being ceded the trumpetership. Soon thereafter, Giuseppe had gone to Ferrara to join the garrison band, apparently to earn a little more money while awaiting a post at Pesaro. In January 1790, Ricci wrote him at Ferrara, urging him to reach Pesaro by early Lent to conclude their business and mentioning that a trumpetership at Pesaro brought in additional fees, reasonably large because they were derived both from playing in churches and from taking part in festivities such as those which would accompany the forthcoming marriage of a nephew of the cardinal-legate, Giuseppe Doria Pamphili.

The commandant of the Ferrara garrison, however, refused to release Giuseppe, who thereupon reacted insubordinately. Imprisoned, he apologized his way to freedom with some difficulty. At Pesaro, he found Ricci adamant about the four additional scudi per year. He thereupon called upon the *gonfaloniere* and told him the whole gritty story. The town authorities found against Ricci, discharging him out of hand for the illegal attempt to sell his position. Then they assigned it temporarily (later permanently) to Giuseppe Rossini, with the stipulation that he was not to pay a single scudo to Ricci: the councilors remarked that the entire stipend was required for the fitting upkeep of a Pesaro town trumpeter. Then or later, Rossini also was given the position of town *donzello,* or ceremonial page. His combined annual stipends and fees amounted to about $630 in today's buying power, according to Padre Giuseppe Albarelli, who in 1939–41 combed the Pesaro town records for references to Gioachino Rossini's childhood and background.*

Released from military confinement at Ferrara, Giuseppe had removed to Pesaro—to which, eight years later, he was to bring his mother and his sister, Giacoma Florida, who married a Pesaro barber named Giuseppe Gorini (or Gurini). His first living quarters in Pesaro were in the Via del Fallo, in a house in which the Guidarini family also lived. He well may have chosen to live there because he already was attracted by Anna Guidarini, then a young seamstress. When she became pregnant by him, they waited some months and then were married—"in a great rush," as Radiciotti wrote—on September 26, 1791, in the old cathedral, before the tomb of the town's patron saint, Terenzio, whose day it was.

After their marriage, Giuseppe and Anna Rossini lived for some time in two rooms in a house at No. 334, Via del Duomo (now Via Rossini), which then belonged to a Spanish Jesuit refugee.* There, in one of the boxlike rooms now open to the public, the composer was born, on February 29, 1792. He was baptized in the cathedral that day, his sponsoring godparents being Conte Paolo Macchirelli and a *"nobile Signora,"* Catterina Semproni-Giovanelli, who had come to Pesaro from Urbino and who was to become notorious for her "inflamed Jacobin speeches." The Rossinis' friendship with members of the local nobility led to gossip about Anna Rossini's morals. But, as Tommaso Casini pointed out, fraternization between classes was common in Pesaro; nothing scandalous was required to explain the presence of a count and a noble lady at Gioachino Antonio Rossini's baptism."

Giuseppe Rossini had acquired the nickname "Vivazza" because of his mercurial liveliness, which in his early youth often had amounted to overexcitability. (No evidence exists, however, for the possibility, sometimes stated as a certainty, that epilepsy "ran" in the Rossini family.) A time-honored anecdote pictures Giuseppe as working himself up into a frenzy during his wife's prolonged, painful labor on that February 29. It depicts him as addressing anguished prayers for a quick, happy delivery to gesso statuettes of the Apostles in the adjacent room. When Anna began to cry out in pain, he is said to have snatched up his walking stick and smashed one Apostle for each scream. Three of the statuettes had been demolished and he was about to smash San Giacomo at the sound of a fourth scream when he heard a faint new cry and relaxed: his child had been born.

Gioachino Rossini's childhood was to be disturbed almost as much by the aftermath of the French Revolution as by the vicissitudes to which need drove his parents. Like many other towns, Pesaro was growing restive under papal rule; many of its citizens dreamed of emulating what had happened in Paris. Late in 1793, some of the "hard-working artisan citizens of Pesaro" sent Pius VI a complaint calling a local magistrate a perjurer who drank the blood of the poor. The town responded wearily to the Pope's demand that it contribute to the troops being mobilized to counter Napoleon's invasion of Italy. When French soldiers entered Pesaro on February 5, 1797, the Pesarese put up no opposition to the occupation of their town; in fact, its civil and ecclesiastical authorities quickly expressed flowery admiration for France and for Bonaparte. A statue of Urban VIII in the Piazza di San Ubaldo was demolished.

Legend had it that when the French took Pesaro, Giuseppe Rossini put on his door a sign reading "Habitation of Citizen Vivazza, a true Republican." He certainly led an orchestra for "tree of liberty" ceremonies in both 1797 and 1800. He lost his trumpetership temporarily: at a town council meeting on December 13, 1797, he was voted out of office, nineteen to fifteen. When, later that month, a group of local patriots (Citizen Vivazza among them) drove out the papal soldiers, arrested the papal governor, and voted to join the Cisalpine Republic, he was restored to the position. What part he played in establishing the local revolutionary government cannot be determined: when, in 1800, he was arrested at Bologna and conducted roundabout to Pesaro for questioning, he testified that he always had done his duty, whatever that duty and for whomever he had performed it.

Giuseppe Rossini was freed after the battle of Marengo (June 14, 1800) turned into a French victory over the Pope's Austrian allies. Control of Pesaro shifted once more. Later that year, Giuseppe and the Cisalpine commander at Pesaro—whose name was G. Verdi!—were granted use of the Teatro del Sole for performances of two *opere buffe* during the Carnival season. Padre Albarelli discovered in the records of the Cisalpine troops the following entries, dated respectively April 6 and April 14, 1798: "As an expense to the civil guard Giovacchino Rossini—30 [bajocchi]" and "To the civil guard Giovacchino Rossini, *listaro* of the band—30 [bajocchi]." Albarelli commented: "The future composer of *Guillaume Tell*, at the age of only six years and two months, belonged to the armed forces of the Pesarese revolution and in them carried out the duties of '*listaro*' of the band, in return for which he received a little stipend, perhaps for the uniform. I have searched the lexicons for the mysterious meaning of the word '*listaro*,' but even today cannot decide whether to see in it the *lista*, the page containing the list or roll of the players, or, rather, the musical instrument made from a rod or strip [*lista*] of steel bent to the shape of a triangle." In a footnote he explained: "Evidently Rossini was the small mascot of the band. The triangle is a percussion instrument normally included in a modern band."

When Pesaro celebrated the ratification of the treaty between the Cisalpine and French republics on June 17, 1798, the *Gazzetta di Pesaro* reported that local patriots had been awakened that day by the sound of a trumpet played by "the excellent patriot Rossini, known by the nickname of Citizen Vivazza." Giuseppe himself claimed authorship of a flaming patriotic hymn beginning "Come, O patriots, let us break the tyrant's chain," but Radiciotti wrote convincingly that he was able to do so only because its true creator was afraid to claim it. Nothing surviving in Citizen Vivazza's script suggests the modest ability that the hymn reveals.

In May 1798, meanwhile, Giuseppe and Anna Rossini had embarked upon an intermittently wandering life as operatic performers, appearing first at Iesi. Giuseppe was in the opera-house orchestra there for Vicente Martín y Soler's *La Capricciosa corretta*,ⁿ in which his wife defied the taboo against women on the public stages of the Papal States. That autumn the Rossinis (or possibly just Giuseppe) took part in perform- ances at Bologna; they also played in Ferrara during the succeeding Carnival. They were back in Bologna for the Lenten season of 1799, but Anna was prevented by a throat complaint from singing until after Easter; thereafter she sang with the company until mid-September. When Count Alexander Suvorov's army reestablished papal rule once again, Giuseppe was arrested at Bologna and borne off to Imola, Forlì, Cesena, Rimini, Cattolica, and finally (early in 1800) Pesaro, where he wriggled out of the charges against him. During her husband's absence, Anna Rossini again sang at Iesi; and when, during the next Carnival season, she again sang at the Teatro Concordia there, she had become so much of a local favorite that a collection of verses in her honor was issued.

Whenever Giuseppe and Anna Rossini were away, their small, good- looking son was left at Pesaro in the care of his maternal grandmother, Lucia Guidarini, and one of her other daughters. During some of these intervals, he attended the community school, which then had three teachers—in reading and writing, elementary grammar, and decorative calligraphy. The young Rossini turns up in two lists of pupils, but no one who has struggled with his script will believe that he learned much in the calligraphy class. Traditions coincide in picturing him as lazy, prankish, and disobedient; he was punished more than once by being sent to pump bellows in a smithy. In 1865, when he was seventy-three, Francesco Genari, one of his childhood friends at Pesaro, wrote to thank him for an autographed photograph, adding: "On the nape of my neck I still bear the healed scar produced by a blow of a stone thrown at me by Your Most Illustrious Excellency at a time when you took delight in raiding sacristies in order to empty the Mass-cruets and when you were a bother rather than a delight to the whole world."

When punishment at a blacksmith's forge failed to improve young Gioachino's deportment and perseverance, he is said to have been boarded out to a Bolognese pork butcher. While there, he apparently had lessons from three priests—in reading and writing, arithmetic, and Latin.ⁿ One

Giuseppe Prinetti of Novara instructed him in the elements of cembalo playing. The adult Rossini thus described Prinetti to Ferdinand Hiller: "He was a strange fellow. He manufactured some brandies, gave a few music lessons, and in that way made ends meet. He never owned a bed —he slept standing up." When Hiller interposed, saying: "Not standing up? You must be joking, Maestro," Rossini insisted: "Just as I said. At night he wrapped himself in his cloak, and slept thus in a corner of any arcade. The nightwatchman knew him and didn't disturb him. Then, at the crack of dawn, he would come to me, pull me out of bed —which I didn't like at all—and then I had to play for him. Sometimes when he hadn't rested enough, he'd go to sleep standing up again while I was working at the spinet. I'd take advantage of that in order to crawl back into bed. On waking up again, he'd look for me there and would be gratified by my assurances that while he had been asleep I had played my pieces without mistakes. His methods certainly weren't very up-to-date: for instance, he made me play scales with my thumb and index finger."[n]

The acme of Anna Rossini's singing career was reached in 1802, by which time she had been dubbed "the [Angelica] Catalani of *seconde donne*." An impresario at Trieste had put together for his spring season at the Teatro Grande (or Comunale) a small company to perform Sebastiano Nasolini's very popular opera *La Morte di Semiramide* and a new opera by Giuseppe Farinelli. To head this troupe, he had captured Giuseppina Grassini, a beautiful young woman from Varese who was already the foremost dramatic contralto of the era and an international courtesan on the highest level, her patrons having included not only members of the English and Italian nobilities, but also Napoleon. Grassini certainly expected to reign undisturbed at Trieste.

But Nasolini, preparing *La Morte di Semiramide* for performance, was dissatisfied with the soprano hired by the impresario for the secondary role of Azema and persuaded him to replace her with "La Guidarini." Anna Rossini responded by going to Trieste with her husband and ten-year-old son. What happened thereafter was picturesquely described by an anonymous chronicler listed as "Un Vecchio Teatrofilo":[n]

"During the course of the performances, disagreement was manifested between old and young habitués. The latter showed a strong preference for La Guidarini, to the point of paralyzing the enthusiasm that the others showed for La Grassini. Whether by chance or by prearrangement, one evening when La Grassini emerged at the point at which, pursued by the shade of Nino, she pronounced the famous 'Lasciami per pietà, lasciami in pace,' a sign of disapproval was heard amid the loud applause. Semiramide fell fainting and the curtain descended. The performance went on with the ballet. This minor episode started litigation between the lawyer Domenico de Rossetti and the management for the demanded refund of forty carantini, the price of admission; but what made the event most memorable was the plotting of the older members of the audience, who wanted revenge on La Guidarini. One evening when she emerged, prolonged whistling broke out." Surprised or aware of the thing, or also out of a spirit of imitation—she permitted herself to fall to the ground in a faint. Even before the stagehands could rush to her, her son, who was near his father in the wings, eluded his father's hands and ran to pick up his mother. While the stagehands were bearing her to the wings, the boy darted disdainful glances at the audience; but the performance proceeded without further incident.

"The parents took stock of the overagitated behavior of their young son, and on their return to Bologna, changed their minds about his career. At first they had wanted to destine him for singing because he possessed a beautiful, strong voice that could be developed better with the progress of the years; but, alarmed by the event at Trieste and by the boy's always-increasing agitation, they presented him to Padre Stanislao Mattei so that he might be instructed in composition. Mattei entrusted him for the first rudiments to Maestro Angelo Tesei of Bologna, and later had him enter the school of counterpoint and composition directed by Mattei himself, where he proved to be a brilliant pupil. Well, this young boy who was so long discussed was no less than Gioacchino Rossini!—He himself recounted the 1823 event to the collector of these memories at Sinigaglia, persuaded that the happening at Trieste could have influenced the changed destination of his career."

Not surprisingly, the boy again proved intractable; he was sent to another smithy. In 1802, however, his parents removed to Lugo (No. 12, Via Poligaro Netto, now Via Eustachio Manfredi), where they somehow managed to maintain a nearly peaceful family life for a year or two. Giuseppe Rossini owned a house in Lugo (No. 580, Via Lumagni), but they could not occupy it because relatives of his were already there. After this house became the composer's property, he several times forwarded sums for its upkeep and restoration and always refused to sell it, though he never had any intention of living in Lugo again. On December 31, 1858, the Lugo authorities placed on it a Latin inscription by Rossini's friend Luigi Crisostomo Ferrucci, beginning: *"Haec domus est Joachim Russini . . ."* That phrase led to persistent misstatements about Rossini's childhood and gave baseless support to a band of odd people who wanted to label him a native of Lugo.[n]

The Rossinis remained in Lugo through 1803 or 1804. One final time, it seems, the overenergized Gioachino proved indifferent to school subjects and was set to bellows pumping. But gradually he came to be dominated by an interest in music, especially after his father taught him to play the horn.[n] He began, too, to form absorbing personal relationships, particularly one with a priest named Giovanni Sassoli, who later acted as his *"mandatorio generale,"* or general agent, in Lugo, and with a new musical preceptor, Giuseppe Malerbi, a canon who belonged to one of the town's rich and prominent families.[n] Malerbi gave the boy singing lessons (Rossini eventually became an excelling amateur *tenore baritonale*). Malerbi's brother Luigi, another musically inclined *canonico* (his compositions struck Radiciotti as original and markedly humorous), unwittingly intensified the boy's innate tendency toward high-spirited talk and caustic or facetious commentary.

Soon the Palazzo Malerbi in the Piazza Padella (now the Largo Galanotti) was always open to the young Rossini. There he was urged to practice on the cembalo[n] and rove through a collection of scores which included music by Haydn and Mozart. The hours spent in the Palazzo Malerbi seconded the influence upon the boy of his father's mercurial personality—and well may have given impetus to his later social and political conservatism, as well as to his lifelong intense interest in good food. To the canons Malerbi we perhaps owe indirectly the existence of *tournedos Rossini.*[n]

The boy's days in Lugo were cut short in 1804, when Anna Rossini's chronic throat ailment forced her to sing less and perhaps to abandon paid performing altogether. Giuseppe's earnings were small; young Gioachino soon was required to supplement them. This necessity —which within a few years became the duty of supporting his parents and even of contributing to the upkeep of aunts, uncles, and cousins —eventually was to drive Rossini into the pell-mell composition of too many operas in too much haste. In 1804, however, it meant no more than a return to Bologna, where father and son would find more opportunity for profitable employment. But before the Rossinis abandoned Lugo, young Gioachino had made his operatic debut. Father, mother, and son had gone to Ravenna for an opera season there. Gioachino, with his piping treble, somehow had replaced an indisposed *basso comico*, Petronio Marchesi, in a role in Valentino Fioravanti's opera *I Due Gemelli*, thus making his first and not quite his last, appearance as a *comprimario*.

By 1805, the Rossinis had settled into second-floor quarters at No. 240, Via Maggiore, Bologna. In that thriving center of Italian musical life,[n] Gioachino received lessons from Padre Angelo Tesei, who had studied under Padre Giambattista Martini at the local Liceo Musicale. These lessons were in singing, solfeggio, figured bass, and cembalo accompaniment, the last described as "practical harmony." The boy also learned to play both violin and viola. Soon he was being sought out as a soprano by Bolognese churches, often receiving three paoli for participating in a service—money that his parents needed badly. He also accompanied operatic recitative in theaters in Ferrara, Forlì, Lugo, Ravenna, and Sinigaglia. For one of these sessions at the cembalo, he was paid twice as much as for singing in a church, about seventy-eight cents.

Rossini told Ferdinand Hiller an anecdote about one of his appearances at Sinigaglia. The leading soprano of the local opera troupe was the very young Adelaide Carpano (who would create the minor role of Zaida in Rossini's *Il Turco in Italia* in 1814). Rossini said: "There I found a lady singer who didn't sing too badly, but certainly was of the unmusical sort. One day, the cadenza that she sang after an aria was of unsurpassably adventurous harmony. I tried to explain to her that she must give some consideration to the harmony held in the orchestra. And, really, she saw the validity of my point to a certain extent. But at the next performance she again succumbed to her inspiration and made such a cadenza that I couldn't help laughing. And the people in the stalls broke into loud laughter too, and the *donna* was enraged. She complained to her special protector, a very rich and respected Venetian who had large estates in Sinigaglia and whom the town had put in charge of the theater.[n] She complained about my ill-mannered behavior, maintaining that I had incited the audience to laughter. I was summoned to the austere gentleman, who stormed at me: 'If you have the nerve to make fun of a first-rank artist,' he raged, 'I'll have you thrown into jail.' He could have done it, but I refused to be intimidated, and so the matter took a different turn. I explained my harmonic complaints to him, convinced him of my innocence, and he took a strong liking to me instead of having me thrown into jail. He finally told me that when I reached the point at which I could compose an opera, I should come to him and he would have me write one." That promise the "austere gentleman" was later to keep.

We have another glimpse of the boy in 1805. Rossini, who at thirteen still had a pleasant soprano voice, was singing the role of Adolfo, the young son of Camilla and Duca Alberto in Ferdinando Paër's opera *Camilla*, at the Teatro del Corso in Bologna.* Because this opera was so popular that it could be performed almost every night, the title role had been assigned to two alternating sopranos. Habitués were entertained to notice that in the scene in which little Adolfo throws himself into his mother's arms, calls her endearing names, and kisses her profusely, the adolescent Rossini reacted much more ardently to the ample Anna Cittadini than to the sparser Chiara Leon. Incidentally, the first line that Adolfo had to utter (Act II, Scene 4) was: "Papa, where are you leading me?"

To 1804 seem to belong Rossini's six *sonate a quattro*, of which Alfredo Casella located a manuscript copy in the Library of Congress, Washington, D.C.* The first page of the violin part contains this inscription by Rossini's widow: "Given to my excellent friend as a token of friendship/O[lympe], widow of Rossini, this March 22, 1872, to Monsieur Mazzoni."* It also contains a note by Rossini, clearly written late in his life, which refers to the work as "six dreadful sonatas composed by me at the country place (near Ravenna) of my Maecenas friend [Agostino] Triossi, when I was at the most infantile age, not even having taken a lesson in accompaniment, the whole composed and copied out in three days and performed by Triossi, doublebass, Morri, his cousin, first violin, the latter's brother, violoncello, who played like dogs, and the second violin by me myself, who was not the least doggish, by God." These sonatas are not string quartets of classical texture, but consist of a chief melody, submelodies derived from or related closely to it, a divertimento, and a restatement of the chief melody.

Rossini's voice was so promising that he was given some supplementary singing lessons by Matteo Babbini,* a renowned tenor. In the minutes of a sitting of the Accademia Filarmonica on June 24, 1806, this appears: "The petition of Signor Gioachino Rossini, Bolognese, approved for his practice of the musical art of singing, in view of which he requests admission to our Academy, was read. The same is admitted by acclamation, being held excused from the burden of any contribution. And this in view of the regard merited by his progress in the profession that he practices to so much praise." This note was subjoined: "The above-mentioned Rossini has for the time being no active voice in the Academy's sittings, considering his minor age of only about fifteen years." When actually only four months past his fourteenth birthday, Rossini thus became a member of the internationally renowned Accademia—in which Padre Martini had secured membership for the visiting fourteen-year-old Mozart only thirty-six years earlier. (Literally, of course, Rossini, having been born on February 29, had a birthday only once every four years, a situation of which he often made his humorous best.)

In April 1806, Rossini entered the Liceo Musicale, then presided over by Padre Martini's pupil and successor Padre Stanislao Mattei. Rossini was to remain at the Liceo for four years, taking classes in singing and solfeggio with Lorenzo Gibelli,[n] in cello with Vincenzo Cavedagna, and in piano with Gian Callisto Cavazzoni Zanotti. On May 20, 1806, he attended for the first time the course in counterpoint to which, under the tutelage of Mattei, he was to devote himself entirely in 1809–10. On August 8, 1806, during a concert of vocal and instrumental music performed by the students, Rossini—now listed as "Accademico Filarmonico" despite his fourteen years—made his final public appearance as a soprano, singing with a pupil named Dorinda Caranti[n] in a duet by Andrea Nencini, also a fellow student; soon thereafter, his voice began to descend toward its later tenor-baritone range.

At least once in later years, Rossini suggested that some thought had been given to the possibility of preserving his boyish voice artificially. In Edmond Michotte's pamphlet *Une Soirée chez Rossini à Beau-Sejour (Passy) 1858*, Rossini is quoted as mentioning that he had composed a single role for *castrato*, that of Arsace in *Aureliano in Palmira* (1813), written for Giambattista Velluti. He then adds:

"Parenthetically, would you believe that I came within a hair's breadth of belonging to that famous corporation—let us rather say decorporation. As a child, I had a very pretty voice, and my parents used it to have me earn a few paoli by singing in churches. One uncle of mine, my mother's brother, a barber by trade [Francesco Maria Guidarini], had convinced my father of the opportunity that he had glimpsed if the breaking of my voice should not be allowed to compromise an organ which—poor as we were, and I having showed *some* disposition toward music—could have become an assured future source of income for us all. Most of the *castrati*, in fact, and particularly those dedicated to a theatrical career, lived in opulence. My brave mother would not consent at any price."

At this point in Michotte's account, one of the other guests asks: "And you, Maestro, the chief interested party?"

"Oh! me," Rossini answers, "all that I can tell you is that I was very proud of my voice. And as for any descendants that I might leave . . ."

Now Rossini's (second) wife interrupts: "Little you cared! Now is the moment to make one of your quips."

"Well, then," Rossini replies, "let's have no half-truths. 'Little' is too much. I didn't care at all."

Probably referring to Rossini's years of study in Bologna, but perhaps to his last days in Lugo, Félix Clément wrote:[n] "He spent considerable patient effort in making arrangements of the Haydn quartets, so that it is fair to say that Rossini was much more a pupil of Haydn than of Padre Mattei."[n] Some of Rossini's Italian contemporaries, alarmed by his "learning" and by the "thickness" of his orchestration, were to call his style excessively Teutonic. He was often referred to as a *tedeschino* (little German). This resistance to change from the complete domination of melody later would bring upon Verdi, with no more justice, the charge that he was imitating Wagner.

On April 11, 1807, a twenty-two-year-old Spanish soprano named Isabella Angela Colbran (often spelled Colbrand) sang at the Accademia Polimniaca at Bologna.[n] On April 19, she took part in a concert in the auditorium of the Accademia Filarmonica. Three days later, she left for Milan, where she made her debut at the Teatro alla Scala on December 26, 1808, in the *première* of *Coriolano* by Giuseppe Nicolini (Niccolini). Colbran's visit to Bologna gave Rossini his first opportunity to see and hear, and perhaps to meet, the magnificently handsome and talented young woman who, at Naples some years later, was to become one of the foremost interpreters of his tragic operas and whom he would marry in 1822 (after a period during which she was very probably his mistress).

During April 1807, the Bolognese journal *Il Redattore del Reno* said: "On April 7 there arrived among us Donna Isabella Colbran, a very celebrated young Spanish woman,[n] at present in the service of His Catholic Majesty. She has the celestial art of singing to such a degree that signs of the liveliest admiration for and purest delight in her have been made clear and manifest in the palaces of the major monarchs of Europe . . . The organ of her voice is truly an enchantment for smoothness, for strength, and for prodigious extension of tones: from the bass G to the high E—that is, for almost three octaves—it makes itself heard in a progression always even in mellowness and energy . . . The method and style of her singing are perfect . . ." Stendhal was to write of Colbran: "She was a beauty of the most imposing sort: with large features that are superb on the stage, magnificent stature, blazing eyes *à la circassienne*, a forest of the most beautiful jet-black hair, and, finally, an instinct for tragedy. As soon as she appeared [on stage], wearing a diadem on her head, she commanded involuntary respect even from people who had just left her in the foyer."

More immediately significant for Rossini's future was his friendship with the tenor Domenico Mombelli (1751–1835), his second wife, Vincenza,ⁿ and two of their ten children—Ester, a mezzo-soprano who could descend well into the contralto register and rise into the soprano, and Marianna (or Anna or Annetta), a contralto who specialized in travesty roles. In recalling the year 1805, Rossini was to tell Ferdinand Hiller: "Mombelli was an excellent tenor; he had two daughters, one a soprano, the other a contralto; they got a bass to join them. As a complete vocal quartet without any outside help, they gave opera performances in Bologna, Milan, and other cities. That was the way they first appeared in Bologna; they gave a little, but very pleasant, opera by Portogallo. . . .ⁿ The manner in which I made Mombelli's acquaintance was delightful, and as you are interested in my little stories, I'll describe it to you.

"Although still a boy (I was thirteen years old at the time), I was already a great admirer of the fair sex. One of my lady-friends, patronesses —what should I call her?—very much wanted an aria from the afore-mentioned opera performed by Mombelli. I went to the copyist and asked him for a copy of it, but he refused me. So I went to Mombelli himself with my request, but he also denied it. 'It won't do you any good,' I told him. 'I'll listen to the opera again tonight, and I'll just write down anything I like from it.' 'I'd like to see that,' Mombelli said. But I, not being lazy, listened to the opera once more, and very carefully. I wrote out the complete piano score and took it to Mombelli. He refused to believe it, raged about the copyist's treachery, and so forth. 'If you don't think me capable of this,' I said, 'I'll listen to the opera a few times more, and then I'll write out the complete score under your very eyes.' My great self-confidence, which was fully justified in this case, tri-umphed over his suspicion, and we became close friends."

Rossini's reminiscences, especially as reported from his conversation many years later, are not always accurate in detail. But in view of his early training and experience and his extremely retentive musical memory, the anecdote is believable. He certainly had the printed libretto of Portogallo's opera in hand while writing out his piano score; filling out an orchestral score from it after one additional listening would not be an incredible achievement. As Rossini himself remarked to Hiller: "It wasn't a score like that of *Le Nozze di Figaro*." And Rossini did become intimate with Mombelli and his family: before entering the Liceo in 1806—near his fourteenth birthday—he had composed for their use most of the numbers of what, to his surprise, later turned out to be a little *opera seria*.[n]

Vincenza Mombelli, who nursed baseless literary hopes, had written a libretto called *Demetrio e Polibio*, an odd farrago retailing passions, disguises, and reconciliation among unlikely royal Parthians and Syrians.[n] It was handed piecemeal to Rossini. He quickly composed several individual numbers for it; when he completed this stint is unclear. The opera was not to be played until 1812 and thus could not figure as his first staged work; indeed, by then it had been preceded by five other operas.

The initial result of Rossini's immersion in Padre Mattei's strict regime had been creative paralysis. He later would tell Hiller that Mattei was all but unequaled in the way in which he could correct a student's exercise, but that any explanation of the corrections could scarcely be dragged from him. Fétis quoted Rossini as having told him that when he had sought such explanations, Mattei's only answer had been: "It is the custom to write that way." Alexis-Jacob Azevedo wrote:[n] "After six months of work in counterpoint class, Rossini, who, before entering it, had composed the delicious quartet ["*Donami omai, Siveno*," in *Demetrio e Polibio*], could not write a single note without trembling." And Rossini would say to Edmond Michotte:[n] "I felt all too clearly that my very exuberant nature was not formed to be subjected to regular, patient labor; and for that reason, even later, the good Padre Mattei hurled anathema against me, calling me 'the dishonor of his school.'" No Rossini composition of any interest survives from 1807.

By 1808, however, the boy had begun to take the academic rules in his stride and to recapture his natural ease in music-making. Although his Liceo studies were being supplemented with lessons in literature with the vernacular writer Jacopo Landoni of Ravenna and with studies of the *Divina Commedia*, *Orlando furioso*, and *Gerusalemme liberata* under Gian Battista Giusti,[n] he found time during 1808 to compose a *Graduale concertato* for three male voices; the *Gradual*, *Kyrie*, and *Qui*

tollis of a Mass that was sung by Liceo students at the Church of the
Madonna di San Luca sul Monte; a *Sinfonia* (known as the "Bologna"[n])
per orchestra; and a cantata, *Il pianto d'Armonia sulla morte d'Orfeo.*
The cantata, with text by the Abbate Girolamo Ruggia, was for tenor
and chorus; it was performed by Liceo students on August 11, 1808,
during prize-day ceremonies at which Rossini was given a medal in
counterpoint. The manuscript displays Padre Mattei's corrections.[n]

Later in 1808, responding to a request from Agostino Triossi, the
Ravenna doublebass player for whom he had composed the six *sonate a
quattro*, Rossini patched together a complete Mass, incorporating into it
the sections of the student Mass composed earlier that year. This Mass
is scored for male voices and chorus, with accompaniment of orchestra
and organ. It was sung at Ravenna while that city was celebrating its
annual fair. Because many musicians were on hand and eager to perform,
the actual forces at the singing of the Mass included no less than eleven
flutes, seven *"clarini"* (either clarinets or high-pitched trumpets), and
nine doublebasses. When, years later, Rossini was asked if he still had
the score of the 1808 Mass, he answered that he had left it, with other
possessions, at Triossi's home in Ravenna, but that as Triossi had gone
into exile at Corfu, possibly the paper on which it had been written had
been used for wrapping salami.

Five so-called string quartets by Rossini, assigned by some writers
to 1808–9, were published by Schott in Paris in 1823–4 and later by
Grua-Ricordi in London. The latter edition is dedicated to Lord Burghersh,[n] who entertained Rossini at Florence in 1830 while British ambassador to Tuscany. In 1954, Alfredo Bonaccorsi, editing the *Quaderni
Rossiniani* at Pesaro, determined that the "quartets" were transcriptions
of five of the *sonate a quattro*. He leaned toward the hypothesis that
someone other than Rossini had done the transcribing "because Rossini,
who had taken into account the characteristics and nature of the doublebass and was composing for a doublebass-player, would not have been
able to give up that instrument's rusty voice, almost that of a *basso
buffo*." Bonaccorsi further noted that the third of the *sonate*, which
includes a set of comic variations for doublebass and gives that instrument special prominence throughout, was precisely the one not transcribed.[n]

Rossini's early vocal pieces were composed either for family friends
(including Luigi Zamboni, for whom he later designed the role of Figaro
in *Il Barbiere di Siviglia*) or for insertion into performances of operas by

others, then a very common method of satisfying the demands of star singers for bravura showpieces. The "Bologna" *Sinfonia per orchestra* was played for the first time at the Accademia Polimniaca on December 23, 1808.ⁿ A writer in *Il Redattore del Reno* said: "The concert was begun with a *sinfonia* expressly composed by Signor Rossini, a member of the Accademia Filarmonica, a young man of whom much is hoped. It was found harmonious beyond all belief. Its type is altogether new, and the composer garnered unanimous applause."

When passing for performance Rossini's cantata *Il Pianto d'Armonia sulla morte d'Orfeo*, the committee remarked that it supplied sufficient reason for his pursuing a musical career. Actually, it is inert and unrewarding. Ruggia's pompous text clearly did not ignite Rossini's imagination; also, he had tried hard to compose in strict accord with academic rules. The cantata consists of a *sinfonia* in two tempos; choruses abounding in crushing sequences of thirds; and two arias in what was then already a museum style. Rossini never was to be at his happiest in occasional pieces.

While still attending classes at the Liceo with some regularity during 1809, Rossini also played recitative cembalo for operas at the Teatro Comunale and at theaters in nearby towns. His energy was boundless: for the annual prize-day festivities at the Liceo, he composed a *Sinfonia a più strumenti obbligati concertata* that was played on August 25. On that occasion too the "Bologna" *Sinfonia* was repeated. The newer piece was to have a prolonged public career: Rossini would use it as the overture for both *La Cambiale di matrimonio* (1810) and *Adelaide di Borgogna* (1817). To 1809 also belongs a set of *Variazioni in fa maggiore per più strumenti obbligati con accompagnamento d'orchestra* which has been published.ⁿ The variations are neither structural nor developmental, but are confined to embellishments of the theme and some adaptation of it for each obbligato instrument.

While playing recitative cembalo at the Comunale during 1809, Rossini very probably heard Isabella Colbran in performances there of Cimarosa's *Artemisia* and Nicolini's *Traiano in Dacia*. The first-string cast of these performances also included the notable tenor Nicola Tacchinardi and the last of the great *castrati*, Giovanni Battista Velluti. These would have been his first opportunities to hear in opera the great soprano for whom he would compose so many roles and the vainglorious *castrato* for whom, in 1813, he would design the only role he ever composed for that artificial voice (Arsace in *Aureliano in Palmira*).

On April 1 and May 28, 1810, Rossini played the piano during programs given at the Accademia dei Concordi. During that year too, while
intermittently attending Mattei's counterpoint class and also earning
small sums by public appearances, he composed a cavatina for tenor and
orchestra (with text beginning *"Dolci aurette che spirate"*) and a set of
*Variazioni in do maggiore per clarinetto obbligato con accompagna-
mento di orchestra.* The varied melody, meditative and lyric, vaguely
suggests latter Rossinian operatic cavatinas.[n]

Rossini's first biographers insisted that during 1810 he abruptly
abandoned his counterpoint studies after a quarrel with Padre Mattei.
Rossini himself gave Ferdinand Hiller an account of his departure which
is closer to the facts recorded in the Liceo's records: "When I had
worked through counterpoint and fugue, I asked Mattei what he would
have me do next. He answered: 'Plain song and canon.' 'How much time
would I have to spend on them?' 'About two years.' But I no longer
could afford that, and I explained to the kind Padre, who understood
completely and always remained kindly disposed toward me. I myself
often have regretted since that I didn't work longer with him."

At first Rossini attended every session of Mattei's counterpoint
class, but as time went on, he increasingly absented himself, and by 1810
he had virtually abandoned the class. The argument carried on by his
biographers and critics as to whether more academic training and practice
would have benefited his techniques or damaged his spontaneity is foot-
less. He was not to be a "learned" composer or even, by academic stand-
ards, a "correct" one. But nothing indicates that he could not have been
rule-abiding if he had wanted to be. His later music testifies to his possession of sufficient knowledge of musical theory and procedure for his
purposes. A Rossini composing with the massive erudition of a Max
Reger or a Ferruccio Busoni is unthinkable. But to regard him as naïve,
as a so-called "natural" composer, is to misunderstand the true character
both of the man and of his music.

A visit to Bologna in August 1810 by two musical friends of Giuseppe and Anna Rossini was to decide Gioachino's immediate activity for
him and to determine the ruling pattern of his next nineteen years. The
couple was Giovanni Morandi (1777–1856) and his wife Rosa Morolli
(1782–1824), who had been colleagues of the Rossinis in provincial
opera troupes. Morandi was an able chorus master and a composer of
both sacred music and operas, the latter chiefly brief farces. Rosa Morandi had a good voice of soprano–mezzo-soprano *tessitura.* In 1804, the

year of her marriage to Morandi, she had made her operatic debut; eventually she would create roles in Rossini's *La Cambiale di matrimonio* and *Eduardo e Cristina* and sing in others of his operas, including *Otello* and *Tancredi*.

When the Morandis stopped at Bologna in August 1810, they were en route to Venice to join a company of singers being gathered together by the Marchese Cavalli to perform at the Teatro Giustinian a San Moisè. Anna Rossini told them about her son's eagerness to compose another opera—*Demetrio e Polibio*, which he had begun four years earlier for the Mombellis, and which was their property for the time being, had not yet been staged. The Morandis promised to find out what could be done for Gioachino at Venice. He was only eighteen, and whatever reputation he had acquired as a composer was almost wholly local. But something more than friendly feelings toward his parents must have motivated Giovanni and Rosa Morandi, both of whom were well equipped to judge musical performance and promise.

The Teatro San Moisè was then specializing in the one-act *opere buffe* known as *farse*. The Marchese Cavalli's season there was to have been made up of an existing opera and four new scores composed expressly for it. The season duly opened on September 16, 1810, with a double bill made up of *L'Infermo ad arte* (1802), an opera by the Neapolitan Raffaele Orgitano which was not liked, and the *première* of Pietro Generali's *Adelina*, which at once promised to become a favorite. Cavalli next tried *Il Prigioniero* by the Paduan Luigi Calegari; it was performed only on October 2 and 3. The third of the little season's new *farse*, by Giuseppe Farinelli, had a resounding title and subtitle—*Non precipitare i giudizi, ossia La Vera Gratitudine*—but produced only an indifferent effect.

At some juncture during the presentation of the four *farse*, Cavalli realized that he was in trouble: a German composer was not fulfilling a promise to provide the fifth offering. Giovanni Morandi recalled the young Rossini to Cavalli, who had been the impresario at Sinigaglia during the contretemps over Adalaide Carpano's "adventurous harmony" and who had kept a pleasant memory of the cheeky boy. Morandi thereupon wrote to ask Gioachino if he would like to come to Venice to try supplying the needed *farsa*. Rossini's answer was to leave at once for Venice. There he was handed a libretto entitled *La Cambiale di matrimonio*, which Gaetano Rossi[n] had adapted either from Camillo Federici's five-act comedy *Matrimonio per lettere di cambio* or from earlier librettos derived from it. Rossini set Rossi's text in a few days, and by the time his score was ready, Cavalli had decided to risk staging it.

At the first rehearsal of *La Cambiale di matrimonio*, some of the cast complained of excessively heavy orchestration and ungrateful vocal lines. Doubtless feeling the handicap of his eighteen years and aware of just how much he and his family needed the promised payment of two hundred lire (about $100 in today's buying power) and of how urgently his own immediate future might benefit from production of his *farsa*, Rossini went to his lodgings and wept. Morandi consoled him by agreeing to make the needed emendations in the score. Tempers were smoothed. Rossini's *La Cambiale di matrimonio*, yoked in a double bill to Farinelli's *Non precipitare i giudizi*, was sung at the San Moisè on November 3, 1810.[n] One of the liveliest, most original, and most delightful of comic-opera composers had made his world debut.

Rossini's originality as a stylist of musical farce lay chiefly in his melodic and rhythmic *brio*, in the disenchanted lack of sentimentality with which he selected from a libretto those story elements which were nonsensical, absurd, preposterous, and then gave them apt musical revelation. Nothing exactly like the dash, the propulsive rhythmic and melodic onrush of *La Cambiale di matrimonio* had been heard earlier. In it, as in his later comic operas, he seized upon every chance for pell-mell involvements, for swift purely musical illustration. In any comparison with such of his predecessors as the Mozart of *Le Nozze di Figaro* and *Così fan tutte*, the Cimarosa of *Il Matrimonio segreto*, or the Pergolesi of *La Serva padrona*, Rossini appears less interested in the complete human qualities of his protagonists, in the range of what they are—and are feeling—as individuals. His attention was on their activities as provokers of laughter. One result was that as early as 1810 reasonable admirers of the older, gentler, more humane style of *opera buffa* found him boisterous and rude, a radical threat to cherished elements of the older, more gallant art.

Buoyed up by the admired performances of Rosa Morandi as Fanny and of Luigi Raffanelli as Sir Tobia Mill, *La Cambiale di matrimonio* succeeded at once: it was sung at the San Moisè twelve or more times between November 3 and December 1.[n] Now, having passed its sesquicentennial, it is a continuing delight. Rossini received the promised two hundred lire from Cavalli: he later told Hiller that they had not seemed a small amount to him at the time. In fact, he had experienced real satisfaction upon receiving those "forty scudi, an amount that I never had seen brought together that way, one on top of the other." He could go back to Bologna hopeful that somewhere another impresario would open a stage door to his next opera. For the audiences of Rossini's opera-composing years were avid for novelties. As Andrea Della Corte noted:[n] "That generation knew only the operas of its own time. The oldest were those of Mozart, from 1786 and 1787—that is, of from thirty to more than forty years earlier." The time of the limited "standard operatic repertoire," lightly skimming the centuries from Gluck's *Orfeo ed Euridice* to the most recently admitted addition (usually at least thirty or forty years old), lay wholly in the future.

CHAPTER II

1810-1813

IN 1808, the Accademia dei Concordi at Bologna had performed
Haydn's *La Creazione* (*Die Schöpfung*) and the audience had unexpectedly received with pleasure this "difficult" German oratorio,
so unlike standard Italian musical fare. The Accademia thereupon also
performed Haydn's *Le Quattro Stagioni* (*Die Jahreszeiten*). In 1811,
Rossini became cembalist and coach of the Accademia—and repeated
Le Quattro Stagioni. In its report of that occasion, *Il Redattore del Reno*
said: "Signor *Gioacchino Rossini, maestro al cembalo,* not to mention
Signor *Giuseppe Boschetti,* first violin and director of the orchestra,
earned particular praise for their tirelessness and precision in leading the
choruses, the players, the singers, and in the difficult concordance of so
many parts and so many instruments." In 1811 too, Rossini composed a
solo cantata called *La Morte di Didone* for Ester Mombelli, who did not
make use of it until 1818.[n]

Late in the summer or early in the autumn of 1811, Rossini was
hired as cembalist and composer by an impresario planning a season of
opera at the Teatro del Corso in Bologna.[n] His first duty at the Corso
was at the cembalo during rehearsals and performances of Portogallo's
L'Oro non compra amore and Stefano Pavesi's *Ser Marcantonio.*[n] He
himself was to receive fifty piastre (about $125 in today's purchasing
power) for a new opera. He accepted, probably in desperation, a rachitic
two-act libretto by Gaetano Gasparri (sometimes spelled Gasbarri),[n]
L'Equivoco stravagante, which tells how one of two rivals for a girl's
hand convinces the other that she is a *castrato* in disguise. Rossini set this
unlikely text with his astonishing swiftness, and *L'Equivoco stravagante*
made its debut at the Corso, with all of the little troupe's leading singers,
on October 26, 1811.[n]

An undated edition of *L'Equivoco stravagante* for voice and piano published by Ricordi (plate numbers and the wording of the Ricordi imprint place it later than 1811) begins with the overture that Rossini used for *Aureliano in Palmira* (1813), *Elisabetta, regina d'Inghilterra* (1815), and *Il Barbiere di Siviglia* (1816). Radiciotti decided that it had been borrowed from a later opera for this edition. Alfredo Bonaccorsi wrote that the *Aureliano* overture shows stylistic signs of having been composed later than *L'Equivoco* and therefore judged that the original overture to *L'Equivoco*, if it ever existed, had been transferred to some other later opera. In fact, however, the *Aureliano* overture preludes a comic opera much more aptly than a tragic one. (Even aside from the overture problem, *L'Equivoco stravagante* adds to Rossini's self-borrowings: a quintet that is its finest single number was taken over in part from the opening and closing of the quartet in *Demetrio e Polibio*—and, in turn, both the first-act trio of *L'Equivoco* and the partially borrowed quintet were to be recalled in *La Pietra del paragone*.)

In an article on *L'Equivoco stravagante*,[n] Adelmo Damerini spoke of "a scintillating and well-developed *Sinfonia*—which offers anticipatory echoes of that to *La Cenerentola* . . . " He was writing, however, of the opera as performed from a score in the library of the Florence Conservatory which is not in Rossini's autograph. The overture in it seems not so much to offer "anticipatory echoes" of the overture to *La Cenerentola* as to quote from it. If this is indeed a faithful copy of Rossini's "lost" overture to *L'Equivoco*, then that to *La Gazzetta* (1816)—the one later transferred to *La Cenerentola*—depended upon it for the skittish middle melody of its allegro.[n]

Several early writers asserted that *L'Equivoco stravagante* was mercilessly whistled down on the night of its *première*. Geltrude Righetti-Giorgi—who greatly admired Rossini and was the first Rosina in *Il Barbiere di Siviglia*—merely wrote[n] that it had been received coldly. What really happened to *L'Equivoco* was made clear by *Il Redattore del Reno* on October 29, 1811: "The music was welcomed with applause, for at every performance the audience has called out onto the stage Signor Rossini, and on that evening the quintet and Signora Marcolini's second-act aria were encored. That the libretto is, permit me, vicious is demonstrated by the resolution taken by the very watchful prefecture, which has forbidden further performances. Only out of regard for the composer had it allowed three performances to be given after having corrected and re-corrected—despite the mutilations thus inflicted—some other [*sic*] expressions that, when sung, produce an impression not to be tolerated, though they would be tolerated in reading. But as the argument of the libretto revolves precisely around a supposed mutilation that necessarily allows room for many equivocal expressions, to mutilate some pieces does not suffice, but [instead it is necessary] to cut the root of the scandal by suppressing the libretto.["] To Rossini's discomfort, then, *L'Equivoco stravagante* was removed from the Corso stage by the police after three performances.

Rossini had to return to his cembalo for rehearsals of *Il Trionfo di Quinto Fabio,* by Domenico Puccini,[n] and of Giovanni Simone Mayr's *Ginevra di Scozia.* At the dress rehearsal of the Puccini opera, some of the choristers so enraged their nineteen-year-old *maestro al cembalo* that he gestured at them with his baton. The choristers reacted so violently that Rossini would have been ejected if the manager had not intervened. The impresario placated the singers by taking Rossini to the police—who set him free because the forthcoming performances at the Corso could not have taken place without him. He was dressed down for reprehensible conduct; the impresario was ordered to keep an eye on the volcanic young man and to report any future eruptions. Soon the downcast Rossini neglected his duties while rehearsing the Mayr opera, thus giving the impresario further reason to complain of him.

Here something must be said about the initial causes of Rossini's long, complex medical history. That he was sexually precocious is confirmed by his own statements, and he almost certainly contracted gonorrhea (not then a clearly differentiated or easily curable disease) in his teens.[n] The ways in which a creative artist's physical health, his mental condition, and his creativity may be related must be largely guessed; they will not support excessive hypothesis. Nor is it possible to date the inception of Rossini's venereal infection. What can be said is that he began to have sexual relations early (note the "lady-friends, patronesses" whom he jokingly referred to in discussing an event that had occurred when he was thirteen). He certainly suffered from gonorrhea for a long time, perhaps from as early as 1807 or 1808, and in later years he succumbed to black moods that seem closely related to his prolonged ill health. Rossini was by no means always the energetic, high-spirited man that he was in his early youth. Nor is it possible to argue with the belief that his long history of illness and his states of abysmal depression, whether caused by illness or not, contributed to his "great renunciation" of operatic composition after *Guillaume Tell* (1829). But to attribute too many or too specific results to these conditions would be to oversimplify Rossini's complex nature.

In 1811, only nineteen, Rossini soared buoyantly over the misfortune of *L'Equivoco stravagante*, over boredom as a *maestro al cembalo*, and, it may be, over continuous physical discomfort. At the time of the ban on his latest opera or shortly thereafter, he agreed to compose another *farsa* for the Teatro San Moisè. He left Bologna in December 1811, having been there about one year, and soon was in Venice at work on a libretto by Giuseppe Maria Foppa[n] called *L'Inganno felice*. With it, he was for the first time composing to a subject that had been used earlier by Paisiello,[n] whose version of *Il Barbiere di Siviglia* (1782) was to cause him difficulties while composing and presenting his own version of it in 1816. *L'Inganno felice* reached its *première* at the San Moisè on January 8, 1812, captured its audience at once, and ran out the season, which closed on February 11—on which day portraits of and verses in honor of Teresa Giorgi-Belloc, its Isabella, were hawked in the theater while doves, canaries, and wild pheasants were let loose from the loges.[n] Although melodic and other gestures in *L'Inganno* were brought over from both Mozart and Cimarosa, it nonetheless presented much of Rossini's future operatic personality as though in dim—and at times rough —preliminary form. For it, Rossini was paid 250 francs (i. e., Lombardo-Veneto lire, about $130 in today's purchasing power).

About two months after that heartening *première* at Venice, the pell-mell Rossini was ready with an *opera seria* (his first except for *Demetrio e Polibio*) in two acts. *Ciro in Babilonia, ossia La Caduta di Baldassare*—deliberately mislabeled "sacred oratorio" or "drama with choruses" so that it could be staged during Lent—used a libretto by Conte Francesco Aventi, a Ferrarese dilettante, which could scarcely be worse. The *première* of the opera was given at the Teatro Municipale (sometimes Comunale), Ferrara, in March (almost certainly March 14), 1812.[n] Discussing *Ciro* with Hiller, Rossini would say: "It was one of my fiascos. When I went back to Bologna after its unfortunate performance, I found an invitation to a meal. I went to the confectioner's and ordered a ship made of marzipan; on its pennant it bore the name 'Ciro'; its mast was broken, its sails were tattered, and it lay on its side in an ocean of cream. Amid great hilarity, the happy company devoured my wrecked vessel." For this "fiasco," Rossini received forty piastre (about $100). *Ciro* never won an international career, but it was sung in Italy for about fifteen years.

The most discussed number in *Ciro in Babilonia* was an *aria del sorbetto* (literally a sherbet aria, intended to be sung by a secondary performer while the audience took refreshments and gossiped). Rossini's own account of the genesis of *"Chi disprezza gl'infelici"* was given thus by Hiller: "For the opera *Ciro in Babilonia* I had a horrible *seconda donna*. Not only was she ugly beyond all description, but her voice too was without any dignity. After the most careful testing, I found that she had a single note, the middle B flat, which didn't sound too bad. I thereupon wrote an aria in which she had to sing just that note. I set it all in the orchestra, and as the piece was liked and applauded, my unitonal singer was delighted with her triumph."[n]

Two days before the Ferrara *première* of *Ciro in Babilonia,* the *Giornale dipartimentale dell'Adriatico,* Venice, had reported: "For the spring season to be inaugurated at the Teatro San Moisè on the second feast-day of Easter, the Signor Maestro Rossini will write a new farce of the poet Foppa." Driven by the need to support himself and contribute to the upkeep of his parents, Rossini had signed a contract with Cera, impresario of the San Moisè, who clearly yearned for another box-office attraction as potent as *L'Inganno felice.* Unhappily, the Foppa libretto entitled *La Scala di seta*[n] was unlikely to evoke the result desired. Rossini, however, had no choice but to accept it: less than two months after the Ferrara *première* of *Ciro in Babilonia, La Scala di seta* was heard at the San Moisè. On that May 9, 1812, it shared a triple bill with one act of Pavesi's endemic *Ser Marcantonio* and a ballet. For it, Rossini was paid the standard San Moisè fee for a *farsa,* 250 francs (about $130).[n]

La Scala di seta, though not approved beyond its merits—which are not myriad after its glinting overture—was played at the San Moisè intermittently for about a month. Foppa was criticized sharply for making use of an intrigue so like that of the libretto of Cimarosa's *Il Matrimonio segreto* (which, in turn, had been extremely close to that of *The Clandestine Marriage,* by George Colman and David Garrick). Rossini was lauded mildly for his agility in making a stale subject seem slightly fresh. Radiciotti was just in calling the score of *La Scala di seta* "faded and banal," but Stendhal's description of it as crowded with deliberately bizarre and extravagant musical effects is incorrect. That he had confused it with *Il Signor Bruschino* is proved by his remark that in its overture the orchestral violinists were required to strike with their bows the tin reflectors behind their candles. In the overture to the later farce, Rossini's instrumentation calls for a related effect, but even *Il Signor Bruschino* is not musically so bizarre as Stendhal mistakenly thought *La Scala di seta.*

Some credibility was lent to Stendhal's criticism by the publication of a letter from Rossini to Cera[n] at the San Moisè. It reads: "Giving me the libretto entitled *La Scala di seta* to set to music, you treated me like a child; in causing you to have a fiasco, I have repaid you with interest. Now we are even." Radiciotti thrice denied the authenticity of this letter; no proof that an autograph of it ever existed has been advanced. It is impossible to believe that Cera, as impresario, would not have attended a single rehearsal of *La Scala di seta*—or that, having done so and discovered the score to be deliberately malformed, he would have risked his enterprise by allowing a performance of it to take place. Yet Francis Toye accepted the letter to Cera as authentic; doing so permitted him to state, without other proof and against Rossini's own statement to the contrary to Hiller (see below), that Rossini went to Rome in the spring of 1812 "to assist his friends, the Mombelli family, in the production of *Demetrio e Polibio*" and wrote to Cera from there.

It is equally unlikely that Rossini would have been permitted to leave Venice for Rome with his remuneration in his pocket before the third performance of *La Scala di seta*: the composer's presence at the cembalo during the first three singings of a new opera was a standard contractual requirement. Unless we can picture Rossini as having left Venice *before* the *première* (May 9), we cannot accept his having referred to the opera as a fiasco, which in fact it was not. Unless a genuine autograph of the "letter to Cera" turns up, Radiciotti's belief that it never existed—which was echoed by Frank Walker[n]—must be shared.

La Scala di seta was played at Sinigaglia in 1813 and at the San Moisè again in 1818; outside Italy, it was heard at Barcelona in 1823 and Lisbon in 1825—after which it remained mostly unheard until a few revivals after World War II.[n] Almost everything after its overture is anticlimactic. That overture is one of Rossini's gayest and most artfully constructed, the earliest of his orchestral pieces presenting him at or near his unique best. Like all Rossini overtures except those for *Le Siège de Corinthe* and *Guillaume Tell* and possibly that for *Semiramide*, this one is distorted by the massive string-preponderance of the modern symphonic orchestra: the performing group must be kept reasonably small and the winds, particularly the woodwinds, must always be given their full intended value if the genuine bouquet of Rossini's extremely individual orchestration is to be evoked.

On May 18, 1812, nine days after the Venice *première* of *La Scala di seta*, Rossini's *Demetrio e Polibio*, in large part six years old, was staged at the Teatro Valle, Rome, under the aegis of an impresario named Rambaldi. The cast included Domenico Mombelli, his daughters Ester and Marianna, and the bass Lodovico Olivieri.[n] Mombelli had prepared and rehearsed the little *opera seria*; Rossini almost certainly was not in Rome for the first performance.[n] When Ferdinand Hiller asked him if he had composed many pieces before studying with Padre Mattei, Rossini replied: "A whole opera, *Demetrio e Polibio*. When my works are enumerated, it is always mentioned later. That is because it was performed publicly only after a few other dramatic attempts, about four or five years after it was written. Originally, I composed it for the Mombelli family without knowing that it would turn into an opera."

Hiller asked: "Then Mombelli commissioned you to write an opera?" Rossini's answer was: "He gave me texts, now for a duet, now for an arietta, and he gave me a few piastre for each piece. That drove me to great activity. Without realizing it, I achieved my first opera that way. While I was doing it, my singing teacher, Babini, gave me many good pieces of advice. As you must know, he was dead set against certain melodic configurations then much in vogue, and he used all his eloquence to get me to avoid them." Hiller remarked that when he had been in Italy, the quartet from *Demetrio e Polibio* still had enjoyed some fame and had been cited as proof of Rossini's early maturity. "Didn't you change anything in the opera when it reached the stage later on?" he asked. "I wasn't even present," Rossini told him. "Mombelli performed it in Milan[n] without my knowledge. What surprised people about that quartet was that it ended without the usual closing cadences, with something like an outcry by the voices. The duet from it also was sung a lot and for a long time: it was very easy, and that was the main thing."

The rather Mozartean quartet *"Donami omai, Siveno"* became the best-known number in *Demetrio e Polibio*. Stendhal, who claimed that he had heard this opera at the opening of a new theater at Como in 1814,[n] wrote of the quartet: "Nothing in the world is superior to this piece: if Rossini had composed only this quartet, Mozart and Cimarosa would recognize him as a peer. It has, for instance, a lightness of touch (what in painting is called making something out of nothing) which I have never seen in Mozart." Less hyperbolic and more germane was Stendhal's appreciation of *Demetrio e Polibio* as a whole: "What augmented still more the charm of those sublime cantilenas was the grace and modesty of the accompaniment, if I may dare to speak thus. These songs were the first flowers of Rossini's imagination; all of them have the freshness of life's morning." He was discussing music mostly composed by a fourteen-year-old boy.

After the May–June 1812 performance of *La Scala di seta* at Venice, Rossini returned to Bologna. There he received his first commission to compose an opera for Italy's leading theater, La Scala, Milan, for what surely seemed to him the large fee of six hundred lire (about $310). Marietta Marcolini and Filippo Galli, both of whom already had sung Rossinian roles, were influential in obtaining this contract for him. The libretto assigned to him was *La Pietra del paragone*, by Luigi Romanelli, a Roman who had become a Scala librettist in 1799 and whose collected librettos eventually filled eight volumes. Although abysmal as verse, this was in some ways the best text that Rossini had faced. It is easily workable on stage and provides a constantly amusing framework for precisely the sort of music he was best prepared to compose: ebullient farce. Happily for him, too, it invited him to echo some of the eighteenth century's "Turkish" or "Janizary" sound effects, which Mozart had used so entertainingly in *Die Entführung aus dem Serail*. Borrowing freely from *Demetrio e Polibio* and *L'Equivoco stravagante*, he composed and put together a brilliant score.

Rossini probably was at La Scala on August 17, 1812, when an *opera buffa* by Giuseppe Mosca, *Le Bestie in uomini*, won the audience's complete approval. That sort of success so shortly before the *première* of his own opera might well have worried him. But when *La Pietra del paragone* was played for the first time, on September 26, 1812, it too was an instantaneous hit. The two-act *melodramma giocoso* was sung fifty-three times that first season—an astonishing record in a city of less than 300,000 people (many members of the audience undoubtedly came to Milan from outlying towns).[n] That sort of acclaim at La Scala transformed the twenty-year-old Rossini into a *maestro di cartello*, a composer whose name would attract the public. Thereafter, he was the leading young composer of Italy.[n]

The venerated Cimarosa had died in 1801; in 1812, the almost equally honored Paisiello, with four meagerly productive years to live, was seventy-one. At sixty-two, Luigi Cherubini had become in effect a foreigner, as had the thirty-seven-year-old Gaspare Spontini. Rossini's chief active colleagues in Italy were Giuseppe Farinelli, Pietro Generali, Giovanni Simone Mayr, Saverio Mercadante, Giuseppe and Luigi Mosca, Giovanni Pacini, Ferdinando Paër, Stefano Pavesi, and Nicola Antonio

Zingarelli—not one of whom was nearly his match. The first major achievements of both Donizetti and Bellini were to postdate Rossini's abandonment of Italian stages in 1823.

Word of Milan's reception of *La Pietra del paragone* brought Rossini orders from Venice for three new operas—two of them for Cera, the impresario at the San Moisè, and one for the foremost Venetian theater, La Fenice. *La Pietra del paragone* proved to be his touchstone in another way: it helped to win for him exemption from military service, to which his age now made him liable.

Circumstantial accounts quoting from spurious documents dot the early biographies of Rossini as they deal with this exemption. The most widespread of them ascribes it to the enthusiasm of Eugène de Beauharnais, the French viceroy at Milan, and quotes a supposed letter from him ordering his minister of the interior to excuse Rossini from army service. Prince Eugène's involvement, in turn, was said to have been brought about by one Olimpia Perticari, a friend (or perhaps more) of Rossini's. Rossini did become friendly with the Pesarese family of Perticari six years later, but no Olimpia Perticari existed, and Beauharnais never wrote such a letter for her. In 1855, Rossini told Hiller: "I had been destined to become a soldier. Because I was a property-owner [the house in Lugo], there was no way to avoid it. And what properties! My manor brought me in forty lire [about $20] a year. But the success of that opera disposed the commanding general kindly toward me. He appealed to the Viceroy Eugène, who was then absent [he was in Russia with Napoleon], and I was permitted to go on with more peaceful occupations." Azevedo wrote that Rossini said to him: "The conscription was the gainer, for I would have been a terrible soldier."

By mid-August 1812, the composer of *La Pietra del paragone* may well have been weary: it had been the fifth new opera by him to be played that year. But he had no time to enjoy resting upon his laurels: he and his parents still had to be fed, housed, and clothed. He went back to Venice to take care of the first of the two new *farse* for the San Moisè. The libretto supplied by Cera was *L'Occasione fa il ladro, ossia Il Cambio della valigia*. This was the work of Luigi Prividali (often spelled Previdali), a shady Venetian scribbler who was to become a trial to Vincenzo Bellini and to many singers. The *Giornale dipartimentale dell'Adriatico* reported, credibly enough, that Rossini composed the score in eleven days, "too narrow a period even for the impulses of a fervent genius." The opera was sung for the first time at the San Moisè on November 24, 1812.ⁿ Received with chill indifference that night, *L'Occasione fa il ladro* pleased its audiences but little more on the four subsequent nights when it was sung. It never became a favorite, but had some scattered stagings elsewhere in Italy and was put on at Barcelona in 1822, St. Petersburg in 1830, and Vienna in 1834.ⁿ It has had few later stagings.

During October 1812, either while Rossini was still in Milan or after his return to Venice, he almost certainly received from Giovanni Ricordi a forwarded letter that pre-echoed one important aspect of his future. On October 8, Giovanni Colbran wrote to Ricordi, complaining that he and Isabella were unable to leave Naples "because the road from here to Rome is full of bandits who are not satisfied with robbery, but also murder all who fall into their hands." At the bottom of her father's letter, this appears in Isabella's script: "My dear Ricordi, I greet you with all my heart and hope to have the pleasure of seeing you soon. Isabella Colbran." Her father states that he is enclosing a letter for Rossini. That enclosure has not survived, but in it he very probably asked the increasingly famous Rossini—whom he could have met in Bologna in 1806 and 1809—to provide Isabella with a role in one of his next operas. She was to have roles in many of Rossini's future operas and to become his wife, but we cannot be certain either of his having replied to her father's letter or of the degree of his friendship with the Colbrans before he saw them again at Naples in 1815.

Rossini was completing his apprenticeship as a composer when his ninth opera, *Il Signor Bruschino, ossia Il Figlio per azzardo,* was staged at the Teatro San Moisè late in January 1813.ⁿ Giuseppe Foppa had borrowed the subject for this *farsa* from a French comedy by Alisan (André-René-Polydore) de Chazet and E.-T.-Maurice Ourry. *Il Signor Bruschino* was not a success. The unexampled burst of glory to be ignited eventually by Rossini's next opera would drive it temporarily from impresarios' minds, but when his name everywhere became a talisman, the work would be revived—at, for example, Milan in 1844, Madrid and Berlin in 1858, Brussels in 1859, and at the Piccola Scala, Milan, in 1957. At the Bouffes-Parisiens on December 29, 1857, a French version, with the music adapted by Offenbach, struck fire. When Rossini, then living in Paris, was asked to attend a rehearsal of this *Don Bruschino,* his reply was: "I have let you do what you wanted to do, but I certainly have no intention of being your accomplice."

Il Signor Bruschino gave rise to one of the most deeply imbedded of the garbled Rossini anecdotes, already referred to in its re-garbled form (see page 28). It reports that when Cera, the San Moisè impresario, denounced Rossini for having accepted a commission from the rival Fenice (or, alternately, consciously assigned him an abominable libretto), Rossini took revenge by filling the score with outrageous extravagances and tricks intended to offend audiences. According to Azevedo, Rossini composed irate music for tender scenes and the softest of strains for moments of wrath; assigned lugubrious music to the most farcical passages and music of the *buffo* sort to the most serious lines; filled with roulades the vocal line of a singer of ponderous voice; gave very high notes to a bass, very low ones to a soprano; composed "the most elegant, delicate, exquisite cantilena" with pizzicato accompaniment for Luigi Raffanelli's gravelly voice; and inserted a very protracted funeral march into this brief one-act *opera buffa*. Azevedo added that Rossini went on passively playing the cembalo while members of the audience privy to the jokes laughed uproariously and the unaware whistled their disapproval.[n]

Luigi Rognoni was accurate when he wrote of *Il Signor Bruschino*: "It should be said that Rossini's biographers (before Radiciotti) had not, however, taken the trouble to read the libretto, which seems no different from many others set by Rossini and peacefully accepted by the public of the time—or, even less, the music, which is among the realistically liveliest and most spirited written by the Pesarese . . ."[n] The proliferating legend probably was started by the measures in the *Bruschino* overture in which the second violinists are directed to strike the wooden parts of their bows rhythmically against the tin covers of the lamp stands before them, thus producing clicking noises suggestive either of a loud clock or of a conductor calling his forces to order. But even that "outrageous" sound does not, as Azevedo asserted, occur at the opening of every measure of the overture: it is asked for four times, for a few measures each time.

The "very protracted funeral march" lasts sixteen extremely funny measures during a scene in which Bruschino *figlio* slinks up to his father with bowed head, making a patter song of the syllables that his stutter drives him to repeat. Except insofar as bizarrerie and outrage were inherent in Rossini's conception of *opera buffa*, nothing in the libretto or music of *Il Signor Bruschino* confirms the legend. The true cause of the unquestioned show of discontent by its first audience probably was the delay of about two hours in opening the doors of the San Moisè for the *première* and the additional delay inside the theater before the overture was begun." In reality, this opera—though not musically on the level of *La Pietra del paragone*, which had preceded it by only four months, and far below the level of *L'Italiana in Algeri*, which followed it by another four—contains music of fresh charm and vivacity and is often both comic and witty. With proper casting and a conductor not willing to inflate, and thus blur and devalue, the delicately balanced sounds of Rossini's orchestra, *Il Signor Bruschino* always stands ready to make its effect.

Not counting the small emoluments that Rossini had received from the Mombellis in 1806 as he delivered separate numbers for *Demetrio e Polibio,* his first nine operas had brought him only a little more than $1,650 in today's purchasing power. Along with other considerations, such as that of his enormous energy and facility in composing, this fact helps to explain why he had been rushing from city to city, composing operas in fretful haste. For on that meager sum, along with amounts earned as coach, conductor, and supplier of occasional numbers for insertion into other composers' operas, he had been supporting himself, paying for his traveling, and contributing largely to the upkeep of his parents. Soon after the production of his tenth opera in February 1813, both his fame and his worldly goods were to begin growing swiftly.

CHAPTER III

1813-1815

ALMOST AS IMPORTANT as a success at La Scala was one at the lead-ing theater of opera-loving Venice, La Fenice, where a Rossini *première* was staged for the first time in 1813. *Tancredi*, the two-act *melodramma* text provided Rossini by the Fenice, was the work of Gaetano Rossi,[n] who had derived its argument from episodes in Tasso's *Gerusalemme liberata* and Voitaire's five-act tragedy *Tancrède*; he may also have been familiar with several earlier librettos dealing with the Tancred story. Rossini, aware of the importance of the Fenice, had asked a fee of 600 francs for *Tancredi*, adducing the fact that it was an *opera seria*. Azevedo wrote that the impresario countered with an offer of only 400; in the end, a compromise at 500 francs (about $260) was agreed upon.

Rossini, who had provided the nearby San Moisè with *L'Occasione fa il ladro* the preceding November and with *Il Signor Bruschino* in January, cannot have spent much time in completing *Tancredi*—a fact that may explain his having borrowed for it the overture to *La Pietra del paragone*, thus demonstrating that, at least under duress, he felt no imperious need for differentiating in musical style between the overture to a farce and one to a serious drama. *Tancredi* received its *première* at the Fenice on February 6, 1813.[n] That performance began as scheduled, but the official local *Giornale* reported that the two leading ladies were unwell, with the result that during both the *première* and the second attempted singing, the opera had to be stopped in the middle of Act II. Only on February 12 was everyone in the cast well and *Tancredi* sung through. It was greeted with many signs of approval, but did not look like a big success. It was sung—with alterations introduced by Rossini along the way—about fifteen times at the Fenice that season. Its wildfire renown was to be sparked by later performances.

Rossi's libretto for *Tancredi* had a happy ending, with Tancredi and Amenaide in each other's arms. But for the second staging of the opera, at Ferrara about March 30, 1813, the text was refashioned nearer to Voltaire's version, in which the wounded Tancredi dies in the presence of Amenaide and Argirio.ⁿ The opera as a whole pleased the Ferrarese audience, but this tragic conclusion upset some of its members, who complained that having to watch such saddening scenes might interfere with their digestion. The original ending had to be restored. The temporary change in the libretto, of course, had necessitated changes in Rossini's music: he had added a new aria (*"Perchè turbar la calma"*), which seems to have been lost along with the new finale after the original ending was restored.

From Venice and Ferrara, *Tancredi* moved south and west to enthusiastic acclaim, thus spreading Rossini's name throughout Italy.ⁿ Beginning with a production in Italian at Munich in August 1817, and then as translated into many languages, *Tancredi* carried his fame across Europeⁿ and to North, Central, and South America, serving to make Rossini a genuinely international figure. But the story that its once internationally popular aria *"Di tanti palpiti"* began its phenomenal, long-enduring success at the first Venice performance is contradicted by contemporary accounts. Only the overture drew separate notice then. But by the time the opera returned to Venice in the autumn of 1815, the lilting aria was well into its extraordinary history. Stendhal probably was reporting sober fact when he wrote that in Venice everyone from gondoliers to the wealthiest gentlefolk was repeating its phrase *"Mi rivedrai; ti rivedrò"*; that sort of universal familiarity was reported from other Italian cities, as well as from Dresden and Vienna.ⁿ

Byron, in Canto XVI of *Don Juan*, attests to Rossini's fame in England:

> . . . *the long evenings of duets and trios!*
> *The admirations and the speculations;*
> *The "Mamma Mia's!" and the "Amor Mio's!"*
> *The "Tanti palpiti's" on such occasions:*
> *The "Lasciamo's," and the quavering "Addio's."*

Byron added a footnote recalling the mayoress of a provincial English town who, objecting to the Italian singing of some performers, had exclaimed: "Rot your Italians! for my part, I loves a simple ballat!" Byron continued: "Rossini will go a good way to bring most people to the same opinion one day. Who would imagine that he was to be the successor of Mozart? However, I state this with diffidence, as a liege and loyal admirer of Italian music in general, and of much of Rossini's, but we may say, as the connoisseur did of painting in *The Vicar of Wakefield*, that 'the picture would be better painted if the painter had taken more pains.' "[n]

Tancredi was not the revolution either in Rossini's musical manner or in Italian opera which it often has been proclaimed to be. The statement has been made that in *Tancredi*, Rossini altogether suppressed *recitativo secco*; he did not, though passages of it are relatively fewer here than in his earlier operas. When *Tancredi* was about to be staged in Berlin in January 1818, Giuseppe Carpani[n] was asked by a journalist about its distinguishing quality. He replied: "Sir, from Berlin, there is cantilena and always cantilena and beautiful cantilena and new cantilena and magic cantilena and rare cantilena. Succeed—with all your precepts about acoustics, esthetics, psychology, and physiology—in inventing just one of those cantilenas *alla Rossini*; discover it and sustain it, *et eris mihi magnus Apollo*. Nature, which had created a Pergolesi, a Sacchini, a Cimarosa, now has created a Rossini."

After the final *Tancredi* of its first Fenice season (March 7, 1813), Rossini dashed to Ferrara to supervise its staging there and to provide the new music already mentioned. But he had little time for Ferrara: he had engaged to supply still another Venetian theater, the San Benedetto, with an *opera buffa* for staging in May. By mid-April, he was again in Venice. Whereas he had been paid 250 francs for a *farsa* at the San Moisè, his fee for the two-act *melodramma giocoso* at the San Benedetto was to be 700 francs (about $360). The libretto supplied him, entitled *L'Italiana in Algeri*, had been based by Angelo Anelli[n] on the legend of Roxelane, the beautiful slave girl of Suleiman the Magnificent.[n] Anelli's text was not new: Luigi Mosca had made it into an opera that had been staged successfully at La Scala, Milan, on August 16, 1808.

Gossip was particularly busy in connecting Rossini's name with that of his San Benedetto *prima donna*, Marietta Marcolini. Stendhal—perhaps on the basis of known facts, perhaps creating fiction—wrote: "It is said that *la M——*, a charming *buffa* singer, then in the flower of her genius and youth, not wanting to be in arrears with Rossini, sacrificed Prince Lucien Bonaparte to him." Stendhal and Azevedo (who perhaps was quoting Stendhal) agreed in picturing Rossini's life in Venice after

L'Italiana in Algeri as a banquet of rich and beautiful women, a time when he could select at will which of the most sought-after invitations to the *palazzi* of the powerful and prominent Venetian families he would deign to accept. These descriptions cannot, of course, be documented. But they invite some discounted belief in view both of Venice's known opera madness and Rossini's known taste for beauty, wealth, good food, and general luxury.

L'Italiana in Algeri aroused noisy enthusiasm at the San Benedetto on May 22, 1813.[n] Then Marcolini (Isabella) fell ill; the second performance had to be postponed to May 29, when she was awarded an ovation. On the next evening, the personal triumph was Rossini's: verses lauding him were floated down into the pit amid acclamations. *L'Italiana*, to then the best of Rossini's comic operas and one of the four or five finest he ever composed, remained on the San Benedetto's boards throughout June. Rossini was reported[n] to have said, the day after its *première*: "I thought that after having heard my opera, the Venetians would treat me as a crazy man; they have showed themselves to be crazier than I am." How astonishingly large the audience for comic opera had become in Venice is suggested by the fact that while these performances of *L'Italiana* continued at the San Benedetto, the San Moisè was basking in thirty-seven performances of Giuseppe Farinelli's *Il Matrimonio per concorso*, another new opera.

The official Venetian *Giornale* reported (May 24, 1813) that Rossini had composed *L'Italiana* in twenty-seven days; the Venice correspondent of the *Allgemeine musikalische Zeitung* (Leipzig) wrote that Rossini had told him that its composition had occupied him for only eighteen days. The *Zeitung* classified Rossini as second among living Italian composers of opera—after Giovanni Simone Mayr (actually a German), who during that year brought out two of his best operas, *La Rosa bianca e la rosa rossa* and *Medea in Corinto*. According to Zanolini,[n] however, it was in view of the spreading popularity of *L'Italiana* that Giuseppe Malerbi asked Padre Mattei what he now thought of Rossini and his works—and received the reply: "He has emptied his sack."

The writer in the Venetian *Giornale* had been correct when noting numerous examples of Rossini's originality in *L'Italiana in Algeri*. But it is easy to agree with Radiciotti (who knew better than most other modern writers the operas of Rossini's now neglected contemporaries) when he wrote: "As with *Tancredi* in the field of *opera seria*, so with

L'Italiana in the field of *opera comica*, Rossini still had not completely acquired his own personality: here and there some trace of imitation still is evident." After detailing passages that owe something to such composers as Mozart (*Die Zauberflöte*), Cimarosa, Pietro Generali, and Pietro Carlo Guglielmi, Radiciotti added: "At least in part, then, we still are in the field of Neapolitan *opera buffa,* but on the verge of coming out of it shortly." Rossini, that is to say, stood almost three years short of *Il Barbiere di Siviglia,* four of *La Cenerentola.*"

Rossini's whereabouts and activities between the performances of *L'Italiana* in Venice in May–June 1813 and December of that year cannot be determined, but he very probably spent much of that interim in Bologna with his parents. Milan, however, had not forgotten the composer of *La Pietra del paragone*: late in 1813, having signed a second contract with La Scala, Rossini set to work on a two-act *opera seria* (or *dramma serio*) for presentation there on Santo Stefano (December 26), the traditional opening night of the winter or Carnival season." This time, his fee was to be 800 francs (about $412). The libretto of *Aureliano in Palmira* long was attributed to Felice Romani; it was almost certainly the product of a much less able librettist named Gian Francesco Romani (or Romanelli)." This time—uniquely—Rossini composed for a *castrato*: the role of Arsace was designed for the vainglorious Giambattista Velluti, who caused trouble during rehearsals by clashing with Alessandro Rolla," the renowned conductor at La Scala, and by so overloading the profiles of his melodies with applause-gathering ornament as to make them unrecognizable to Rossini, who was scandalized.

Aureliano in Palmira had an agitated first performance at La Scala on December 26, 1813, and was coldly received." The *Giornale italiano* blamed the unfavorable reception of the opera upon the singers. The *Allgemeine musikalische Zeitung* said: "It does not please, but for various reasons apart from the music, which contains many beauties; but in it one senses the lack of inner vitality." *Il Corriere milanese* called *Aureliano* boring, the performance extremely sluggish, and said that Rossini, "on whom so many good hopes have been placed, has slept this time like the good Father Homer, with the difference, however, that the Greek singer rested from time to time, whereas the Pesarese composer now has been sleeping for a long period. . . ." *Tancredi* is the most beautiful musical composition of our times; as regards effect, *Aureliano* does not seem to be an opera by Rossini." The opera nonetheless ran up fourteen performances at La Scala that season." Nor did the coolness of the first, strict Milanese audience toward it discourage the impresario of La Scala: on an undetermined date in the spring of 1814, he signed Rossini to a contract for a two-act *opera buffa* (or *dramma buffo*) for the 800-franc fee, the new work to be ready to open the autumn season in August.

This time Rossini was at last handed a libretto by Felice Romani.[n] It rang an inverted change on the outline of *L'Italiana in Algeri*, setting a Turk down in Italy for the winningly absurd events of *Il Turco in Italia*. Rossini, who almost certainly had returned to Bologna after the first performances of *Aureliano in Palmira* that winter, was in Milan again in April. He was at the Teatro Re on April 12 for that theater's first performance of *L'Italiana,* and had to appear onstage with the singers at the close of both acts to acknowledge the audience's enthusiasm.

Although *Il Turco in Italia*, first heard at La Scala on August 14, 1814,[n] would be sung there twelve times that season, it was regarded as having been a disaster. A lively writer in *Il Corriere milanese* said that after listening to several numbers, "I examined, took thought, recognized, and said into the ear of my neighbor, a most discreet man: *'C'est du vin de son cru.'* 'An indecent new edition,' he added, rather loudly. A third man, having heard him, began to shout in a stentorian voice: *'Potpourri, potpourri! . . .'* " Evidently disturbed by the mirror resemblance of the plot involvement of *Il Turco in Italia* to that of *L'Italiana in Algeri*, that first Milanese audience imagined that Rossini was repeating —even quoting—himself, warming over the earlier opera; actually the two operas are little more alike than *Le Nozze di Figaro* and *Così fan tutte.*

Il Turco in Italia not only has a distinct musical personality—largely because of Rossini's intense imaginative reaction to the character of Prosdocimo the Poet as a sort of teasing Greek chorus—but is much more completely Rossini's own than *L'Italiana.* As soon as its complete separateness from the earlier opera was recognized, it became a Rossini success. Stendhal, and others who depended upon his book, said that the Milanese themselves began to appreciate *Il Turco* four years after its *première*, but in fact it was not sung in Milan again for nearly seven years. Then, in the season of 1820-1, it was received enthusiastically at both the Teatro Lentasio and the Teatro Carcano.[n]

Although early Rossini letters are scarce, his whereabouts and professional activities can be traced through accounts of first productions of his operas, references to him in periodicals and the letters and diaries of others, and autograph datings on his compositions. We know, for example, that in Milan in 1814, he composed and dedicated to a Principessa Belgiojoso a cantata for two voices entitled *Egle ed Irene*.* By mid-November 1814, however, he was once more in Venice, this time under contract to the Teatro La Fenice for a two-act *opera seria* (or *dramma*) to a text by Giuseppe Foppa entitled *Sigismondo*. His fee was to be about 600 francs (roughly $310), less than he had received for his last *opera buffa* at La Scala. Foppa's libretto very probably was the worst that Rossini ever was cornered into composing.* The *Nuovo Osservatore Veneto* said of it (December 27, 1814): "The libretto is the unhappy child of a writer who now submits the hundredth proof of his ineptitude." Radiciotti called Foppa an *abborracciatore* (bad bungler). Rossini's setting of this hackwork, which both showed stigmata of weariness or boredom and lacked an overture, received its *première* on the opening night of the Fenice's season, December 26, 1814.*

Azevedo reported that the Fenice orchestra had applauded at rehearsals of *Sigismondo*, declaring it Rossini's best opera.* "Despite the favorable predictions of the Fenice musicians," Azevedo added, "*Sigismondo* produced general ennui and was greeted with a unanimous yawn. Rossini, leading the performance, was himself seized by this boredom: never, he said later, had he suffered so much at a first performance as at that of *Sigismondo*. . . . To some friends placed near the orchestra who attempted to applaud, he said in a loud voice: 'But whistle, whistle!' He felt that only memories of *Tancredi* and *L'Italiana* were saving him from hostile manifestations by the audience; he did not want to owe anything to such considerations."

Sigismondo failed. Geltrude Righetti-Giorgi wrote that when Rossini sent notice of that fact to his mother, he drew on the outside of the letter a fine *fiasco*.* He told Hiller: ". . . one evening I was really touched by the Venetians. That was at the *première* of *Sigismondo*, an opera that bored them mightily. I could see how gladly they would have given vent to their annoyance; but they restrained themselves, kept quiet, and let the music pass by them without disturbance. That kindness made me go quite soft!" With *Eduardo e Cristina* (1819), another opera that Rossini put together for Venice, *Sigismondo* remains the least known of his stage works.

Sigismondo, probably never staged outside Italy, achieved few productions inside it: it never was sung at La Scala or in Naples, and it had all but disappeared by 1827. It marked a minatory decline in Rossini's inventiveness and workmanship. He clearly stood in need of new impulses, new scenes, new audiences—and of a less constantly peripatetic life. With the opera after *Sigismondo*, fortunately for him and his admirers, his Neapolitan period would begin. He had composed (not counting *Demetrio e Polibio*) thirteen operas in four years for Venice, Bologna, Ferrara, and Milan; of the twenty Italian operas that he would write in the next nine years, exactly half would be for Naples.

From Bologna on May 15, 1815, Rossini wrote to the Venetian librettist Prividali: "Have you yet selected the subject for the oratorio? I beg you not to waste so fine an opportunity, one so dear to me: grant the prayers of your friend, who desires to clothe your beautiful words in his *divine music* (this is known as giving merit its due)."" This suggests that he had promised to provide someone in Venice with an oratorio to a text by Prividali. But he appears never to have set any Prividali text but *L'Occasione fa il ladro,* and he never composed a true oratorio, though that superscription was often lent to operas (as with *Ciro in Babilonia*) given pseudo-Biblical subjects to make them available for Lenten performance.

Rossini's first direct contact with the Bonaparte family occurred early in 1815, at Bologna, when he gave some music lessons to Napoleon's niece, the daughter of Elisa Bacchiocchi, ex-Grand Duchess of Tuscany. Napoleon's vicissitudes now began to affect Rossini directly. Joachim Murat, the Emperor's brother-in-law, who had been King of Naples, had taken Napoleon's abdication in April 1814 as the signal to ally himself with the confused forces struggling to unite an independent Italy. When Napoleon escaped from Elba in March 1815, Murat tried to lead uncommitted troops against the Austrians, but most of the soldiers deserted and went home. In the continuing course of his maneuvers, Murat issued at Rimini on April 5, 1815, a proclamation of Italian independence; it, in turn, led to an uprising at Bologna, which temporarily succeeded. That success clearly demanded a patriotic celebration with music—and Rossini was at hand. He was provided with a flatulent text by Giovanni Battista Giusti, with whom he had read Dante, Ariosto, and Tasso a few years before. Giusti had produced this doggerel at the request of the patriot Pellegrino Rossi, who also had drawn up Murat's *Proclama di Rimini*. It was headed *Agli italiani*, but became known as the *Inno dell'indipendenza*. It could not raise Rossini out of the slough of more or less automatic composing into which providing an occasional piece almost always drove him. His *Inno* was sung for the first time at the

Teatro Contavalli, Bologna, on April 15, 1815, in Murat's presence. Received with feverish enthusiasm as conducted by Rossini, it was at once
dubbed "the Italian *Marseillaise*."

Unhappily, the Austrians retook Bologna the next day; then or
at some time later the score of Rossini's *Inno dell'indipendenza* appears
to have been destroyed or lost. The Austrian authorities, having become
aware of Rossini's "revolutionary" effusion, put him down in their
black books as a subversive fellow. Although a less likely revolutionary
could scarcely be conceived, he was kept under surveillance for several
years.[n] A story that he refitted the score of the *Inno dell'indipendenza*
to a pro-Austrian text and presented the result to the commanding
Austrian general tied up in yellow and black ribbons probably was
concocted by a curious Frenchman named Charles-Jean-Baptiste Jacquot,
who, under the pseudonym Eugène de Mirecourt, published at Paris in
1855 a tortuous and defamatory booklet entitled *Rossini*. The tale was
repeated by Enrico Montazio in his *Giovacchino Rossini* (Turin, 1862)
and, surprisingly, even by Zanolini in the 1875 edition of his book,
originally written in 1844. ("Eugène de Mirecourt" at one point was
imprisoned by the Paris police for having printed libels on several noted
personages.)

Rossini twice denied the story, but in doing so himself made a
mistake that also became imbedded in legend. On the occasion of the
first denial, he told Hiller: "There's not a word of truth in it. I remained
calm; I had no wish to jest with those severe gentlemen." That appears
to have been the truth. But more than fifty years after the events at
Bologna, he wrote a letter (June 12, 1864) to his Palermitan friend
Filippo Santocanale. In it, he said that "some of my miserable fellow-
townsmen have given me the reputation of being a *reactionary*, those
unhappy fellows being unaware that in my artistic adolescence, I set
to music with fervor and success the following words:

> See that for all of Italy
> Examples are born anew
> Of valor and of daring!
> In the battle they will see
> What we Italians are worth![n]

and later, in 1815, when King Murat came to Bologna with sacred
promises, I composed the *Inno dell'indipendenza*, which was performed
under my direction at the Teatro Contavalli. In this hymn is found
the word *indipendenza*—which, though it is not very poetic, aroused

lively enthusiasm as intoned by me in my then resonant voice and repeated by the people, choruses, etc.

"A little story that was invented about this hymn offended me a
little; a lovely biographical soul asserted that I had offered this hymn
([reset] to another poem)[n] to the Austrian General Stef[f]anini in celebration of his return! He had wanted to give the color of a pleasantry
to this joke, but it would have been a cowardice of which Rossini is
incapable.

"I am gentle in character but brave of soul: when the Austrian
general returned to Bologna, I was in Naples concentrating on the composition of an opera for the Teatro San Carlo: see how history is
compiled ! ! !'"

But Rossini was in Bologna, not Naples, when General Steffanini
reached Bologna on April 16, 1815. Louis Hérold, the twenty-four-year-
old future composer of *Zampa* and *Le Pré aux clercs*, was there from
April 12 to 24, 1815; he wrote that during those days he met several
Bolognese music lovers and musicians, among them Rossini, "a young
composer who at that moment was making a devil of a reputation in
Italy." Rossini was at times subject to neurotic cowardice; his description of himself as "brave of soul" needs careful interpretation. Eager to
scotch an unfounded story, he had confused the timetable of events
blurred by passage of half a century—which certainly does not mean
that he carried out the rear-guard action attributed to him by Eugène de
Mirecourt.

Rossini's existence now was being sharply altered by the intervention of Domenico Barbaja, one of the most interesting figures in early-
nineteenth-century Italian theatrical life. Whether the two men met in
Bologna, as early biographers insisted, or whether Rossini went to Barbaja's Neapolitan fief in response to a letter summoning him there,
or whether both meetings occurred cannot be determined. He seems to
have reached Naples for the first time early in the spring of 1815, to
have remained there only a few weeks, then to have returned to Bologna,
and then to have gone back to Naples: in the letter to Prividali cited
above, he said, "I shall leave the day after tomorrow [May 16, 1815]
for Naples." When Rossini saw the great Bay of Naples for the first
time, fourteen operas lay in his past, twenty-five in his future. He was
only a little past his twenty-third birthday.

CHAPTER IV

1815-1816

WHEN ROSSINI reached Naples in the spring of 1815, the city was emerging from a series of political vicissitudes. During the Napoleonic interregnum, with Murat as King of Naples from 1808 to 1815, the Bourbon Ferdinand IV[n] had been reigning in Palermo as *de facto* king of only one Sicily. In 1815, with the aid of English ships, Naples was recaptured by Austrian troops and returned to Bourbon rule. On May 22, almost at the time of Rossini's arrival in Naples, Prince Leopold of Salerno—a younger brother of Ferdinand—rode into the city flanked by Austrian generals and was greeted with undecipherable enthusiasm by large throngs of Neapolitans. Ferdinand himself returned to Naples in triumph in June, to reign there for another ten years as Ferdinand I, King of the Two Sicilies, before being succeeded in 1825 by his son Francis I. Only anti-Bourbon Neapolitans, their numbers increasing slowly, thought of themselves as Italians: Ferdinand's subjects usually spoke of people coming from the north, for example, as having "arrived from Italy."

Fervently operatic, Naples was enjoying several lyric theaters, the three leading ones being the San Carlo, the Fondo (more recently known as the Mercadante), and the Nuovo; opera was also staged at the Teatro dei Fiorentini until 1820, and occasionally until 1849 at the San Carlino. The living composers chiefly represented on these stages were Valentino Fioravanti (1764–1837), now remembered mostly for *Le Cantatrici villane* (1799); the greatly prized Giovanni Simone Mayr (1763–1845); Giuseppe Mosca (1772–1839), and Ferdinando Paër. Giovanni Paisiello (1740–1816) had, at seventy-five, only one year more to live. Domenico Cimarosa (1749–1801) and his best operas were alike regarded as classics.

Neapolitans generally considered their city to be the operatic—and therefore the musical—capital of the Italian peninsula, and therefore of Europe. They thought their own special type of opera the finest product of eighteenth- and nineteenth-century musical civilization. For some time, first under the aegis of Paisiello, then under that of Nicola Antonio Zingarelli (1742–1837), conservative Neapolitan musicians and opera lovers had been warning against the threat "from Italy" implicit in Rossini, his operas, and his imitators.

Paisiello had called Rossini a "licentious" composer who paid little attention to the rules of his art, a debaser of good taste, a man whose great facility in composition was in part the result of a very tenacious memory. Zingarelli, who had become director of San Sebastiano (the Royal School of Music),[n] was commonly said to have forbidden its students even to read the scores of Rossini's operas. In a footnote to his book on Rossini, Zanolini reported that Zingarelli once listened with Rossini to a student's opera at the Conservatory. At the end of it, he turned to Rossini to say: "You see? Another new *maestro* who is imitating you!" "He is doing the wrong thing," Rossini replied, "but I can't stop him." What should be realized is that Paisiello and Zingarelli were not jealous or mean-spirited nonentities: they were highly trained, expert musicians. From their point of view, they were entirely right: Rossini was the most advanced threat at that hour to the remarkable, dying operatic style of which they were among the last practitioners.

But the most important individual in operatic Naples was the former Milanese scullion and *caffè* waiter Domenico Barbaja (1778–1841[n]). Very intelligent, poorly educated, shrewd, and energetic, Barbaja had amassed the beginning of a large fortune by catering to the passion for faro and other games which had ruled the Milanese, the members of Napoleon's and other armed forces stationed in Lombardy, and the businessmen who battened upon them. He not only gambled successfully, but also operated tables in the foyer of La Scala at which others gambled to his profit. Removed to Naples and—on October 7, 1809—having initiated his almost uninterrupted thirty-one-year reign as chief impresario of the city,[n] he received from the Bourbon government both a subsidy and a license to operate theater gaming tables as he had at Milan. A *bon vivant* and gourmet,[n] this "prince of impresarios" moved with aplomb through all strata of society, royalty included. During various overlapping periods, he presided over the San Carlo, the Fondo, and other Neapolitan theaters and also—at times in association with others—over La Scala and the Teatro della Canobbiana at Milan (1826–32) and the Kärnthnertortheater and Theater an der Wien at Vienna (1821–8). In 1823, he commissioned Weber to compose *Euryanthe* for the Kärnthnertortheater.

When the Teatro San Carlo was ruined by fire on February 12–13, 1816, Barbaja promised to have it rebuilt in record time, and he reopened it on January 13, 1817. When Ferdinand I, fulfilling a vow made on his return from Palermo in 1815, ordered a church erected west of the Royal Palace, Barbaja became in effect the contractor, worked with the architect Antonio Niccolini on an adaptation of the Pantheon at Rome, and in 1835 saw completed the Church of San Francesco di Paola, still the central landmark of the hemicycle in the Piazza del Plebiscito. By 1843, Barbaja's renown had reached Paris: in that year, he was represented, at the Opéra-Comique, as a character in *La Sirène*, an opera by Auber to a Scribe text.

Barbaja was to be extremely influential in Rossini's career (he was present in somewhat smaller roles in the careers of Weber, Donizetti, and Bellini). He was directly responsible for the staging of ten of Rossini's operas. Moreover, Isabella Colbran, who was generally believed to be Barbaja's mistress at this time, later became Mme Rossini. Naturally, no documentary proof of the Barbaja-Colbran relationship survives; nor can the inception of Colbran's intimacy with Rossini be dated, though it seems certainly to have predated their marriage in 1822. Many people said that Rossini stole Barbaja's mistress. Significance was read into the fact that her marriage to Rossini occurred exactly one month after *Zelmira*, the last of Rossini's Neapolitan operas, was staged at the San Carlo for the first time. But the Rossinis went directly from their wedding to Vienna—where they were eagerly awaited by Barbaja, who was impresario of the Kärnthnertortheater, where he at once re-staged that same opera, with Mme Colbran-Rossini in its title role. Rossini and Barbaja certainly indulged in no enduring dispute over Colbran.

This was the man with whom, after some haggling over details, Rossini signed a contract binding him to act as musical director of the San Carlo and the Fondo and to compose two operas for Naples each year. Looking back upon this agreement long after, Rossini said: "If he had been able to, Barbaja would have put me in charge of the kitchen too!" Their contract, intended to become effective in the autumn of 1815, provided Rossini with an annual stipend that has been reported at figures rising from the 8,000 francs mentioned by Rossini himself to Hiller to the 12,000 francs specified by Stendhal. It provided that Rossini occasionally would be free to produce new operas elsewhere and that during such absences from Naples, his payments from Barbaja would lapse."

That Rossini left Naples after being there for a (second?) short stay in the spring of 1815 is suggested by an article in the *Giornale del Regno delle Due Sicilie* (hereinafter referred to as the official *Giornale*) for the following September 25: "From everywhere, conductors, singers, dancers of every sort are arriving. In a few days, the arrivals have included [Salvatore] Viganò, renowned creator of ballets; Signora [Antonia] Pallerini and Signor Le Gros, *primi ballerini*; Signor [Luigi Antonio] Duport and his young wife, both of them so much applauded on our stages; Signor [Giovanni Battista] Rubini, destined to sing at the Teatro dei Fiorentini; and, finally, one Signor Rossini, *maestro di cappella*, who, it is said, has come to give one of his operas, *Elisabetta, regina d'Inghilterra*, on the stage at the Teatro San Carlo, which still echoes to the melodious accents of the eminent Signor Mayr's *Medea* and *Cora*."" The opera that Rossini was finishing for the San Carlo—the largest opera theater in Europe—used a feverish pseudohistorical libretto by Giovanni Federico Schmidt" which reflected the post-Waterloo popularity of English stories by retailing supposed incidents in the love life of Queen Elizabeth and the Earl of Leicester. Nothing else about *Elisabetta, regina d'Inghilterra* was as important for Rossini as that he composed its title role for Isabella Colbran.

Colbran had evolved into a true dramatic soprano capable of the most elaborate coloratura. Besides singing in all of Rossini's Neapolitan *opere serie* and numerous operas by others, Colbran herself composed songs. Stendhal and others wrote that her voice began to give serious warnings of deterioration about the year of Rossini's introduction into her life, but she sang steadily until 1822, when she was thirty-seven. This tall, beautifully proportioned, greatly talented Spanish woman would directly influence Rossini's acceptance of librettos and the sort of music that he would compose from 1815 to 1823. She was never a comedienne; her penchant for grand, tragic roles led Rossini to compose only one true comic opera between *La Cenerentola* (composed for Rome in 1817) and *Le Comte Ory* (1828, written for Paris in Rossini's post-Colbran, post-Italian period). Any expression of bitterness against Barbaja and Colbran for having deprived posterity of the *opere buffe* that Rossini might have composed during those years betrays our century's lack of familiarity with his "Colbran" operas and our lack of the means to perform them adequately. In 1858, asked who had been the greatest female singer of his early years, Rossini replied: "The *greatest* was Colbran, who became my first wife, but the *only* was Malibran."

Elisabetta, regina d'Inghilterra reached its *première* at the San Carlo on October 4, 1815.[n] The occasion was doubly gala: it opened the San Carlo's autumn season and, as the printed libretto states, honored the name day of Francesco, Hereditary Prince of the Two Sicilies. It was therefore unrolled in the presence of Ferdinand I, Maria Carolina, the Hereditary Prince, and the Court. It marked an important change in Rossini's composing: for the first time, he altogether dispensed with *recitativo secco*. Nor was that all: it also marked his first effort to force virtuoso singers to perform the notes that he composed for them—the vocal ornaments were autographed as integral parts of the score. The care and comparative richness with which he had orchestrated *Elisabetta* reflected Rossini's reaction to the excellent San Carlo orchestra and its conductor, Giuseppe Festa. The carefully annotated florid vocal line for Elisabetta represents his exploitation of Colbran's special, rare capabilities and of their assured welcome from the *fioritura*-loving Neapolitan audience.

Those who purchased printed librettos for the *première* of *Elisabetta* could read the following "*Avvertimento*" by its librettist, Giovanni Federico Schmidt, an enlightening comment on the casual operatic usages of the time: "The unpublished subject of this drama, written in prose by the *signor avvocato* Carlo Federici and taken from an English romance [Sophia Lee's *The Recess*], was presented last year at the Teatro del Fondo. The fortunate success that it obtained resulted, at the request of the management, in my having had to arrange it for music. The original manuscript [of Federici's play] was not available (it belongs to the company of actors, which left Naples some months ago). Having attended various performances of it, I have imitated it insofar as my memory could help me, reducing five very long acts in prose to two very short ones in verse. As a result, I do not call myself the author except of the words and of some slight alterations to which the laws of our present-day operatic theater constrained me. Giovanni Schmidt, poet employed by the Royal Theaters of Naples."

Received with ecstatic enthusiasm from the night of its first performance on, *Elisabetta* brushed aside much of the entrenched Neapolitan resistance to a composer coming highly praised from the north. Simultaneously with the first performances of *Elisabetta* at the San Carlo, the Fiorentini was pleasing other Neapolitan audiences with *L'Italiana in Algeri,* which also helped. It ran at the San Carlo through October and was brought back on December 26 to open the winter season. King Ferdinand was said to have liked the opera so well that he commanded Zingarelli to rescind the ban against the reading of Rossini scores by students at San Sebastiano. *Elisabetta,* then, brilliantly justified Barbaja's having attracted Rossini to Naples. But it did not become one of Rossini's most frequently staged or most enduring operas, in part because no second Colbran appeared to sing and act its title role.

On August 18, 1838, less than twenty-three years after the *première* of *Elisabetta* (by when it had been staged in at least thirty Italian and foreign cities), Rossini answered from Bologna an impresario named Bandini who had written him from Florence for advice about staging it at the Teatro della Pergola there: "I shall not be able to give you any instructions about *Elisabetta,* as all memory of the costumes, decoration, etc., has been canceled from my mind. These are operas to be left at rest. Give modern music to the public, which loves novelty, and do not forget an oldtime composer who is your friend." Bandini disregarded Rossini's advice: the Pergola presentation took place. But by 1840, *Elisabetta* had all but disappeared from the operatic stage.

The overture used for *Elisabetta, regina d'Inghilterra* was that of *Aureliano in Palmira,* its orchestration reinforced to fit the size of the San Carlo and the abilities of its musicians. The big crescendo in the overture reappears in the opera itself, as the termination of the first-act finale. The orchestral prelude to the prison scene in Act II was borrowed from *Ciro in Babilonia.* Elisabetta's first-act cavatina, imported from *Aureliano,* later was to become the second section of *"Una voce poco fa"* in *Il Barbiere.* This makes clear once again that Rossini had no strong sense that an *opera seria* constantly required music different in kind from that of *opera buffa*: often a mere change of tempo would in his eyes transform one sort into the other.

For an undetermined reason—perhaps because Rossini earlier had agreed to supervise the staging of one of his operas for Pietro Cartoni and Vincenzo De Santis, co-impresarios of the Teatro Valle at Rome— he did not at once begin to fulfill that part of his contract with Barbaja which required him to compose two new operas each year for Naples: his second Neapolitan opera, *La Gazzetta,* was not to be staged until nearly a year after the *première* of *Elisabetta.* By late October or early

November 1815, he was in Rome, a city that had displayed highly approving interest in *Demetrio e Polibio, Il Naufragio felice (L'Italiana in Algeri), L'Inganno felice,* and *Tancredi.* There he supervised the mounting of *Il Turco in Italia* at the Valle, where it was received so warmly that it was sung throughout November and into December.

Rossini also had promised to compose a new opera for the Valle. Cartoni and De Santis supplied him with a two-act *dramma semiserio* libretto entitled *Torvaldo e Dorliska,* the first text by a young Roman dilettante named Cesare Sterbini,[n] who, Radiciotti wrote, "was going to add to the unfortunately exorbitant number of those abortions which then infested the Italian musical theater." His *Torvaldo e Dorliska* really is an *opera seria* into which a single character intrudes an element of supposed comic relief. The opera was sung for the first time at the Teatro Valle on December 26, 1815,[n] less than two months before Rome also heard the *première* of *Il Barbiere di Siviglia.* These were Rossini months in Rome: *L'Inganno felice* also was sung at the Valle during this Carnival season.

Geltrude Righetti-Giorgi wrote that when Rossini sent his mother news about the reception of *Torvaldo e Dorliska,* the *fiasco* he drew on the outside of it was much smaller than the one with which, exactly a year before, he had told her of the failure of *Sigismondo.* A writer in the *Notizie del giorno,* Rome, for January 18, 1816, said: "The reception of the *opera semiseria* called *Torvaldo e Dorliska,* new music by *signor maestro* Rossini, has not lived up to the hopes that were reasonably conceived for it. It should be said that the subject of the very dismal and uninteresting libretto has not waked Homer from his sleep; for which reason it was only in the introduction and in the inception of a trio that the famous composer of *Tancredi, La Pietra del paragone,* etc., was recognizable."[n]

Azevedo first recorded an anecdote that has survived in many books on Rossini. According to it, Rossini, after his 1815 arrival in Rome, had been shaved in his quarters several times. When time for the first orchestral rehearsal of *Torvaldo e Dorliska* was at hand, the departing barber said to Rossini: "Until we meet again." When Rossini, surprised, probed for an explanation, the barber's reply was: "I am the first clarinet of the orchestra." Rossini then realized that he might, at the rehearsals, have risked mortally offending a man who each day held a cutting edge against his throat, and "only the next day, after his beard had been shaved, did he point out [his instrumental errors] to the man; and the poor man, touched by a procedure so delicate and so rare, put himself out to satisfy his illustrious client."

Eleven days before the first singing of *Torvaldo e Dorliska* at the Valle," Rossini signed a contract for a new opera with Duca Francesco Sforza-Cesarini, owner-impresario of the Teatro di Torre Argentina, who was intensely devoted to opera and lavished large portions of his own substance on his theater each year. Several terms of this contract —and, even more, their implications—now seem extraordinary, but were not so in 1815." Rossini's fee, equivalent to about $1,250 in today's purchasing power, was high for the period, but the Argentina account books for 1816 show that three of the singers (Righetti-Giorgi, Manuel Garcia, and Luigi Zamboni) received more, the very renowned Garcia receiving about $3,800. The contractual provisions that the composer accept any libretto handed him by the impresario, compose the opera in five weeks, adapt its music to the voices and demands of the singers, preside at rehearsals, and act as *maestro al cembalo* during the first three public performances would strike a twentieth-century composer as demented. Little wonder that a decade later Donizetti would write to Mayr: "Well, I have known from the start that the profession of the poor composer of operas is of the unhappiest, and only necessity keeps me tied to it."

When Sforza-Cesarini signed the contract with Rossini, he was feeling a need to retrench, his personal fortune not being limitless. Audiences were used to an evening's entertainment that added a ballet to an opera; they were extremely critical of singers. The Duke felt unable to provide the expected ballet troupe and had reason to fear that the absence of dancing (perhaps even more of female dancers) would reduce the sale of tickets. That possibility, in turn, led him to engage singers who did not demand excessive sums—though, of course, he had to have one first-magnitude star, in this instance Garcia. Not until five days after the date of the contract with Rossini could Sforza-Cesarini sit back to wait, secure at last in the knowledge that he had a company to perform the opera. That opera was scheduled to be on the boards of his theater in about seven weeks (actually, sixty-seven days elapsed between the date of the agreement and the *première*).

Sforza-Cesarini first approached Jacopo Ferretti for a libretto for the new Rossini *opera buffa*. Ferretti submitted a text dealing with the loves of an officer and an inn hostess, with a lawyer added to form a triangle. Having rejected that as too ordinary,

Sforza-Cesarini turned to Cesare Sterbini,[n] who accepted the task of
grinding out a libretto, but only after considerable urging from both
Rossini and the impresario. The subject, drawn from Beaumarchais's
Le Barbier de Séville,[n] was easier to refashion as a libretto because
Beaumarchais himself had thought of it as an *opéra-comique* text (he
had staged it at least once as an *opéra-comique*, adapting for it songs that
he had collected in Spain). Thus it could be parceled out among arias,
duets, other ensembles, and recitative. Also, a renowned opera on the
same subject already existed: Paisiello's *Il Barbiere di Siviglia*, first
played at St. Petersburg on September 26, 1782, and later staged in
many Italian opera houses, elsewhere in Europe, and in America.[n] Its
libretto, by Giuseppe Petrosellini, was available in printed form to
Sterbini and Rossini, providing them with hints for procedure and warnings of what not to repeat.[n]

Rossini, it was said, aware of the aged Paisiello's strong *amour
propre* and wanting to disarm the *paisiellisti* in advance, wrote the older
composer in very respectful terms, explaining why and how he was
using a subject already operatically immortalized—and Paisiello supposedly replied that he took no offense and wished the new opera well.
Righetti-Giorgi wrote: "Rossini did not write to Paisiello, as is supposed, having in mind that a single subject could be treated by various
artists." Her explanation not only disregarded the central fact that
Paisiello and his opera were regarded by many Italians as sanctified
classics, but also was based on insufficient information. On April 22,
1860, Rossini himself wrote to a French admirer named Scitivaux: "I
wrote a letter to Paisiello, declaring to him that I had not wanted to
enter into a contest with him, being aware of my inferiority, but had
wanted only to treat a subject that delighted me, while avoiding as
much as possible the exact situations in his libretto . . ."[n] A further
attempt to forestall anger by the *paisiellisti* took the form of the *Avvertimento al pubblico* printed as a preface to the first libretto of the
opera, originally entitled *Almaviva* rather than by the name of Paisiello's
opera.

Sterbini kept his promise to deliver the libretto within twelve days.
Setting to work on January 18, 1816, he completed Act I on January
25, Act II on January 29. Rossini delivered the completed Act I to the
maestro concertatore of the Argentina on February 6. The parts then
were copied out overnight in the belief that the first rehearsal would
occur the next day. But during the night of February 6–7, tragedy was

added to confusion: Sforza-Cesarini, aged only forty-four, died of a stroke that well may have been induced by the strains under which he had been working. His immediate successor, Nicola Ratti, and Rossini and the others involved could set aside little time for mourning: the new opera had to be mounted as swiftly as possible, not only for the sake of the Argentina and its artists (and also to fulfill the contract, which the impresario-owner's death did not nullify), but also for that of Sforza-Cesarini's widow and children, whose thinned-down pocket-book some proceeds of the performances were to nourish.

Numerous versions exist of the story that Rossini composed and orchestrated *Il Barbiere di Siviglia* in eight days (Joseph-Louis d'Ortigue, quoting, he said, Manuel Garcia); eleven days (Montazio); thirteen days (Félix Clément); or fourteen days (Lodovico Settimo Silvestri).[n] The documented dates show only that Rossini did not, as Righetti-Giorgi said, spend "a long time at work on it." As Radiciotti wrote:[n] "Accepting the hypothesis that in order to save time, the librettist passed on the pages of his manuscript to the Maestro one by one as he completed them, exactly one month (January 19–February 19) would have elapsed between delivery of the first pages and the staging of the score; but from that we must subtract a dozen days required for rehearsals and *concertazione*;[n] so that Rossini could not have had available more than nineteen or twenty days for composition. Thus it is demonstrated that the six hundred immortal pages of this masterpiece were conceived and composed [i.e., written down] in a period of time which would be needed by a swift amanuensis for re-copying them! A real prodigy!"

Sixty-nine years after the Rome première of *Il Barbiere di Siviglia*, Verdi, starting to compose *Otello*, wrote to Giulio Ricordi: "Perhaps they will say that Meyerbeer was slow; but I answer that Bach, Handel, Mozart, Rossini, etc., etc., wrote *Israel in Egypt* in fifteen days, *Don Giovanni* in a month, *Il Barbiere* in seventeen or eighteen days! But add: that those men, besides their imagination, did not have exhausted blood, were well-balanced natures, had their heads on squarely, and knew what they wanted. They had no need to take inspiration from others, nor to do as the moderns do, *alla Chopin, alla Mendelson* [*sic*], *alla Gounod*, etc. They wrote spontaneously, as they felt; and they made masterpieces that—it is true—had inequalities, defects, even incorrectnesses, which at most times were traits of genius . . . Amen." And in 1898, writing to thank Camille Bellaigue for a copy of his *Les Musiciens*, Verdi said:

"You say many things about Rossini and Bellini, and they may be true, but I confess that I cannot help believing *Il Barbiere di Siviglia*, for abundance of ideas, for comic verve, and for truth of declamation, the most beautiful *opera buffa* in existence."[n]

Chroniclers doubting that Rossini could have composed so much music of such quality in so short a working period have pointed out that some of his apparent swiftness can be explained by his having made use of an already existing overture and having interpolated music from earlier operas into the new score. But the surviving 600-page manuscript score in the Conservatorio G. B. Martini at Bologna includes no overture: as is well known, the overture now played before *Il Barbiere di Siviglia* had been used for *Aureliano in Palmira* in 1813; with very slight alterations for *Elisabetta, regina d'Inghilterra*, in 1815[n]—and possibly for *L'Equivoco stravagante* in 1811. The assumption has been that an overture that Rossini composed expressly for *Almaviva* on Spanish melodies given him by Manuel Garcia has been lost. That Rossini composed or adapted for that opera an overture other than the one used with it now is certain.

Rossini gave the autograph score of the opera to a Professor Baietti; when Léon Escudier wanted to publish it in Paris, Rossini wrote from there to his friend Domenico Liverani, asking him to try to locate the missing overture and Lesson Scene in Bologna. On June 12, 1866, having heard from Liverani that the missing pieces could not be found, Rossini wrote him[n]: "Here am I to thank you for the trouble you went to in trying to locate (in my so-called autograph of *Il Barbiere*) the original of my overture and of the concerted pieces for the Lesson. Who could be the possessor of them now? Patience—Escudier wanted, as a pendant to the *Don Giovanni*, to do a complete edition of *Il Barbiere* according to my original, and I was hopeful that I could help him by obtaining the replaced pieces. But it will have to be less because Fate wants it that way."[n]

The borrowed music in the body of *Il Barbiere di Siviglia* is chiefly the following:

1. from *La Cambiale di matrimonio*: from the end of Fanny's aria "*Vorrei spiegarvi il giubilo*," a melody used in the cabaletta of the first-act Rosina-Figaro duet "*Dunque io son, tu non m'inganni*," at the words "*Ah, tu solo Amor tu sei*";

2. from *Il Signor Bruschino*: four and a half measures of a melody in the bass-soprano duet "*È un bel nodo che due cori*," a motive used

for orchestra alone during Bartolo's "*A un dottor della mia sorte,*" to the text words "*I confetti alla ragazza; il ricamo sul tamburo*";

3. from *Aureliano in Palmira*: the first eight measures of Arsace's rondo "*Non lasciarmi in tal momento,*" in Rosina's "*Io sono docile*" ("*Una voce poco fa*"); also the first six measures of the priestly chorus "*Sposa del grande Osiride,*" in Almaviva's "*Ecco ridente in cielo*"; also a figure from the Arsace-Zenobia duet, at the beginning of Basilio's "*La calunnia è un venticello*";

4. from the cantata *Egle ed Irene*: a melody with echo response in the allegro section ("*Voi che amate, compiangete*"), in the second-act trio "*Ah qual colpo,*" at Rosina's words "*Dolce nodo avventurato, Che fai paghi i miei desiri*";

5. from *Sigismondo*: a motive from the introductory chorus to Act II ("*In segreto a che ci chiama*"), as the motive of the introductory chorus, "*Piano, pianissimo*"; also the motive treated crescendo in the Ladislao-Aldimira Act I duet, in the crescendo of "*La calunnia*";

6. "reminiscences" from other composers (pointed out by Radiciotti): from Haydn's *Die Jahreszeiten*, a motive from Simon's aria, in the allegro section of the second-act trio, at Figaro's words "*Zitti, zitti, piano, piano*"; from Spontini's *La Vestale*, a melody from the second-act finale, in the Act I finale at the words "*Mi par d'esser colla testa in un'orrida fucina.*" Radiciotti noted that the Spontini melody also had been quoted in Nicola Antonio Manfroce's opera *Ecuba* (San Carlo, Naples, 1813).

Because that amount of "borrowing" would not suffice to explain the rapidity with which Rossini composed *Il Barbiere*, writers have speculated on his having summoned a collaborator, perhaps to supply the recitative. The candidates most often named have been Manuel Garcia, Luigi Zamboni, and Pietro Romani. But the Bologna autograph score is wholly in Rossini's script and displays clear indications of having been composed consecutively. Further, the collaborator most often put forward has been Romani, described as *maestro concertatore* of the Argentina when *Almaviva* was being prepared there. But he was not: Camillo Angelini was. Nor was any Romani on the payroll of the Argentina that season. What Romani actually composed was "*Manca un foglio,*" the aria that long was substituted for Rossini's more difficult aria for Bartolo, "*A un dottor della mia sorte.*" Romani composed that substitute for the special limitations of the *buffo* Paolo Rosich at performances of *Il Barbiere* given at the Teatro della Pergola, Florence, in November 1816, nine months after Rossini's "*A un dottor della mia sorte*" had been sung handsomely in Rome by Bartolommeo Botticelli, the original Bartolo.

We must accept the fact, astonishing rather than incredible, that Rossini composed and orchestrated *Il Barbiere di Siviglia* in less than three weeks.

Rossini, Sterbini, and probably the new impresario of the Argentina were apprehensive of the audience's reaction to the new setting of the subject of Paisiello's beloved opera. The printed libretto issued for sale to its first audiences therefore contained this *Avvertimento al pubblico*:

"*Almaviva, or The Futile Precaution*, comedy by Signor Beaumarchais, newly and completely versified and adapted to the use of today's Italian musical theater by Cesare Sterbini, Roman, to be staged at the Noble Theater of the Torre Argentina during the Carnival of the year 1816, with music by Maestro Gioachino Rossini. Rome. . . .

"The comedy by Signor Beaumarchais entitled *The Barber of Seville, or The Futile Precaution*, is being presented in Rome, adapted as a *dramma comico* under the title of *Almaviva, or The Futile Precaution*, this for the purpose of convincing the public fully of the sentiments of respect and veneration which animate the creator of the music of the present *dramma* toward the greatly celebrated Paesiello, who dealt with this subject under its original title.

"Called upon to take up the same difficult task, the *signor maestro* Gioachino Rossini, wishing not to incur the accusation of a temerarious rivalry with the immortal composer who preceded him, expressly asked that *The Barber of Seville* be *re-versified completely* and that some new situations for musical pieces be added, and he further asked that these be to the modern theatrical taste, so much altered since the epoch in which the renowned Paesiello wrote his music.

"Some added difference between the text of the present *dramma* and that of the Comédie-Française mentioned above was caused by the need to insert choruses into the subject itself, either because they are required by modern usage or because they are essential for producing a musical effect in a theater of notable capacity. And thus the courteous public will be informed, also on the responsibility of the writer of the new *dramma*, for without the concurrence of such influential circumstances, he would not have dared to introduce the slightest change into the French product, now consecrated by theatrical applause throughout all of Europe."

The first performance of *Almaviva, ossia L'Inutile Precauzione* took place at the Teatro Argentina, Rome, on February 20, 1816.ⁿ Its cast was: Geltrude Righetti-Giorgi (Rosina), Elisabetta Loyselet (Berta), Manuel Garcia (Almaviva), Luigi Zamboni (Figaro), Bartolommeo Botticelli (Bartolo), Zenobio Vitarelli (Basilio)—reputed to be a *jettatore*, one who has the evil eye—and Paolo Biagelli (Fiorello).ⁿ What occurred at the Argentina that night has become so entangled in legend that a factual account of it will always remain impossible to construct.

On March 22, 1860, Rossini wrote to a French admirer named Scitivaux who had asked for a short account of the conception and first performance of *Il Barbiere*: "I was called to Rome in 1815 to compose, at the Teatro Valle, the opera of *Torvaldo e Dorliska*, which had a good success; my interpreters were Galli, Donzelli, and Remorini, the most beautiful voices I have ever heard. The Duca Cesarini, proprietor of the Teatro Argentina and its director in that same Carnival season, finding affairs sad in his enterprise, proposed to me that (in haste) I make an opera for the end of that season. I accepted, and I associated myself with Sterbini, a treasury secretary and poet, in searching for a subject for the poem that I had to set to music. The choice fell on *Le Barbier*, I set to work, and in thirteen days it was finished.ⁿ I had as my interpreters Garcia, Zamboni, and Giorgi Righetti, all three of them valiant. I wrote a letter to Paisiello, declaring to him that I had not wanted to enter into a contest with him, being aware of my inferiority, but had only wanted to treat a subject that delighted me, while avoiding as much as possible the exact situations in his libretto. That disclaimer having been made, I believed myself sheltered from criticism by his friends and legitimate admirers. I was wrong! On the appearance of my opera, they rushed like wild beasts upon the beardless little *maestro*, and the first performance was one of the most tempestuous. I, however, was not troubled, and while the audience whistled, I applauded my performers. That storm having passed, by *Barber*, who had an excellent razor (Beaumarchais), shaved the beard of the Romans so well that I was borne in triumph (a theatrical phrase)."

According to Azevedo,ⁿ laughter, catcalls, and whistling broke out when Rossini appeared in a hazel-colored Spanish-style habit with gold buttons given him by Barbaja to wear on this occasion: "The progeny of the oldtime *maestri* of the world were men too common-sensical to believe that a man wearing a coat of that color could have the slightest spark of genius or that his music deserved to be listened to for a single instant." But that was only the beginning. When Vitarelli came onstage in highly original makeup on which he was counting heavily, he tripped over a trapdoor and fell painfully. When he picked himself up, his face was badly scratched, his nose almost broken. "The good public, like its ancestors in the Colosseum, viewed that flow of blood with joy," Azevedo wrote. "It laughed, applauded, demanded a repetition—in a word, made an abominable hubbub. Some people, thinking that this fall was an integral part of the role, cried out against the bad taste and gave signs of the most intense anger.

"Under such encouraging conditions, the wounded Vitarelli had to sing the incomparable 'Calumny' aria." In order to staunch the blood from his principal wound, he had every moment to raise to his nose the handkerchief that he carried in his hand," and each time that he allowed himself that motion, so necessary in a like situation, the whistles, catcalls, and laughter came from all parts of the hall. . . . As a climax to the disaster, a cat appeared during the superb finale, mixing among the performers. The excellent Figaro, Zamboni, chased it off to one side; it returned from the other and hurled itself into the arms of Bartolo-Botticelli. The doctor's unfortunate pupil and the respectable Marceline [Berta], fearing scratches, evaded with the greatest liveliness the prodigious leaps of the distracted animal, which respected only the sword of the chief of the patrol; and the charitable audience called out to it, imitated its miaowing, and encouraged it by voice and gesture to proceed with its improvised role."

Righetti-Giorgi reported that the audience whistled at her after her first brief appearance to say "Segui, o caro, deh, segui così," did not listen to Zamboni's performance of Figaro's cavatina or the duet as he sang it with Garcia (Almaviva), honored her with three outbursts of applause after "Una voce poco fa," and thereby led her to believe that all was well. "Zamboni and I then sang the beautiful Rosina-Figaro duet, and jealousy, turning still more rabid, unloosed all its tricks. Whistled at from every part [of the audience], we reached the finale . . . Laughter, shouts, and the most penetrating whistling; no silence except that in which they could be heard louder." After the "Quest'avventura" unison, someone shouted: "Here we are at the funeral of D[uke] C[esarini]!" She found it impossible to describe "the insults to which they subjected Rossini, who sat at his cembalo undaunted and seemed to be saying: 'Pardon these people, O Apollo, for they know not what they do.' When the first act was over, Rossini applauded with his hands —not his opera, as was commonly believed, but the singers . . . Many people were offended. That suffices, too, to give a notion of the outcome of the second act. Rossini left the theater as though he had been an indifferent onlooker. My spirit full of what had happened, I betook myself to his house to comfort him; but he had no need of my consolations; he was sleeping tranquilly."

"The next day, Rossini removed from his score whatever seemed culpable; then he feigned illness, perhaps so as not to have to appear at the cembalo." In the meantime, the Romans got back their senses and decided that at least they should listen to the whole opera and then judge it fairly. They returned to the theater on the second evening and remained intensely quiet. The opera was crowned with general applause. Afterwards, we went to the pretended sick man, who was in bed surrounded by many distinguished Romans who had gone to compliment him upon the excellence of his work. The applause increased at the third singing."

The details of Rossini's behavior on the second night were reported by Salvatore Marchesi di Castrone, who quoted Rossini as saying: "I had stayed at home alone. I tried to distract myself by writing, by composing music; but my head was elsewhere. With a watch in hand, counting the minutes, agitated, feverish, I had sung and played to myself the overture and the first act. Then irresistible curiosity and impatience took hold of me. I burned with the desire to know how my music had been received at the second performance. I had decided to dress myself and go out when I heard down the street a devil of a hubbub." If the "hubbub" was being created by the "many distingushed Romans" coming to compliment him, he may have climbed back into bed, a "sick man" again, to receive them—and have been there, surrounded by flattery, when his Rosina arrived.

A different account of what occurred at Rossini's hotel on the night of the second performance of *Il Barbiere* is given—purportedly in Rossini's own words—in Edmond Michotte's pamphlet *Une Soirée chez Rossini à Beau-Sejour (Passy) 1858*: "I was sleeping peacefully when I was awakened suddenly by a deafening uproar out in the street, accompanied by a brilliant glow of torches; as soon as I got up, I saw that they were coming toward my hotel. Still half asleep, and remembering the scene of the preceding night, I thought that they were coming to set fire to the building, and I saved myself by going to a stable at the back of the courtyard. But lo, after a few moments, I hear Garcia calling me at the top of his voice. He finally located me. 'Get a move on you; come now; listen to those shouts of *bravo, bravissimo Figaro*. An unprecedented success. The street is full of people. They want to see you.' 'Tell them,' I answered, still heartsick over my new jacket gone to the devil, 'that I f—— them, their bravos, and all the rest. I'm not coming out of here.' I don't know how poor Garcia phrased my refusal to that turbulent throng—in fact, he was hit in the eye by an orange, which gave him a black eye that didn't disappear for several days. Meanwhile, the uproar in the street increased more and more. Next, the proprietor of the hotel arrived, breathless. 'If you don't come, they'll set fire to the building. Now they're breaking windows . . .' 'That's your affair,' I told him. 'All you have to do is not stand near the windows . . . Me, I'm staying where I am.' Finally I heard some panes crashing. Then, battle-weary, the crowd dispersed at last. I left my refuge and went back to bed. Unhappily, those brigands had defenestrated two windows opposite my bed. It was January [*sic*]. I'd be lying if I told you that the icy air penetrating into my room gave me a delicious night."

Il Barbiere di Siviglia had a maximum of seven performances in Rome during 1816: the Argentina closed for the season on February 27. It was not heard in Rome again for five years. In that interim, however, it was sung with constantly increasing success elsewhere. At Bologna in September 1816, it was billed for the first time under its present title; it was sung later that year at Florence. Thereafter, it spread swiftly along the length of Italy. Beginning at Her Majesty's Theatre, London, on March 10, 1818, it moved abroad. By the time of its return to Rome in 1821, it already was well into its history of thousands of performances throughout the world.

One early reaction to *Il Barbiere* remains fascinating because of its source. On April 19, 1820, Stendhal wrote to his friend Baron Adolphe de Mareste:[n] "Rossini has done five operas that he always copies; *La Gazza ladra* is an attempt to break out of the circle; I shall see. As for the *Barbiere*, boil up four operas by Cimarosa and two by Paisiello with a symphony by Beethoven; put it all in lively measures by means of eighth-notes, lots of thirty-second-notes, and you have *Il Barbiere*, which is not worthy to untie the strings for *Sigillara* [*La Pietra del paragone*], *Tancredi* and *L'Italiana in Algeri* . . . " These sentences were written less than four years before Stendhal published in volume form his worshipful *Vie de Rossini*.

During the last rehearsals of *Almaviva* at the Argentina, Rossini must have heard that at Naples on the night of February 12–13, the Teatro San Carlo had been gutted by fire. But he cannot have known how that conflagration would influence his own future or his status vis-à-vis Barbaja when, on February 29—his twenty-fourth birthday— he signed an agreement with Pietro Cartoni to compose for the Teatro Valle, Rome, an opera that would turn out to be *La Cenerentola*. Having appointed that rendezvous for the next Santo Stefano (December 26, 1816), he could return to Naples, to his contractual duties there, and —in all likelihood—to the arms of his imperious, beautiful, difficult Spanish soprano mistress, Isabella Colbran.

CHAPTER V

1816-1817

A<small>T</small> N<small>APLES</small> on April 24, 1816, a marriage contract was signed between Carolina Ferdinanda Luigia, eldest child of the Hereditary Prince of the Two Sicilies, and Charles-Ferdinand, Duc de Berry, second son of the future Charles X, King of France. The Teatro San Carlo lay in charred ruin; the first singing of Rossini's unusually extended and elaborate marriage cantata, *Le Nozze di Teti e di Peleo,* therefore took place at the Teatro del Fondo. Long presumed lost, the autograph of this cantata was found in the library of the Naples Conservatory by Philip Gossett, who reported[n] that even within the one aria not in Rossini's hand, autograph indications occur. Mr. Gossett wrote: "There are no characters, no events, merely a succession of pastoral scenes, and Rossini obligingly supplies pastoral music. In general, the quality of the music is high, although much of the thematic material is derivative. Indeed the extent of self-borrowing in this cantata is quite remarkable. Of the eleven distinct musical numbers, eight are in whole or in part borrowed from earlier compositions." He then lists the sources as including eight operas, from *L'Equivoco stravagante* to *Il Barbiere di Siviglia,* as well as the 1810 tenor aria, *"Dolci aurette che spirate."*

On April 30, 1816, Antonia Olivieri Rossini, mother of the composer's father, died at Pesaro at eight-one. She had been the boy's substitute mother at intervals when his parents had been traveling the provincial operatic circuit. But it is unlikely that he went to Pesaro for her funeral: he would have been unable to absent himself from Naples for the several days required for the round trip. During the succeeding months, he was occupied at the Teatro del Fondo with the *concertazione* of the first Neapolitan performance of *Tancredi.* Also, he had agreed to compose a two-act *opera buffa* for the Teatro dei Fiorentini; this would be staged as *La Gazzetta, ossia Il Matrimonio per concorso.* Its libretto, which Giuseppe Palomba had based upon Goldoni's *Il Matrimonio per concorso,* had been touched up for Rossini by Andrea Leone Tottola.[n] Early in August 1816, the official *Giornale* said of the promised new Rossini opera: "Everyone asserts that it is just about to appear; everyone is eager for it, but unhappily it still is not ready to respond to the unanimous desires of a public irritated by interminable repetitions of old rigmaroles."[n] The same paper, reporting later that month on the preparations for *Tancredi* at the Fondo, added: "We hope that now Signor Rossini, freed of that task, will want to turn his most careful ministrations to *Il Matrimonio per concorso,* promised to the Teatro dei Fiorentini, which has been asking for some new musical composition for a long time now."

The *première* of *La Gazzetta* occurred at the Fiorentini on September 26, 1816.[n] Listed as a *dramma per musica,* it was nonetheless in effect an *opera buffa.*[n] A failure, it was sung for only a few evenings. It never was remounted at Naples; nor was it staged elsewhere during Rossini's lifetime.[n] But *La Gazzetta* does not altogether lack Rossinian attractions: of particular charm are Lisetta's aria *"Presto dico,"* one aria for Madama La Rosa, and much of the music for Don Pomponio Storione, including an aria in which he doggedly, thunderingly enumerates the rulers of the countries of the world.

The failure of *La Gazzetta* proved to be merely a short sag in the rapidly reascending line of Rossini's career. Before going back to Rome to fulfill his contract with the Teatro Valle, Rossini had to go on carrying out his arrangement with Barbaja, this time by composing a three-act *opera seria* with a role for Colbran. Its libretto, a bowdlerizing of Shakespeare's *Othello,* was the careful if mistaken labor of an interesting man, the Marchese Francesco Berio di Salsa, who would also supply Rossini with the text for *Ricciardo e Zoraide* two years later.

Berio di Salsa was a wealthy literary dilettante belonging to the Neapolitan nobility. He was said to know by memory much of Homer, Sophocles, Terence, Corneille, Alfieri, and Shakespeare. Stendhal wrote of him: "Very charming as a man in society, he was without talent as a poet." Lady Morgan, describing Neapolitan salons that she had visited during the Winter of 1820, said:[n]

"The saloons of the Marchese Berio present another aspect of society equally favourable to the impressions previously received of Neapolitan intellect and education. In Rome a *conversazione* is an assembly where nobody converses, as in Paris a *boudoir* is a place '*où l'on ne boude pas!*' The *conversazione* of the Palazzo Berio, on the contrary, is a congregation of elegant and refined spirits, where every body converses, and converses well; and best (if not most) the master of the house.

"The Marchese Berio is a nobleman of wealth, high rank, and of very considerable literary talent and acquirement, which extends itself to the utmost verge of the philosophy and belles-lettres of England, France, Germany, and his native country. He has read every thing, and continues to read every thing; and I have seen his sitting-room loaded with a new importation of English novels and poetry while he was himself employed in writing, *al improvviso*, a beautiful ode to Lord Byron, in all the first transports of enthusiasm, on reading (for the first time) that canto of Childe Harold, so read and so admired by all Italy [Canto IV]. Time, and a long and patiently endured malady, have had no influence over the buoyant spirit, the ardent feelings, the elegant pursuits, of this liberal and accomplished nobleman; his mind and manners are beyond the reach of infirmity; and the *ci-devant jeunes hommes* of other countries might purchase his secret at any price, were such a secret (which Nature only communicates) purchaseable.

"Of the *Conversazioni of the Berio Palace*, it is enough to say, that its circle comprised, when we were at Naples—Canova, Rosetti (the celebrated poet and *improvisatore*), the Duke de Ventignano (the tragic poet of Naples), Delfico (the philosopher, patriot, and historian), Lampredi and Salvaggi (two very elegant writers, and accomplished gentlemen), Signore Blanc (one of the most brilliant colloquial wits of any country, which the author of this work 'ever coped withal'), and the Cavaliere Micheroux, a distinguished member of all the first and best circles of Naples." While *Duchesse* and *Principesse*, with titles as romantic as that which induced Horace Walpole to write his delightful romance of 'Otranto,' filled up the ranks of literature and talent,—Rossini presided at the piano-forte, accompanying alternately, himself, Rosetti in his *improvisi*, or the Colbrun, the *prima donna* of San Carlos, in some of her favourite airs from his own Mosé. Rossini, at the piano-forte, is almost as fine an actor as he is a composer. All this was very delightful, and very rare! . . ."

Berio di Salsa, despite his erudition, social charms, and conversational accomplishments, was a feeble dramatist. His exceedingly free adaptation of *Othello* has made him a figure of fun, particularly since the appearance of Boito's strong, Verdian libretto from the same play. As Vincenzo Fiorentino wrote: "It is true that the demands of Italian opera of the period did not leave him [Berio] full freedom of action, but Shakespeare's sublime masterpiece emerges excessively disfigured, unrecognizable, from this, his reduction. Byron was scandalized." Writing a letter from Venice to John Murray on February 20, 1818, Byron added as a postscript: "To-morrow night I am going to see Otello, an opera from our Othello, and one of Rossini's best, it is said. It will be curious to see in Venice the Venetian story itself represented, besides to discover what they will make of Shakespeare in music." Eleven days later, writing to Samuel Rogers, he said: "They have been crucifying *Othello* into an opera (*Otello*, by Rossini): the music good, but lugubrious; but as for the words, all the real scenes with Iago cut out, and the greatest nonsense inserted; the handkerchief turned into a *billet-doux*, and the first singer would not *black* his face, for some exquisite reasons assigned in the preface. Scenery, dresses, and music very good."

This was the text to which Rossini, in a brief but undeterminable length of time, composed *Otello, ossia Il Moro di Venezia,*[n] one of the most popular and longest-lived of the operas in which he expressly designed a leading dramatic soprano role for Colbran. His nineteenth completed opera, *Otello* was given its first performance at the Teatro del Fondo, Naples, on December 4, 1816,[n] thus closing for Rossini a year of three new operas which had begun in February at Rome with *Il Barbiere di Siviglia*. Although many Neapolitans were dismayed (some of them were angered) by the opera's tragic denouement, *Otello* was a success; its real triumph, however, would date from singings at the San Carlo beginning in 1817.[n]

In 1817, a book entitled *Rome, Naples et Florence* was issued under the new pseudonym Stendhal: it was the third published work of the thirty-four-year-old Henri Beyle. We read in it, under the date February 17, 1817: "I shall hurry through in very few words what I have to say of the music heard at the San Carlo. I came to Naples transported with hope . . . I began at the San Carlo with Rossini's *Otello*. Nothing colder. It must have taken a lot of *savoir-faire* on the part of the writer of the libretto to render insipid to this degree the most impassioned of all dramas. Rossini has seconded him well . . ."[n] By the time of the 1826 edition of his book, however, Stendhal was touching it up and even redating his diary-like entries. Now, under date of March 17, 1817, we read: [n]

"My first experience at the *San-Carlo* was Rossini's *Otello*. I can conceive nothing more chilling. [Stendhal's footnote adds: "To punish myself for having entertained such unworthy thoughts in 1817, I am resolved to leave this epithet exactly as it stands. At the time, I was carried way, albeit unconsciously, by the tempest of my wrath against the *marchese* Berio, the author of that unspeakable *libretto* which turns Othello into a *Blue-Beard*! In the portrayal of the gentler emotions, Rossini (who has by now written himself out) never rose to within a thousand leagues of Mozart or Cimarosa; in compensation, however, he conceived a style so swift and glittering as these great masters never dreamed of."] The wretched librettist must have needed something very near to genius to reduce the most powerful tragedy that ever was on any stage to such a tasteless mess of insipidity. On the other hand, Rossini has aided and abetted him in every way he knew. The overture, admittedly, is of an astonishing originality, entrancing, easy to grasp, and full of irresistible charms for the unmusical, yet never tending to banality. Yet when the subject of the tragedy is Othello, the music may have all these qualities, and still be hopelessly, shamelessly inadequate. Neither in the whole life's-work of Mozart, nor yet in Haydn's *Seven Last Words of Christ*, is there any music too profound for such a subject. Indeed, the most satanic discords of enharmonic writing, would scarce suffice to portray the villainous Iago (*cf.* Pergolesi, *Orfeo*,[n] first recitative). Rossini, so I suspect, is himself insufficiently master of his own idiom to describe such things. Furthermore, he is too good humoured, too merry, too fond of his food. . . ." And, under the date March 18: "This evening, the *San-Carlo* company gave a performance of *Otello* at the *teatro del Fondo*. I picked out quite a number of attractive themes, hitherto unsuspected: among others, the duet for two female voices in Act I ["*Inutile è quel pianto . . . Vorrei che il tuo pensiero . . .*"][n]

Giacomo Meyerbeer was in the audience at the Teatro San Benedetto, Venice, when *Otello* was sung there. On September 17, 1818, he wrote from Venice to his brother Michael Beer in Berlin:[n] "Soon after your departure, Rossini's Otello was staged in Venice. The first act was totally unsuccessful, and truly it is very weak with the exception of a very lovely canonlike adagio in the finale, which he took from his oldest *farsa, Il Matrimonio per stravaganza* [*L'Equivoco stravagante*] (composed in Bologna) and inserted into *Otello*. In the second act, the *stretta* of a duet drawn completely from an aria in *Torvaldo e Dorliska* was pleasing, as were the *stretta* of a trio copied almost complete from *La Gazza ladra* and twelve measures of a cabaletta in an otherwise barbarous aria for Festa. With the last, he closed the second act, and the thinking part of the audience openly expressed its displeasure over this unheard-of plagiarism. The old theater habitués actually uttered the word 'fiasco,' particularly as it was known that the last act contained only three pieces, of which two (a romance and a prayer) were quite small. And yet those two small pieces not only saved the opera, but also elicited a furor the like of which has not been heard in twenty years, and which was so great that after thirty performances, all sold out, the enthusiasm was so enormous that Tacchinardi and Festa were granted very large sums to play a continuous three-month run this coming autumn. The third act of *Otello* established its reputation so firmly that a thousand blunders could not shake it. But this third act really is godlike, and what is so extraordinary is that its beauties are absolutely anti-Rossini-ish. First-rate declamation, ever-impassioned recitative, mysterious accompaniment full of local color, and, particularly, the style of the oldtime romances at its highest perfection."

The gigantic Verdian *Otello* has made the onetime universal popularity of Rossini's opera all but incredible to some twentieth-century operagoers. Beginning in 1818, it started to spread rapidly in and out of Italy;[n] within a decade, it was very widely established. Thereafter, it held the world's stages until late in the century. Both Giuditta Pasta and Maria Malibran incredibly essayed the role of Otello, having found Desdemona too pallid. After the Second World War, concert performances of *Otello* began to occur. A staging of it, with costumes and scenery by Giorgio de Chirico, was greeted enthusiastically at the Teatro dell'Opera, Rome, during its 1963–64 season (and repeated in 1964–65), when sophisticated listeners shed their Shakespearean and Verdian preconceptions to accept the Berio di Salsa–Rossini *Otello* for its own musical and operatic beauty.

Only with *Otello* safely on the stage at the Teatro del Fondo could Rossini concentrate upon the two-act *opera buffa* that he had agreed to deliver to Cartoni in Rome. By their contract of February 20, 1816, he was required in Rome not later than the end of October: the new opera was supposed to be staged on December 26. That Rossini reached Rome in October is barely possible, but that he took any step toward composing the new opera then is extremely unlikely: the *première* of *La Gazzetta* occurred in Naples on September 26, that of *Otello* there on December 4. Actually, he appears to have gone to Rome in mid-December.[n] On December 23, three days before the date originally foreseen for the first performance of the new opera, its libretto had not yet been chosen. As Cartoni and Rossini were close friends, the composer stayed in the impresario's apartment in the Palazzo Capranica, hard by the Teatro Valle. The plan had been for him to take his meals there too, but he later told Zanolini that he found the Cartoni food so overloaded with spicy, highly aromatic condiments that he decided to eat elsewhere. In no case can the possibility have arisen that Cartoni might invoke the contractual clause providing a penalty for late delivery.[n]

In 1898, Alberto Cametti, an admirable chronicler, published a book about the librettist Jacopo Ferretti.[n] In it, he quoted from a memoir left by Ferretti upon his death in 1852 a passage dealing vividly with the belated selection of a libretto for Rossini to compose for Cartoni:

"Just two days before Christmas in the year 1816, the placid impresario Cartoni and Maestro Rossini invited me to a meeting with the ecclesiastical censor. The subject was the considerable modifications to be made in a libretto written by [Gaetano] Rossi for the Teatro del Valle which Rossini was to compose as the second Carnival opera. The title read '*Ninetta alla corte*,' but the subject was *Francesca di Foix*, one of the least moral comedies of the French theater at a time when it had begun to change into the notorious school of libertinism which it later, without tinsel or any veil of shame, showed itself to be.

"The modifications reasonably desired by the provident Cato would have denatured the comic farce of its story. The ecclesiastical censor, who did not go to theater, was not persuaded by me, but Rossini was painfully convinced; thereupon he begged me, I say—and the phrase is exact, because of a little injury that he had inflicted upon me.[n] But an inability to say no, combined with an ambition to write with this distinguished Pesarese, drove me to torment my imagination and kept us drinking tea at Cartoni's home that very cold evening. I proposed twenty or thirty subjects for a *melodramma*, but one was visualized as too serious *for Rome then*, at least during Carnival, when they wanted to laugh; one was too complex; one would have cost the impresario too much—and an impresario's views on economy always must be respected docilely by poets; and, finally, one would not fit the virtuosos who had been designated.

"Weary of making suggestions, and half falling asleep, in the middle of a yawn I murmured: *Cinderella*. Rossini, who had climbed into bed so as to concentrate better, sat up as straight as Alighieri's Farinata."ⁿ 'Would you have the courage to write me a Cinderella?' And I, in turn, asked him: 'Would you have the courage to set it to music?' And he: 'When [can I have] the outline?' And I: 'If I go without sleep, tomorrow morning.' And Rossini: 'Good night!' He wrapped himself up in the bedclothes, stretched out his limbs, and, like Homer's gods, fell into the most blessed sleep. I took another glass of tea, agreed to a price, shook Cartoni's hand, and rushed home.

"There, good mocha coffee replaced the Jamaica tea. I paced up and down and back and forth across my bedroom with folded arms, and when God willed it and I saw the picture before me, wrote the outline of *La Cenerentola*.ⁿ And the next day I sent it to Rossini. He was satisfied with it.

"I had called the opera *Angiolina, ossia La Bontà in trionfo*. But the censorship deleted the Angiolina because an Angiolina was wrecking hearts with two most beautiful eyes at that time, and they suspected an allusion. Had I thought of making such an allusion, I would not have put *bontà* into the subtitle, but beauty—or, better, flirtatiousness—in triumph!

"Rossini had the introduction on Christmas Day; Don Magnifico's cavatina on Santo Stefano [December 26]; the duet for the *donna* and the soprano on San Giovanni [December 27]. In short, I wrote the verses in *twenty-two days* and Rossini the music in *twenty-four*. It is known that except for the Pilgrim's aria, the introduction to the second act, and Clorinda's aria—which were entrusted to Maestro Luca Agolini, called Luchetto the Lame—all the rest was composed by Rossini."ⁿ Four days before he was to have the whole score completed, Rossini had realized that he could not complete it in time, and therefore had turned to the Roman composer Agolini for assistance. The same pressure probably drove him to borrow the overture from *La Gazzetta*, an opera unknown in Rome and showing no likelihood of continued life anywhere.

Besides obtaining contributions from Agolini, Rossini borrowed two numbers for *La Cenerentola* from earlier operas of his own: the overture and Angiolina's pyrotechnical concluding rondo "*Non più mesta accanto al fuoco.*" The overture is that written for *La Gazzetta*. Angiolina's rondo had been sung earlier in another key and somewhat simpler form by Almaviva in *Il Barbiere di Siviglia*, to the words "*Ah!*

il più lieto, il più felice."[n] Cametti quotes Ferretti as writing: "That magnificent Cimarosian duet between the two buffos, '*Un segreto d'importanza,*' was completed the night before the opera's first performance and was rehearsed the next morning and then between one act of the opera and the next, while the Bazzi comedians played the second act of Goldoni's *Il Ventaglio.*"

Geltrude Righetti-Giorgi, the first Angiolina, wrote: "At Rome I saw him [Rossini] composing *La Cenerentola* amid the greatest hubbub. 'If you leave me,' he often said, 'I have no inspiration and lack all support.' A singular peculiarity! They laughed, talked, and even sang pleasant ariettas, but off to one side. And Rossini? Rossini, helped by his genius, made all his puissance felt from time to time, taking the happiest sections to the piano." But Louis Spohr recorded in his journal,[n] under the date January 8, 1817, that when he went to call upon Rossini, Cartoni refused him entrance to the workroom and would not bring Rossini out to meet him, saying that he did not want to interrupt the composer's work. Rossini's fee for that work, the *concertazione* of the opera, and his duties at the cembalo during its first three performances had been set by contract at 500 scudi (about $1,575).

The basic materials used by Ferretti in his hastily prepared libretto had originated in "*Cendrillon, ou La Petite Pantoufle,*" one of Charles Perrault's *Histoires ou contes du temps passé* (1697). Ferretti very probably had more direct recourse to an adaptation of the tale by Felice Romani, who had written a Cinderella libretto for Pavesi's 1814 opera *Agatina, o La Virtù premiata,* which was being sung at La Scala in April 1814, when Rossini was in Milan to sign the contract for *Il Turco in Italia.* Rossini is likely to have heard Pavesi's opera, and Ferretti certainly knew Romani's libretto: in it appeared for the first time the non-Perraultian characters of Dandini and Alidoro, who reappear in Ferretti's text. Also, Cinderella's slipper, replaced by a rose in Romani's *Agatina,* was changed into a bracelet by Ferretti. Mario Rinaldi[n] has called Ferretti's libretto "a true and genuine plagiarism."

Of the *première* of *La Cenerentola* at the Teatro Valle, Rome, on January 25, 1817, Ferretti wrote:

"The virtuosos who performed this opera were Geltrude Giorgi-Righette [Angiolina-Cenerentola], rich in a voice classic for its extraordinary range; Andrea Verni [Don Magnifico, a role that he also had sung in Pavesi's *Agatina*], who was in the evening of his glory; Giuseppe De Begnis [Dandini], who had only shortly before torn himself from the first conjugal embraces of Giuseppina Ronzi, and who had the system, when singing, of shouting like a man possessed; Giacomo Guglielmi [Don Ramiro], whose beautiful voice was beginning to deteriorate and often seemed a shopful of wrong notes [*spaccio di sincopate*]; the pretty Caterina Rossi [Clorinda], sister of the distinguished *concertatore* Lauro Rossi; Teresa Mariani [Tisbe], and Zenobio Vitarelli [Alidoro].[n]

"Except for the *maestro*, who on all of his most tempestuous first nights had applied to himself the Horatian *adversis rerum immersabilis undis*, all those taking part in the performance of the *melodramma* on that fatal first night had rapid pulses and the sweat of death dripping from their pallid foreheads.

"And solemn reasons existed for that fever and that icy rain. What was being presented was an opera difficult of musical execution and a drama largely not understood. But the Carnival was short and the impresario's interests required it thus. To be feared was a cabal by all the acerb and immature little *maestri* and all the semi-retired little *maestri*, who hated the new *maestro* to death, like pygmies at war with the sun. They had to deal with that pretty little head of Rossini's, which did not have to sweat in order to hit upon cold sarcasms or ironic applause sufficient to give a singer an apoplectic convulsion, and which had happily indulged in more than one such sally during the few rehearsals. To lessen the terrors of the virtuosos, there descended into the prompter's sepulchral grotto, giving the rarest example of self-effacement, the not-mediocre *maestro* [Pietro] Romani, who in that same theater had staged his own new *melodramma*, *Il Qui pro quo*,[n] which had been applauded up to the preceding day; and himself prompted with precision, accent, and energy and heartened him who, *pallidus morte futura*, by then was certain that he would leave for funeral pyre or pillory rather than in a triumphal car.

"On that first, extremely stormy evening, nothing escaped the shipwreck but the largo and *stretta* of the quintet, the final rondo, and the sublime largo of the sextet: the rest went by unobserved, and here and there even whistled at. But Rossini, not having forgotten the temporary downfall of *Il Barbiere di Siviglia* and being conscious of the magic with which he had largely infused *La Cenerentola*, bewildered and saddened by that fiasco, afterward said to me: 'Fools! Before Carnival ends, everyone will be enamored of it. . . . Not a year will pass before it will be sung from the Lilibeo to the Dora, and within two years it will please in France and be considered a marvel in England. It will be fought over by impresarios, and even more by *prime donne*.' "[n]

Rossini's prophecy proved substantially correct. On February 8, only twelve days after that dismal *première*, the *Notizie del giorno* said: "Well-earned applause continues to [be given to] the *signor maestro* Rossini at the Teatro Valle for his most beautiful *Cenerentola*." The *Galleria teatrale* noted that the singers, exhausted by rehearsals of this "difficult" score, had not been in good voice on the first four nights, but that thereafter they had been capable of giving their best, thus evoking general enthusiasm—for which the writer assigned special credit to Righetti-Giorgi. *La Cenerentola* was played at the Valle not less than twenty times before the season ended on February 18. Of a performance of it at the Teatro Tordinona, Rome, on October 26, 1818, Cametti wrote: "At the Tordinona, the eternal *Cenerentola* was performed; and it was on this occasion that Ferretti amended his *melodramma* at many points at which phrases sinned by triviality; and this also is clear from the libretto, which was republished by De Romanis in large format."

By the time Rossini was twenty-five, in 1817, his career as a composer of *opere buffe* for Italian opera houses was over," though he would compose nineteen more operas during the succeeding twelve years. He had left Rome on February 11 with his wealthy young Bolognese composer-friend the Marchese Francesco Sampieri; he was going to Milan to compose for that city's strict audience its first new Rossini opera since *Il Turco in Italia* two and a half years before. The two men stopped off at Spoleto on February 12. Learning that *L'Italiana in Algeri* was to be performed there that evening, they obtained the local impresario's delighted consent to indulge in a lark: throughout the performance, Sampieri acted as *maestro al cembalo* while Rossini played a doublebass. From Spoleto they went on to Bologna.

How long Rossini stayed in Bologna with his parents cannot be determined, but he was in Milan by late February or early March 1817. He had contracted to compose for La Scala a two-act *opera semiseria* that would turn out to be *La Gazza ladra*. Writing from Milan to his mother on March 19, he told her that he had lodgings in "the house in which [Maffei-]Festa lives and her very amiable husband, from whom I receive endless politenesses." This was Francesca Maffei-Festa, who had created the role of Fiorilla in *Il Turco in Italia*. Now, too, Rossini became acquainted with the German composer Peter von Winter. This sixty-two-year-old former pupil of the Abbé Vogler had made a resounding name for himself with his operas, particularly with *Das unterbrochene Opferfest*, first staged at Vienna in 1796. His *Maometto*

II, composed to a Felice Romani libretto, had had an intensely applauded *première at* La Scala just before Rossini's arrival in Milan.

Rossini went to hear *Maometto II*. He later told Hiller: "There were several very pleasant things in that opera; I especially recall one trio, in which one personage had a broadly conceived cantilena back-stage while two others performed a dramatic duet onstage. It was excellently done, and very effective. My chief objection to Winter was his unsavoriness. He was a man of very imposing exterior, but cleanliness was not his forte. . . . One day he invited me to dinner. We were brought a big dish of meatballs, and he proceeded to serve himself and me in the Oriental manner, with his fingers. As far as I was concerned, that ended the meal."

The libretto supplied to Rossini by La Scala had been written the preceding year for Paër, who however, had not used it. The work of Giovanni Gherardini,[n] this text was based on *La Pie voleuse*, a *"mélodrame du boulevard"* by Jean-Marie-Théodore Baudouin d'Au-bigny and Louis-Charles Caigniez which had been staged successfully in 1815 at the Théâtre Porte-St. Martin, Paris. Rossini demanded some changes in the story, which had had its origin in a curious French legal case. Azevedo reported that before accepting it, Rossini, smiling but in earnest, said to Gherardini: "Because of your wide experience at the bar, I leave you entirely free to deal as you see fit with the courtroom scene. But I want you to follow my suggestions about the rest." For this opera, Rossini's remuneration was to be 2,400 lire (about $1,235).

Conscious that he had not won a first-night battle at La Scala since that of *La Pietra del paragone* in 1812, and perhaps having noted some musical pro-Germanism in Austrian-controlled Milan, Rossini lavished every care on the score of *La Gazza ladra*, taking special pains with its orchestration, which he wanted fully capable of filling the large expanse of the theater. The first performance took place on May 31, 1817.[n] The audience showed that in its view that care had been effective. This opera, which even German critics came to call the best of Rossini's non-comic works up to 1817, was greeted with almost hysterical delight. (One may wonder if some of that glee did not represent relief from the diet of non-Italian operas by such composers as Joseph Weigl, Adalbert Gyrowetz, and Joseph Hartmann Stuntz with which La Scala recently had been favoring its audiences.) When the *première* was safely over, Rossini is said to have admitted that he was exhausted—though more from the very numerous bows he had had to make than from the intoxicating emotions of success. The success of *La Gazza ladra*, given powerful impetus by the season's twenty-seven performances at La Scala,[n] was to continue for half a century.

The Milan correspondent of the Leipzig *Allgemeine musikalische Zeitung* found only one quintet good in *La Gazza ladra*, and even that flawed; in the overture he heard only noise. On the other hand, the *Corriere delle dame* (Milan) one week after the *première* reported (June 7): "*La Gazza ladra* now supplies the favored pastime of those who go to the Real Teatro alla Scala. We gladly forgive Rossini for having made us crave a little excessively this product of his, which brings us delight and demonstrates that, despite the death of a Cimarosa, a Paisiello, a [Pietro Carlo] Guglielmi, etc., etc., *la bella Italia* still can brag of being the mother of Classic Masters and of maintaining herself as the champion of the most beautiful of the fine arts." Clearly, nationalistic and political prejudices were involved in both the German and the Italian reactions.

Azevedo told an anecdote of Rossini's experience with a frenzied pupil of a violinist at La Scala. This young man objected so violently to the presence of drums in the orchestra for *La Gazza ladra* that he went about stating publicly that Rossini must be killed to save the art of music, and that he felt himself chosen to deliver the required stiletto thrust. Rossini heard about him, and asked the would-be assassin's teacher to see that an introduction be arranged. The teacher demurred, not wanting Rossini to be (at the least) insulted. "I'll repay him in kind," Rossini replied. "My supply isn't exhausted. But I do at all costs want to talk with a man who wants to stab me because of the drum."

Face to face with his enemy Rossini attempted to vindicate the drums. "Are there—yes or no—soldiers in *La Gazza ladra*?" he asked. "They are only gendarmes," the young man answered. "Are they on horseback?" Rossini asked next. "No, they are on foot." "Well," Rossini said reasonably, "if they are on foot, they will have drums, which, in common with all foot soldiers, they need. Why, then, do you want to stab me for not having deprived them of their drums? The use of the drum in the orchestra was demanded by dramatic verisimilitude. Stab the libretto as often as you like. I'll not oppose you in any way. It's the real culprit. But don't spill my blood if you wish to avoid remorse." He then promised with mock solemnity that he would never employ the drum again in the orchestra. This story made the rounds of the Milan *caffè* world, and Azevedo asserted that it increased the success of *La Gazza ladra*.

Stendhal, who thought the subject of *La Gazza ladra* "dismal and grossly unsuitable for musical treatment," said that during the period of its composition, Rossini was accused of being an idler, a man who cheated impresarios, who even cheated himself. In view of statements in letters that Stendhal wrote to his friend Baron Adolphe de Mareste in 1820, little doubt is possible that he himself had a hand in spreading, if not in creating, the very gossip that he publicly pretended to disparage. Pushkin, on the other hand, hearing *La Gazza ladra* in Odessa during the 1823–4 season, became much interested in it. Vladimir Nabokov, in a note to his English translation of *Eugene Onegin*, quotes a demonstration by Boris Viktorovich Tomashevski that Pushkin borrowed from Act I, Scene 8 of *La Gazza ladra* the idea of having the false Dimitri in *Boris Godunov* misread aloud a description of himself in an arrest warrant, thus throwing suspicion onto someone else."

By the time of *La Gazza ladra*, Rossini had become the musical paladin of the Italian romantics, the principal target of the beleaguered classicizers. Hard as it may be to think of *La Gazza ladra* as in any sense revolutionary or even radical (we cannot be sufficiently familiar with performances of operas by Rossini's Italian predecessors), it undoubtedly had become a storm center on the weather front separating the eighteenth century from the nineteenth. An article published in 1822 in *Il Giornale teatrale*, Venice, summarized the charges against Rossini and the tone of the defense. The writer imagines a dispute between a classicist and a romanticist which is interrupted by "a man of venerable aspect, skilled in technique," who tries to arbitrate the dispute:

"As for Rossini, ringleader of the musical romantics, I'll set forth the good and the bad that I think of him, not pretending to judicial infallibility. Rossini is accused of plagiarizing himself; it is my belief that this does not result from any poverty in his vein, but from haste in composing; all the *maestri di musica* assert with one voice that his compositions overflow with contrapuntal blunders; but that unfavorable opinion, in part just, is not completely devoid of jealousy. Rossini has spoiled the true forms of harmony, overwhelming vocal music with instrumental; but the purpose of this art is pleasure, which must come chiefly from the poetry; but how could this *maestro* achieve that end if in today's theaters what is listened to least is the word? He therefore replaces it with a perpetual battle of musical phrases of all colors, one after the other, rarely presenting a melody conducted from beginning to end in unity of thought. Thus it happens that he forgets that simplicity is the first element of beauty, that the instrumenal part is nothing but a support for the voice, and that the listener must be refreshed, not oppressed.

"Therefore it comes about that after an opera by one of the classicists of the last century, each person leaves the theater with his spirit in repose, serene, and with the desire to hear it again, whereas the music of Rossini, all of which seems blithe, only rarely evokes the feeling of that compassion which is the source of inexhaustible beauty for delicate spirits. Take, for example, *La Gazza ladra;* the crowding one upon the other of so-called 'character' actions, the tempest of notes not leaving you a moment to breathe, the timpani, the pipes, the trumpets, the horns, and the entire family of the noisest instruments assault you, transport you, trick you, intoxicate you, and many times transmute a sort of tragedy into a bacchanalia, a house of mourning into a festivity. Despite these censures, it would be unjust to deny Rossini a great abundance of harmonic prerogatives; perhaps no one else ever had so many of them; and, furthermore, one must admit that not the least of the reasons for his straying from the proper road is the abundance with which Nature was so generous to him. But his impatience while composing, his wish to please, his mixture of a hundred heterogeneous elements, the turgidity of his style, his lack, finally, of that sobriety so dear to the old *maestri*, the inseparable companion of the beautiful, has distorted the happiest genius that ever issued from the hands of harmony."

Those paragraphs, if nicely interpreted in view of the lapse of time, supply just and accurate criticism of the Rossini who had composed the operas up to and including *La Gazza ladra*. He did plagiarize himself because he composed in too great haste. His "contrapuntal blunders" did exist—from the point of view of the *"maestri di musica,"* whether jealous of his success or not. He did overwhelm vocal music with instrumental, again from the point of view of Paisiello and the unmodernized partisans of Pergolesi and Cimarosa. We may not want to agree that the "pleasure" of opera must come chiefly from the libretto, but we cannot deny that Rossini sought chiefly to supply pleasure— or that the "poetry" he set to music was infrequently of a quality to attract attention to itself or increase "pleasure."

Rossini was never (at least not until his Paris days) a full-blown romantic composer looking upon each new effort at composition as one to which he was being driven by his "demon"; one that therefore must be his great and unique work, as nearly perfect as he could make it. Composing operas was his *métier*, his way of earning a livelihood; he had to make operas in haste in order to live at all, and he naturally—and unthinkingly—made them as attractive as possible to their potential audiences. No different from the majority of his Italian colleagues in these attitudes, he altered them only when composing for Paris rather than for Italy later in his career. What the writer in *Il Giornale teatrale* was lamenting was that Rossini's relation to his art was not that which we associate with Beethoven or Wagner. In truth, during the first fourteen years of his operatically active career, his attitude toward composing was closer to that of Haydn the symphonist and that of such a latter-day composer for the musical-comedy stage as George Gershwin.

We do not know when Rossini left Milan or where he passed the time between the first performances of *La Gazza ladra* (May–June) and August. Probably he stopped off at Bologna again, spent a lazy holiday with his parents and friends, and then went south. On August 12, the official *Giornale* at Naples spoke of him as being in that city, at work on a big three-act spectacle opera to be staged at the San Carlo that autumn. This would prove to be one of the most singular and, in several senses, least Rossinian of his operas: *Armida*.

CHAPTER VI

1817-1819

Rossini must have accepted with reluctance the libretto for his next opera, *Armida*, for it included sorcery and supernatural occurrences, forms of theatrical fiction which he particularly disliked. He was to write to the Turinese librettist Conte Carlo Donà in April 1835: "If I should counsel you, it would be to return within the limits of the natural rather than go farther into the world of wild fancies and *diablerie* from which modern philosophers say that they have worked so hard to free a too credulous humanity." But Tasso's epic *Gerusalemme liberata*, from which Giovanni Federico Schmidt had derived his faulty text,ⁿ could not, in Italy, be tampered with as cavalierly as Perrault's *Cendrillon*, and so Tasso's "wild fancies" remained. Also, Rossini was bound by custom to accept whatever libretto Barbaja might assign to him.

Armida, a three-act *opera seria*, reached its *première* at the San Carlo on November 11, 1817.ⁿ Sumptuously staged, it displayed, as Radiciotti put it: "Armida's palace and enchanted garden, appearances and disappearances of demons, furies, specters, chariots pulled by dragons, dances of nymphs and *amorini*, characters swept up into the sky and descending from artificial clouds." It thus harked back to the "machinery" operas of the two preceding centuries, but even more clearly foretold the stage manners of French grand opera, which already had been prefigured by Spontini's *La Vestale* (1807) and *Fernand Cortez* (1809) and which would be set in most of its usages by Auber's *La Muette de Pòrtici* (1828) and Rossini's *Guillaume Tell* (1829). Alone among Rossini's Italian operas, *Armida* originally provided music for ballet; like only *Otello* and *Mosè in Egitto* among his Italian operas, it was in three acts.

Despite the lavishness with which Barbaja had staged *Armida,* neither its first San Carlo audiences nor the Neapolitan journalists approved of it. Because Rossini's own lavishness had extended to unwonted density of instrumentation and harmony, as well as to the most carefully elaborated recitatives and choruses, the score was deplored as "too German" and was compared very unfavorably with the unencumbered "native" Italian melody that had made the immediate fortune of *Elisabetta, regina d'Inghilterra* two years before. In a turgid review, the official *Giornale* (December 3, 1817) accused Rossini of choosing "to erect his glory upon the century's corruption," of "preferring his intellectual combinations and calculations to that sacred fire by which he is animated." This writer believed that Rossini had been "born with the spirit of Cimarosa and Paisiello," but had labored untiringly "to repress the impulses of his inner nature so as to appear adorned in barbaric [read "Germanic"] styles, either because he has been seduced by the giddiness of a fashion or because he has been nourished immoderately on the literature of the foreign classics." This variety of reactionary jingoism was to be spewed at both Donizetti and Verdi within a few decades, and not in Naples alone.

That *Armida* never became an enduring repertoire opera was owing more to the difficulties of casting and staging it than to any stylistic differences in texture from earlier and later Rossini operas that became widely popular. It requires, besides a spectacularly agile soprano actress, three extremely accomplished tenors and an equally able bass. The wonder is that despite those prerequisites, *Armida* won later stagings even in Naples, where it was revived in a two-act version in 1819 and again in 1823. By the latter year, Neopolitan ears had begun to catch up with Rossini's so-called "Germanizing"; Mme Fodor-Mainvielle garnered a personal triumph as Armida at the San Carlo.[n]

Twenty-four days after the first performance of *Armida,* the official *Giornale* (December 5, 1817) mentioned that Rossini was about to absent himself from Naples for a long period: he was going to Rome, where he was under contract to Pietro Cartoni to supply the Teatro Argentina with a new opera. On December 27, the paper stated that he had left Naples "some days earlier" so as to attend the first performance of that new opera. The phrase "some days earlier" must be interpreted very loosely. As Cametti noted, Rossini must have been in Rome by December 9 or 10. The new opera, *Adelaide di Borgogna, ossia Ottone, re d'Italia,* was to be given its *première* at the Argentina on the very day of the paper's publication (December 27),[n] and even if, as seems very likely, Rossini carried its almost completed score with him from Naples to Rome, he still would have had to be in Rome a minimum of two weeks for *concertazione* and rehearsals.

Many writers have attributed the libretto of *Adelaide di Borgogna* to Jacopo Ferretti; unhappily, it was another botch by the egregious Giovanni Federico Schmidt. Rossini, unquestionably and understandably weary (he had composed *La Cenerentola*, *La Gazza ladra*, and the three elaborate acts of *Armida* within one year), saw the new opera only as a way to earn 300 Roman scudi (about $950). *Adelaide di Borgogna* reveals all the signs of debilitating haste and lack of real involvement. He summoned his friend Michele Carafa[n] to prepare some of the less noticeable arias; he slid back to using only *recitativo secco*; and he borrowed for this darkly serious opera the gleaming overture to *La Cambiale di matrimonio*, the student *sinfonia* that he had composed more than eight years earlier.

The respectful Radiciotti called *Adelaide di Borgogna* "the worst of Rossini's *opere serie*" and added that in it "we find nothing but banality from start to finish." Rossini probably had known well in advance that Cartoni was signing up a largely indifferent company of singers for this opera and had compounded its score cynically without serious thought (it is notable that the secondary characters express themselves entirely in recitative).[n] *Adelaide di Borgogna* received its first performance, at the Teatro Argentina, on December 27, 1817.[n] Audience and press alike were unfavorable toward it. The Rome correspondent of the *Nuovo Osservatore Veneto* wrote (December 31, 1817): "*Adelaide di Borgogna*, poem by Schmidt, was seen to live and die within a single evening at the Teatro Argentina"—actually it played there into mid-January. The *Notizie del giorno*, Rome, remarked that even a reputation as big as Rossini's would not suffice to rescue "a production that does not satisfy the audience's taste."

Back in Naples, on January 27, 1818, Rossini wrote to Antaldo Antaldi, *gonfaloniere* of Pesaro, to discuss the forthcoming reopening of his native town's Teatro del Sole, which had been rebuilt after having fallen into advanced disrepair.[n] Conte Giulio Perticari, one of the prominent Pesarese who had sponsored the rehabilitation of the theater, was to become very friendly with Rossini. "I love and venerate you as one of the great glories of our country," Perticari wrote him, "and am boastful about being your fellow townsman. Allow me also to boast of being your friend." (It should be remembered that the man Perticari was addressing was not yet twenty-six years old.) Rossini was to stage and conduct *La Gazza ladra* for the festive reopening of the theater. An earlier letter that he had sent to the *gonfaloniere* had not been answered; Rossini now restated his wish to engage Isabella Colbran and Andrea Nozzari for the planned performances.

Rossini repeated the proposal in another letter to Antaldi on March 10. Somewhat later, writing to Luigi Achilli in Rome, he reported that the *gonfaloniere* had sent a kindly but inconclusive reply. "I cannot ask the singers to be at my disposition for six months in the hope of singing in a town where they can pay very little," he told Achilli. "I have dickered with these people. But Nozzari, the tenor, is engaged for Naples; Mme Colbran cannot hold herself at my disposition any longer. The bass [Raniero] Remorini, whom you will have heard in Rome, is at my disposition, and I have brought him down to 300 scudos [about $950] of payment. [Alberico] Curioni, the tenor, wants 400 scudos, which is what he gets in Milan. Meanwhile, I advise you to send the agreements for the above-mentioned Curioni to Milan so that he may not escape us, he being, in the scarcity of tenors in which we now find ourselves, one of the good ones. You should send the contract for Remorini to Bologna, addressed to my father, who will be able to hand it to him when he passes through, as we have agreed. I am trying to engage la Sciabran [Margherita Chabrand], la [probably Ester] Mombelli, and la Beloc [*sic*, for Teresa Giorgi-Belloc], and I should have final answers from them soon."

A *prima donna* for the Pesaro season still had not been found on April 29; on that day, Rossini wrote to Rosa Morandi, inviting her to sing in *La Gazza ladra*: "Signor Remorini, [Michele] Cavara, Curioni will round out the opera troupe. Signor Panziere[n] will give *Ulisse*, a *gran ballo*, and you will find yourself, dear Rosina, among people of merit—and I too (mark my modesty) will be among them, I who wish to see and hear you." But Rosa Morandi did not accept the invitation; Rossini finally engaged Giuseppina Ronzi De Begnis to be his Ninetta.

During these protracted negotiations, Rossini was composing and preparing for the San Carlo his twenty-fourth opera. Andrea Leone Tottola[n] supplied the libretto, *Mosè in Egitto,* which he said he had based upon a well-known tragedy by Padre Francesco Ringhieri.[n] Called an *azione sacra* because of its Biblical subject (chosen so that the opera could be staged during Lent), *Mosè in Egitto* was often referred to as an oratorio, though in style it is a three-act proto-grand opera. Because Carnival ended very early in 1818 (Easter fell on March 22), Rossini once more had to compose in a rush. He again summoned Carafa to his aid, this time to compose only one aria: Faraone's "*A rispettarmi*," frequently omitted in performance. He nonetheless produced one of the biggest and most carefully elaborated scores he had thus far composed, completing it about February 25.

Mosè in Egitto was sung for the first time at the San Carlo on March 5, 1818.[*] It did not contain what later became its universally familiar choral prayer "*Dal tuo stellato soglio*," which was to be added to it for Lenten performances at the San Carlo in 1819. It was an immediate, resounding success. A typically vivid passage in Stendhal's *Vie de Rossini* describes the results of the first efforts of the San Carlo's stage machinist to present the dividing of the Red Sea in Act III of *Mosè*: "In the third act, I no longer remember how, the poet Tottola had brought in the passage of the Red Sea without considering that the passage was not so easy to stage as the plague of shadows [which opens this opera]. Because of the way the parterre is situated, one cannot, in any theater, perceive the sea except as from afar; here, because it had to be passed through, it necessarily had to be on a raised level. The San Carlo machinist, wanting to solve an insoluble problem, had done ridiculously incredible things. The parterre saw the sea raised from five to six feet above its shores; the loges, gazing down upon the waves, clearly perceived the little *lazzaroni* who made them open at the voice of Moses. . . . There was a good deal of laughter; the hilarity was so spontaneous that no one could get angry or whistle. The end of the act was not heard at all; everyone thought only of discussing the admirable production . . ."

When Rossini had returned to Naples from Rome after the staging of *Adelaide di Borgogna*, he had been faced with a barrage of new attacks by conservatives and reactionaries. Much of the cast that he was to have for *Mosè in Egitto* had aroused great enthusiasm at the San Carlo on January 3, 1818, in Francesco Morlacchi's *Boadicea*. The anti-Rossinians had taken up *Boadicea* as a club with which to belabor the "pernicious innovations" introduced into opera by Rossini "and his followers." The official *Giornale* for February 13 had referred to Morlacchi as a composer "who prefers the Muses to the Sirens and replaces vain, false ornaments with that noble and precious simplicity which, in the arts, as in literature, shapes the character of what is true, great and beautiful. . . . What new prodigies," the writer then asked, "would not music produce today if others would set to work to follow Morlacchi's example?"ⁿ

One month later, the same journal said: "Rossini has won a new triumph with his *Mosè in Egitto*. A very simple songfulness, natural, always animated by true expressiveness and the most grateful melody, the grandest effects of harmony soberly used for the terrible and the pathetic; a rapid, noble, expressive recitative; choruses, duets, trios, quartets, etc., that are equally expressive, touching, declamatory: here are the rewards of this new music, for which he is deeply indebted to the poet." This writer had evolved an unbeatable system for being right: he liked only what was "simple" and whatever he liked thereby became so. That Rossini had won a new triumph, however, was a fact: *Mosè in Egitto* helped to blot out poor Morlacchi, his *Boadicea* (probably a charming old-fashioned *opera seria*, as he was a composer of considerable lyric talent), and the moans, threats, and alarums of the anti-Rossinians.ⁿ

Lady Morgan,ⁿ who gave an extended, vivid account of operatic life in Naples at the time (1819–20) of an early revival of *Mosè in Egitto* at the San Carlo, wrote:

"But whether the opera of Naples be sacred or profane, serious or comic, the only composer still received with endless applause is Rossini. His MOSÈ was performed at the San Carlos during the whole of our residence; and though we heard it almost as often as it was played, we attended to its splendid *scenas* with unabated delight and gratification.

"The opera of 'Moses' is strictly conformable to the most noted events of that warrior-prophet's mission, as related by himself; but is told with such amplifications as may tend to heighten the dramatic effect of the several characters. When the curtain rises, the divine mandate has just gone forth, by which the heart of Pharaoh was hardened; but in a royal theatre every possible delicacy and indulgence were shewn to the King of Egypt, as if he were rather the victim than the enemy of that power, which withdrew from the sovereign his divine right of volition. While the heart of Pharaoh hardens through a fine solo, the heart of his son softens in an exquisite duo with a pretty Israelitish girl (an episode introduced *à plaisir*, and one rendered exceedingly affecting by the struggles of the young Egyptian prince and his Jewish love, who is a protegée of Moses). The *gran scenas* are all between the prophet and the king. Moses is always stern, despotic, and audacious, and threatens, in his deep double bass, the obstinate Pharaoh with those plagues, which are exhibited from time to time in the scene. The Israelites, however, are at last permitted to depart; and as they range themselves at the gates of the city to commence their miraculous march, they really exhibited a most effecting sight. . . . The scenery and choruses at this moment were magnificent and melodious beyond description. . . . At the moment that Aaron is about to give the word, and Moses has secured his fair young ward (whom he forces to accompany her unhappy compatriots), the young, enamoured Prince of Egypt rushes forward—seizes his mistress—and, by his father's orders, arrests the flight of the Jews; Moses, who 'never knew what love was,' as the Prince tells him, enraged beyond further endurance at this new act of tyranny, falls on his knees, invokes the wrath of the Most High, and calls down fire from heaven, which consumes the devoted Prince under the eyes of his mistress, who goes instantly mad, and sings a frantic requiem over the body of her lover. Moses listens to her with the composed air of an amateur; then gives the word to march, and moves his wand—the sea opens, and he leads his followers over the dry sands, amidst the plaudits of an audience, who retire from this fine opera, vociferating through the streets, *'Mi manca la voce,'* ["My voice fails me," Lady Morgan adds in a footnote] the popular quartetto of the piece, and a chef-d'œuvre of Rossini."

On May 2, 1818, at the Teatro San Benedetto, Venice, Ester Mombelli sang the first performance of *La Morte di Didone,* the *"monologo sceneggiato"* that Rossini had composed for her in Bologna some seven years earlier. It was her benefit night. The *Gazzetta privilegiata di Venezia* was pitiless: "Poetry beneath criticism, music nothing, performance indifferent. Vergil, describing the death of the superb Dido in the fourth book of the *Aeneid,* wrote: *'Quesivit coelo lumen, ingemuitque reperta.'* The same can be said of this cantata, for which it would have been better to have left it in Signora Mombelli's strongbox than to have disclosed it to the light of day, only to return it there, moribund and wailing." Nothing more was to be heard of performances of *La Morte di Didone.*

With *Mosè in Egitto* safely establishing itself at the San Carlo, Rossini could turn some of his attention to the forthcoming Rossinian season at Pesaro. In an undated letter to Conte Perticari, he said: "Here is the completed company; nothing is lacking but your approval to make final this difficult affair, which absolutely must take place during the current month of June and be over by the 10th or 12th of July, as many of the people have engagements at that time. Remorini, who is in Milan, now is following my instructions to set out, and should be there within three days, bringing the score of *La Gazza ladra* with him: the tenor Curioni is here, having arrived yesterday. The *prima donna* Ronzi has started on her way and will reach there in two days; she has a husband [Giuseppe De Begnis] who sings, and as *La Gazza ladra* was composed for three *primi buffi*, I shall be able to induce him to lend himself for a small payment and thus have another *primo buffo* in addition to Remorini and Cavara. Besides, we shall have a *prima donna* who plays male roles, and thus the duets will be sung by two white voices, as is the usage for *opera seria*. In so brief a time, we could not have been luckier, for we have assembled a company that is excellent and best adapted to the music and the characters that they must represent. Enclosed you will find a note of the settings both of the opera and of the ballet. Panzieri proposed an excellent painter, who is at Brescia. In case you do not already have one, I beg you to give me the right to engage him. I should like to be sure that the man handling the stage machinery is capable and clever. . . . Bring the members together, then, and give me the full right to make the contracts so that I shall be able to start the rehearsals in advance, at Bologna. . . . It seems to me that we should not promise the public more than twenty-four performances, as any sort of mishap could occur; but now I have calculated that thirty could be given easily.

"Payments for the singers: *prima donna*, 400 scudi; *primo buffo*, 300; another *primo*, 300; another *primo*, —; *primo tenore*, 300, *secondo tenore*, 100; *musico*," 150; total 1,500(?) [*sic*]. As soon as you give me your final answer, I shall go to Ravenna to fill out the orchestra. Send me, therefore, the note about musicians to be found in the Marches, and their abilities."

Perticari had invited Rossini to be his guest while in Pesaro. Rossini declined the invitation, writing: "And then regarding your kind offer to me to make use of your house, if I should listen to my heart, I should embrace it with rapture. But discretion and reason absolutely will not allow me to cause that much disturbance." But Perticari insisted, and by early June, Rossini was in his natal city as the Perticaris' guest. He later told Filippo Mordani that Perticari was very well disposed toward him, but that his wife, the Contessa Costanza Perticari (daughter of the poet Vincenzo Monti), was the most bizarre woman he had ever known. During his visit in her home, she flew into disordered rages and fought violently with her husband—who thereupon begged Rossini to placate her. Gossip soon was saying that Rossini had become her lover. Giulio Vanzolini related[n] that one day "Costanza told her maidservant to watch and to tell her when Rossini rose from bed and left the house; and, learning that he had gone out, she got naked into that bed and wrapped herself up so as to *absorb* by that contact (as she said) a small particle of his *genius*."

The libretto printed for the Pesaro performances of *La Gazza ladra* states that the opera has been "revised and enlarged." The first performance in the rebuilt opera house took place on June 10, 1818. When Rossini, dressed in high fashion, appeared at the cembalo, he was greeted with prolonged applause. Superbly mounted, with sets by Camillo Landriani and the famous Alessandro Sanquirico, and well sung by the laboriously assembled troupe, *La Gazza ladra* aroused immediate and prolonged enthusiasm among the Pesarese and the many visitors who had come to their city for this occasion. Then followed Panzieri's ballet *Il Ritorno d'Ulisse*, with spectacular scenic effects, ten couples dancing, eighty extras, and an orchestra on the stage. The double bill held that excited audience in the theater until dawn.

A conspicuous member of that audience was Caroline of Brunswick, already separated from the future George IV of England, upon whom she had been forced as a wife in 1795 by George III, who was her uncle and his father.[n] The fifty-six-year-old Princess of Wales was living just outside Pesaro with her lover, a violent, shady young Italian named Bartolomeo Bergami. A flurry of flattered welcome had greeted her arrival in Pesaro, but by 1818 she was being ostracized by more conservative Pesarese, who could not stomach Bergami and others of her courtiers. Among those who no longer favored her were the Perticaris, who probably influenced Rossini against her. She several times invited him to her evening receptions, but he refused the invitations, at least once declaring that he suffered from rheumatic pains that had so reduced the elasticity of his knees that he no longer could bow as prescribed by court etiquette. He would have reason the next year to regret having snubbed Caroline of Brunswick.

After twenty-four performances in *La Gazza ladra*, Alberico Curioni refused to participate in two supplementary performances of *Il Barbiere di Siviglia*. Given without him, the opera appears to have been poorly sung; also, no ballet was provided with it. The all-Rossini season, begun

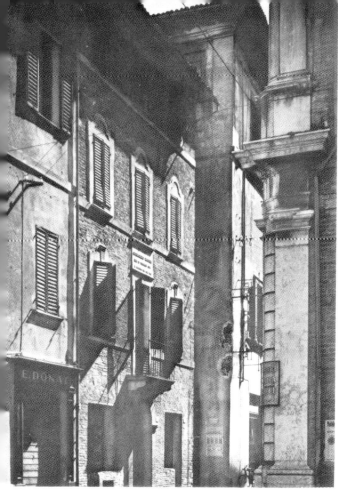

A. ROSSINI'S BIRTHPLACE, PESARO

B. ANNA GUIDARINI ROSSINI, THE COMPOSER'S MOTHER

C. GIUSEPPE ROSSINI, THE COMPOSER'S FATHER

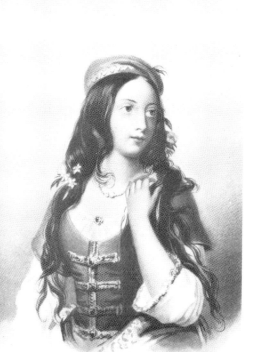

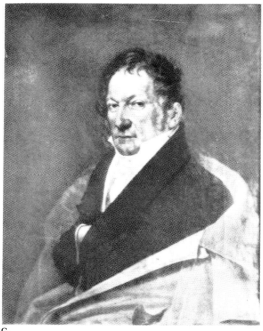

C.

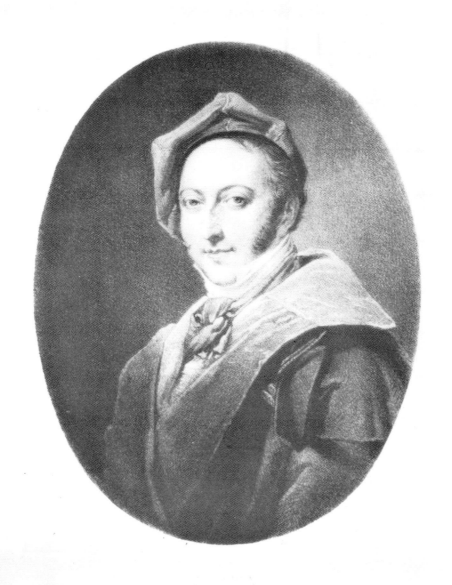

Vivace

A.

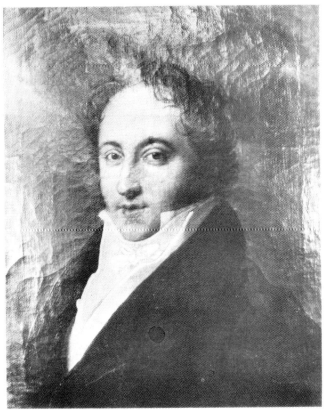

B.

A. ROSSINI IN 1820

B. ROSSINI IN 1831

C. ISABELLA COLBRAN

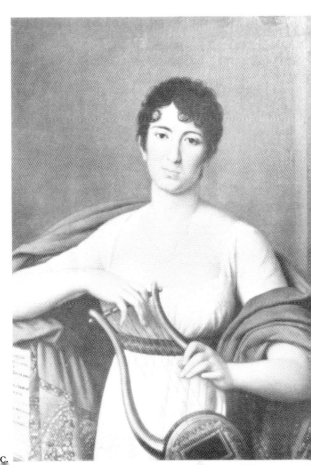

C.

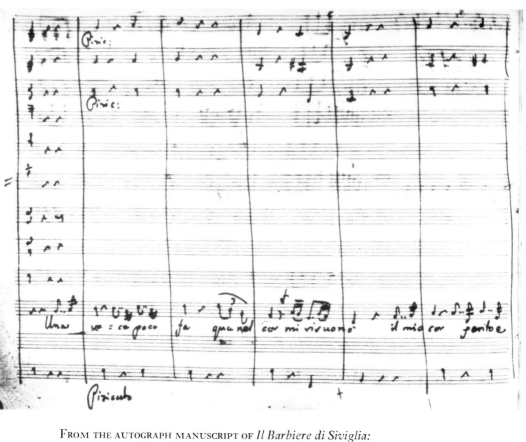

FROM THE AUTOGRAPH MANUSCRIPT OF *Il Barbiere di Siviglia:*
FIRST PAGES OF "*Una voce poco fa*" AND "*La calunnia è un venticello*"

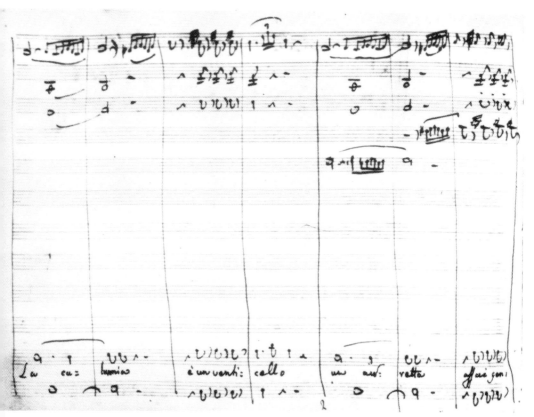

so brilliantly, ended in near-disaster. It also came close to proving fatal to Rossini: after the first few performances of *La Gazza ladra* he had fallen ill with what was called "a very grave throat inflammation." Put to bed, he soon was so ill that his life was feared for. His death was reported in both Naples and Paris. Then *Le Moniteur* (Paris) announced solemnly that he still lived and the official Naples *Giornale* (July 9, 1818) said: "Letters from the very famous Maestro Rossini, from Pesaro, under date of the 2nd of this month, give the lie to notices of his death. Rossini has been dragged to the edge of the sepulcher by a grave malady, but is now out of danger . . ." Before his departure for Bologna near August 1, the Perticaris gave a banquet in his honor. Writing to Conte Gordiano Perticari from Paris more than forty-five years later (January 15, 1864), Rossini would say: "I shall never be able to forget the generous and affectionate hospitality that I received from the Perticaris on the occasion of the opening of the new theater in Pesaro."

Back in Bologna, Rossini received a curious commission. A son of the Lisbon prefect of police and inspector of theaters invited him to compose a one-act *opera-buffa* to be staged there. When and where Rossini completed the resulting *farsa*, *Adina, o Il Califfo di Bagdad*, is unclear, but he is likely to have begun work on it in Bologna in that August of 1818. Its libretto was a revision by his painter-friend the Marchese Gherado Bevilacqua-Aldobrandini of a text by Felice Romani entitled *Il Califfo e la schiava*, some verses of which it quoted intact.[n] Rossini apparently completed *Adina* that summer and sent it off to Portugal. For reasons not known, its production was delayed for nearly eight years: it would not reach its *première* at the Teatro São Carlos, Lisbon, until June 22, 1826.[n]

A letter[n] that Giacomo Meyerbeer wrote from Milan to his brother Michael Beer in Berlin on September 27, 1818, gives a strangely accurate foretaste of events that were not to occur until 1823–4: "Also, he [Rossini] is conducting serious negotiations with Paris to compose for the big French Opera there. The Italian Opera has devolved to the administration of the Grand Opéra since the departure of the Catalanis[n] (which is about equal to confiding the care of the chicken to the fox or of the canary to the cat). They already have robbed the poor Italiens [Théâtre-Italien] of their three best singers, Lipparini! ! ! Ronzi! ! and De Begnis! ! ! ! ! ! ! I have it from the mouths of two emissaries themselves that they have made a number of propositions to Rossini in the name of the French Opera. His conditions (and they are said to be *oltremodo stravagante e forte*) already have been sent to Paris. If they are accepted, he moves to Paris, and we shall witness strange things."

With quaint Bourbon sententiousness, the official Naples *Giornale* said (September 3, 1818): "Rossini is expected from upper Italy today ... He could not arrive at a better moment [Cimarosa's *Il Matrimonio segreto* was being sung at the Teatro del Fondo] ... Will he go to hear the Cimarosa? Oh, certainly! ... And will he attend its counsel docilely? We hope so for our own good, for the glory of the composer of *Elisabetta*, for the good fortune of Italy's degenerated music." We do not know if Rossini then heard *Il Matrimonio segreto*, but what is certain is that shortly he was at work on another opera for Barbaja—and that it shows no signs of his having accepted posthumous advice from Cimarosa. That opera was *Ricciardo e Zoraide*.

The libretto for *Ricciardo e Zoraide* was a poor thing by the Marchese Berio di Salsa—who this time had for bowdlerizing no such resilient original as *Othello*, but only a *Ricciardetto* by Niccolò Forteguerri.[n] Nonetheless, the opera, first heard at the San Carlo on December 3, 1818,[n] was an unclouded success, and would be revived at the San Carlo in May 1819 to continued applause. It shows Rossini integrating the instrumental prelude into the score and the performance. The opening largo of its introduction lasts only eleven measures. Then the curtain parts and a *tempo di marcia* follows, played by a stage band. Next comes an *andante grazioso con variazioni*, after which the march is repeated and the chorus joins in. This extended four-section introduction differs greatly from the discrete overture that could be transferred from opera to opera without noticeable irrelevance.

Seeming inactivity on Rossini's part during the months following the *première* of *Ricciardo e Zoraide* was only seeming. He was refashioning *Armida* in the two-act form in which it was to be restaged at the San Carlo in January 1819; he was composing a cantata for soprano solo, dancing, and chorus to welcome Ferdinand I back to the San Carlo after an illness;[n] he was also at work on the revision of *Mosè in Egitto* for its second season at the San Carlo. For this production, he composed and fitted into the score the later universally familiar prayer "*Dal tuo stellato soglio*." Edmond Michotte told Radiciotti that Rossini said that he had composed the prayer without having a text: he had turned over to Tottola the scheme of the musical meter and the number of verses required, on the basis of which the librettist had written the words. Stendhal, who believed incorrectly that the prayer was added for the third rather than the second season of *Mosè* at the San Carlo, told a different story." His version has Tottola appearing unexpectedly to say that he has written a prayer for the Hebrews to chant before the passage of the Red Sea, a labor that has occupied him a full hour. "Rossini looks at him: 'It was an hour's work, eh? . . . Well, then, if it took you an hour to write this prayer, I must do the music in a quarter of an hour,'" and he proceeds to do exactly that amid the noisy talk of several friends. The story is too good to be either ignored or credited.

Louis Engel" told another anecdote about the *Mosè* prayer; it may well be true. "I asked him [Rossini] was he in love, or very hungry and miserable, when he wrote that inspired page; for hunger as well as love has the power of making people write with lofty inspiration. 'I will tell you,' he said, and from his ironical smile I saw some fun was coming: 'I had a little misfortune; I had known a Princess B—g—e, and she, one of the most passionate women living, and with a magnificent voice, kept me up all night with duos and talking, etc. A short time after this exhausting performance, I had to take a *tisane*, which stood before me, while I wrote that prayer. When I was writing the chorus in G minor I suddenly dipped my pen into the medicine bottle instead of the ink; I made a blot, and when I dried it with sand (blotting-paper was not invented then), it took the form of a natural, which instantly gave me the idea of the effect which the change from G minor to G major would make, and to this blot is owing the entire effect—if any.'"

The remounting of *Mosè* had to be postponed because Colbran was suffering from a severe sore throat. Two other members of the cast also sang despite passing indispositions when *Mosè in Egitto* finally was represented at the San Carlo on March 7, 1819. The official *Giornale* was quick to congratulate "the imaginative Rossini for original new beauties with which he has enriched this work of his, and above all for the pathetic, sublime religious canticle with which the Hebrew people, pursued by Pharaoh, implore the assistance of their fathers' God and then, full of hope and faith, prepare to pass through the divided waters of the Red Sea." Stendhal asserted that a Dr. Cotugno had told him of treating young ladies who were so overexcited by this prayer that they were seized by fever and violent convulsions. No opera but *Mosè* was heard at the San Carlo until after March 22. Rossini's twenty-fourth opera had become what we could call a smash hit.

Meanwhile the apparently inexhaustible Rossini was occupied with preparing one new opera each for Naples and Venice. The earlier of them, *Ermione*, was composed to a two-act *azione tragica* that Tottola had based, somewhat remotely, on Racine's *Andromaque*. It had its indifferently received *première* at the San Carlo on March 27, 1819.[n] A deal of critical nonsense has been published about the score of *Ermione* in attempts to show it as a successful essay by Rossini at adopting the severest manner of Gluck. In fact, however, it differs little from the floridly ornamented operas that preceded or followed it. True, Rossini here again introduced the stage chorus into the orchestral introduction, this time having it sung from behind the still-unparted curtain. *Ermione* was unique among Rossini's operas only in that no later performances of it have been traced either in Italy or elsewhere.

The new "opera" for Venice, a strange *pasticcio* or *centone* called *Eduardo* [sometimes *Edoardo*] *e Cristina*, was staged for the first time at the Teatro San Benedetto on April 24, 1819. Rossini had arrived in Venice on April 9, probably in time to attend one or more performances of his *Otello* there, a likelihood that makes possible a meeting between him and Lord Byron and the Contessa Teresa Guiccioli. Leslie A. Marchand wrote of Byron:[n] "Whatever he may have thought of the libretto [for *Otello*] (for which Rossini was in no way responsible), Byron was captivated by the composer's melodies, particularly after he had heard them in the company of the Countess Guiccioli, to whom he became romantically and passionately attached in the course of a few days in the spring of 1819. When, at the end of ten days of their liaison, Teresa's aging husband announced that they must return to Ravenna the next morning, she rushed to the theater and went boldly into Byron's box, where she told him of her chagrin. Rossini's *Otello* had just begun as she entered. 'It was in the midst of that atmosphere of passionate melody and harmony,' Teresa recalled years later[n] when Byron was dead, 'which by a language far superior to words had already put their souls in communication and had made them feel all that they had found, that they were now made to feel all that they were going to miss and to lose.' "

When Rossini realized that the *concertazione* of *Ermione* would hold him in Naples too long to leave him time for composing an entirely new opera for Venice, he arranged with the San Benedetto impresario that the contracted opera be made up in part of existing music. The numbers, he promised, would be selected to fit as well as possible the dramatic situations and characters in the new libretto. This libretto, which Tottola first and then Bevilacqua-Aldobrandini stirred together and called *Eduardo e Cristina*, was an only partial rewriting of one that Schmidt had prepared in 1810 for Pavesi's opera *Odoardo e Cristina* (San

Carlo, Naples, 1810).* What the two men mostly did was adapt verses from Schmidt's text to music from three Rossini operas unfamiliar to Venetians: *Adelaide di Borgogna, Ricciardo e Zoraide,* and *Ermione.* Rossini supplied new cembalo-accompanied recitatives and seven wholly new numbers. For this *centone,* his fee was 1,600 lire (about $825).

Poetic justice was not served by the outcome, for beginning on its first night—April 24, 1819—*Eduardo e Cristina* was a raging success, in some part because of the highly praised performances by the most important members of its cast.* The official Venetian *Gazzetta* reported: "It was a triumph like no other in the history of our musical stages. The first performance, begun at eight in the evening, ended two hours after midnight because of the enthusiasm of the audience, which required repetition of nearly all of the numbers and summoned the composer out onto the stage many times." *Eduardo e Cristina* ran up twenty-five performances at the San Benedetto that season, the last of them on June 25.* Writing to John Cam Hobhouse on May 17, 1819, Byron said: "There has been a splendid opera lately at the San Benedetto, by Rossini, who came in person to play the harpsichord. The people followed him about, cut off his hair 'for memory'; then he was shouted, and sonnetted, and feasted, and immortalized much more than either of the Emperors. In the words of my Romagnola [Teresa Guiccioli] (speaking of Ravenna, and the way of life there which is more licentious than most here), 'Cio ti mostri un quadro morale del' Paese; e ti basti [That gives you a picture of the morality of the place; and it ought to be enough for you].' Think of a people frantic for a fiddler, or at least an inspirer of fiddles."

In mid-April, 1819, Giacomo Meyerbeer, then twenty-seven, returned to Venice for the staging of his new opera, *Emma di Resburgo,* at the San Benedetto. He had visited Venice four years before, and what he had heard in opera houses there had taught him that one way toward operatic success lay in becoming Rossinian. His familiarity with some of Rossini's music had been evidenced in his first Italian opera, *Romilda e Costanza* (Padua, 1817), which had reached Venice in October 1817, and equally by his second, *Semiramide riconosciuta* (Turin, January 1819). He now had written a third Rossinian score, *Emma di Resburgo,* to a libretto by Gaetano Rossi. Meetings between him and Rossini certainly took place: Meyerbeer's opera was staged at the San Benedetto one day after the final performance of *Eduardo e Cristina* there. In later years, and particularly in Paris, the two composers became warm friends.

Meyerbeer's opera was received well by the San Benedetto audience.

The local critics praised it for its meticulous workmanship (always a Meyerbeer characteristic), but found it overprecious and much too close an imitation of Rossini. The Venice writer for the *Allgemeine musikalische Zeitung* went his usual way, stating that anti-Rossinians in Venice hoped that Meyerbeer would stay in Italy for some time, this in the "hope that he would succeed in obscuring the fame of the lucky composer"—a darkly prophetic remark in view of what would take place in Paris a decade later.

Perhaps meaning to display publicly his gratitude for the way that Pesaro had received him and *La Gazza ladra* the preceding year, Rossini left Venice about May 20 and returned to his birthplace for what proved to be his final visit there. Now the bravos and thugs surrounding the Princess of Wales would make him pay for having snubbed her by refusing to attend one or more of her soirées. What happened at the Teatro del Sole on the evening of May 24, 1819, was described in a letter written three days later by Conte Francesco Cassi, a friend of both Rossini and the addressee, Conte Giulio Perticari, who was then in Rome:"

"On the evening of May 24, the Pesaro theater should have been gladdened by the presence of our fellow townsman, Gioachino Rossini, who was on his way back from Venice . . . But the evening of May 24 was very sad for the Pesaro theater, for the people who had gathered there in a large number to celebrate the arrival of this illustrious fellow townsman had to endure the shame that Rossini's entrance through the door of the orchestra pit of the theater was awaited in ambush by thugs of the Princess of Wales, who, seeing Rossini first, were able to forestall the citizens' applause and to greet him with the most horrible whistling, which threw the people into the greatest disorder and instilled a feeling of terror into everyone, as the thugs also were scattered about in various parts of the theater and gave signs that they were ready also to use their knives and pistols, which, as you know, they never travel without.

"In a few moments, however, the people conquered their surprise and fear, and the whistling of this rabble was drowned out by universal and repeated hand-clapping and by shouts of *Viva* which avenged that insult. And though, not content with the first outrage, Pergami [*sic*] and his vile mercenaries tried to produce a second one and to terrify the good Pesarese again by their ugly shouting and assassins' whistling, their further efforts were nullified. . . .

"Alone in the situation, Councilor Arminelli proved himself worthy of praise, for he rushed to the pit to lead Rossini from among the crowd of whistling and applauding people and conducted him to Signora Belluzzi's loge, where he remained until the ballet was over. . . .

"Rossini left the theater after the ballet, but he was cleverly passed through the director's small door, thus going out to Signora Belluzzi's carriage and returning to the Posta, where he was staying. This baffled the double watch of those awaiting his return to the loge so that they could renew the injuries and of those waiting to honor him with fresh applause and accompany him to the hotel with torches. The latter, however, were not wholly disappointed, for, learning in time of Rossini's secret departure, they were able to join him and pay him the desired honor. A few hours later, Rossini left Pesaro, and a crowd of citizens accompanied him beyond the Fano Gate with increasing cries of *Evviva* and with torches. But because the outraged citizens interspersed their shouts of applause with 'Death to the whistlers,' they had the grim experience of being arrested by the police as they came back into the city."

The next morning, Conte Cassi resigned as a theatrical deputy and sent the *gonfaloniere* a strong protest against the "most unjust, vile insult that the Pesarese suffered yesterday from non-Pesarese and the mercenaries in this theater."[n] In solemn conclave, the local Accademia then decreed that a marble bust of Rossini should be installed in its meeting hall and that a gala evening should be arranged in his honor. Cassi prepared a speech to read to the town council, this in the hope of enlisting its participation in the festivities. But Bergami and his bravos had not been forgotten by Rossini's admirers: Cassi counted fourteen bloodthirsty and "plebeian" satires circulating as attacks on the Princess of Wales, Bergami, and her other courtiers—who, in turn, began to threaten with disfigurement and even death those preparing to honor Rossini. At this juncture, the Pontifical Delegate intervened, forbidding both Count Cassi's speech to the council and the gala at the Academy.[n] Only the subsequent departure of the Princess for England completely restored local peace. Rossini never again visited his birthplace.

By June 1, 1819, Rossini was back in Naples. That city had not forgotten him during his absence. On May 9, a gala at the San Carlo in honor of a visit by the Emperor Francis I (Ferdinand I's father-in-law) had been marked by the singing of a Rossini cantata. That untitled piece, a setting of verses by Giulio Genoino, had been sung by Colbran, Giovanni Battista Rubini, and Giovanni David, with chorus. Also, the official *Giornale* had reported on May 18: "Real Teatro di San Carlo.

[Ricciardo e] Zoraide returned to supply delight to the stage and to receive new applause. Its appearance has been of happy augury: in it, Nozzari returned to the theater after having been ill for several days."

Among musicians whom Rossini saw in Naples at this time was Désiré-Alexandre Batton (1798–1855), a young *prix de Rome* who had studied at the Paris Conservatoire under Cherubini.[n] Batton later told Radiciotti that one day in 1819, a conversation between him and Rossini had run like this:

" 'Are you looking for a subject?' the young prize winner said to the Pesarese. 'I too am looking for one for my return to Paris, and I think that I found one in a little book that I read yesterday: it is a translation of an English poem, the author of which, if I remember correctly, is Walter Scott, and which is entitled *The Lady of the Lake*; the action takes place in Scotland and the situations please me greatly.'

" 'Lend me the little book,' the other replied. 'I want to see if it will do for me.' The prize winner hastened to satisfy the desire of the Maestro, who, meeting him again two days later, took his [Batton's] head between his two hands and said to him very happily: 'Thanks, my friend! I read the whole poem, and I like it a lot. I'm going to turn it over to Tottola right away.' "[n] Like Byron, Scott was then in the European air, bringing news of British romanticism across the Channel.[n] Tottola had the grace, when publishing a preface to his libretto based on *The Lady of the Lake*, to express hope that Scott would understand that reducing the poem to a libretto had necessitated changing it arbitrarily. These alterations are notable in the brief Act II of *La Donna del lago*, which is inferior to Act I in both text and music. Some of Scott's wild, pathetic emotionality nevertheless suffused both acts of Rossini's opera. On February 25, 1832, Giacomo Leopardi was to write to his brother from Rome: "At the Argentina we have *La Donna del lago*, which music, performed by astonishing voices, is something stupendous, so that even I might weep if the gift of tears had not been denied me."

Rossini completed *La Donna del lago* in time for it to be presented at the San Carlo on September 24, 1819.[n] The report in the official *Giornale* stated that only Colbran's final rondo had caught more than half of the audience's attention: that audience did not like what was to become one of Rossini's most popular operas. One anecdote, often repeated, concerning the first performance of *La Donna del lago* is almost certainly untrue. Azevedo[n] reported that Rossini went to Colbran's dressing room to congratulate her. A functionary of the theater burst in to insist that he return to the stage to acknowledge shouts for the composer from the audience. Rossini made no verbal reply, but gave the man such a punch that he reeled from the room. Rossini, this unlikely tale has it, then rushed from the theater, dashed into his carriage, and hurried away. Stendhal originated another story: that the relative failure of the *première* of *La Donna del lago* so affected Rossini that he fainted; Azevedo said that he asked Rossini if that particular story was correct, and was answered in round terms that it was not. In view of Rossini's physical timidity and lack of pugnacity, the story of the assaulted functionary is no more believable.

The indifference of that first Neapolitan audience resulted in large part from its hearing an opera very unlike the one that it had expected and wanted to hear. What a sizable portion of it really desired had been indicated by the official *Giornale* when announcing Rossini's arrival from Venice: "We would like to know whether in this new opera he has contained himself within the boundaries preserved by [*Ricciardo e*] *Zoraide*, or whether he has abandoned himself unrestrainedly to the impetus of his imagination. In the first case, we congratulate ourselves and Rossini for having become worthy of the Delphic crown and, with the Venetians, a defender of Italian glory; in the second case (for this manner depraves public taste), we shall dare to ask if the decadence for which music is criticized should be blamed on the composers or on the listeners." As Radiciotti suggested, the audience may have been so stunned by what seemed to it "that unwonted luxuriance of orchestral and choral sound, by the clangor of trumpets on the stage, by the ingenious numbers, now lyric, now epic, now dramatic" that it roused from its comatose condition only when Colbran, displaying all her agility, sang the old-fashioned concluding rondo.

The second audience for *La Donna del lago* was much more responsive: perhaps it included a larger scattering of receptive music lovers. Also, as a precaution, the number of trumpets played on the stage had been halved. From that second night on, the opera made its career swiftly. At a performance of it heard at the Teatro Argentina, Rome, on January 23, 1823, a custom was inaugurated of inserting into Act II a duet beginning "*Nel rivederti, o caro,*" the work of a Roman singer, singing teacher, and composer named Filippo Celli. That duet (sung that night by Rosmunda Pisaroni and Santina Ferlotti Sangiorgi) thereafter often was included in performances of *La Donna del lago*—and sometimes was inserted also into Morlacchi's opera *Tebaldo e Isolina*.

Again Rossini followed an opera of high quality with one of his poorer works, this one unhappily composed for La Scala. He was in Milan on November 1, 1819: under the date November 2, Stendhal wrote to Mareste (to whom he was likely to tell the truth): "I saw Rossini yesterday on his arrival"; this was almost certainly their first meeting. On that same day, Giacomo Meyerbeer wrote from Milan to Franz Sales Kandler in Venice: "*Rossini ist gestern hier angekommen.*" The libretto handed Rossini was by Felice Romani, who had derived it from Alessandro Manzoni's drama *Il Conte di Carmagnola*. *Bianca e Falliero, o Il Consiglio dei tre* was one of the expert librettist's least viable texts. Rossini put together for it a score excessively marked by musical ideas that he had used before.[n] For this two-act *melodramma* or *opera seria*, he was to be paid 2,500 lire (about $1,290).

Bianca e Falliero reached the stage of La Scala on December 26, 1819;[n] it was received indifferently by an audience capable of detecting that much of the music was not new—and perhaps aware that Rossini, rushing to complete the score on time, had fallen back again on *recitativo secco* (as he had under similar circumstances earlier that year for *Eduardo e Cristina*) after having mostly dropped it from his *opere serie* since 1814. Despite that languid initial reception, *Bianca e Falliero* held the stage of La Scala through thirty-nine performances that season and went on to many other stagings elsewhere.

When *Bianca e Falliero* was first heard at Milan in 1819, Rossini was not yet quite twenty-eight. He had composed thirty operas and considerable nonoperatic music in thirteen years. If the juvenile *Demetrio e Polibio* is not counted, he had in fact written twenty-nine operas—some of them enduring pleasures—in nine years. But many of those twenty-nine were structurally shoddy, inferior operas starred with self-borrowings; they had served Rossini's exchequer but not his enduring reputation. He would compose only four more operas for Italy—one each in 1820, 1821, 1822, and 1823. All of them rank high among his works for the care with which he conceived and executed them. They were to be *Maometto II, Matilde Shabran, Zelmira,* and *Semiramide.*

CHAPTER VII

1820-1822

A<small>T</small> B<small>OLOGNA</small> on January 4, 1820, Giuseppe Rossini, the composer's father, noted: "At the hour of one-thirty at night, our Maestro Rossini left for Naples . . ." Returning to Barbaja-land from Milan, he stopped off at Rome, sitting to Adamo Tadolini for the portrait bust that had been commissioned by the Pesarese Accademia. Somewhat later the official Neapolitan *Giornale* reported: "Rossini has been among us since the 12th of the current January. Since that day he has dedicated himself entirely to the rehearsals of [Spontini's] *Fernando Cortez*. The loving care with which he is trying to assure good results for a product of the composer of *La Vestale* is worthy of the composer of *Elisabetta*." (It is interesting to note that Rossini, who by January 1820 had composed eight operas for Naples, remained for that journalist the composer of the first of them, staged more than four years before.) Spontini's "Mexican" opera, despite the benefits of Rossini's *concertazione* and of a cast including Colbran and Nozzari, was too "Teutonic" for the audience at the San Carlo, where it was received with indifference on February 4.

During that February, Rossini was honored spectacularly *in absentia* at Genoa, where the choreographer Domenico Grimaldi arranged a *"gran festa teatrale"* at the Teatro San Agostino in connection with a very successful staging of Rossini's *Otello*. The manifesto issued by Grimaldi asserted that he had created the *festa* expressly for that night (February 12). That morning, an inscription decorated with flowers and musical emblems was placed in the Piazza de' Bianchi. That evening, the inscription was illuminated with torches, which also lighted up the Stradone di San Agostino and the façade of the theater. All the loges were "elegantly adorned with garlands of myrtle and golden branches," and the auditorium was magnificently lighted. The *festa* consisted of a performance of *Otello*; a ballet by Grimaldi; and a symbolic musical performance entitled *L'Apoteosi di Rossini*. It was liked well enough so that it was repeated the next year at the Teatro Carcano, Milan.

At Naples in March, the Arciconfraternità di San Luigi invited Rossini to compose a Mass to be sung in the Church of San Ferdinando on the 19th of that month. He accepted the commission while fully aware that he lacked time for composing a whole Mass. He called in Pietro Raimondo (in Naples to supervise the staging, at the San Carlo, of his opera-oratorio *Ciro in Babilonia*) to work with him on it. Apparently Rossini provided the solos and choruses and entrusted the connective recitative to Raimondi." Their collaborative *messa di gloria* was duly sung in San Ferdinando on March 24.

The official *Giornale* judged the music of the Mass "learned, grave, sublime." Stendhal may have given a more judicious notion of what actually had occurred at San Ferdinando: "It was a delightful spectacle: we saw pass before our eyes, and in a slightly different form that lent piquancy to the recognition, all the great composer's sublime arias. One of the priests cried out in all seriousness: 'Rossini, if you knock on the gate of Heaven with this Mass, St. Peter will be unable to delay opening it for you despite all your sins!' "

Carl von Miltitz, who was in San Ferdinando on March 19, 1820, wrote:" "Who would not have been very eager to hear the favorite of the Italian (I could almost say of the European) stages in a holy place, and to admire as well his fecund individuality in the worthiest employment of all musical means? But little was to be hoped for, as it is impossible to have any notion of the decadence and disgusting neglect into which this part of the service had fallen in Italy. I learned from Rossini himself that he composed this Mass in two days, and I later heard him say that he had Maestro Raimondi as a collaborator. What a botched work!

"The Mass was preceded by a Mayr overture with a dance theme. Then an interval. After this introduction, so well adapted to the Feast of the Sorrows of the Divine Mother, they played the overture to *La Gazza ladra*. I confess that such profanation of the holy place and its solemnity hurt my soul profoundly.

"After the second intermission, the *Kyrie* (in E-minor) began very sadly, with harsh dissonances, conducted without a shadow of art or of knowledge of the ecclesiastical style, but still with a certain dignity. If it had continued like that, one would at least have been able to say that the Mass did not lack value entirely.

"The succeeding *Gloria*, which the Neapolitans began to applaud as though they were in a theater, was, as the composer had conceived it, a chorus of angels sung against the rejoicing of shepherds: not an entirely new piece, but pleasing. The first twenty measures made one hope for an original work; its flight rose to a discreet altitude, but toward the close, it fell to earth.

"The *Credo* and the *Offertory* were a ragout of phrases from Rossinian opera jumbled together without intention or purpose and mixed higgledy-piggledy like meat in a sausage: a procession of all the figures most in vogue to be found in Rossini's thirty-two [actually thirty] operas, in part stolen from German masters and in part heard from the mouth of the famous [Giambattista] Velluti.

"I do not know whether the *Sanctus* and *Agnus* were composed by Rossini or Raimondi; I can say that they were not worth much. There was a sort of fugue, the sobbing themes of which coursed through all twelve notes of the tonality.

"During the rite, the organ was played in a way that aroused pity. At the same time, the orchestra tuned up its instruments while Rossini, in a loud voice, so as to be heard, gave orders to this one and that one! It is easy to imagine how the sanctity of the place was respected. In spite of all that, the public went into ecstasy, and I am sure that one week later, in the macaronic parties of high and low Neapolitan society, the favorite melodies from a Mass composed in two days for the *festa dell'Addolorata* were to be heard being hummed."

That amusing description is malicious and—perhaps knowingly—false. For, being a *messa di gloria*, the Rossini-Raimondi Mass would not have included some of the sections described so circumstantially by Miltitz. To question his account, however, is not to deny that by 1820 church music had sagged to very low estate, not only in Naples, but throughout Italy.

In April 1820, Giovanni Colbran—Isabella's father—died at his villa at Castenaso, outside Bologna; had he lived two years longer, he would have become Rossini's father-in-law. Rossini, by now almost certainly Isabella's lover, wrote to Adamo Tadolini about a sculptured monument to be placed at her father's tomb as a surprise for her. In a later letter to Tadolini, Rossini said: "The thought, in the monument in question, would be as follows: the daughter at the foot of the tomb weeping over the loss of her father; at the other side, a singer chanting his glories. I don't know how to draw, but I nonetheless make for you here two sketches from which you, with your genius, will be able to work it out. . . . As of now, I foresee that the two figures should be two portraits, if this is possible."[n]

Rossini still was under contract to Barbaja to supply operas for the Neapolitan theaters, and the official *Giornale* for May 25, 1820, announced that he was then setting a new libretto. This was a two-act *dramma* or *opera seria* entitled *Maometto II*. It had been extracted and reduced from Voltaire's *Mahomet, ou Le Fanatisme* (1742) by Cesare della Valle, Duca di Ventignano.[n] The original date set for the *première* of this opera is not known, but it clearly was earlier than that of the December night on which it was first sung at the San Carlo. Nor do we know how much, if any, work Rossini did on the score of *Maometto II* immediately after receiving the libretto.

In June 1820, the fact that an uprising against the Bourbon regime of the Two Sicilies was brewing appears to have become obvious to everyone but Ferdinand I, his family, and his closest advisers. On July 1, a miscellany of army deserters, leaders of the Carbonari, and disaffected priests marched on Avellino, some twenty-five miles east of Naples. On July 5, five of the Carbonari demanded to be received by the King, to whom they announced that if he did not at once proclaim a constitution like the one granted in Spain in 1812, revolution would ensue. The King gave in, issuing the required proclamation the next morning. Troops loyal to General Gugliemo Pepe, a leader of the Carbonari, entered Naples on July 9. The new constitution was promulgated. Then things went swiftly wrong. From Vienna, Metternich threatened to intervene in support of absolutism. On October 6, two British frigates sailed into the Bay of Naples. On November 20, the Emperor, the King of Prussia, and the Tsar sent King Ferdinand what amounted to an order to come to Laibach (Ljubljana) to confer with them.

Ferdinand embarked on December 13 and reached Laibach on January 8, 1821, there to find the Holy Alliance determined to restore the Neapolitan *status quo ante*, by force if necessary. When news of this determination reached Naples, the parliament, controlled by General Pepe and the Carbonari, decided to fight for the constitution. Some scattered engagements with Austrian troops followed—and by March 23, the Imperial army was able to enter Naples amid cheers from large

throngs of Neapolitans. Ferdinand, however, cautiously delayed returning to his capital until May 15.

Activities in the theaters having been interrupted, Rossini appears
to have had to serve briefly in the *guardia nazionale* during the disorders,
perhaps in a musical capacity. But his days probably were passed partly
in idleness that may well have benefited his overworked art, however
they may have irritated his restless spirit. At some time, he went ahead
with the composition of *Maometto II*. Stendhal and others listed among
Rossini's works an *Inno di guerra dei costituzionali*, supposedly written
to verses beginning "*Chi minaccia le nostre contrade*"; a diary quoted in
1905 in the *Archivio storico per le provincie napoletane* also mentioned
this hymn. Stendhal placed its singing after that of an opera at the San
Carlo on February 12, 1821—by which date Rossini had left for Rome.
Newspaper reports of that San Carlo performance do not mention a
Rossini *Inno* (no manuscript of which is known); its existence remains
doubtful.

On November 28, 1820, the singer Filippo Galli, who was to create
the role of Maometto II, wrote from Naples to a music publisher (probably Giovanni Ricordi): "Regarding the *Maometto*, then, I can tell you
that from what I have heard of it up to now, it seems to be a masterpiece,
but that he [Rossini] still has not completed it; they hope to be on stage
next Saturday, but I can't assure you of that . . ." *Maometto II* was in
fact ready for its *première* at the San Carlo on December 3, 1820." As
first presented, it had no overture, but when it was staged at Venice
during the Carnival season of 1823, Rossini not only supplied it with an
overture and a new trio, but also substituted for its original tragic ending
the rondo finale of *La Donna del lago*, thus both delighting Colbran
(again the Anna) and sending his audiences away happy.

Maometto II was not well liked at Naples in 1820, its earliest audiences having realized quickly that it was not couched in the older style
that many of them still cherished: in fact, the opera shows unmistakable
signs of Rossini's having absorbed aspects of Spontini's grand, mar-
moreal manner while preparing the San Carlo staging of *Fernand Cortez*.
At Milan, *Maometto II* racked up fifteen performances beginning on
August 16, 1824, but it was not so well liked there as another opera on
the same subject (but to a Felice Romani libretto): Peter von Winter's
Moametto II, which had had its *première* at La Scala on January 28, 1817.
All in all, this was not a Rossini success. That fact well may have in-
fluenced his decision to quit Naples shortly after its *première* there—

and it certainly led him to rescue large portions of its score by putting them into *Le Siège de Corinthe* at Paris in 1826.[n]

By mid-December 1820, Rossini was in Rome, staying with Pietro Cartoni in the Via del Teatro Valle; he was not to return to Naples until mid-March 1821. Announcements of the Carnival season at the Teatro Apollo soon were specifying that it would begin with a new Rossini opera entitled *Matilde* (for which he was to be paid 500 Roman scudi, about $1,575). Because of the shortness of the time he would have in Rome for composing the new opera, Rossini originally had commissioned a libretto from a Neapolitan writer, who was to derive it from a French play called *Mathilde de Morwel*, whence the early announcement of it simply as *Matilde*. But, finding that he was obtaining a poor text much too slowly, Rossini went to Rome determined to locate another librettist, though he already had composed Act I of *Matilde*. He approached Jacopo Ferretti.

Ferretti had supplied librettos for two new operas to be staged in Rome that season.[n] He was unwilling to undertake a third immediately. At home, however, he had five scenes of a play entitled *Corradino il terribile*, which he had been adapting in his spare time from the five-act libretto that François Benoît Hoffman had derived from Voltaire for Méhul's opera *Euphrosine et Coradin, ou Le Tyran corrigé* (1790). He showed the scenes to Rossini, who begged him to make a libretto from the play. To this text, Rossini and Ferretti gave the name *Matilde Shabran*,[n] *ossia Bellezza e Cuor di Ferro*. How that title came about was explained by Ferretti in 1829 in a letter to the *Nuova Biblioteca teatrale*:

"I did not want to place a weapon in the hands of the enemies of the management [of the Teatro Apollo]: and those enemies were numerous, artful, rich, and powerful. So, as the subject was not historical and the lovely enchantress who softened Ironheart [Cuor di Ferro] in the old comedy was called Isabella Shabran, I took the liberty of changing the title and of calling my *melodramma Matilde Shabran*. All those who did not know this secret story believed that I had been engaged before the prospectus was issued: but in fact, that happened many weeks later, and I was engaged not by [Luigi] Vestri,[n] but by Rossini, who brought with him from Naples the complete first act of *Matilde* [*de Morwel*] as rewritten by one of the poets there." The resulting Ferretti libretto, though in only two acts, too plainly shows the stigmata of its five-act origins.

Having to get *Matilde Shabran* composed to the new libretto, Rossini both raided some of his earlier operas[n] and called in as a collaborator Giovanni Pacini,[n] then in Rome following the successful *première* at the Teatro Valle on January 25, 1821, of his opera *La Gioventù di Enrico V* (the libretto of which was also by Ferretti, who had derived it from Shakespeare's *Henry V*). According to an account published by Francesco Regli,[n] "One fine morning toward the end of Carnival," Rossini sent Pacini this note: "My dearest Pacini! Come to me as soon as you can, for I need you. In these circumstances, one knows one's friends." Regli added: "As can be understood easily, Pacini was there very quickly, and Rossini said to him: 'You know that I am composing *Corradino* for the Tordinona;[n] we have reached the last days of Carnival, and I still am short six pieces of music . . . The old Duca Torlonia[n] is tormenting me, and he is right. For that reason, I thought of dividing the effort with you: that is, you will compose three of the pieces and I'll compose three. Here is paper and a chair—write!' Pacini said nothing, but set to work."[n]

Azevedo wrote that Rossini's emphasis on ensemble numbers in *Matilde Shabran* reflected his awareness that the troupe of singers at the Apollo was mediocre; other writers have said that he skimped on effort while composing the opera because of that awareness. And certainly the mixed reception awarded the opera at its Apollo *première* on February 24, 1821,[n] was in part attributed by the reviewers to flaws in the singing. Applause was mixed with whistling that evening; fights raged between Rossinians and the myrmidons of the older style, then most recently incarnated in Pacini's *La Gioventù di Enrico V*. Azevedo said that a street brawl took place outside the theater after the performance. Rossini's detractors soon were retailing the story that the *première* of *Matilde* had been delayed in the first instance by his laziness and that its first performance had been a disaster.

What really happened at the first performance of *Matilde Shabran* was clarified by a writer in the *Notizie del giorno* for March 1, 1821: "Long awaited by the impatient lovers of musical beauty, delayed only by the usual theatrical circumstances, despite whatever may be said to the contrary by certain people . . . the *opera semiseria* entitled *Matilde Shabran, ossia Bellezza e Cuor di Ferro* (that is to say, *Corradino*) has made its appearance. . . . The merit of the music is remarkable. The quintet in the first act and the sextet in the second act surprise and enchant; Ambrogi's introduction, Moncada's aria, the duet for Lipparini and Parlamagni touch the hearts of the most backward spirits. The re-

ception of the opera nonetheless clearly presents a picture of two opposed factions. On one side fights a group of people inflamed with a
spirit of innate contradictoriness and aroused by a collection of reflected
details rather than moved by the judgment of their inner sense; on the
other side are the dispassionate lovers of harmonic beauty.

"During Act I, the outcome remained doubtful, but in the second,
the former found themselves driven into voluntary retirement while the
latter unfurled the banner of complete victory, courteously welcoming
a good portion of the enemy faction too under their flag. In the meantime, the impartial Genius who repays virtue has added a new leaf to
the crown encircling the youthful brow of Maestro Rossini, which is,
one notices, mixed with the diverse laurels that bind the honored foreheads of Mozart, Mayr, Paër, Paisiello, and Cimarosa. While the hymn
to his triumph goes on being intoned from evening to evening with
ever-increasing applause, however, we shall not refrain from exhorting
the victor to abstain in the future from further repetitions of a single
musical phrase of which he was more than a little prodigal in *Matilde*."

Relations between Rossini and the owner-impresario of the Teatro
Apollo had been strained severely during the preparation of *Matilde
Shabran*, perhaps because Torlonia had not been pleased to learn that
the score was neither all new nor all Rossini. After the mixed reception
of the *première*, he refused to pay Rossini the contractual 500 scudi.
Rossini thereupon gathered up the score and orchestral parts, removed
them from the Apollo, and on February 27, 1821, wrote the following
letter to Cardinal Bernetti, Governor of Rome and Chief of the Pontifical Delegation in charge of public spectacles:

"EXCELLENCY: The attitude held toward me for some weeks by the
signor duca Torlonia, and much more his having given me to understand
that he has no intention of replying to a letter that I wrote him yesterday
—in which, according to precise clauses in the agreement that he signed,
I demanded the sum of 500 scudi, the amount still due me for my opera
Matilde—have obliged me to take an action as energetic as it is just,
besides being imposed by the circumstances and being the only one that
can effectively guarantee my interests during the brief time remaining
of my stay in this city. Making use, therefore, of my proprietary right in
the score, a right guaranteed to me by the aforementioned agreement,
I have retired both the above-mentioned score and the orchestral parts
for it, in the firm intention of not handing them over until payment of
the aforementioned sum has been effected. I believe it my duty to inform

Your Excellency of my action so that you, in your wisdom, will be pleased to provide for an emergency in view of the fact that, starting this evening, performance of the aforementioned *dramma* at the Teatro d'Apollo must cease.

"I beg Your Excellency to receive with favor the feelings of profound respect with which I have the honor to declare myself Your Excellency's humble servant, GIOACHINO ROSSINI."

Alberto Cametti, who discovered this letter and published it in his valuable book *La Musica teatrale a Roma cento anni fa* (1916), reported that it bore a marginal endorsement stating that it had been attended to. As *Matilde Shabran* appears to have been sung at the Apollo until the season closed on March 6, Torlonia evidently paid Rossini the 500 scudi.

Rossini's undeserved reputation as a dangerous political revolutionary had not died out in 1821. A document found among secret papers of the Austrian police at Venice reads: "Venice, March 3, 1821, D. R. To the Signori Chief Inspectors. The famous composer of music Rossini, who is now in Naples, is indicated as strongly infected by revolutionary principles. I promptly inform the Signor Chief Inspector, not only so that he may direct the most rigorous surveillance toward him should he appear in that province, but also in order that he may pay the most careful attention to the relations that Rossini may have in order to express his political enthusiasm. He will then give me quick and precise information about everything that he may discover in this emergency. Kubeck."

This document can be attributed to nothing but nervousness on the part of the Austrian authorities: Rossini's sense of nationalism never was vivid and his political attitudes were rapidly becoming conservative enough to please even the secret police. Nor should Kubeck's statement that Rossini was in Naples on March 3, 1821, be taken literally: he was lingering in Rome because he was enjoying himself there. Pacini wrote:[n] "During the last days of Carnival, Rossini concocted with a group of friends (I too was of that goodly number) the performance of a masquerade. We prepared ourselves and dressed in the style of oldtime *maestri*—that is, with black togas and with large wigs on our heads, altering our faces a little with black and red marks. We memorized a chorus from *Il Pellegrino bianco*,[n] which had so delighted the spirit of the Roman audience. Thus transformed, we proceeded toward the Corso, each with a piece of sol-fa in his hand and singing the aforementioned chorus full-throatedly. And when we reached the Caffè Ruspoli, we stopped. The crowd of curious onlookers kept growing. Suddenly, many people, supposing (I leave the truth untouched) that by our masquerade we meant to ridicule Maestro Grazioli and his music, addressed a quantity of improprieties at us and threatened us with arguments that we found sufficiently persuasive so that one by one we prudently slipped away." Pacini also reported[n] that at one of Pauline Bonaparte Borghese's Friday receptions, "Rossini sang the famous cavatina from *Il Barbiere di Siviglia*, '*Largo al factotum della città*'; and in truth he could have said: 'I am not the factotum of Rome alone, but surely that of the whole world, for in Caesar's manner I could repeat the *veni, vidi, vici!*' "

Also of that early part of 1821, the politician-writer Massimo d'Azeglio wrote:[n] "Paganini and Rossini were in Rome. Lipparini was singing at the Tordinona, and in the evening I often found myself with them and their mad contemporaries. Carnival was approaching, and one evening we said: 'Let's arrange a masquerade.' 'What to do?' What not to do! Finally we decided to mask as blind people and sing requests for charity as they do. We put together four lines of verse which said:

> " '*We are blind. We were born*
> *To earn our living from kindness.*
> *On a happy day,*
> *Do not refuse charity.*'

"Rossini quickly set them to music.[n] They were rehearsed and re-rehearsed, and finally we decided to go on stage on the last Thursday before Lent. We decided that we should wear very elegant clothes beneath a top covering of poor, patched rags. In short, an apparent but clean misery.

"Rossini and Paganini had to act as the orchestra, strumming two guitars, and they decided to dress as women. Rossini filled out his already abundant form with bundles of straw, looking absolutely nonhuman! Paganini, as thin as a door, and with a face that seemed to be the handle of his violin, appeared twice as thin and loose-limbed when dressed as a woman.

"I ought not to say so, but we created a furor, first at two or three homes where we went to sing, then in the Corso, then on the festal night."

Some time in March, Rossini returned to Naples. There he received for the second time an invitation to compose an opera for the King's Theatre, London. In a letter of which the date probably is April 23, 1821, and of which the addressee is uncertain, but is very likely to have been Giovanni Battista Benelli, impresario of the King's Theatre, he said that it was essential that everyone believe that he would be going to London the next April. "I beg you, in the name of the friendship that has reigned between your family and mine for so many years, that in all the business letters that you send to Naples you will predict and convince everyone, and Barbaja in particular, that I am definitely signed up for London." He was, then, engaged in playing one future possibility against another. Or, perhaps, two future possibilities against another: Hérold, then in Italy, said in a letter to his mother from Naples on April 10, 1821, that Rossini was "burning to come to Paris." In the French capital, his reputation was soaring despite productions of his operas which fluctuated between indifferent and bad, especially in the matter of the texts used.

During April, Rossini directed a performance at the San Carlo of his old favorite, Haydn's *Die Schöpfung* (in Ignaz Pleyel's Italian translation). Hérold, in the letter just quoted from, said: "*The Creation of the World*, by Hadyn, is being given this evening, and Rossini had me come to the rehearsal so as to ask my advice." At some later date during this year, Rossini must have begun to realize that his Neapolitan period was drawing to its close. Barbaja was negotiating to take over the Kärnthnertortheater at Vienna as impresario. His doing that would not necessarily mean that he would give up the Neapolitan theaters, but it clearly might affect Rossini's future. Also, Rossini now became certain that he wanted that future to include activities outside Italy, and particularly in Paris.

Barbaja signed a contract with the Kärnthnertortheater on December 1, 1821. Soon thereafter, he made a new agreement with Rossini, freeing him to travel to Vienna, London, and Paris—after which it was foreseen that he would return to Naples for some additional years there. The official *Giornale* for January 5, 1822, said: "Rossini, a name in itself worth a thousand eulogies, the honor of Pesaro, the ornament of Italy— Rossini is about to abandon our precincts. During his six-year stay here in Naples as director and composer for the Royal Theaters, he wrote *Elisabetta, Otello, Armida, Zoraide, La Donna del lago, Ermione, Maometto II*, and *Mosè* [the writer omitted *La Gazzetta*], operas of which just one would have sufficed to consecrate his name in the Temple of Immortality; and here, too, he has set to music *Zelmira*, which we shall hear at the beginning of next month. . . .

"In Vienna, he will give *La Donna del lago*,[n] and from Vienna, at the onset of good weather, he will pass over to England, then to Paris, and then, returning from the banks of the Seine, will stay among us again for further years, according to an agreement reached with the impresario of the Royal Theaters."

Before Rossini could devote himself entirely to his final Naples opera, he had to prepare a cantata to be sung at the San Carlo on the benefit night to which he was entitled by contract. Taking a verse text by Giulio Genoino, he produced *La Riconoscenza*, a cantata for chorus and four solo voices. King Ferdinand permitted the suspension of ticket subscriptions for the night of December 27, 1821, so that it could be a gala for Rossini's benefit. First heard that night in the presence of the King, the royal family, all the ministers, and a large section of the nobility,[n] *La Riconoscenza* was to be repeated at the Teatro del Fondo in the spring of 1822, when a fifth character, Silvia, was introduced. This cantata had a longer active life than most of Rossini's occasional pieces: it was repeated during the summer of 1829 at the Teatro Communale, Bologna, as *Il Serto votivo*, on the occasion of the welcome to a new papal legate.

The box-office receipts to which Rossini was entitled for the December 27 gala amounted to about 3,000 ducats (approximately $720)—"a handsome sum," Radiciotti wrote, adding: "Here is another proof of the falsity of certain information propagated by some biographers, according to which Rossini had inspired an infinity of apathies and enmities in Naples during his sojourn in that city." Naples, however, was a large city; it almost certainly contained both people who disliked Rossini (who was a very definite personality and, what is more, successful) and a large number who admired him, as well as many who merely enjoyed gala nights at the San Carlo in the presence of their King and his court.

With the benefit out of the way, Rossini could concentrate on completing the new opera, intended by Barbaja for a sort of trial-run production at the San Carlo, after which it would serve to introduce Rossini in person to the impresario's new Vienna public. The libretto by Tottola was based on a tragedy by Dormont de Belloy (pseudonym of Pierre-Laurent Buyrette). This *Zelmira*, as Rossini surely did not fail to notice, is an abomination, no improvement over the original French *Zelmire*, which Radiciotti well called "a collection of false concepts, commonplaces, and forced situations which certainly did not improve while passing through the hands of the Neapolitan librettist." Rossini nonetheless composed the opera with special care and deliberation: it was to launch his personal career in Vienna, recently the home of Mozart and Haydn, still the home of Beethoven. He gave much more than his wonted attention to purely musical considerations—harmonic variety, contrapuntal accuracy, richness of modulation—as well as to relating the music expressively to the text. Radiciotti felt that in the resulting score "preoccupation with appearing accurate and learned has at times been injurious to the composer's spontaneity and melodic fluidity." *Zelmira*, certainly, reaches no summits as high as those in *Otello, Mosè in Egitto,* and two or three others among Rossini's earlier operas. But, in compensation, it has a unity of style and of musico-dramatic texture which demonstrates what its twenty-nine-year-old composer was capable of when he worked long and hard enough over a score.

Zelmira reached its *première* at the Teatro San Carlo on February 16, 1822,[n] thirteen days before Rossini's thirtieth birthday. Warmly welcomed by public and press, it remained on the San Carlo stage until March 6, on which evening King Ferdinand graced the theater with his presence. The official *Giornale* reported: "His Majesty gave the departing *maestro* and the singers flattering signs of his gratitude at the close of the performance; all of that huge auditorium then echoed to *viva* and continuous applause; the actors were recalled to the stage, and obtained from the approving audience that farewell which is the dearest and most wished-for recompense of generous spirits . . ."

Six days after the *première* of *Zelmira*, the official Naples *Giornale* announced that one of the new operas to be staged during the summer season would be "a production of Signor Gaetano Donizetti [who] is a young pupil of one of the most valued *maestri* of the century, Mayer [Mayr] . . ." And in fact, on May 12, 1822, Donizetti's *La Zingara* (a two-act setting of the usual Tottola screed) was staged at the Nuovo, the first of the numerous operas that he would compose for Naples, which soon became his temporary home. When Donizetti first reached Naples, in February 1822, he was twenty-five years old—not quite six years Rossini's junior.

On March 4, 1822, Donizetti wrote from Naples to Mayr in Bergamo to report on a performance of Mayr's oratorio *Atalia* at the San Carlo under Rossini's direction: "It will be enough for you to know that the role of David is being done by [Domenico] Donzelli, that of Natan by Cicimarra, and that of Atalia by Fabbré [Giuseppina Fabré], who has not sung for two years and is not good enough; she has a very dark contralto voice, for which reason Signor Rossini has had to edit the entire part. At the rehearsals, he lazes along Jesuitically with the singers, who don't follow him well, and then, at the orchestra rehearsals, there he is, gossiping with the *prime donne* instead of conducting. . . . If that isn't enough, I'll tell you that Dardanelli doesn't sing the first-act aira, that they have deleted recitatives, choruses, the little second-act finale after Atalia's aria, etc., etc. Really, I don't know whether by doing it they are doing well or badly, for they are such dogs that they ought to be out hunting bones rather than performing this music . . . ; that is the gratitude of la Colbran after you favored her so. As for me, I don't care to watch any more of this, and that's what I told myself this morning. But Barbaja says that he will give it later at Vienna, and that there it will be what it really is."[n] Naples, then, was about to acquire one of the leading opera-composers of the era while losing another. For Rossini's departure proved final: he would visit Naples later, but never would live or compose there again.

A few months before, on December 14, 1821, Rossini had written to his uncle, Giuseppe Guidarini, to say that he had need of a baptismal certificate and of proof of his bachelorhood: he was going to marry Isabella Colbran. Later, he would say that he would have preferred to remain single, but had married to please his mother—who may well have been disturbed by gossip about his liaison with Colbran, and perhaps about other affairs. In view of his having asked his uncle to keep secret the news of his forthcoming marriage (he also arranged for non-publication of the usual banns), it is likely that he had decided to surprise his parents.

On March 7, 1822, the day after the last *Zelmira* at the San Carlo, Rossini left Naples with Colbran and three of the other singers whom Barbaja had been awaiting in Vienna since December: Ambrosi, David, and Nozzari. At Castenaso,[n] a few miles east of Bologna, on March 16, the parish priest of the local church married Rossini and Colbran. The record in the Castenaso church reads:

"Year 1822, the 16th of the month of March, I, the undersigned parish priest of San Giovanni Battista, also as delegated, have joined in matrimony in the Sanctuary of the Blessed Virgin of the Pillar, according to the prescript of the Council of Trent, Signor Giovacchino Rossini, professor of music, son of the living Giuseppe and of the living Signora Anna Guidarini, with Signora Isabella Colbran, daughter of the late Giovanni and of the late Signora Teresa Ortola, a native of Madrid and at present of this parish of San Giovanni Battista. Witnesses, Signori Luigi Cacciari, living at No. 142 of this parish, and Francisco Fernandes,

servant of the aforementioned Signora Isabella. This marriage was celebrated without the publication of the customary Conciliar banns."

By the marriage settlement, Colbran brought Rossini the entire
usufruct, as well as half of the rights, of her possessions, which consisted
of lands and loans or mortgages in Sicily (including a "castle" at Modica)
and the Castenaso villa. The dowry's value was estimated at 40,000 Roman
scudi, about $126,000 in today's purchasing power. The considerable
size of that dowry soon unloosed malicious tongues. Knowingly, many
professed to see the Rossini-Colbran marriage as a good business deal on
Rossini's part, adding that it certainly was no love match. They also
blackened Colbran's less than pure-white character. Stendhal, for example, described her as "forty or fifty years old" when she married
Rossini—she was only thirty-seven—and said that Barbaja had presented
Rossini "gratis, a carriage, food, lodgings, and his mistress. The divine
Colbran . . . had been the delight of Prince Wablonowski, of the millionaire Barbaglia [*sic*], and of the Maestro."[n]

No documentary evidence for or against these charges and insinua-
tions exists; judgments of the true situation must be based upon estimates
of the known characters of Rossini and Colbran, upon their known
future behavior, and upon some awareness of the mores of the time
and the place—and particularly those of theatrical life. Colbran almost
certainly was sexually permissive when young: she would have been
a notable exception among successful *prime donne* had she not been.
She was almost certainly Barbaja's mistress for a time, and then Rossini's. Nor is it unlikely that Rossini, whatever his physical and emotional (not to mention artistic) attitudes toward her may have been
in 1822, knew that she was well-to-do. She was seven years his senior
and clearly nearing the end of her singing career.

Nothing discoverable about either Rossini or Isabella Colbran suggests that theirs was a prolonged, impassioned romance. Nor was their
marriage to endure. For better or for worse, however, they lived together for about eight years after their wedding. Their eventual separation was brought about, in part, by Rossini's prolonged absences,
during which Isabella, then no longer an operatic star, was left either
alone or in the company of her aged father-in-law. Meanwhile, she had
developed a passion for gambling and had become insistently, if fruit-
lessly, demanding. But Rossini, even when irritated by the sharp edges
of her later character and by her often rash behavior, treated her
respectfully. She never lost her steady affection for him. On the whole,
their marriage was a calm and dignified one. It faded out rather than

foundering during a tempest. To picture Rossini as having married an aging nymphomaniac so as to acquire her money is nonsense. His motives—and hers—were humanly mixed.

Some days after their wedding, the Rossinis left Bologna for Vienna in the company of Ambrosi, David, and Nozzari. That even early in 1822 they had no intention of returning to Naples is indicated by a letter that Rossini wrote from Vienna on March 22 to Benelli in London. After apologizing to the impresario for a delay in writing, Rossini went on: "I am now Colbran's husband. I entered into this marriage a few days ago at Bologna in the presence of my parents. To put things briefly: I do not want to return to Naples after Vienna, nor do I want my wife to return there. If you have no *prima donna* for next year, if you can offer me an advantageous contract, I will undertake a campaign in London and oblige myself during the contract to compose an opera and to stage all the others that you want. Make me an offer for both of us. Tell me the obstacles and the advantages, all this in secret for the time being, as I have other negotiations under way and you know well how badly it works out to run with the hare and hunt with the hounds. I will have my wife make her debut with the opera *Zelmira*, which was the last that I gave at Naples, which I am giving now at Vienna, and which is my property."

On March 27, 1822, Rossini was at the Kärnthnertortheater to hear Carl Maria von Weber conduct a performance of *Der Freischütz*, which had been sung at Berlin for the first time the preceding June 18 and now had as its Agathe the renowned Wilhelmine Schröder-Devrient. The two composers appear not to have met in Vienna, however, and Weber—who nursed a self-protective distaste for current Italian opera—shortly developed an understandable intense jealousy of Rossini's conspicuous success in Vienna. Some years later, in Paris, Weber and Rossini met on friendly terms.

Vienna—which had heard *L'Inganno felice* and *Tancredi* in 1816; *L'Italiana in Algeri* and *Ciro in Babilonia* in 1817; *Elisabetta, regina d'Inghilterra* and *Demetrio e Polibio* in 1818; and *Il Barbiere di Siviglia* and *La Gazza ladra* in 1819—had succumbed to the Rossini magic despite the anti-Rossinian writings of jingoistic, anti-Italian, pro-Teutonic critics. In late March 1822, it was awaiting with intense excitement a new Rossini opera and personal acquaintance both with several of his other operas and with the nimble thirty-year-old composer himself. Rossini already was the Austrians' favorite purveyor of operas.

CHAPTER VIII

1822-1823

ROM APRIL to July 1822, the Kärnthnertortheater presented a Rossini festival. It was initiated on April 13 with the first extra-Neapolitan singing of *Zelmira*.ⁿ An indisposed Isabella Colbran was not vocally at her best; also, she found difficulty in adjusting her voice—which she had been used to letting swell out in the Teatro San Carlo—to the comparatively small auditorium of the Vienna theater.ⁿ *Zelmira* itself, however, delighted the Viennese, and the enthusiasm increased at later singings. Rossini, who had staged and prepared the opera for Barbaja, had preferred to leave the conducting to the theater's regular chief conductor, Joseph Weigl. An operatic composer, Weigl (1766–1846) was reputed to be envious of the much-feted Italian. But he devoted himself fanatically to the success of *Zelmira*. Rossini told Ferdinand Hiller: "He knew that he had been described to me as one of my enemies. To convince me of the contrary, he rehearsed the orchestra for *Zelmira* with such care as I have never experienced in myself or anyone else. At times, I felt like asking him not to carry his exactness to such extremes; but I must admit that it went off wonderfully."

At Leipzig, the *Allgemeine musikalische Zeitung* published a very long, generally laudatory essay on *Zelmira* by the Beethoven partisan Friedrich August Kanne. Giuseppe Carpani, then Caesarean poet to the Austrian court (and thereby a successor to Apostolo Zeno and Metastasio), added his praise in a dispatch to *La Biblioteca italiana* (Milan), during the course of which he said: "*Zelmira* is an opera in only two acts which lasts almost four hours, but does not seem long to anyone, not even to the musicians, and that says everything." Thereupon,

Carpani swooped off into fantastic exaggerations,[n] drawing down upon his head censure from *L'Osservatore veneziano*. When a writer in *La Gazzetta di Milano*, while admitting that he had only read through a score of *Zelmira* at the piano, attacked it and pointed out the superiority of Morlacchi's *Tebaldo e Isolina*, Carpani became enraged. He sent the *Gazzetta* another farrago of nonsense in defense of Rossini, propounding claims for the eternal greatness of *Zelmira* and fulminating against all who disagreed.

In the Rossini festival at the Kärnthnertortheater, *Zelmira* was followed by *La Cenerentola* (March 30) and then by *Matilde di Shabran* (May 7). Rossini had prepared *Matilde* for Vienna so that it too lasted four hours. On the night of its first Vienna singing, a heat wave combined with the opera's unusual length to reduce the audience's enthusiasm during Act I to indifference as Act II stretched on into the night. Rossini at once abridged the score; on the second evening (May 11) of its run, it was an uninterrupted success. The *Allgemeine musikalische Zeitung* said of *Matilde di Shabran*: "Again the music is pure Rossiniana. We find ourselves in a circle of dear acquaintances: if we wanted to greet each of them we should never have done with bows and reverences . . . Rossini, then, has stolen, but from a musical millionaire: himself." This accusation was much closer to the truth than Carpani's repeated insistence that Rossini had not borrowed from his older operas to fill out the scores of new ones.

Later in May, the Rossinian attraction at the Kärnthnertortheater was *Elisabetta, regina d'Inghilterra*. "Signora Colbran performed the protagonist's role superbly," the *Allgemeine musikalische Zeitung* stated, "and she was truly the queen of the evening." *La Gazza ladra* followed (June 21), bringing to a boil Viennese excitement over matters Rossinian. This time the Leipzig periodical reported: "The fanatics raised stentorian shouts. The Maestro had to show himself onstage at the end of the overture—and four or five times for each number that was applauded! . . . This is a true epidemic, against which no physician could discover a preventive."

The season's farewell performance, Rossini's benefit night, was reached on July 8. He had prepared a one-act condensation of *Ricciardo e Zoraide*, doubtless excising from it those numbers which Viennese audiences already had heard in other operas. Its performance became an almost unbroken ovation for him, for Colbran, and for the other principal singers, who later joined the Rossinis in their rooms for supper, it being Colbran's name-day. A throng gathered beneath the windows, attracted by a rumor that Vienna's leading artists would serenade Rossini there that night. According to the *Allgemeine musikalische Zeitung*, Rossini at first was perplexed when he learned the reason for the crowd down below. Then he exclaimed to his guests: " 'Don't let it ever be said that these fine people went away unsatisfied. As they are expecting a concert—courage, my friends! We'll give them one *ex abrupto!*' And, the piano having been opened, he began the ritornello of an aria from *Elizabetta*, which his Isabella performed stupendously.

"From the street arose shouts of joy and calls of *'Viva, viva! Sia benedetto! Ancora, ancora!'* The tenor David and Fräulein Eckerlin then sang a duet; new *vivas*, new requests. Nozzari, with his formidable voice, sang the tenor's entrance in *Zelmira*; then Colbran, as a finale, cooed with her Rinaldo the voluptuous notes of the famous duet from Armida, *'Cara, per te quest'anima.'*

"By then the audience's enthusiasm was unbounded. The entire street was jammed with people: 'Come outside! Come outside! Maestro!' a roaring unison thundered. The Maestro went to the window, bowed, and thanked them. Then the shouting grew louder still: *'Viva, viva! Sing, sing!'* All smiles, the Maestro accepted the invitation, and in his charming manner sang the aria from *Il Barbiere*: *'Figaro qua, Figaro là'*; then he saluted again, with a very distinct 'Good night'; but the pit, which would have liked to prolong that artistic feast until dawn in the Italian way, demanded that it be continued.

"Then Rossini and his guests—who, having performed a long opera in the theater and having given this little *ex abrupto* concert in addition, thought themselves entitled to rest, the second hour after midnight having sounded—rose from the table, extinguished the lights, and went away.

"Upon this unforeseen departure, there came from the audience a dull, disdainful murmur that gradually grew with a formidable crescendo of the sort of which the Maestro offers many examples in his operas; a din and insults followed; perhaps such generosity would have been repaid with a stoning if many police guards, who had been circulating unobserved through the throng for some time, had not taken the precaution of ordering the fanatics to retire."

Rossini had become so attractive to Imperial Vienna that people followed him whenever he appeared in the streets; faces were pressed to windows as he passed. Nor did the Viennese popularity of his operas prove fleeting: they remained standard fare for the city's operagoers for many years. In September 1824, apparently after hearing *Otello* at the Kärnthnertortheater, Hegel wrote to his wife:[n] "As long as I have money to go to the Italian opera and to pay for my return trip, I shall remain in Vienna!" A few days later, the philosopher added: "I have heard *Corradino* [*Matilde di Shabran*] performed by Dardanelli and David: what a duo! These artists have voices, spirit, and warmth that are theirs alone. Now I understand clearly why Rossini's music is denounced in Germany, and especially in Berlin: that is because it is made for Italian throats, just as velvets and silks are made for elegant young women and Strasbourg pâtés for gourmets. This music must be sung as the Italians sing it, and then no other music excels it."

Berlin was not the only Germanic city in which anti-Rossinian voices were raised. In Vienna, admirers of Weber and other German composers became relentless in attacks on this foreign music. So vituperative did some of them sound that the correspondent of the *Allgemeine musikalische Zeitung* sent from Vienna an enthusiastic biographical sketch of Rossini in which he compared the detractors to dogs barking around the feet of a monument to his fame. Beethoven's friend Anton Schindler said mournfully that the Viennese taste for Rossini had become a delirium and that the city appeared bereft after the troupe of Italian singers had departed. Although Schindler said that these "scandalous" successes had been owing entirely to those singers, the Rossini operas remained favorites when inferior casts sang them—though, of course, they might not have become so firmly entrenched in Vienna's affections if they had been sung first in Vienna by such inferior casts.

On July 27, 1823, Beethoven, writing to Louis Spohr, referred to the Rossini craze in punning terms: "I have little news to send you from here, except to tell you that we are having a rich harvest of raisins [*i.e., Rosinen*, dried or pressed grapes]." As the composer of *Fidelio*, which had failed in 1805, failed again in a revised version in 1806, and had not become a craze even after its better reception in 1814, Beethoven understandably was irritated by the Italian invasion. But when a composer-pianist named Theophilus Freudenberg asked him for his opinion of Rossini's music, Beethoven replied: "It is the translation of the frivolous spirit that characterizes our times, but Rossini is a man of talent and an exceptional melodist. He writes with such ease that for the composition of an opera he takes as many weeks as a German would take years."

Rossini, on his part, felt profound admiration for his great German contemporary. He knew several Beethoven piano pieces as early as 1817; while in Vienna in 1822, he heard several other Beethoven compositions, including string quartets and the *"Eroica"* Symphony. His desire to meet their composer increased steadily. In one of Beethoven's conversation books, used by the deaf man's interlocutors to communicate with him, an entry by his brother Jonathan reads: "Today I met Maestro Rossini, who greeted me very affectionately and made clear to me his wish to meet you. If he had been sure of finding you at home, he would have come with me then to pay you a visit." Rossini asked one of the music-publishing Artarias to arrange a time for him to call upon Beethoven. The answer came that Beethoven was suffering from a severe "fluxion of the eyes" and could receive no one that day. Then Rossini enlisted the good offices of the septuagenarian Antonio Salieri, Mozart's onetime rival, who had given Beethoven some instruction in writing for the voice. Salieri finally arranged the meeting through Giuseppe Carpani.

Rossini's call upon Beethoven took place in late March or early April 1822. He described it to Richard Wagner in 1860.[n] Thanks to the meticulous note-taking of Edmond Michotte, who was present at the meeting as a friend of both Wagner and Rossini,[n] we have a preponderantly reliable detailed report of the entire Wagner-Rossini conversation, which took place in Rossini's Paris apartment in the rue de la Chaussée d'Antin. It was carried on in French, which Rossini by 1860 spoke fluently. Michotte noted that Wagner, less familiar with the language, several times repeated phrases with slight alterations, hoping to improve the exactness with which he was expressing his thoughts and propounding his theories.[n]

In the course of their conversation, Rossini mentioned that upon seeing Weber for the first time, he had felt much as he had felt "earlier upon finding myself in the presence of Beethoven."[n] He then tried to go on to other subjects, but the fascinated Wagner soon brought Beethoven's name up again.[n] "Need I tell you?" Rossini said. "As I went up the stairs leading to the poor lodgings in which the great man lived, I had some difficulty in containing my emotion. When the door was opened, I found myself in a sort of hovel, so dirty as to testify to frightening disorder. . . .

"The Beethoven portraits that we know render the whole of his physiognomy faithfully enough. But what no burin would know how to express is the undefinable sadness spread across all his features, so that from under heavy eyebrows there shone, as if from the depths of caverns, two eyes which, though small, seemed to pierce you. The voice was soft and very slightly fogged."

"When we first entered, he paid no attention to us, but for some moments remained bent over a piece of printed music, which he was finishing correcting. Then, raising his head, he said to me brusquely in Italian that was comprehensible enough: 'Ah, Rossini, you are the composer of *Il Barbiere di Siviglia*? I congratulate you; it is an excellent *opera buffa*; I read it with pleasure, and it delights me. It will be played as long as Italian opera exists. Never try to do anything but *opera buffa*; wanting to succeed in another genre would be trying to force your destiny.'" When Carpani, who had accompanied Rossini in order to present him to Beethoven, pointed out that Rossini had written a large number of *opere serie* and mentioned *Tancredi*, *Otello*, and *Mosè in Egitto*, Beethoven said:

"In fact I have looked through them. But, look, *opera seria*—that's not the Italians' nature. They don't have enough musical science to deal with real drama; and how could they acquire it in Italy. . . . In *opera buffa*, nobody would have the wit to match you, you Italians. Your language and your vivacity of temperament destine you for it. Look at Cimarosa: how superior the comic part of his operas is to all the rest! It's the same with Pergolesi. You Italians, you make a great thing of his religious music, I know. I agree that there is very touching feeling in his *Stabat*, but its form lacks variety . . . the effect is monotonous; whereas *La Serva padrona*—"

At this point, Wagner interrupted Rossini's narrative: "We must agree, Maestro, that happily you refrained from taking Beethoven's advice . . ." Rossini replied:

"To tell you the truth, I really felt more aptitude for *opera buffa*. I preferred to treat comic rather than serious subjects. But I never had much choice among librettos, which were imposed upon me by the impresarios. I can't tell you how many times it happened that at first I received only one part of the scenario, an act at a time, for which I had to compose the music without knowing what followed or the end of the subject. To think of it . . . what I had to do was earn a living for my father, my mother, and my grandmother! Going from town to town like a nomad, I wrote three, four operas a year. And don't think for a moment that all that earned me the means to act the *grand seigneur*. For *Il Barbiere* I received 1,200 francs paid all at once, plus a hazel-colored suit with gold buttons which my impresario gave me so that I would be in a decent state to appear in the orchestra. That suit, it is true, may have been worth one hundred francs. Total: 1,300 francs. It had taken me only thirteen days to write that score. . . ."

Again Wagner interrupted: "Thirteen days! That fact surely is unique. But, Maestro, I wonder how, under such conditions, shackled to that *vie de bohème*, which you have described, you were able to write those pages of *Otello*, of *Mosè*, superior pages that bear the mark, not of improvisation, but of thought-out labor after a concentration of all your mental forces!"

"Oh!" Rossini interjected. "I had facility and lots of instinct."[n]

Later in the conversation, Rossini said: "Ah! If I had been able to take my scholastic studies in your country, I feel that I should have been able to produce something better than what is known of mine!"

Wagner: "Surely not better—to cite only the scene of the shadows in *Moïse*, the conspiracy in *Guillaume Tell*, and, of another sort, the *Quando Corpus morietur* [in the *Stabat Mater*]. . . ."

Rossini: "I'll have to concede that you have mentioned some happy episodes of my career. But what is all that alongside the work of a Mozart, of a Haydn? I wouldn't know how to tell you strongly enough how much I admire those masters for that supple science, that certainty which is so natural to them in the art of composing. I have always envied them that; but it must be learned on the school benches, and one must also be a Mozart to know how to profit by it. As for Bach—not to leave your country—he is an overwhelming genius. If Beethoven is a prodigy of humanity, Bach is a miracle of God! I subscribed to the great publication of his works [the edition of the Bach Gesellschaft, founded in 1850]. Look, you'll see it there on my table, the last volume to appear. Can I tell you? The day when the next one arrives, that too will be an incomparably happy day for me. How I should like to hear a complete performance of his great [*Matthäus-*] *Passion* before leaving this earth! But here, among the French, that's not to be dreamed of."

After some talk about Mendelssohn, Wagner once more returned to Beethoven, asking Rossini how the visit had ended.[n] Rossini answered:

"Oh, it was short. You understand that one whole side of the conversation had to be written out. I told him of all my admiration for his genius, all my gratitude for his having allowed me an opportunity to express it to him.

"He replied with a profound sigh and exactly these words: '*Oh! un infelice!*' After a pause, he asked me for some details about the

Italian opera houses, about famous singers, whether or not Mozart's operas were performed frequently, if I was satisfied with the Italian troup at Vienna.

"Then, wishing me a good performance and success for *Zelmira*, he got up, led us to the door, and said to me again: 'Above all, make a lot of *Barbers*.'

"Going down that ramshackle staircase, I felt such a painful impression of my visit to that great man—thinking of that destitution, that privation—that I couldn't hold back my tears. 'Ah!' Carpani said, 'that's the way he wants it. He is a misanthrope, morose, and doesn't know how to hold on to a single friendship.'

"That very evening, I attended a gala dinner given by Prince Metternich. Still completely upset by that visit, by that lugubrious *'Un infelice!'* which remained in my ears, I couldn't, I assure you, protect myself from an inner feeling of confusion at seeing, by comparison, myself treated with such regard by that brilliant Viennese assemblage; that led me to say stoutly and without any discretion at all what I thought about the conduct of the court and the aristocracy toward the greatest genius of the epoch, who needed so little and was abandoned to such distress. They gave me the very reply that I had received from Carpani. I demanded to know, however, if Beethoven's deafness didn't deserve the greatest pity, if it was really charitable to bring up again the weaknesses with which they were reproaching him, to seek reasons for refusing to go to his assistance. I added that it would be so easy, by means of drawing up a very small subscription, to assure him an income large enough to place him beyond all need for the rest of his life. That proposal didn't win the support of a single person.

"After dinner, the evening ended with a reception that brought to Metternich's salons the greatest names in Vienna society. There was also a concert. One of Beethoven's most recently published trios figured on the program—always he, he everywhere, as was said of Napoleon. The new masterpiece was listened to religiously and won a splendid success. Hearing it amid all that worldly magnificence, I told myself sadly that perhaps at that moment the great man was completing—in the isolation of the hovel in which he lived—some work of high inspiration which was destined, like his earlier works, to initiate into beauties of a sublime order that same brilliant aristocracy from which he was being excluded, and which, amid all its pleasures, was not at all disquieted by the misery of the man who supplied it with those pleasures.

"Not having succeeded in my attempts to create an annual income for Beethoven, I didn't lose courage immediately. I wanted to try to get together sufficient funds to buy him a place to live. I did succeed in obtaining some promises to subscribe; but even when I added my own, the final result was very mediocre. So I had to abandon that second project. Generally I got this answer: 'You don't know Beethoven well. The day after he became the owner of a house, he would sell it again. He never would know how to adjust himself to a fixed abode; for he feels the need to change his quarters every six months and his servant every six weeks.' Was that a way of getting rid of me?"

Thus ends[n] that part of Michotte's text which reports Rossini's interview with Beethoven in 1822. What must Rossini have thought about Beethoven's urgent advice to "make more *Barbers*" and not attempt *opera seria?* By the time of that Vienna meeting of which he told Wagner, thirty-two of his operas had been staged. Although twelve of them could be classified as *opere buffe,* twenty of them were *opere serie* or *opere semiserie.*[n] Not counting *Adina* (which still had not been performed in 1822), he had not composed an *opera buffa* since *La Cenerentola,* which had been produced at Rome in January 1817. But during the five years since that *première,* he had composed twelve *opere serie.*

The bachelor Beethoven probably would not have understood or sympathized with perhaps the chief reason for the existence of most of Rossini's *opere serie*: the great talent of Isabella Colbran for singing and acting roles of high tragedy. Almost certainly, Colbran had altered the course of her husband's career as a composer of opera. That Rossini's career was to end before their marriage failed—and that Rossini would compose only one more true comic opera, *Le Comte Ory,* not intended for an Italian theater but for the Paris Opéra—is significant. Had Colbran not been thrust into Rossini's path, we might have been given more *opere buffe* such as Beethoven wanted, as swift and glinting as those we have. But then we should probably not have had those *opere serie*: *Elisabetta, regina d'Inghilterra, Otello, Armida, Mosè in Egitto, Ricciardo e Zoraide, Ermione, La Donna del lago, Maometto II, Zelmira,* and *Semiramide* (in all of which Colbran created the leading female role). Without the special experience that composing and preparing them had brought Rossini, he could not have composed (or arranged) *Moïse, Le Siège de Corinthe,* or *Guillaume Tell.*

Either for the banquet tendered by Metternich or for a similar festivity, Rossini composed *Addio ai viennesi*, a song or concert aria to stumbling verse that he may well have written himself.[n] The *Allgemeine musikalische Zeitung* reported that at the close of the banquet at which it was sung, Rossini was handed on a silver salver a gift of 3,500 ducats "with a prayer that he not disdain its smallness, as a token of appreciation for his inestimable merit and in recognition of the delightful evenings that he has provided . . . by his music." Unless he continued to muse darkly over the disparity between his own estate and Beethoven's, his feelings about Vienna must have been happy when he and Isabella left for Bologna on July 22. He was never to revisit Austria.

Stopping en route at Udine on July 25, the Rossinis went to the local opera house to attend a performance of *Matilde di Shabran*. He was recognized and became the focus of an excited ovation. Before the end of that month, he and Isabella were enjoying the comfort and quiet of the Castenaso villa. There they signed a contract promising their joint services to the Teatro La Fenice, Venice, during the forthcoming 1822–3 Carnival season.[n] At Castenaso, too, he worked at what he then referred to as his *"studio di canto,"* which later became the *Gorgheggi e solfeggi per soprano* (*Vocalizzi e solfeggi per rendere la voce agile ed apprendere a cantare secondo il gusto moderno*)—"Exercises and Solfeggios for Soprano (Vocalizations and Solfeggios to Render the Voice Agile and to Learn to Sing According to the Modern Taste)"—which was published in Paris by Antonio Pacini in 1827.[n] The contents were eighteen *gorgheggi*—that is, technical vocal exercises—and four solfeggios, all of which probably owed much to advice from Isabella. While in Bologna, finally, Rossini instituted negotiations toward acquiring a *palazzo* at No. 243, Strada Maggiore (now No. 26, Via Mazzini).[n] In November, he would purchase it for 4,150 Roman scudi (about $13,100); he would begin its restoration and extensive alteration in 1824, and would be living in it by the late autumn of 1829.[n]

In the summer of 1822, the Rossinis received an invitation to come to Verona, where he was to compose ceremonial pieces for festivities planned in connection with the congress to be held there in mid-October. The invitation was from Metternich, as Rossini later told Hiller.[n] "Seeing that I was '*le Dieu de l'harmonie*,' he wrote, would I come there, where harmony was needed so badly?" By mid-October, Rossini and Isabella were in Verona. Almost immediately, he was honored by a visit from Chateaubriand, chief of the French delegation to the congress. During the nearly two months of his stay in Verona,

Rossini was to be presented to the Emperor Francis I, Tsar Alexander I, the Duke of Wellington, and many lesser luminaries.

When telling Hiller about the letter of invitation from Metternich, Rossini said: "Had it been possible to achieve that [harmony] with cantatas, I certainly should have been able to do it: within the briefest time, I had to compose five[n] of them—for the businessmen, for the nobility, for the Festa di Concordia, and God knows what else. . . . In part, I made use of earlier things, just giving them a new text; besides, I could hardly finish the task. It happened that in a chorus in praise of Concord, the word '*Alleanza*' coincided with the most pitiful chromatic sigh. I had no time to change it, but I thought it necessary to inform Prince Metternich in advance of this sad stroke of chance . . . He at least accepted it in good humor. But the celebration, which took place in the Arena, was beautiful, and I recall it vividly. Only one thing upset me on that occasion: while conducting my cantata, I had to stand under a tremendous statue of Concordia, and I was frightened the whole time that it was going to fall on my head."

The occasional verses for that cantata, *La Santa* (sometimes *Sacra*) *Alleanza*, were forced labor by the Veronese librettist Gaetano Rossi,[n] who had to make three separate versions of them (for which he was paid six luigi, about $76) because—in a text purportedly dealing with the Holy Alliance—the governor of the Veneto insisted upon the removal of all references to war, politics, and peace. Rossini's remuneration for putting the music together was fifty zecchini (about $332). The *podestà* of Verona had agreed with the commission of public spectacles that the Festa should also include Salvatore Viganò's ballet *Il Convito degli dei*. But Metternich intervened to point out that use could be made of singers (including the *castrato* Giambattista Velluti) at the Teatro Filarmonico who were performing Morlacchi's *Tebaldo e Isolina*.[n]

The choreographer Giovanni Galzerani devised a spectacle built around a bardic country dance with choruses. Rossi produced the first version of his verses; Rossini set to work. The third, final version of the text was ready on November 20, four days before the Festa: Rossini, receiving it that evening, had the needed emendations in the music ready for rehearsal the next day. One hundred dancers and mimes were to be used during the singing of *La Santa Alleanza*;[n] the orchestra, made up of members of local and nearby military bands, swelled to 128 players; the chorus enlisted twenty-four singers. From early morning on

Sunday, November 24, 1822, people poured into the vast Roman Arena. By noon, it was full; outside, an equal number of would-be spectators was packed into the Piazza Brà.

The *podestà* had warned that the proceedings must move along rapidly lest the august guests should murmur: *"Longueur, ennui!"* Also, Francis I liked to be at luncheon by one thirty, and the Veronese were used to eating between two and three. The ceremonies began with the awarding of the first twelve of twenty-four lottery prizes (clothes, bolts of cloth, watches). Then the Festa itself began. As Radiciotti noted, the journalists who described its visual aspects at some length said nothing whatever about Rossini's music.

Another Rossini cantata, *Il Vero Omaggio*, was sung in the presence of visiting sovereigns and other dignitaries at five o'clock on the afternoon of December 3 at the Teatro Filarmonico,[n] which was illuminated by 472 Venetian wax candles and four torches. Reporting on this illumination and the fact that the garden of the Museo Lapidario, through which the guests were escorted into the theater, was lit by 575 pitch torches, Vittorio Cavazzocca Mazzanti remarked:[n] "Probably there was more smoke than light." The Royal Chamber of Commerce had commissioned the cantata and arranged its performance at the Filarmonico. Rossi again ground out appropriate verses, to which Rossini hurriedly attached music.

The stage of the theater first showed the banks of the Adige near the Church of San Zeno. From there, a group of shepherds moved toward a palace (Scene 2), where the Genius of Austria handed out palms, laurel wreaths, and olive branches.[n] *Il Vero Omaggio* was followed by a *pas de deux* and by Act II of Morlacchi's *Tebaldo e Isolina*. After the cantata, Rossini was summoned to the Imperial loge to receive the congratulations of Francis I. While he was thus occupied, the chief organizer of the performance approached the orchestra librarian, who was busily collecting the parts from the musicians' stands, and demanded the autograph score of the cantata. The librarian replied that Rossini had given very specific instructions that the score be returned directly to him. In a rage, the functionary threatened both the librarian and a musican seated at the cembalo, at the same time denouncing Rossini.

When Rossini learned of this incident, he wrote a letter to express his displeasure and to state clearly that the autograph score was his property. Further, he said, he had left the vocal and instrumental parts behind: a score could be compiled from them. If, however, the organizer wanted a copy of the score, he would have one prepared in Venice, whither he was going shortly. He also asked the organizer to reassure the two men whom he had terrified by his behavior. The reply was a threatening letter. Receiving, it, Rossini in turn replied: "The naïveté with which you treat the affair of the Cantata makes me laugh. I repeat to you for the last time that the original is mine and always will be mine; that I contracted no commitment to the Chamber [of Commerce] beyond that of composing and conducting the Cantata, which I have done; that there was no agreement between us by which I ceded either the proprietary right in or the use of this Cantata.

"I beg you to drop your vehemence and avail yourself of reason if it is your wish that I continue always to be at your service. Your devoted servant, Rossini.

"P. S.: If the Chamber should be displeased over going to the expense of putting the Cantata into score, I think myself sufficiently solvent for such an expenditure—which, furthermore, I shall contract on my own account."

The Chamber of Commerce insisted that by paying Rossini for *Il Vero Omaggio*, it had acquired proprietary rights on the autograph score. The ensuing dispute continued at least until April 1823, though Rossini was within his rights both legally and by custom. Exactly because he had foreseen trouble of this sort with the Chamber, he had demanded and received his remuneration (2,400 lire, about $1,237) in advance and had instructed the librarian to release the autograph score to nobody but himself. He was acutely aware, as the men at the Chamber of Commerce probably were not, that the score was a patchwork of borrowings from his earlier works.

If, when, and under what conditions the two other Verona cantatas listed by Ricordi (*L'Augurio felice* and *Il Bardo*) were compounded and performed is not known. What is known is that while Rossini remained in Verona, he supervised stagings at the Teatro Filarmonico of *La Donna del lago* and *L'Inganno felice*[n] and that he himself sang at reception-concerts given by both Metternich and Wellington. But by December 9, he and Isabella were in Venice,[n] where they were guests of the wealthy, world-traveling pharmacist Giuseppe Ancillo. By Rossini's contract with La Fenice, he was to receive 5,000 francs (about $2,575) for preparing a version of *Maometto II* adapted to the capabilities and requirements of La Fenice's roster of singers and for composing a new opera with a leading role for Colbran.

The time during which Rossini had planned to revise *Maometto II* was truncated when he had to conduct two court concerts before Francis I and Alexander I, who stopped off at Venice on the way from Verona to their capitals. At the second concert, the Emperor, the Tsar, and Prince Metternich asked Rossini to sing: he joined Filippo Galli in the duet from *La Cenerentola* and then sang his personal warhorse, Figaro's cavatina from *Il Barbiere di Siviglia*. Azevedo wrote that the two emperors smiled their thanks and that Alexander I sent Rossini a valuable diamond ring a few days later, whereas Francis I did not go beyond the imperial smile.

The first performance of the slightly revised *Maometto II* occurred at La Fenice on December 26, 1822, with Colbran in the role of Anna, which she had created at Naples two years before. The opera was received coldly. Colbran was unwell and sang at less than her remaining best: one evening she was whistled at. La Fenice retired *Maometto II*, substituting for it an entertainment made up of its Act I and the single-act version of *Ricciardo e Zoraide*. That combination was liked no better. Thus, 1823 began under unhappy auspices for the Rossinis. For him, however, it was to be a decisive year.

The libretto supplied to Rossini for the new Fenice opera was again the work of Gaetano Rossi, whose *La Cambiale di matrimonio* he had set for Venice twelve years earlier. Called *Semiramide*, it was based on Voltaire's *Sémiramis* (1748) and was a two-act *opera seria* or *"melo-dramma [sic] tragico."*[n] Rossini seems to have had much or all of the text in hand the preceding autumn; he may even have composed two or three numbers for it at Castenaso. His actual time for completing the unusually long score was thirty-three days. Azevedo quoted him as saying: "It is the only one of my Italian operas which I was able to do at my ease; my contract gave me forty days. . . . But I didn't put in forty days at writing it."

Not quite all of the libretto of *Semiramide* was the work of Gaetano Rossi. Rossini's friend the Marchese Gherardo Bevilacqua-Aldobrandini —who had written the libretto of *Adina* and collaborated on that of *Eduardo e Cristina*—published in 1839 an article[n] in which he said: "One evening I found myself in Rossini's lodgings when two very exalted personages came there to see him compose. Rossini did not know what to write so as to satisfy the curiosity of these two important men. I suggested a new piece [for *Semiramide*]. In this opera, made up wholly of arias and duets, there was not, as there was in all of Rossini's other operas, a trio or a quartet. 'A trio, then,' one of those exalted personages said. 'But where? but how? . . .' The unhappy Queen of Babylon and her son meet in the underground vault: there is a situation . . . 'Well, then,' Rossini added, 'give me the words.' The poet Rossi was not there: I improvised '*L'usato ardir*,'[n] and in less than three quarters of an hour Rossini had composed the music, which was quickly performed by Colbran, [Rosa] Mariani, and [Filippo] Galli."

When *Semiramide* was given its *première* at La Fenice on February 3, 1823,[n] its first act lasted two and a half hours, its second an hour and a half (the opera was shortened for later performances).[n] Between the acts, furthermore, a ballet entitled *Adelaide di Guesclino* by the choreographer Francesco Clerico was danced. The musical style of the opera perplexed most members of that audience, which blew hot and cold during Act I. Then, perhaps because the first act had acquainted them somewhat with Rossini's changing, more complex manner, Act II won them over. Enthusiastic applause followed. *Semiramide* was performed twenty-eight times at La Fenice by March 10.

The frequently cited statement (probably made first by Azevedo) that Rossini was so upset by Venice's poor reception of *Semiramide* that he resolved never to compose another note for Italy cannot be squared with the record. His reasons for abandoning Italian stages after 1823 lay in his interpreting as promises of larger remuneration and easier working conditions invitations that he had been receiving from London and Paris—as well, in all likelihood, as in disillusionment with Isabella Colbran as both wife and singer. But that he never wrote another opera for Italy was the result of happenings that he could not have foreseen in 1823.

After the first performances of *Semiramide*, the Rossinis left Venice on March 17 and returned to Bologna. Nothing indicates that either of them understood that she had sung in Italy for the last time. Later in 1823, they both signed contracts with Giovanni Battista Benelli, impresario-director of the Italian Opera at the King's Theatre, London.[n] Colbran agreed to sing there; Rossini promised (according to Azevedo) to compose an opera to be called *La Figlia dell'aria*,[n] for which Benelli was to pay him an amount equal to about $3,100 in today's purchasing power. This payment was to be effected in three installments: the first third on Rossini's reaching London, the second third on his delivery of the first half of the new opera, the final third on his delivery of the rest of the score.

During his otherwise apparently inactive sojourn in Bologna from March to October 1823, Rossini carried out a promise to provide an occasional cantata for the inauguration at Treviso of a memorial bust of Canova, who had been born near there in 1757 and had died at Venice on October 13, 1822. The orchestral score of this *Omaggio pastorale* in the Biblioteca Comunale at Treviso states that the cantata was "especially composed by the celebrated Maestro" for the occasion, but Radiciotti properly doubted "that it *all* had been written for that circumstance." *Omaggio pastorale*, for three solo voices, was sung at the Treviso unveiling on April 1, 1823.

On October 20, 1823, Rossini and Colbran started out from Bologna en route to England. They were in Milan on October 27, when the Duke of Devonshire gave Rossini letters of introduction to important people in London. From Geneva on November 4, Rossini sent a letter to an unidentifiable "dear friend," asking him to forward copies of the score and parts of *Semiramide* to Benelli and promising the friend that if he would but ask a reasonable price for them, he would in return receive a copy of the new opera to be composed in London. The Rossinis left Geneva on November 5 and had reached Paris by the evening of November 9. All unaware, the thirty-one-year-old composer had for the first time entered the great capital with which his final fame was to be connected.

CHAPTER IX

1823-1826

W HEN ROSSINI reached Paris in November 1823, twelve of his operas had been staged there by the Théâtre-Italien, which had been alternating its performances between the small Salle Louvois and the Salle Le Peletier (then the home of the Académie Royale de Musique or Opéra). Its director was Ferdinando Paër,[n] who was often accused of being maliciously jealous of the younger Rossini. Radiciotti was so convinced of the director's interference with Rossini's career that he asserted that Paër had staged *Torvaldo e Dorliska* in 1820 because he deemed it an inferior opera and sure to fail. Paër well may have been obliged to stage Rossini operas in response to popular demand, but what remains unexplained is how he could have hindered their success deliberately without realizing that he would be simultaneously hindering his own and that of his company.

Certainly Paër had presented several Rossini operas in bastardized versions, but such texts were frequently employed when a composer was not on hand to restrain the pretensions of singers, conductors, impresarios, and directors, as Rossini—and, after him, Donizetti, Bellini, and Verdi—learned by experience. The long endurance of the legend that Paër had been willing to damage his own directorship of the Italien in order to prevent Rossini's operas from gaining a secure toehold in Paris was in part owing to Stendhal. But even Fétis, in his *Biographie universelle des musiciens*, said of Paër: "It is noticeable that he delayed as long as he could the moment of the appearance of Rossini's operas in Paris and that when he was obliged to stage *Il Barbiere di Siviglia* for [Manuel] Garcia's debut and to follow it with some other works by the same composer, he employed certain underhanded maneuvers to hinder their success." What Stendhal, and even Fétis, failed to take into account was that by 1823 Paër had staged no less than twelve Rossini operas at the Italien."

Beginning the day after the Rossinis reached Paris, the press devoted a large portion of its limited space to the renowned Italian visitor. Soon it was announced that a group of his Paris admirers was planning a grand banquet for him. His daily activities, what he said, which salons he graced—it was all reported like the schedule of a visiting head of state. He took part in a musicale at the Duchesse de Berry's, seating himself at the piano to sing some of his arias. The great actress Mlle Mars gave a resplendent party for him at which she and the tragedian Talma spoke two scenes from *L'École des vieillards* and he again sang. At the salon of the Comtesse Merlin," he was introduced to many leaders of the Parisian artistic world, including the tenor Gilbert-Louis Duprez. The Comtesse and Duprez, with Rossini at the piano, sang a duet from *Ricciardo e Zoraide*. At the Théâtre-Italien on November 11, Manuel Garcia's benefit performance of *Il Barbiere di Siviglia* took place. Rossini attended; after the performance, Gambaro, the noted first clarinetist of the orchestra, led the band of the Garde Nationale to the rue Rameau—where the Rossinis were staying as guests of the Genoese writer Nicola Bagioli—there to tender the composer a serenade.

By general agreement, however, the real *clou* of Rossini's first visit to Paris was the banquet given on Sunday, November 16, 1823, at the Restaurant du Veau Qui Tette, in the place du Châtelet. *La Gazette de France* called it "a colossal picnic": more than 150 guests assembled in a room decorated with flower-encircled medallions bearing in golden letters the titles of Rossini's operas. As Gambaro led an orchestra in the overture to *La Gazza ladra*, the guest of honor was conducted to a seat above which his initials gleamed brightly. He was seated between Mlle Mars and Giuditta Pasta; opposite them, the composer Jean-François Lesueur was flanked by Mme Colbran-Rossini and the actress Mlle George. Many facets of artistic endeavor were represented: the composers present included Auber, Boieldieu, Hérold, and Panseron; the singers were headed by Pasta, Laure Cinti-Damoreau, Manuel Garcia, Jean-Blaise Martin, and Henriette Méric-Lalande; the stage people by Mlles George and Mars, Joseph de Lafont, and Talma; the painters by Horace Vernet. Piquancy is added to the meeting of Rossini and Vernet by the fact that at this time Vernet's mistress was Olympe Pélissier, who was later to become Rossini's second wife.

While the repast was being served, numbers from Rossini operas were played and (according to newspaper reports) listened to. The speeches began with the second course. Nicola Biagoli, the Rossinis' Paris host, recited verses of his own entitled "*La Nascita del gran Rossini*," which Talma then repeated in French. The toasts waited for the fruit. Lesueur lifted his glass: "To Rossini! His ardent genius has opened a new road and signalized a new epoch in the art of music." Rossini replied: "To the French school and the prosperity of the Conservatoire!" Lesueur's rejoinder to that was: "To Gluck! Rich in the resources of German theory, he grasped the spirit of French tragedy and set forth the model!" Succeeding toasts were to Grétry, Mozart, Méhul, Paisiello, and Cimarosa, "the precursor of Rossini." During this neap tide of good will, the orchestra tried to play at least one snippet of music by each composer toasted.

In the coffee room, Talma recited Macbeth's dream and a poem about the Alps by Jean-François Ducis. A medal struck off in honor of the occasion was handed to each guest. As the evening wound to its conclusion, the announcement was made that subscriptions to the banquet had more than covered its cost: the excess amount was to be donated to needy artists. The company's departure was accomplished to the "*Buona sera*" from *Il Barbiere*.

But that was not the last heard of the famous dinner. On November 29, the Gymnase-Dramatique presented a one-act "*apropos-vaudéville*" entitled *Rossini à Paris, ou Le Grand Dîner*. Its text was a collaboration by Scribe and Edmond-Joseph-Ennemond Mazères—who, not wishing to alienate the noted visitor, invited him to a rehearsal of their farce, asking him to point out anything in it which he found offensive. Rossini was not offended, but when a cancan was sung to the words "Rossini! Rossini! Why aren't you here?" he turned to say: "If this is the French national music, I can pack my bags: I'll never succeed in such a genre."

Rossini à Paris alluded tangentially to the disapproval, envy, and aroused jingoism with which some Parisian critics and musicians—most vocally, Henri-Montan Berton[n]—had been reacting to the near-deification of the Italian invader. In its issue of November 1, 1823, *La Pandore* had made play with Rossini's reputation for noisy orchestration: "Rossini has arrived in Paris. One can be sure that the trumpets, the trombones, the basses, the doublebasses, the oboes, and the flageolets of the capital will have to be assembled to give him a concert in which nothing but music of his own composition will be played." In 1827, the anti-Rossinian Jean-Toussaint Merle would say: "Since Rossini's arrival . . . I remember often having laughed with you at this doubling of dilettantism, at this paroxysm of Italian fever which lays hold of all heads; the delirium was stronger than at the first appearance of the Bouffons in 1752 and during the musical war of 1778. At the moment of the attack, it would have been dangerous to pronounce at the Salle Louvois the name of Boyeldieu [*sic*], Berton, Méhul, or d'Alayrac during a performance of *La Gazza* or *Il Barbiere*."[n]

Boieldieu, who remained on the friendliest footing with Rossini, stated his position in a letter of December 16, 1823, to Charles Maurice:[n]

"First, I am as much of a Rossinist as all the fanatical howlers, and it is because I really love Rossini that I dislike seeing his style used in bad copies.

"Second. I believed that it is for want of means that in music one can love only one style at a time; and I am very content to have found enough to be completely transported when I hear *Don Giovanni*, completely intoxicated when I hear *Otello*, and completely moved when I hear *Nina* [Dalayrac or Paisiello].

"Third. I believe that one can make very good music by copying Mozart, Haydn, Cimarosa, etc., etc., and that one always will be no more than an ape when copying Rossini. Why? Because Mozart, Haydn, Cimarosa, etc., etc., always speak to the heart, to the intelligence. They always speak the language of feeling and of reason. Whereas Rossini is full of strokes, of *bons mots* in his music. One cannot copy this style; one must either steal it whole or keep silent when one cannot invent new *bons mots*, which would be new creation.

"Fourth. I find it maladroit to risk making much less effect than Rossini when one borrows the same means, the same dispositions of the orchestra, etc., etc. To do that is to invite being defeated by him on his own terrain, which is always humiliating. Then one is the aggressor and all the glory goes to him . . ."

At a meeting of the Académie des Beaux-Arts in December 1823, its musician members opposed the nomination of Rossini; however, by acclamation of the painter and architect Academicians, he was voted an "*associé étranger*." When royal and other lofty favor helped to solidify Rossini's reputation in Paris, many French musicians abated their opposition to him. Some of it, however, was to survive until, after 1829, Rossini's abstention from operatic composition removed him from active competition with native composers.

On November 25, Rossini and Colbran had attended Garcia's benefit performance of *Otello* at the Italien. The audience had recognized the composer, who had gone to the stage to acknowledge its applause, standing between Garcia and Pasta. At about this time, Jacques Law, Marquis de Lauriston, Minister of the Royal Household, offered Rossini in the name of Louis XVIII a proposition that would have tied him to Paris. But, probably wanting to discover what London had to offer, he left Paris on December 7 with Isabella without having entered upon any arrangement with the French government. The Rossinis reached London on December 13, putting up in rooms at No. 90 Regent Street, in Nash's Quadrant, which was ornamented with a colonnade. A tradition developed that Rossini soon fell into the habit of taking a magnificent parrot and going to sit on top of the colonnade to watch in fascination the constant flow of the London throng. The Rossinis were to remain in England until July 26, 1824.

Rossini had suffered acutely from seasickness and fear while crossing a rough English Channel. For a week after reaching London, he remained in bed recovering from exhaustion and nervous debility. When, therefore, Count de Lieven, the Russian ambassador (whose wife Rossini had met in Verona), called upon him with an invitation from George IV to present himself at court (which then meant the Pavilion at Brighton), Rossini had to decline. He sent thanks and word that he would request the honor of presentation to His Majesty as soon as he had recovered. The King was said thereafter to have sent a chamberlain each day to the Quadrant to inquire about the state of the Italian composer's health.

Rossini's fame was scarcely smaller in London than in Paris: *Il Barbiere di Siviglia* has been sung at the King's Theatre on March 10, 1818, and had been followed by twelve other Rossini operas.[n] The company that Benelli had assembled for the 1824 "Rossini" season was so notable that the remunerations paid to its members would contribute critically to the downfall of his regime: at the end of the season he would find himself £25,000 in debt. He had engaged two composers: Rossini (£1,000) and Carlo Coccia[n] (£500). The mighty battalion of singers included Colbran (£1,500), Pasta and Giuseppina Ronzi De Begnis (£1,450 each), Lucia Elizabeth Vestris (£600), Maria Caradori-Allan (£500), Manuel Garcia (£1,000), Alberico Curioni and Giuseppe De Begnis (£800 each), Raniero Remorini and Matteo Porto (£700 each), and six dimmer luminaries: the total for vocal attractions came to £10,950.[n]

On December 29, 1823, Rossini was borne to the Pavilion at Brighton in a vinaigrette (a two-wheeled Bath chair) to be presented to George IV. The court wind band played the overture to *La Gazza ladra* as he was brought into His Majesty's presence, the usual "*Buona sera*" as he was ushered out.[n] At the King's express wish, Rossini accompanied himself at the piano in one of his *buffo* arias and (apparently singing falsetto) in Desdemona's "*Assisa al piè d'un salice*" from *Otello*. "He has a clear and limpid tenor voice," the *Morning Post* (London) of January 1, 1824, reported; but *The Musical Magazine* was scandalized because Rossini had imitated the voice of one of the *castrati*, who had been "banished from the stage for many years because they offended the humanity and modesty of the English." The King, however, had "honored him several times with signs of royal approbation"; the two men were to meet again.

Social success thus guaranteed, Rossini devoted much of the rest of his stay in London to arranging and conducting his operas at the King's Theatre, directing concerts, and making lavishly remunerated appearances as accompanist and lion at the homes of the royal, the noble, and the merely wealthy. All of these activities were undertaken at such high fees that during seven months in England, Rossini amassed the equivalent of $90,000 in today's buying power. This sum laid the solid basis of the personal fortune that he invested in well-selected shares, which in turn (as combined with later earnings, inheritances, and an annuity from the government of France) put him in a comfortable financial position for the remaining forty-four years of his life.

At the King's Theatre, however, things did not go well. The first performance that Rossini conducted there—*Zelmira*, on January 24, 1824[n]—suffered unmistakably from Colbran's rapid vocal decline and the notable deficiences of the Emma, Lucia Elizabeth Vestris. Also, the opera itself appealed only to a small group of dedicated Rossinians, failing to attract a larger public. We catch a glimpse of Rossini a few weeks after this failure in Thomas Moore's journal (March 7, 1824): "Thence on to call on [Henry] Luttrell . . . Lady Caroline Worsley and her son came soon afterwards; and we joined in the choruses of 'Semiramide'. Rossini, a fat, natural, jolly-looking person, with a sort of vague archness in his eye, but nothing further. His mastery over the pianoforte miraculous."

Of the eight operas that Rossini conducted at the King's Theatre, *Il Barbiere di Siviglia* fared no better than *Zelmira*: Mme Vestris, the

Rosina, again was found insufficient, and Figaro was sung poorly by Benelli himself. But Pasta and the elder Garcia made the fortunes of *Otello* and *Semiramide*: evidently it had been decided belatedly that Colbran was in no condition to sing. When Benelli's finances nonetheless began to worry him acutely, he called in Angelica Catalani, then forty-four, to save his season. After a decade's absence from London, Catalani still exercised considerable hold upon its audiences. Her inescapable demands for half of the box-office receipts and a share of the subscription fees for the boxes, however, merely deepened Benelli's troubles."

The finances of the King's Theatre were, for the moment, of only secondary account to Rossini, who continued to earn fat fees by seating himself at the pianos of lordly mansions to accompany himself, Colbran, or another singer in music of his own. The newspapers said that in return for such an appearance, he often received a superb gift in addition to his stipend. A "Lord A." was said to have paid him £200 for one such appearance, a "rich Jew" to have presented him with shares of stock which he was able to dispose of for £300. He himself later told Ferdinand Hiller: "I never earned enough from my art to be able to save anything except for my stay in England. And in London I made money not as a composer, but as an accompanist. . . . I may have been prejudiced, but in a way it went against my grain to let myself be paid as a piano accompanist; and I did it only in London. But they wanted a chance to see my nose and to hear my wife. I charged the rather high fee of fifty pounds for our participation in musical soirées; we took part in about sixty of them, and that, after all, was worth the bother. By the way, in London musicians will do anything and everything to make money. I experienced the oddest things there. . . .

"For example, the first time I undertook to accompany at one of those soirées, I was told that the famous horn player [Giovanni] Puzzi and the famous contrabass player [Domenico] Dragonetti would also be present. I thought that each of them would play solos. Not in the least! They were to support my accompaniment. 'But do you have separate scores for all these pieces?' I asked them. 'God forbid!' was the answer, 'but we get well paid and accompany as we think best.' Well, those improvised attempts at instrumentation seemed to me a little too dangerous, and so I begged Dragonetti to satisfy himself with a few *pizzicati* each time I winked at him, and I asked Puzzi to reinforce the final cadence simply with a few tones, and he, as a good musician,

did so with ease. Consequently there were no bad accidents, and everyone was satisfied."

Azevedo stated that Rossini played at Thursday-morning musicales
at the palace of George IV's son-in-law, Prince Leopold of Saxe-Coburg,
the future Leopold I of the Belgians. The Prince, who had a fair voice,"
enjoyed singing solos and sharing duets with his sister, the Duchess of
Kent, already the mother of the future Queen Victoria. Rossini sometimes joined in the singing, as did George IV when he could bring
himself to visit London. The King's bass was worse than mediocre, and
Rossini suffered while accompanying him and taking the tenor line in
semi-royal duets. On one of these odd occasions, a *buffo* duet was in
progress when His Majesty stopped singing, saying that he had made
a mistake in the time and that Rossini should begin the duet again.
Rossini replied: "Sire, you have every right to do what pleases you.
Do it, then, I'll follow you to the grave!""

Manuscript notations made by Rossini in the *Almanack and Cash
Account* now in the library of the Conservatoire Royal at Brussels
show that he taught singing to many noble and rich ladies and a few
of their husbands and brothers while in London. He was said to be
trying to limit their number by asking exorbitant fees. When a friend
later asked him how he dared to demand so much for a lesson, he
answered: "Because not even £100 per lesson could compensate me
for the tortures that I suffer while listening to those ladies, whose
voices creak horribly.""

Early in May 1824, the *Harmonicon* (London) reported sarcasti-
cally that members of the high aristocracy, wanting "to compensate the
Maestro for the sufferings borne and for the dangers undergone in
crossing the execrable Straits of Dover," had formed a committee of
patronesses to organize two grand concerts for Rossini's benefit at
Almack's Assembly Rooms. Rossini had to pay only for the orchestra
and chorus and for the copying-out of the music: many of the most
conspicuous artists then in London contributed their services, and the
concert room was given him gratis. A ticket for the two events was
priced at £2, the committee having hoped that so high a price would
keep out undesirable commoners. But the demand for tickets for the
second concert was such that plebeians had to be admitted. The sum
that Rossini earned from the two concerts, as reported in the *Allgemeine
musikalische Zeitung*, was equivalent to about $21,000 in today's pur-
chasing power.

The first of the two Almack's concerts occurred at nine o'clock on the evening of May 14, 1824. For the second concert, Lord Byron having died at Missolonghi on April 19, Rossini put together a cantata in his honor entitled *Il Pianto delle muse in morte di Lord Byron*, which was sung on July 9. This was written for tenor (Apollo) and mixed chorus, with orchestral accompaniment." Rossini sang the role of Apollo —and had to repeat his line in the face of insistent applause. A writer in the *Morning Post* said of this "Frenchified . . . extravagant" composition that it "would have seemed ridiculous had not respect toward the dead suppressed the desire to laugh." The *Morning Post* and the *Harmonicon*, as Michael Bonavia remarked, evidently expressed the anti-Rossinian feelings of some local musicians.

Early in July, Rossini went to Cambridge to take part in the annual University Music Festival, then under the direction of John Clarke-Whitfeld. Sacred music was performed in Great St. Mary's Church, profane music in the Senate House. Rossini played on the Great St. Mary's organ, accompanying a singing of the quartet "*Mi manca la voce*" from *Mosè in Egitto*, evidently deemed "sacred." At the Senate House, he joined Angelica Catalani in the duet "*Se fiato in corpo avete*" from Cimarosa's *Il Matrimonio segreto*, which had to be repeated; then he sang the inevitable "*Largo al factotum*" from *Il Barbiere*. When he also made his voice heard in the terminal *God Save the King*, he was complimented upon his unexpected command of English, whereupon he was reported to have replied, "Very well indeed."

Apparently the final social event that the Rossinis attended in London was a large rout given by the Duke of Wellington (whom Rossini had met at Verona) at the behest of George IV, who attended it. On July 26, the Rossinis left London behind, heading for Paris. In the generally reliable *Seven Years of the King's Theater*, published in 1828, John Ebers reported that during 1824, public dissatisfaction at the failure to present the promised new Rossini opera had been swelled by repeated announcements that his *Ugo, re d'Italia* would indeed be staged soon, whereas at the end of May, the reports had it that only half of the opera was composed and that Rossini "had quarrelled with the management, and had accepted the situation of composer to the Académie Royale—an engagement that was to commence in a month or two."

In fact, Rossini had not presented the new opera that he had contracted to compose, and which had been referred to in the beginning as *La Figlia dell'aria*. Azevedo said that Rossini completed Act I of that opera, deposited it with Benelli at the King's Theatre, and vainly waited for the promised payment—and, further, that he had empowered some-one to claim the score and the payment after he left England in July 1824, but had heard nothing further of either. Zanolini also asserted that Act I of *La Figlia dell'aria* lay in the archives of the King's Theatre. Both of those statements now appear to have been erroneous.

Andrew Porter,[n] having consulted documents in the archives of Barclays Bank Ltd., has clarified most details about Rossini's "London opera," but not the most tantalizing of them: what became of the score. On or about June 5, 1824, perhaps having abandoned—because of time-consuming social and money-earning activities—an original intention to set a libretto entitled *La Figlia dell'aria*,[n] Rossini signed a new arrangement with Benelli. This guaranteed that he would have ready for rehearsal by January 1, 1825, an opera to be called *Ugo, re d'Italia*, "then commenced and in great part finished." Before leaving for Paris, he was to deposit the existing portion of this new opera with Messrs. Ransom, bankers, together with a £400 bond, which was to be forfeited if he failed to complete his undertaking. Benelli and a Mr. Chippendale of Messrs. Yallop & Chippendale, his solicitors, promised that if the completed opera was delivered on time, they would pay Rossini £1,000: £600 on February 1, 1825, and £400 on March 1, 1825.

Rossini deposited both an operatic score and the £400 bond with Messrs. Ransom: John Ebers reported (1828) that *Ugo, re d'Italia*, largely complete, remained in their hands. Ebers's other statement—that before leaving London in 1824, Rossini had signed an agreement to compose exclusively for the Paris Opéra (Académie Royale de Musi-que)—also was correct. At the French Embassy in London in February 1824, Rossini had signed a promise to compose only for the Opéra for one year to begin in July (after, that is, he would have completed *Ugo, re d'Italia*). In Paris in August, however, he would discuss (and on November 27 would sign) a different arrangement with the royal gov-ernment of France.

Complicating all matters related to the Rossini opera was the fact that after the 1824 season at the King's Theatre ended, Benelli left Eng-land. A "Commission of Bankrupt" was issued against him on January 18, 1825. His interest in the King's Theatre was mortgaged for £15,000 to Rowland Yallop of Yallop & Chippendale, his solicitors. Ebers there-after purchased the lease and the theater's physical properties from Yal-lop for £5,500, persuaded Benelli's assignees to settle their claims on the theater for £1,500, and himself planned and carried through the 1825 season. On or about March 21, 1825, Benelli's assignees laid formal claim to the Rossini score, thus in effect impounding it at Ransom's.

Messrs. Ransom certainly held two packets of Rossini score and the £400 bond. As Mr. Porter pointed out, this could mean simply that Rossini had left an incomplete *Ugo* in their custody. As against that presumption of its incompleteness, however, Mr. Porter cited the phrasing of a letter that Rossini sent to Ransom's on December 18, 1830:[n] "I have been favoured with a communication from my Friend Mr. Obicini[n] relative to my Opera of Ugo Ré d'Italia now in your hands, I request that you will have the goodness immediately to deliver that opera to Mr. Obicini (to whom I have written on the business) on my account. I beg to add that much as I should regret to be myself the cause of litigation, yet in case that you should still[n] decline to restore to me the Opera, I have requested Mr. Obicini to give directions that proper legal measures be taken without delay, to compel the restitution of my Property, the withholding of which, Gentlemen by You, had in fact occasioned me considerable loss."[n]

Across the bottom of that letter, someone at Messrs. Ransom wrote: "Rogers & Son, Manchester Buildings" (Rogers & Son were the solicitors for Benelli's assignees). And on February 2, 1831, Mr. I. W. Rogers of that firm wrote a letter to "Messrs. Kinnaird & Co.,"[n] instructing them to release the Rossini manuscript score that they were holding. Mr. Yallop, who some time earlier had instructed Messrs. Ransom not to repay the £400 to Rossini before his own claim against Benelli had been considered, wrote the bank again on November 27, 1830, to say that he had no further interest in the score. Messrs. Ransom then drafted a long letter of bond, dated March 23, 1831; it recounted many details of the Rossini-Benelli controversy. By it, Rossini agreed to indemnify the bank for any claims that either Mr. Yallop or Benelli's assignees might in the future lodge against them regarding it. Rossini appears to have recovered the £400 deposit. And on April 9, 1831, one James Kemp signed a receipt reading: "Received of Messrs. Ransom & Co. two Packets of Music purporting to be the Opera of Ugo Ré d'Italia deposited with them by Signor Rossini one packet only sealed (with the seal of A. Obicini) for Fyson & Beck/Jas. Kemp."

"Later in the century," Mr. Porter wrote, "Fyson and Beck passed to the firm of Tathams & Pym. Mr. Pym became sole partner; he suffered from heart trouble, and arranged with a former partner of the present firm of Maples, Teesdale & Co., who occupied the office opposite him in Old Jewry, that were he to die suddenly they would take over Tathams & Pym. He died in 1896; Tathams & Pym were run from, and eventually absorbed in, Maples, Teesdale & Co., but there was no formal take-over or checking of documents. Messrs. Teesdale & Co., who supply me with this information, have 'made a search in our records but were unable to find any trace of the two packets of music . . . We think it unlikely that Messrs. Tathams & Pym held the two packets in 1896 as we can find no record of them.' In the hands of James Kemp on 9 April 1831 we catch our last glimpse of Rossini's lost London opera."

James Kemp or someone else may, of course, have forwarded the two packets of score to Rossini. But as Rossini composed no operas after 1829 and could not have received the packets until April 1831, it is extremely unlikely that parts of *Ugo, re d'Italia* were used in *Il Viaggio a Reims* (1825), *Le Siège de Corinthe* (1826), *Moïse* (1827), *Le Comte Ory* (1828), or *Guillaume Tell* (1829). Also, following his long-established custom, he had put together *Il Pianto delle muse in morte di Lord Byron* in part from earlier music; very possibly he had done the same in *Ugo, re d'Italia*, especially as many of his existing operas had not been heard in London, so that quotations from them would not have been identified easily by listeners there. If, therefore, he recovered the score, he may simply have destroyed it as not being, by 1831, an opera that he wanted to complete (or, if it was completed, to produce) for Paris, where the press had speculated about a staging of it early in 1826. Unless sections of it were incorporated into the *Stabat Mater*, the *Petite Messe solennelle*, or the many small pieces that Rossini composed during the rest of his life, *Ugo, re d'Italia* has vanished completely."

When Rossini returned to Paris on August 1, 1824, he was under contract to the Ministry of the Royal Household. The arrangement had been initiated during his first visit to Paris, in 1823, when he had been asked to designate terms under which he would enter into such an agreement. He had outlined them on December 1, 1823," saying that he would obligate himself to compose a *grand opéra* for the Académie Royale de Musique and either an *opera semiseria* or an *opera buffa* for the Théâtre-Italien—and to stage for the Italien one of his existing operas, probably *Semilramide* or *Zelmira*, as adapted to the circumstances of its troupe. He would ask in return for 40,000 francs (about

$23,740) and a benefit performance. The negotiator representing Louis XVIII had hesitated in the face of so large a demand. When, however, word had reached Paris that Rossini might be entertaining handsome invitations to remain in England (no trace of any such invitations has survived), Prince de Polignac, the French Ambassador to England, had been ordered to conclude the proposed contract with him. Signed at the French Embassy in London on February 27, 1824, by Rossini and Comte de Tilly, Chief of the Second Division of the Ministry of the Royal Household, the contract was made up of ten articles.[n] It fleshed out and slightly altered the terms he had proposed in December 1823.

Neither Rossini's preliminary proposition nor the agreement signed in London on February 27, 1824, had mentioned his becoming director of the Théâtre-Italien, though that possibility had been mentioned. Shortly after his return to Paris on August 1 (he took up temporary quarters at No. 28, rue Taitbout), he was received with every sign of royal favor by Louis XVIII and was urged by Vicomte Sosthène de La Rochefoucauld, the King's Director of Beaux-Arts, to accept the Italien directorship. Demurring at first, Rossini finally agreed to become, in effect, co-director with Paër, whom he still had no wish to displace. No agreement formalizing this arrangement had been signed, however, when Rossini and Isabella left Paris for Bologna, which they reached on September 4.

Rossini at once set about arranging his affairs for a one-year absence. Then, having visited with his parents and his Bolognese friends,[n] he set out again with Isabella for Paris. Soon after arriving there, he completed negotiations for a new contract to replace that of February 27. Louis XVIII having died on September 26 while the Rossinis were in Italy, the new contract was signed in the name of the as yet uncrowned Charles X.[n] Thereafter, having moved with Isabella into No. 10, boulevard Montmartre—a house in which Boieldieu and Carafa also lived—Rossini quickly took up his new duties.

Paër, offended at being subordinated to the newcomer, tendered his resignation, but withdrew it when told that it would also terminate his appointment as the King's *maître de chapelle*. Thereafter, he contented himself with performing exactly the duties to which he was bound, holding onto his post until 1826. Of the peculiar conditions under which Rossini set to work, Castil-Blaze wrote in *L'Opéra-Italien*: "By a stroke of good fortune which all Europe envies us, the first musician of the world, Rossini, just has come to rest in our Théâtre-

Italien as its director. But this director, who is second to none, has to be in leading-strings, has to be governed by a chief who recently ran a troupe of mendicants [one M. Duplantys, who had been running a poorhouse when he succeeded François-Antoine Habeneck as administrator of both the Opéra and the Italien], which brother of charity receives orders from M. le Vicomte de la Rochefoucauld, Director of Beaux-Arts, under the tutelage of the minister, his father, M. le Duc de Doudeauville. What a general staff! What a trio to hover over the modest sublieutenant Rossini!"

Six days after the new contract became effective, the Théâtre de l'Odéon inaugurated the career of a prolonged operatic success. Called *Robin des bois, ou Les Trois Balles*, this was Weber's *Der Freischütz* in an extremely free adaptation by Castil-Blaze and Thomas-Marie-François Sauvage. This distortion of Weber's opera was to run for more than three hundred performances, becoming a rallying point for Parisian anti-Rossinians.[n] The *Gazette de France* gave them their signal: "Unquestionably, the hearing of this opera will oblige the partisans of Rossini to reflect seriously. In M. de Weber's music one would look in vain for that miserable luxury of deafening notes, that chattering of ritornellos, that uniform sequence of suborned crescendos which so uselessly inflates the scores of the Italian Orpheus. The musical edifice of the German master is everywhere solidly based, and all its parts, even those which escape the ears of the multitude, are conscientiously elaborated."

Rossini was entirely aware of the opposition to him. He was equally conscious of French sensitivity about the use and musical setting of the French language. He therefore approached the composition of an opera for the Académie by slow, carefully graded steps. At the beginning, indeed, he set not a French but an Italian text. Charles X was to be crowned at Rheims; a ceremonial pseudo-opera by the new director of his Italian Opera was called for. To a properly indifferent text by Luigi Balocchi,[n] stage director of the Italien, he put together a one-act, two-part *cantata scenica* of fifteen or sixteen numbers entitled *Il Viaggio a Reims, ossia L'Albergo del giglio d'oro*. For this semicomical gallimaufry of old and new music, Rossini refused a sizable special honorarium, but did accept, as a token of royal gratitude, a Sèvres dinner set.

The text of *Il Viaggio a Reims* appears not to have survived intact; nor is it now possible to reconstruct the score as it was performed. For after the three-hour *première* at the Italien on Sunday, June 19, 1825,[n] and one or two later performances, Rossini retrieved the score." For even the admiring Castil-Blaze, after writing that *Il Viaggio* proved that "Rossini possessed in supreme degree the knowledge of voices and of the art of grouping them so as to produce the most splendid and picturesque results," felt forced to add: "One should not judge M. Rossini by this first work; it is an occasional piece written in a few days. The text is without action and without interest. We await his French grand opera . . . *Il Viaggio a Reims* is an opera in one act that lasts three hours, and the lack of action makes it seem even longer than it really is."" Rossini, wisely having withdrawn the score, thereafter understandably refused good-sized offers for it.

A few numbers in *Il Viaggio a Reims* had been welcomed with audible pleasure (though not, it would seem, by the bored King): a ballet, with variations for two clarinets; the finale of a hunting scene; and—especially, according to the Paris press—the grand finale, an arrangement of national anthems and songs from several European countries, among them *Vive Henry IV* (with solo harp) and *La Belle Gabrielle* for France; *Gott erhalte Franz den Kaiser* for Austria; *God Save the King* for England, and comparable numbers for Russia and Spain. Castil-Blaze's critique, published in the *Journal des débats* of June 19, 1825, stated that *Il Viaggio* lacked an overture, but among manuscripts that Rossini or his widow left to the Liceo at Pesaro, one not in his autograph bears the superscription *"Gran Sinfonia scritta per l'Opera Reale, nel Melodramma Un Voyage à Reims."* The work also contained one number for fourteen real parts; after praising that, one journalist concluded that "the rest is noise, crescendos, and the other culminating forms that now are used and abused to satiety."

A few days after the *première* of *Il Viaggio a Reims*, Rossini took to his bed, seriously unwell; he was unable to resume his activities again for almost three months, but the nature of his ailment is nowhere mentioned. As soon as he was able again to supervise the Italien, he devoted his full energy to staging the first Paris performance of an opera by Giacomo Meyerbeer. This was *Il Crociato in Egitto* (Teatro La Fenice, Venice, March 7, 1824). Its reception (first Paris performance September 22, 1825, with Pasta, Ester Mombelli, Schiassetti, Donzelli, and Levasseur) was enthusiastic enough to initiate what would unroll as the most brilliant career ever made in Paris by an operatic composer. Rossini had called Meyerbeer to Paris for the production of *Il Crociato*, inviting him to direct the last rehearsals. The friendship of the two men, begun at Venice in 1819, was strengthened; it was to endure until Meyerbeer's death thirty-nine years later.

On October 6, 1825, the Théâtre-Italien presented Rossini's own production of *La Cenerentola*, in which the tenor Giovanni Battista Rubini made his Paris debut and dazzled the audience by his unrivaled ability swiftly to diminish and swell the volume of his sensuously seductive voice. Next Rossini put on *La Donna del lago*,[n] with Amalia Schütz-Oldosi and Rubini (who interpolated a cavatina from *Ermione*), and *Otello*, with Rubini in the title role that Donzelli had sung the preceding April 26 in his Paris debut. The Italien had begun to approach the days of its greatest glory.

Only after *La Donna del lago* did Rossini introduce to Paris a Rossini opera that it did not yet know: *Semiramide*, on December 6, 1825—not with Colbran in what was pre-eminently her role (though she was in Paris), but with the thirty-six-year-old Mme Fodor-Mainvielle, supported by Schiassetti, Bordogni, and Filippo Galli. When the brilliant, very popular Fodor-Mainvielle appeared on the stage as Semiramide, she was greeted with noisy enthusiasm.[n] For a time, all went as had been foreseen. Then her tones began to emerge hoarse and strangled and she could be seen to struggle. The orchestra fell silent; the curtain was closed. A functionary announced that the performance had had to be interrupted because Fodor-Mainvielle was suffering a temporary indisposition. The wait lengthened.

The scene in the star's dressing room was of consternation, as she alternately wrung her hands and struck them against her face. Rossini wept, fearing the worst. The nightmare fear of singers had become a reality for Fodor-Mainvielle: her voice somehow had been damaged irreparably. After a period of rest, she attempted to sing opera again at the San Carlo, Naples; Mendelssohn, who heard her in 1831, praised her singing in a letter dated April 27 of that year. But she never recovered fully: she sang for the last time at Bordeaux in 1833, thereafter abandoning the stage. She lived forty-four years after her disaster at the Italien, many of them on the friendliest terms with Rossini.

Mme Fodor-Mainvielle's tragedy suspended the run of *Semiramide* until January 2, 1826, by when Giuditta Pasta was ready to sing the title role, doing so with such success that the opera became a longtime favorite with Parisian audiences. Eugène Delacroix, who heard a performance of it on March 31, 1853, wrote in his journal: "The memory of that delightful music (*Semiramide*) fills me with satisfaction and gentle thought on this next day, April 1. What remains in my mind is simply the impressions of the sublime which abound in that work. On the stage, the padding, the transparent planning, and the routine of the Master's talent chill the impression; but when I am away from the actors and the theater, memory melts the general effect into an ensemble, a few divine passages transport me, and, doing so, remind me of my character when I was young. . . . One thing that no one thought of when Rossini appeared—and for which they forgot to criticize him after awarding him so much criticism—is the point to which he is romantic. He breaks with the ancient formulas that were illustrated by the greatest exemplars down to his time. Only in him does one find those pathetic introductions and those passages which, though often very fast, summarize a whole situation for the soul and do it outside all the conventions. That is indeed one part, and the only one, in his talent which is protected from imitation. He is not a colorist in the manner of Rubens. I still am speaking of those mysterious passages. Elsewhere, he is more crude or more banal, and then he resembles the Fleming; but everywhere in him there is Italian grace, and even abuse of that grace."

Rossini got around to *Zelmira*, at the Italien on March 14, 1826, with a cast headed by Pasta, Rubini, and Bordogni. Not very well liked at first, it too nonetheless won its audiences. Thereafter, the frequenters of the Italien soon began to complain vigorously over the poverty of a repertoire that threatened to consist indefinitely of Meyerbeer's *Il Crociato in Egitto* and five Rossini operas with which it already was familiar. Where was the new opera that Rossini had promised to compose for them? The press, guessing, several times announced that the Italien soon would offer Rossini's *Il Vecchio de la montagna*, his *Ugo, re d'Italia*, his *L'Oracolo di Delfo*—even his *Don Giovanni*. In fact, Rossini, never composed another opera to an Italian text.

En route to London to supervise the first production of his *Oberon*, Carl Maria von Weber stopped off at Paris on February 25, 1826. In the *Courier des théâtres* two days later, Charles Maurice said: "M. Weber, author (except for the poem) of *Robin des bois*, recently arrived in Paris. M. Rossini—will he allow him to stage his work? No!" What "work" Maurice meant is unclear, but he went on belaboring Rossini and his maladroit direction of the Italien, rising on June 13 to this denunciation: "Let the director of another of our theaters permit himself half of the infractions, a quarter of the impertinences, a tenth part of the laziness equivalent to the laziness, impertinences, and infractions of M. Rossini, and one would find the voice of the public and the government raised everywhere, united to put a stop to such culpable abuses."

Weber himself had publicly attacked Rossini's operas, in part because their aesthetic was antipodal to his, in part because—and particularly in Vienna—Rossini's "foreign" operas were crushingly and obstructively popular. In 1875, Max Maria von Weber, the composer's son, who had visited Rossini in 1865 and 1868, published reminiscences of his father and of Rossini.[n] He quoted Weber as having said that whereas a critic must be receptive to everything, an artist must insist that his own approach is the only correct one, and therefore may reject even the sublime works of other creators: he gave this as his reason for thinking Rossini the "Lucifer of music." After hearing the second act of *Mosè*, Weber had said: "He is able to do everything, good things also, but Satan is not always willing." Also, he had left a performance of *La Cenerentola* midway, saying: "I am running away. Now I'm beginning to like the stuff myself!"

Of *Euryanthe*, Weber had felt that it was "no more than dreamy moonlight as compared with the brilliant day" of Rossini's operas. Max von Weber, felt that his father also had been self-conscious about his rather unattractive physical presence in contrast to Rossini's good looks. He explained Rossini's more tolerant attitude toward his father as "the charity of the more fortunate," adding that his father had lost some of his feeling of animosity as he grew older and less well. It had been, Max von Weber commented, an honorable struggle between equals, both of whom had been in the right.

Immediately after reaching Paris, in 1826, Weber called upon Cherubini, Hérold, Boieldieu, and other leading musicians, but felt some doubt as to how Rossini might receive him. Ignaz Moscheles later said[n] that Rossini had remarked of Weber: "He has talent enough, and to spare . . ." Moscheles said, too, that Rossini had told him "that when the part of 'Tancred' was sung at Berlin by a bass voice,[n] Weber had written violent articles not only against the management, but also against the composer, so that when Weber came to Paris, he did not venture to call on Rossini, who, however, let him know that he bore him no grudge for having made those attacks; on receipt of that message, Weber called and they became acquainted."

In Michotte's report of the Wagner-Rossini conversation, Wagner is quoted as saying:" "Weber, oh! I know, he was very intolerant. He became intractable above all when it was a question of defending German art. That could be forgiven him; so—and this is understandable— you did not have friendly relations with him during your stay in Vienna? A great genius, and he died so prematurely!" To that, Rossini's reply, in part, was:

"A great genius, certainly, and a *true* one, he was, for being creative and strong within himself, he imitated no one. In fact, I didn't meet him in Vienna; but, you see, as a result of those circumstances I saw him later in Paris, where he remained for a few days before starting for England . . . Not having foreseen his visit, I must admit that when I found myself unexpectedly facing that composer of genius, I felt an emotion not unlike the one that I had felt earlier upon finding myself in the presence of Beethoven. Very pallid, breathless from having climbed my stairs (for he was already very ill), the poor fellow thought it necessary, as soon as he saw me, to tell me—with an embarrassment that his difficulty in finding French words increased even more—that he had been very hard on me in his critical articles on music . . . but . . . I didn't let him finish . . . 'Look,' I told him, 'let's not discuss that. To begin with,' I added, 'those articles—I've never read them; I don't know German . . . the only words of your language—which is devilish for a musician—which I was able, after heroic application, to remember and pronounce were *ich bin zufrieden* [I am delighted]. . . .'

" 'Furthermore,' I continued, 'you have done me too much honor by discussing my operas, I who am such a small matter alongside the great geniuses of your country. And I want to ask you to permit me to embrace you; and believe me that if my friendship has any value in your eyes, I offer it to you completely and with all my heart.' I embraced him effusively and saw a tear appear in his eyes." At this point Wagner interrupted to say that Weber was then already suffering from the consumption that would kill him a short time later. "Exactly," Rossini said. "To me he appeared to be in a pitiable state: with livid coloring, emaciated, racked by the consumptive's dry cough . . . limping, too. It hurt one to see him. He came back to see me a few days later to ask for some introductions for London, as he was about to go there. I was appalled by the idea of seeing him undertake such a journey [Rossini had not forgotten the English Channel]. I tried very energetically to dissuade him, telling him that he would be committing a crime . . . suicide! It did no good. 'I know it,' he answered, 'my life will end there

. . . But I must do it. I must go to produce *Oberon*, my contract obliges me to, I must, I must . . .'

"Among other letters for London—where I had formed some important relationships during my stay in England—I gave him a letter of presentation to King George [IV], who, being very gracious to artists, had been particularly affable with me. With a broken heart, I embraced that great genius for the last time with the foreboding that I should never see him again. That was only too true. *Povero* Weber!" (Weber died in London during the night of July 5–6, 1826, aged thirty-nine, less than three months after the Covent Garden *première* of *Oberon*.)

The continuing war for Greek independence from Turkey was much in the French public mind, and on April 3, 1826, Rossini conducted a Paris concert given to raise funds for the patriots. Tickets, announced at twenty francs each, were disposed of for as much as 150 francs. The socially and artistically most eminent musical dilettantes in the city contributed their services; the Greek cause was enriched by about 30,000 francs ($17,800). That cause was very fashionable—and the fact that the Duca di Ventignano's original libretto for Rossini's *Maometto II* showed Greeks fighting Turks for freedom (three centuries earlier) was to contribute largely to the good fortune of Rossini's 1826 recasting of that opera as *Le Siège de Corinthe*.

On June 22, 1826, at the Teatro São Carlos, Lisbon *Adina*, the *farsa* that Rossini had composed to order in 1818, received its first performance.[n] Judged too short to supply an entire evening's entertainment, it was supplemented with the second act of *Semiramide* and a ballet. Beyond an undocumented assertion that *Adina* was sung only once at Lisbon, nothing is known of its reception by the Portuguese. No other production of its seems to have taken place until September 1963, 137 years after its *première*, when it shared a double bill at the Teatro dei Rinnuovati, Siena, with Donizetti's *Le Convenienze ed inconvenienze teatrali*. It was thus unique among Rossini's operas in that he never saw it staged. It was, however, published in piano score by Ricordi; the autograph manuscript also survives in the Library of the Pesaro Conservatory. It has no overture, a fact that was said to have irked its Portuguese patron, particularly after Rossini was asked to compose one and refused, saying that the original contract for the opera had not specified an overture.

Some months after the performance of *Zelmira* at the Théâtre-Italien, Rossini resigned his directorship of that house.[n] Press criticisms may have stung his pride, but, in any case, he had been finding the work there too confining. For the rest of his life, he kept a paternal eye on the troupe's activities. He was to be on terms of the closest friendship with its later co-directors Édouard Robert and Carlo Severini, and he was instrumental in attracting to the Italien, to the delight of its adherents, Maria Malibran, who made a resounding official Paris debut there as Desdemona in his *Otello* on April 8, 1828; Henriette Sontag and Rosmunda Pisaroni, who were heard in his *Tancredi*; and Ester Mombelli, Filippo Galli, Luigi Lablache, Antonio Tamburini, Domenico Donzelli, Giovanni Battista Rubini, Carlo Zucchelli, Felice Pellegrini, and Francesco Graziani. He also helped to further the success of Giulia Grisi, who sang with notable results at the Italien in *Il Barbiere di Siviglia* and *La Donna del lago*. But he not only brought a clutch of the greatest Italian singers of the era to the Italien; he also improved matters vocal there by appointing Hérold to coach its singers.

Having lost whatever interest he may originally have felt in composing for the Italien, Rossini was bent upon approaching step by step the composition of a big *grand opéra* for the Académie Royale de Musique. It is not unlikely that he was looking ahead to that opera as the culmination and finale of his career as a theatrical composer. When his Royal Household contract of November 26, 1824 (or, at least, that part of it which bound him to direct the Italien) was terminated amicably, a new agreement was drafted between him and Charles X's government. By its terms, Rossini was to receive 25,000 francs (about $14,840) annually from the Civil List. As Azevedo wrote, this stipend was merely a means of keeping Rossini in Paris. Vicomte Sosthène de La Rochefoucauld is said to have advanced the suggestion that Rossini be designated *Premier Compositeur du Roi* and *Inspecteur Général du Chant en France*. The royal appointment, including those titles, was dated October 17, 1826.

Rossini, highly entertained at the notion of using his new titles to disguise a sinecure, occasionally was to be seen on a Paris street listening attentively to strolling singers or to revelers indulging in song. If asked what he was doing there, he liked to answer that he was carrying out his duties as Inspector General of Singing in France, and that in this way, lacking a better one, he at least could find something to mention in his official reports. Others, however, took the ostensible significance of his inspectorship as its real one. Cherubini saw in it a threat to the freedom of the singing teachers at the Conservatoire: a letter from La Rochefoucauld to the edgy Italian survives in which every attempt is made to calm his nerves by assuring him that in accepting the position, Rossini had wanted to play no other part than that of an adviser vis-à-vis the Conservatoire.

While Rossini was transforming *Maometto II* into a French opera, a strange *pasticcio* of his music was strung together with his permission and staged at the Odéon on September 15, 1826. Reflecting the continuing attraction of Scott's writing, it was called *Ivanhoé*.[n] Its libretto was the joint product of Émile Deschamps (who later collaborated with Scribe on the text for Meyerbeer's *Les Huguenots*) and Gabriel-Gustave de Wailly; the music had been selected and arranged by the music-publishing musician Antonio Pacini, who had put it together from bits of *La Cenerentola*, *La Gazza ladra*, *Mosè in Egitto*, *Semiramide*, *Tancredi*, and *Zelmira*.[n] Radiciotti said of *Ivanhoé* that it was "a sort of magic lantern by means of which fragments of the Rossinian operas could be seen parading by, very ably stitched together by Pacini, but without any dramatic significance; which made Rossini say that they had dressed him up as Harlequin and that the Odéon had anticipated Carnival." *Ivanhoé* was a mild success.[n]

Meanwhile, Rossini was studying the French language, French prosody for singing, and the desires of the Opéra audiences. He was coaching the excellent young French tenor Adolphe Nourrit. He had had the Opéra take over from the Italien both Laure Cinti-Damoreau and Nicolas-Prosper Levasseur. These were all preparations for his next step toward composing directly for the French-language stage: the production of *Le Siège de Corinthe*, so complete a refashioning of *Maometto II* that it properly is listed as a new opera. With its three-act libretto (*Maometto II* is in two acts) by Luigi Balocchi and Alexandre Soumet, with its recasting of several leading characters, and with its much expanded musical richness, particularly in ensemble numbers, *Le Siège de Corinthe* was what the hastily contrived (and Italian) *Il Viaggio a Reims* could not have been: a dependable vehicle for Rossini's debut as a French composer.

CHAPTER X

1826-1829

THE FIRST PEFORMANCE of Rossini's first French opera, *Le Siège de Corinthe*, took place on October 9, 1826,ⁿ at the Salle Le Peletier, to which the Opéra's activities had been transferred from the Salle Favart, in 1822. All of it pleased; its success was immediate and enduring. The grandly designed act finales moved the audience to prolonged shows of enthusiasm. Of the finale to Act III, Léon Escudier wrote: "The hall, which had remained as if petrified during the performance of this number, as new in form as original and elevated in thought, leaped to its feet as one man at the final notes of the chorus and gave vent to a long shout of admiration." A writer in *La Quotidienne* said: "Nothing was lacking from the composer's triumph: not only was every number saluted by a triple salvo of applause, but also after the performance the entire audience wanted to enjoy Rossini's presence. For almost half an hour, the Maestro was called persistently onto the stage; finally the call-boys appeared to announce that he had left the theater, whereupon the audience decided to follow his example. During the night, a large group of musicians played the finale of Act II of his opera under the illustrious Maestro's windows . . ."ⁿ

The second singing of *Le Siège de Corinthe* had to be postponed several days because Henri-Étienne Dérivis, the Mahomet II, had injured himself painfully in a fall at the close of the *première*. Thereafter, the opera imbedded itself so deeply in the repertoire that its one-hundredth performance was sung at the Salle Le Peletier on February 24, 1839; it was heard intermittently until 1844. Rossini, who had not sold any of his earlier operas to a publisher, accepted an offer of 6,000 francs (about $3,560) for *Le Siège de Corinthe* from Eugène Troupenas, thus initiating a friendly relationship that lasted until the publisher's death in 1850." He dedicated the published score to his sixty-eight-year-old father.

Not everyone in musical Paris was reconciled to the *grand opéra* manner, of which *La Siège de Corinthe* provided an almost fully ripe example. More conservative musicians and opera-lovers were beginning to object vigorously both to the unwonted length of many of the new operas and to the "noisiness" of their orchestral writing. Curiously, one of the complainers was Berlioz. In an article published in the *Journal des débats* as late as February 6, 1852, he accused Rossini of one of the sins of which he himself often was accused: "Rossini just had given *Le Siège de Corinthe* at the Opéra. He had noticed, not without chagrin, the somnolence of our large theater's audience during performances of the most beautiful works . . . and Rossini swore not to suffer such an affront. 'I know very well how to keep you from sleeping,' he said. And he put the big drum everywhere, as well as the cymbals and the triangle, and the trombones and the ophicleide for bundles of chords; and, coming down mightily on sudden rhythms, not to mention harmonies, with such thunderbolts that the audience, rubbing its eyes, took delight in a new sort of emotions, livelier if not more musical than those which it had felt up to then.

"Be that as it may, from the date of Rossini's arrival at the Opéra, the instrumental revolution in theater orchestras was accomplished. The big noises were used for every purpose and in all works, whatever style was imposed upon them by their subject. Soon the kettledrums, the big drum, and the cymbals and triangle no longer sufficed; a snare drum was added to them; then two cornets came to the aid of the trumpets, trombones, and ophicleide; the organ was installed in the wings, along with the bells, and one saw military bands emerge onto the stage; and finally Sax's instruments, which are to the other voices of the orchestra what a cannon is to a musket."

Auguste Laget, a former singer, published a series of articles on singing in which he summed up the anti-Rossinian point of view of the late 1820's." He wrote, for example, "Who would ever have said that it would be Rossini, the king of melody, who, having formed so many illustrious singers, would react against his own school and sacrifice to false gods at one instant, one fatal instant, so that from then on, several composers would follow his example and others erect into a system what on his part had been nothing but an incident, a caprice? . . . In a critical revue played in Paris in 1827, the author had introduced onto the stage a melomane enthusiastic about Rossini; being unable to get into the auditorium of the Opéra, he sang, out in the public *place*, a *couplet* that ended with these significant words:

> "'*What am I saying! Great Rossini!*
> *I hear you very well from here!*'

"And one heard in the corridor the march in *Le Siège de Corinthe*," with its accompaniment of bass drum, trumpets, cracked brasses, etc." Laget was to make even more deprecatory remarks about the loudness of *Guillaume Tell*."

Adolph Nourrit, the Néoclès of these first performances of *Le Siège de Corinthe*, reacted humorously to the opera itself and to the critics' attitude toward it. On November 13, 1826, he wrote to a friend:" "I have had to buoy up *Le Siège de Corinthe* & the journalist Turks dealt us out plenty of difficulty; happily, the public has been Greek & some outbursts of drums and trombone—I should say even of cannon—have not prevented it from coming thrice weekly to admire the denouement of these unhappy Hellenes, who get killed by my chromatic scale & died on an A-flat roulade . . ."

On October 14, 1826—five days after the *première* of *Le Siège de Corinthe*—*Le Moniteur* had announced that Charles X, "desiring to give Rossini proof of his satisfaction over the new masterpiece with which he has enriched the French stage," had made him a *chevalier* of the Légion d'honneur. Eight days later, however, the journal stated that the information had been incorrect. Rossini, learning that this honor was about to be conferred upon him, had gone to La Rochefoucauld to say that he did not want to accept it for the revision of an old opera and moreover that many French composers who deserved it—and particularly Hérold —still did not have it (Hérold received it on November 3, 1828). He may have felt that the hour at which he was abandoning the direction of the Théâtre-Italien and being appointed First Composer to the King and Inspector-General of Singing in France was not a good one for also accepting the Légion d'honneur."

In November 1826, furthermore, Rossini was entertaining a proposal made to him by John Ebers that he return to London. On November 24, writing to Ebers," he mentioned a proposed agreement and added: "I am taking the necessary steps to obtain my leave, and I shall send you the copy of this agreement as soon as I have obtained permission to go to

London." In retrospect, England must have seemed an Eldorado to
Rossini. But nothing came of these negotiations; he never revisited
London.

Rossini meanwhile was at work on a second project of the sort that
had transmuted *Maometto II* into *Le Siège de Corinthe*. To a four-act
libretto by Luigi Balocchi and Victor-Joseph-Étienne Jouy (called
Étienne de Jouy), he was reshaping *Mosè in Egitto* into a French grand
opera, *Moïse et Pharaon, ou Le Passage de la Mer Rouge.*[n] He labored
over this extensive refashioning for less than two months. When the
result was heard at the Opéra on March 26, 1827,[n] it was greeted with
almost hysterical enthusiasm. Most of the singers now used the open-
voiced, sensuous manner inculcated in them by Rossini, which frequenters of the Opéra greeted as a new dispensation. *Moïse* was to be
sung at the *Opéra* one hundred times by August 6, 1838.

The Paris press, even publications that had been taking a strongly
anti-Rossinian attitude, now chanted the praise of *Moïse*, calling it great
music, a laudable defense of the admired Greeks against the hated Turks,
and an infusion of fresh singing sufficient (as *Le Globe* put it) to re-
juvenate "that old and feeble remnant of the *ancien régime* which is
called the Opéra." The writer added: "Maestro Rossini has transformed
a young artist's sublime sketch into the perfect composition of a mature
genius which has enchanted the ignorant stalls and found ardent partisans
also among the Conservatoire professors, and particularly in the talented
man [Cherubini] who directs it." That the severe Cherubini would admire the ethical loftiness of *Moïse* could have been predicted.

Aside from exalted praise for the score of *Moïse*, the chief burden of
the Paris critiques was delight that real singing, of the sort long familiar
at the Théâtre-Italien, at last had breached the defenses of the Opéra's
traditional prosodic declamation. The change, which would not have
pleased Lully, Rameau, or Gluck, really meant the readmission of sensuously winning virtuoso singing, without which the four-decade flowering
of grand opera—from Auber's *La Muette de Portici* in 1828 to Meyerbeer's *L'Africaine* in 1865—could not have occurred. The mid-nine-
teenth-century renaissance of *bel canto* found one of its homes in Paris
because of the Théâtre-Italien and because of Rossini's direct influence
upon the style of singing there and at the Opéra. Radiciotti was right
when he wrote: "Rossini, then, did not Gallicize himself, as many have
asserted and still assert, but French music, responding to the fascination
of his genius, Rossini-ized [read Italianized] itself . . ."

The apparent novelty of the vocal sounds being heard in *Moïse* was summed up by the *Gazette de France*: "Immense results if they be considered under the heading of technique, for this means nothing less than a lyric revolution carried through in four hours by M. Rossini. From now on, the French shouting[n] is banished without possibility of return, and at the Opéra they are going to sing as they sing at the Favart [then the home of the Italien]. *Vive* Rossini! . . . The audience, after learning how to pronounce M. Rossini's name, shouted: 'Rossini! Let him appear!' Touched by these signs of esteem and interest, the illustrious composer came forward a few steps, less accompanied than led by Dabadie and his wife."

On the night of *Moïse*'s debut at the Opéra, Rossini was in the grip of his first grief over an irreparable loss. During the earliest rehearsals of the opera, he had been told by his friend Dr. Gaetano Conti, just arrived from Bologna, that his mother was gravely ill. The fifty-five-year-old Anna Rossini had been suffering from a heart ailment for some time; an aneurism that Giuseppe Rossini had described in a letter to her brother Francesco Maria as "one of the most horrible ailments of the world, which is called *ereonisma* [*sic*], or a dilated vein in the breast" had become very painful and alarming. Rossini decided to leave for Bologna at once, but Conti forbade him to go: on an earlier occasion, his unexpected return home had so excited his mother that she had to stay in bed for two weeks, and it now seemed certain that his appearance would frighten her and might even cause her death.[n]

Anna Rossini died on February 20, 1827. Her husband was so weakened by sorrow and the strain of her illness that, after asking someone else to send the awful news to Gioachino, he himself took to his bed for several days. Rossini, in a transport of grief as all his old emotional attachment to his mother rose to the surface, managed to write consolingly to his father,[n] ordering Masses to be said for his mother and urging his father to come to Paris to spend some time with him. Giuseppe at first resisted leaving Bologna. On March 20, writing in his warm, colorful, often ungrammatical way, he told his son: "You can well believe that I would be very happy to fly to your arms so that we could blend our pains and sorrows together. For the moment I am held back by my age [sixty-eight], by being slightly constipated, by the weather, which has turned bad, and by the difficulty of the journey. If, however, it would please you, I shall do it and gladly, but, however, you will have to tell me frankly, also assure me that you will be staying in Paris when I set out [for there] on the long road." On March 28, he wrote his late wife's sister Annunziata Ricci: "Tuesday I leave for Paris with my manservant," whom Gioachino sent from there to fetch me."

From Paris on July 24, 1827, Giuseppe wrote to Francesco Maria Guidarini: "The other day, a banker, who is called by the name Signor Aguado," ordered from him [Rossini] a cantata in music, which he wrote in six days, where it was performed at the country home of the afore-mentioned by the Signore [Virginia De] Blasis and Pisaroni and the Signori Donzelli, Bordogni, Zucchelli, and Pellegrini." He added that a grateful Aguado had sent Rossini a heavy gold neck-chain worth 1,000 napoléons d'argent (about $1,035). Calling this "truly a king's gift," Giuseppe contrasted it with the ring that Alexander I had given Rossini at Verona in 1822. The score of the cantata, which Rossini had prepared for the baptism of Aguado's son on July 16, 1827, and which he accom-panied at the piano, appears not to have survived.

During his father's visit to Paris, Rossini was seeing Domenico Bar-baja, who had come from Italy to try to assert his right to the services of Donzelli—whom Rossini was advising on ways to evade the terms of his contract with the impresario. Rossini's role in these maneuvers speaks rather for his strong feeling of friendship for Donzelli than for his sense of fairness or justice or even honesty of statement: in the role of "medi-ator" between singer and impresario, he acted wholly to the singer's ad-vantage. Nonetheless, that Rossini's friendly relationship with Barbaja was not damaged is proved by the survival of at least three letters of recommendation which he sent the impresario at later dates," as well as by other indications.

For his first opera after his mother's death, Rossini anomalously was to prepare a ribald comedy, his first comic opera since *Adina* (1818). Borrowing much of its score from *Il Viaggio a Reims*, he put together *Le Comte Ory* to a libretto by Scribe. That he could compose a comic opera in 1828 in part meant that he no longer was designing tragic roles for Isabella; it may also have reflected a need on his part not to deal, for the time being, with serious or tragic matters. While waiting for Scribe to complete the text, he himself prepared for publication by Antonio Pacini the *Gorgheggi e Solfeggi* that he probably had worked out at Castenaso in 1822: they were published before the end of 1827.

On November 21, 1827, Rossini wrote to Dr. Conti at Bologna to say that he and Isabella had been at Dieppe, "where I was horribly bored," and to thank Conti for having sent him a report on the work proceeding on his Bologna *palazzo*: ". . . and I beg you to tell Professor [Francesco] Santini that I am completely desolated to learn that he has not yet finished painting the bottom part of the staircase and that I adjure him to bring to an end something that I had thought completed long since." That Rossini had begun to yearn for the easy, comparatively quiet life of Castenaso and Bologna is demonstrated by another letter from Paris to Dr. Conti (July 24, 1827): "Embrace all our friends for me and tell them that your departure [from Paris] has brought to life in me more than ever the need to repatriate myself; and I'll do it sooner than you believe." Eight years before that, to be sure, Stendhal, writing from Milan to Baron Adolphe de Mareste, had said: "I saw Rossini when he arrived yesterday; next April he will be twenty-eight, and he is eager to stop working at thirty. This man, who four years ago had not a penny,″ has just invested one hundred thousand francs with Barbaglia [*sic*] at seven and a half per cent."

Confirmation of Stendhal's remark is found in a passage in a letter written by Giuseppe Rossini from Paris on the very day (July 24, 1827) of his son's letter to Conti quoted above. This throws a strong, different light on Rossini's so-called "great renunciation" of opera after 1829. Writing to Francesco Maria Guidarini, Giuseppe said: "Gioachino has given me his word that he wants to retire home from everything in 1830, wanting to enjoy acting the gentleman and being allowed to write what he wishes, as he has been exhausted enough (may Heaven desire it, as I want it in my heart!)." Rossini himself would see to it that Heaven granted his father's wish.

Rossini's intention to withdraw from operatic combat had become public property too: in April 1828, *La Revue musicale* (Paris) said: "Rossini has promised to write a work: *Guillaume Tell*, but he himself has asserted that he will not go beyond the promise that he has made; and that this opera will be the last to come from his pen." His decision to retire, then, apparently was firm at least four months before the *première* of *Le Comte Ory*, sixteen months before that of *Guillaume Tell*. What even those closest to Rossini seem not to have realized was that in his mid-thirties he was rapidly becoming a prematurely middle-aged man, though one in whose future lay a rejuvenation so strange and remarkable that it would look much like a reincarnation.

The first performance of *Le Comte Ory* occurred at the Opéra on August 20, 1828.″ Its libretto (described alternately as *opéra-comique* and *opéra-bouffe*) originally had been a one-act vaudeville written in

1817 by Scribe and Charles-Gaspard Delestre-Poirson, who had derived
it from an old Picard Crusaders' ballade collected in 1785 by Pierre-
Antoine de La Place. Scribe later had extended the text to two acts for
Rossini. Except for an unyielding review in the anti-Rossinian *Le Constitutionnel*, the published critiques of *Le Comte Ory* testified to the
entire happiness of those who first heard it. Later, however, Adolphe
Adam was to say in *La France musicale*, the very pro-Rossinian weekly
of the Escudier brothers: "*Le Comte Ory* was not understood, and it
was only at the sixtieth performance that the public began, after a year,
to perceive that it was hearing a masterpiece." It is impossible to believe
that an opera could reach sixty singings in one year at the Opéra without
having enlisted understanding—or at least pleased—audiences, but the
truth is that *Le Comte Ory*, more notable for musical beauties than for
the sort of comic energy which propels *Il Barbiere di Siviglia* or *L'Italiana in Algeri*, always has appealed most directly to a small, devoted group
of connoisseurs (of whom Adolphe Adam and Berlioz were among the
first) than to audiences in general.

Le Comte Ory nonetheless proved very profitable to everyone connected with it. Troupenas was willing to pay Rossini 16,000 francs
(about $9,500) for it, and the Opéra took in about 7,000 francs ($4,155)
each night that it was sung. It remained in the Opéra repertoire for
twenty years. Then it was revived in 1853, first at a special performance
to honor the newly married Napoleon III and Eugénie. Restored to the
Opéra's stage again in 1857, it went on being sung there for another
six years. On January 18, 1884, it was heard for the 433rd and last time
at the Palais Garnier.

After the second performance of *Le Comte Ory*, Rossini went to
Petit-Bourg, a chateau on the Fontainebleau route belonging to Aguado,
there to work in quiet on his major effort in French opera, which he
intended to be his last opera of any sort. He had rejected two workable
librettos by Scribe. One of them was later used by Auber for his
Gustave III and (as awkwardly adapted by Antonio Somma) by Verdi
for *Un Ballo in maschera*; the other was used by Fromental Halévy for
La Juive. Having settled upon an adaptation of Schiller's *Wilhelm Tell*
by Étienne de Jouy,[*] Rossini may have begun to work on the score even
before going to Petit-Bourg. He soon was encountering difficulties with
Jouy's monumental four-act tragedy of more than 700 verses, which he
rightly thought excessively long. What now would be called a play
doctor was summoned: Hippolyte-Louis-Florent Bis, who recast Jouy's

second act almost completely and succeeded in reducing the prolix text to practical size. Rossini then found the second-act scene of the gathering of the Three Cantons too brief; one day he described in the presence of young Armand Marrast, Aguado's secretary, the added material that he needed. Marrast set to work and shortly produced a versified version of the scene as Rossini had outlined it; his lines joined those of Jouy and Bis in the completed opera,[n] though he never is listed as a co-author of it.

In September 1828, the Paris press reported that Rossini was forging ahead with the eagerly awaited new opera; on October 15, it gave currency to a rumor that he had returned to the city and would institute rehearsals of *Guillaume Tell* on November 1. Fifteen days later, one Paris paper announced that some of the music was in the copyist's hands and said: "*Tell* is the first [*grand*] *opéra* that Rossini has written expressly for the French stage, and perhaps it will be the last of his compositions, he having manifested the intention of discarding his pen and retiring to Bologna to enjoy in peace his glory and his well-earned fortune."

Rossini had been intending the role of Mathilde for Laure Cinti, who recently had married the tenor V.-C. Damoreau, and who was pregnant. To replace her temporarily at the Opéra, the Austrian soprano Annetta Maraffa-Fischer was summoned; when she was not well liked by Opéra audiences, the *première* of *Guillaume Tell* was delayed. Rossini took advantage of this postponement to finish the score at a more leisurely pace. By early May 1829, however, rehearsals were being held, and in June the Paris papers were saying that *Tell* would be staged at the Opéra in July and that Rossini planned to leave for Italy by the middle of that month. Full rehearsals were under way by July 5, when it was said that the opera would be heard at the end of that month. Scheduled for Friday, July 24, and then for Monday, July 27, it had to be delayed again, this time because the returned Cinti-Damoreau had become hoarse.

At about the time when *Guillaume Tell* was put into rehearsal, Rossini thought it necessary to make regular and formal his arrangement with the Royal Household. On April 13, 1827, he had written a long letter to La Rochefoucauld to acknowledge receipt of a draft of a supplementary letter of agreement which the official had proposed to send to Baron de la Bouillerie, General Intendant of the Royal Household, in the belief that it would suffice to amend and make permanent Rossini's position:[n]

"Assuredly, the projected letter includes all the details needed to make positive the conditions of the contract under which I have the honor of submitting my objections to you; but supposing that M. the General Intendant wished to accept them, I ask myself if a letter emanating from him would be sufficient to assure the future carrying-out of an arrangement that has been drawn up in phraseology so unclear as to require interpretation. Without question, I shall always be disposed to commit myself confidently to the loyalty of people who, like M. le Baron de La Bouillerie, never hesitate about keeping even a simple promise. But this is a question of my future. Men do not always remain in the same position; other men may neither think nor act like them. I ought, therefore, to desire to place myself in a fixed and assured situation, and for that purpose it is impossible for me to accept simple statements recorded in a correspondence in lieu of a contract including clear and positive conditions not susceptible to discussion.

"Please, M. le Vicomte, weigh with the feelings of friendliness with which you honor me the comments that I submit to you, not in defiance, but with the thought of avoiding the discussions that an insufficiently clear contract could give rise to one day. If you will agree to put yourself in my position for a moment, I am deeply convinced that your solicitude will lead you to share my fears and will inspire you with my wish to free myself of them.

"Concerned wholly with my art, and wanting to think of the future only in the interest of my reputation, it will seem very simple to you, I hope, that my desire is not to prolong any doubt about the carrying-out of the conditions that the King, you, and M. de La Bouillerie clearly intend to grant me and to maintain.

"To achieve that purpose, I shall wish, then, M. le Vicomte, that the contract may be concluded with the terms that I have submitted to you, and above all that a new royal ordinance, more explicit than the first one, may assure me in an absolute and definitive manner the lifetime annuity of 6,000 francs [about $3,410] independent of the circumstances and conditions that the contract itself may include."

Rossini was foreseeing three months of each year in Bologna, during which, on his own schedule, he might compose—to a libretto of his own choosing, in effect—a new opera if and when he liked. During a year in which he might compose such an opera, he would spend nine months in Paris putting it on and enjoying Parisian life. He was prepared, at a vague future date, to compose for the French state theaters, that is, but only on condition that he be granted in all clarity a lifetime income from the royal purse which should be in no way tied to the terms of any working contract. He had proposed that those terms provide that he compose five operas in ten years, at the rate of one every two years; that *Guillaume Tell* be deemed the first of those five; that the librettos should be selected by agreement between himself and the Direction Générale de Beaux-Arts; that in payment he should receive 15,000 francs [about $8,515] for each opera, as well as a benefit performance for each; and that the lifetime annuity of 6,000 francs thenceforth should be looked upon as recompense for services that he already had rendered to the Opéra and as encouragement for him to work further toward its improvement.

Charles X had let it be known that he was agreeable to meeting Rossini's terms. But up to early 1829, nothing had been done to produce the proposed contract, almost certainly because the royal advisers understood that Rossini's acceptance of it would be at cross-purposes with his by then well-known determination to retire from operatic composition. They made the tactical mistake, that is, of thinking that he was bluffing. The question of the lifetime annuity hung unanswered in the Paris air. On April 10, 1829, however, Rossini addressed La Rochefoucauld again:

"It is not self-interest that guides me, and this you cannot doubt: much more advantageous conditions have been offered me repeatedly by England, Germany, Russia, and Italy;" I have refused them. My musical career is in all respects sufficiently advanced so that I have no need to prolong it, and nothing would stop me from going to enjoy a sweet repose in my own country if I were not animated by the most ardent wish to offer proof of my lively gratitude to His Majesty the King of France, who has constantly honored me with his august good will, and that by continuing to devote my labors to the great theater that this magnanimous prince protects and by using all my efforts to contribute to the prosperity and glory of this magnificent establishment, unique in Europe.

"There you have my only wish and my only purpose. It is evident that the new arrangement will be more advantageous than the old one to the King's Household and the Administration [of the Opéra], seeing that it fixes the number of works to be composed and the times when they will be performed, matters indicated only vaguely in the first contract."

What Rossini was saying in flowery, disingenuous language was that his personal fortune now would support him in comfort in Bologna and that he felt no urge to go on composing operas; he would, however, agree to compose four operas after *Guillaume Tell* for a total fee for it and the four future works of something like $44,500—plus the proceeds from five benefit nights at the Opéra—and a perpetual annuity of about $3,560, if he could be allowed a decade in which to provide the four unwritten operas. He was tired; he wanted to rest—but he also liked money. And when nothing happened, Rossini became angry. He then let Émile-Timothée Lubbert, director of the Opéra, know that unless he received the contract at once, he would call off the rehearsals of *Guillaume Tell* and not hand the third and fourth acts of it to the copyist. He meant what he said: when the contract was not forthcoming, he forced suspension of the rehearsals. This was not Rossini at his most attractive.

It was now Lubbert's turn to address La Rochefoucauld:

"The administration of the theater has done everything that it has been possible to do: scenery, costumes—everything is ready; only the musical preparation is being delayed and, I repeat, will not be rebegun until Rossini has been satisfied. It is not for me to judge Rossini's conduct under these circumstances; but I can assure you that he will not alter it . . . The situation is becoming still more critical because the Maestro has let it be known that if the conclusion of his affair should be delayed further, he will withdraw the opera!"

On April 14, La Rochefoucauld placed the dilemma before the highest royal authorities. On May 8, 1829, the contract that Rossini had been demanding was put through. Charles X signed it in person, with the result that the July Revolution of the next year, which removed him from the throne, did not alter the fact that Rossini held a contract with a ruler of France. That fact finally was to weigh decisively in his favor in the protracted litigation in which he later was to involve French officials and courts with regard to the perpetual annuity. He had been extremely shrewd, too, in insisting that payment of the annuity be independent of the other terms of the contract. It is possible, of course, that he at no time intended to compose the four post-*Tell* operas; in any case, he never wrote them."

The new contract having been signed and Cinti-Damoreau restored to good health, at seven p.m. on Monday, August 3, 1829, François-Antoine Habeneck raised his hands to begin the overture to *Guillaume Tell* at the Opéra before an audience dotted with famous men and women." That audience received the opera respectfully—even, during the first two acts, with some show of enthusiasm, but with sparse signs of pleasure during the other two. The critics, however, rolled forth paeans of mighty praise, perhaps best summed up in one sentence from *Le Globe* of August 5: "From that evening dates a new era, not only for French music, but also for dramatic music in all countries." Perhaps influenced by the press, audiences kept coming. In the August issue of *La Revue musicale*, Fétis could say: "*Guillaume Tell* pursues the course of its success—or, rather, sets out upon it; for the public now understands this music, which was too strong for it at first. As for us, who have had a little more experience, at each performance we discover a hundred beauties that had escaped us even in numbers that cannot be singled out. In this opera there is enough to make ten very beautiful operas full of ideas." Troupenas gladly paid Rossini 24,000 francs (about $13,630) for the right to publish the score.[*]

By July 1830—the time of the overthrow of Charles X—*Guillaume Tell* would have been sung forty-three times at the Opéra. Beginning at the second or third performance, however, Arnold's tremendous fourth-act aria "*Asile héréditaire*" and the succeeding cabaletta "*Amis, amis, secondez ma vengeance*" had been omitted as beyond Nourrit's powers; they seem not to have been heard to full effect until sung by Duprez in 1837. With the July Revolution over and Louis-Philippe on the throne, *Tell* reached its fifty-seventh singing on June 1, 1831. By then, however, it had been contracted to three acts: the third act now began where the fourth began in the score.[*] "But that was only the timid beginning of the mutilations," Azevedo wrote; "with our own eyes we have seen, and often enough, the prodigious second act of *Guillaume Tell* performed alone by the troupe's secondary and tertiary singers and made to serve as a curtain raiser for some ballet. And during the three years that preceded the debut of M. Duprez, the public was unable to hear more than that sole fragment of so beautiful a work."[*]

One of the most frequently repeated of Rossini anecdotes pictures him, after the telescoping of *Guillaume Tell* had been proceeding for some time, as encountering in the street one day Charles Duponchel, then director of the Opéra. "I hope," Duponchel is said to have told him, "that you will have no reason to complain about the Opéra directorate: this evening we're giving Act II of *Guillaume Tell*!" And Rossini is said to have replied: "Ah! Really? *All* of it—the *whole thing?*"[*]

On April 17, 1837, Gilbert-Louis Duprez sang Arnold at the Opéra for the first time. The unique combination of his wide-ranged voice (he sang high C as a chest tone and soared to the E above it in falsetto) and his handling of the role at once re-established *Guillaume Tell* as a public favorite. Of this revival, Charles de Boigne wrote:" "Rossini had not been too bad a prophet when, asked about what success Duprez might obtain in Paris, he answered: 'Duprez! He doesn't sing my little music too badly, but I don't know how he'll sing the big.' '*The big*!' Thus Rossini designated the music of Meyerbeer. He had never forgiven his rival the glory of the three or four hundred performances of *Robert le Diable*, a little weakness that has cost us dear," one that penetrates all his words. He was approached at Bologna by directors begging him to break a silence as obstinate and unfortunate for the art as for their interests. 'Do what I am doing,' he told them. 'Wait, wait; me, I wait well . . .' 'But what are you waiting for?' one of them asked. 'I am waiting until the Jews have finished their Sabbath.' ""

What Rossini had required orchestra and singers to accomplish while performing *Guillaume Tell* naturally did not escape excoriation by lovers of other, older styles, particularly the earlier manner of *bel canto*. Auguste Laget went on from his listing, quoted on page 155, of the instrumental horrors of *Le Siège de Corinthe* to deal with *Tell*: "Rossini did not stop there. Having unloosed the bellowings of the brasses and the fracas of the percussion, he composed his immortal masterpiece, *Guillaume Tell*, that destructive opera which has exterminated three generations of tenors in twenty years . . ." Not being aesthetic philosophers or historians, Laget and those who agreed with him did not realize that what they were inveighing against was erosion of the past caused by the full tide of theatrical romanticism. Andrea della Corte, looking back almost a century, could discover what really had happened to the operatic manner that the younger Rossini had evolved from that of his immediate precedessors:"

"The tendency to force the voice represents the culmination of the vocal crisis between 1820 and '40, and also an element in the crisis of musical taste imposed by artistic expressions of the fullness of romanticism. In Italy, in France, in Germany, the very cultivators and worshippers of a way of singing which was, above all, delicate, soft, shaded, which had preserved the best part of the singing of the eighteenth century—that is, its substance—these very men observed that one of the strongest of spiritual evolutions was in progress and that the feeling of life and art was promoting manners different from and daily more antithetical to their predecessors. Faced with romanticism, which invaded and transformed everything, Rossini abandoned the field. The singer was one of the many instruments of the new expression. The libretto, the scenography, the melody, the harmony, the orchestration, the dramatic and operatic conception—everything was changing. Impetus, vehemence, pathos, which were pushed—as happened in the corruption that was not long in accompanying and damaging the new ideas —which were pushed to exaggeration, to exasperation, characteristics of the romantic sensibility, were put at the service of the new democratic public that could throng the large theaters. Loud playing and singing became the most banal expedient. In what earlier period had the tenor had occasion, let us say the pretext, to attempt the emission, the launching, the explosion, of high sounds of unprecedented violence, sufficient, as Rossini ironically said, to break glasses and mirrors? An investigation of the factors in the crisis, lighting up the reciprocal accusations of orchestration and singing, the brutality of the effects that pleased and excited the crowd, the adherence of composers to the new mode, and so forth, would be interesting nevertheless. In the end, as we have said, they would be accepted as corruption and at the same time as inescapable necessity."

Rossini, that is to say, composed operas as long as—perhaps somewhat longer than—the general social and artistic environment, particularly in Italy and in France, demanded and supported the evolved eighteenth-century operatic style for which he was natively gifted and, by experience, superbly trained. In his French-revised Italian operas and in *Guillaume Tell*, he mixed that manner with some of the more obviously accepted aspects of the new. But even if elements in his character and events in his life had not persuaded him to compose no opera after *Tell*, nothing about him suggests that he could have competed—or would have wanted to compete—with the composer of *Les Huguenots* and *Le Prophète* and the composer of *Nabucco* and *Ernani* in order to supply audiences whose taste he did not share with operas that he could not wholly like. By 1829, the Rossinian operatic world no longer existed."

On August 7, 1829, four days after the *première* of *Guillaume Tell*, Charles X conferred the Légion d'honneur upon its composer. That evening, Rossini dined with friends. Returning home, he found musicians and other people clogging the street outside No. 10, boulevard Montmartre: a serenade in his honor was being made ready. He tried to enter the building, but a police guard stopped him. "I am Rossini!" he was reported as saying. "It can't begin without me. Let me pass!" The officer replied: "You Rossini! Eh, get along with you, joker!" An elderly functionary, finally convinced that Rossini was indeed Rossini, ordered the guard to stand aside. A firsthand report of the serenade was given by François-Joseph Méry:[n] "The conductor Habeneck went with his army at nine in the evening to the boulevard Montmartre to perform the overture to *Tell*. Soulier, the elegant writer for *La Quotidienne*, had led to the same spot a crowd of Realists: Armand Marrast, [Armand] Carrel, Rabbe; I represented the party of the Left. People applauded in a way to make the boulevard windows tremble; the enthusiasm became frenzied when Levasseur, Nourrit, and Dabadie intoned the oath-swearing trio. Maître Boieldieu, a musician of genius and heart who also was a tenant at No. 10, went down to Rossini's apartment and embraced him. Paër and Berton, who were taking an ice at the Café des Variétés, exclaimed: 'The art is lost!' "

With *Guillaume Tell* still intact at the Opéra, the Rossinis left Paris for Bologna on August 13, Isabella for the last time. Rossini, having arranged to give up his apartment in the boulevard Montmartre, that very day composed a farewell to the Parisians; it was published in September by Pacini as *Addio di Rossini, Cavatina da lui composta il giorno della sua partenza*. After crossing the Alps, the Rossinis stopped in Milan. There, on August 26 and 27, Rossini went to the Teatro della Canobbiana to hear performances of Bellini's 1827 opera *Il Pirata*. Word had spread that he would be in the theater, and the crowd attending was unusually large on both nights. On the first of them, Rossini remained hidden in the back of a loge; the audience saw Isabella, but only a few old friends went to greet him.

On August 28, Bellini wrote from Milan to his uncle Vincenzo Ferlito in Catania a letter that includes this description of his first encounter with Rossini:[n]

"The celebrated Rossini, after having created a furor with *Guglielmo Tell* in Paris, now is passing through here, betaking himself to Bologna; paying a visit to the proprietress of this house, he learned from her that I was living in the same house, and then begged her to take him to me. In fact, I saw the door open and a servant enter to announce a visit from Rossini, who had reached Milan the evening of the 26th. And the first to see him was the proprietress of the house, and for that reason no one knew that he was in Milan. You can imagine my surprise, which was such that I was all atremble with contentment. Not having had the patience to put on a jacket, I went to meet him in my shirtsleeves, and therefore begging his pardon for the indecent manner in which I was presenting myself to him, justified only by the sudden pleasure of getting

to know so great a genius. He replied that it was of no importance, adding many, many compliments regarding my compositions, which he had
come to know in Paris.

"And then, continuing, he said to me: 'I have recognized in your
operas that you begin from where the others have stopped.' I answered
that such praise from him would serve to make me immerse myself more
in the career that I had taken up and that I considered myself fortunate
to have elicited a compliment from the musical man of the century. That
evening, he came to hear *Il Pirata*; then he returned the next evening,
which was the last performance of the season, and he has said to all Milan
that he found in the whole of the opera a finish and an organization
worthy of a mature man rather than a young one, and that it was full of
great feeling and, in his view, carried to such a point of philosophic
reasoning that at some points the music lacked brilliance.

"That was his feeling, and I shall go on composing in the same way,
on the basis of common sense, as I have tried to do it that way in my
enthusiasm. Yesterday, then, I was invited to dinner by the Cantùs,"
where I found Rossini and his wife. He repeated his compliments to me,
but said nothing of feeling and brilliance; but at our first meeting he said
to me that from my music he understood that I must love a lot, a lot,
because he found great feeling in it. etc., etc.

"So in Milan now they talk of *Il Pirata*, of Rossini, of Rossini and
Il Pirata, because each one says the thing that pleases him, and the same
thing of the singers. Meanwhile, I consider myself fortunate for this incident because I made the acquantance of so great a man." Bellini was
to see much more of Rossini and to obtain both detailed advice and encouragement from him in Paris in 1834 while completing his final opera,
I Puritani di Scozia.

From Milan, Rossini and Isabella went on to Bologna, arriving there
on September 6 and going almost at once to the villa at Castenaso. Paris
was not to see its favorite composer again until September 1830.

CHAPTER XI

1829-1837

DURING THE SUMMER of 1829, Bologna celebrated the arrival of a new papal legate. In honor of that event, a Rossini cantata entitled *Il Serto votivo* (sometimes *I Tre Pastori*) was sung at the Teatro Comunale, where it was followed by a Rossini aria and a Rossini quartet. The cantata was a revised version of *La Riconoscenza*, first sung at Naples in 1821 (see page 110)." Rossini's only operatic activity during the rest of 1829 consisted of helping in the preparation of *Tancredi, Otello,* and *Semiramide* for staging that autumn as starring vehicles for Giuditta Pasta at the Comunale. Otherwise, he was supervising agricultural activities at Castenaso and being very sociable and social.

Winter set in early in 1829, and the Rossinis soon moved from the Castenaso villa into the spacious Bologna *palazzo* that he had owned for seven years. There he devoted himself to the pleasures of domestic idleness with Isabella and his father, family friends, and cronies. In March 1830, Édouard Robert, co-director of the Théâtre-Italien with Carlo Severini, since October 1, 1829, stopped off at Bologna to consult Rossini, whose desires and advice still counted heavily in the theater's affairs. When, during May, to celebrate the name-day of the Marchese Francesco Sampieri," Rossini conducted in the Marchese's private theater at the Villa Casalecchio a performance of a one-act condensation of *Il Turco in Italia*, Robert took the role of Geronio." A chorus in honor of Sampieri, which Rossini had prepared for the occasion, also was sung.

Robert complained of Rossini's gregariousness, writing: "I cannot keep the Maestro's attention for more than a moment at a time, and it is much harder to talk to him about affairs here than in Paris, as he amuses himself too much here with these cursed Bolognese loafers—may the Devil take them! They come to bother him at his house from noon on, when he has scarcely awakened, and they never leave him until one o'clock in the morning . . . When I go out with him in the hope of having him in my company for at least a short while, more often than not it happens that he slips away behind the columns of an arcade—and once he has begun gossiping with his friends, it no longer is possible to settle anything with him."

When warmer weather permitted the Rossinis to return to Castenaso in the spring of 1830, Rossini—less occupied there with familial and social matters—began, despite his earlier decisions, to feel some itch to compose an opera. He began to bombard Paris with demands that he be sent a libretto for the second opera foreseen in the new contract. On May 4, 1830, he wrote to La Rochefoucauld:[n] "I still have not received my poem, which I have been awaiting over the past nine months since I left Paris. I should have liked above all to profit from the beautiful spring days and my stay in the country, where I have been installed for a short time, to push the opera along rapidly; for I should like my labor and my zeal to prove to you my desire to please you. But I cannot work without a poem." And on July 7, after returning to Bologna from a visit to Florence, he wrote to Severini:[n] "We are in the country, and I still am idle, waiting for this famous libretto. It seems to me that Lubbert is resting on his oars." He himself had roughly sketched out a scenario based on a reading of Goethe's *Faust* in Italian: in Florence in 1854, he was to tell the French architect Doussault that he had wanted "to try myself at composing a fantastic opera, but leaving out the specters, demons, and lugubrious fantasms, having the fates and genii sing instead."

Discussing *Faust* with Hiller in 1855, Rossini said: "For a long time, it was one of my pet schemes, and I already had outlined a whole scenario with [Étienne de] Jouy. Of course, it would have been based upon Goethe's poem. But at about that time a veritable *Faust*-fury raged in Paris: every theater had its own private *Faust*. That spoiled it for me. Then there was the July Revolution, and the Grand Opéra, formerly a royal institution, then came under private management. My mother had died, and a continued stay in Paris was intolerable to my father because he did not speak French. And so I dissolved my contract, which had obligated me to compose four more big operas. I preferred residing in my native country, where I hoped to cheer my father's last year. I had been far away during my mother's last hours; that had grieved me, and I was awfully afraid that the same thing might happen with my father." No record of the dissolution of Rossini's contract has been located, but he almost certainly was reporting a fact. Fascinating to speculate upon is what a *Faust* by Rossini, composed after *Guillaume Tell*, might have been and the effect it might have had on the careers and fame of Gounod and Boito.

Rossini's visit to Florence had extended from June 11 to June 22, 1830. He was at the Teatro della Pergola there on the nights of June 12 and 13, seemingly as a guest of the British ambassador, Lord Burghersh,[n] who also invited him to one or more lavish banquets. While in the grand-ducal capital, Rossini sat to the sculptor Lorenzo Bartolini,[n] who made a sketch of him from which he later carved in marble a portrait that was considered very handsome, but which later was lost (lithographs of it survive).

Rossini was back at Castenaso when thunderous news arrived from France: on July 27, 28, and 29, a revolution had taken place in Paris. Charles X had been dethroned. Profound political changes were taking place and, most important for Rossini, the royal Civil List had been suspended. If Rossini really had been planning to return to Paris, he now dropped the notion: he was not, as later events in Bologna would prove, a man exhilarated by rioting, gunfire, or streetfighting. He remained in and near Bologna through August. During that time, he was the guest of honor at an elaborate entertainment given by Sampieri at Casalecchio which was reported in extraordinary detail by the local press of August 25. Of a musical party given by Rossini himself that summer, Gaetano Fiori wrote in his paper, *Teatri, arte e letteratura*:

"Besides various pieces of music which were admirably sung under

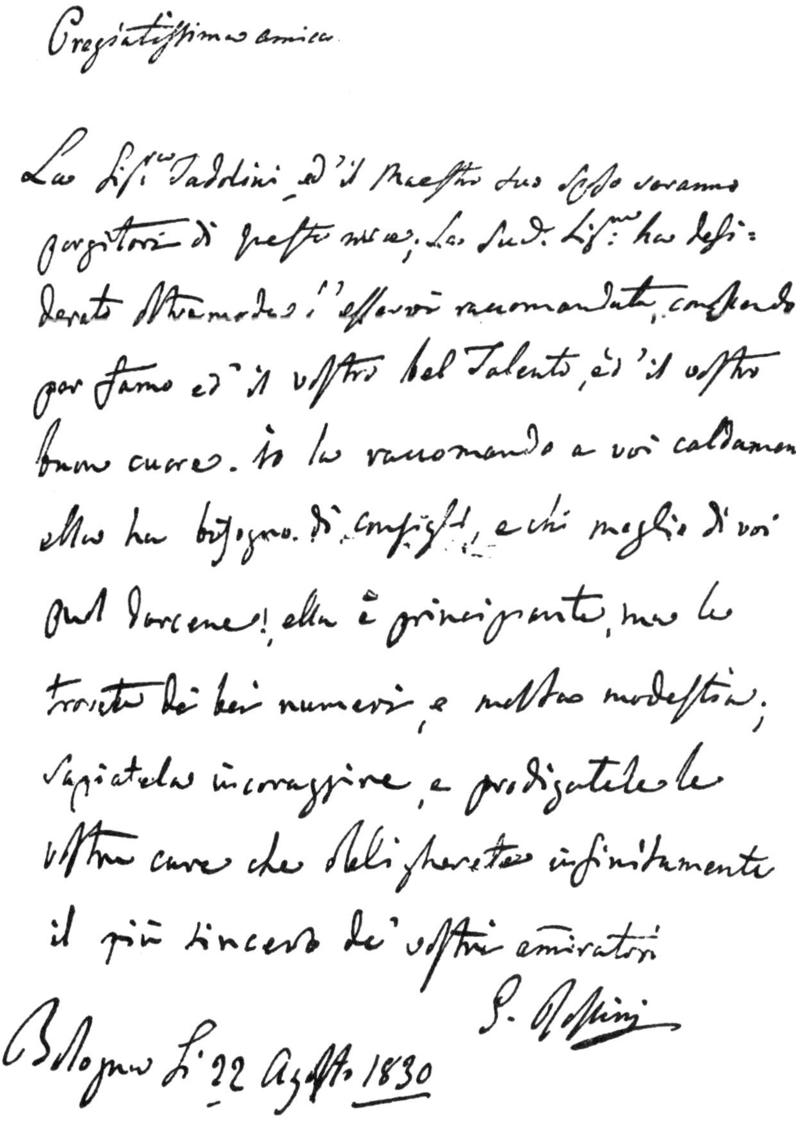

[handwritten letter in Italian]

LETTER FROM ROSSINI TO MARIA MALIBRAN, AUGUST 22, 1830

his [Rossini's] direction by the illustrious artists *madamigella* [Costanza] Tibaldi and Mme [Eugenia] Tadolini, there were also performed in chorus with them, by various music-loving ladies and gentlemen, the very famous choruses from his renowned recent score *Guglielmo Tell*, which were heard with enthusiasm; so much did the excellence of the composition and the merit of the performance shine forth. Then, ceding to the prayers of the gathering, the *cavaliere maestro* himself and his very able wife sang a most graceful duet, in which he constantly showed himself at his best and she recalled effectively that she was the Colbrand [*sic*] who had gathered so many and such illustrious laurels in the foremost theaters of Europe. . . .

"Finally, not knowing how to resist the prayers of all his most noble guests, he agreed to sing his very famous entrance aria of Figaro from *Il Barbiere di Siviglia*, and confirmed the fact that nobody, not even among the most celebrated living artists, sang or ever will sing better than he this truly classical piece, it being given only to him to feel and set forth the truth of the ideas that his music includes."

On September 4, Rossini set out for Paris with a manservant. This time he was not taking Isabella with him: he believed that he would be back in Bologna in a month. Also, his relations with Isabella had begun to cool toward strained formality. Some time before, her extravagances had driven her secretly to give singing lessons in an attempt to restore her fortune. She had told Rossini that she had entered upon this activity merely out of friendship for her students. But stories were circulated in Bologna that she had been driven to teaching by Rossini's niggardliness. When these rumors reached him, he confronted her, learned the truth, and was sharply offended. Isabella understandably was not finding retirement from the opera stage easy after having been a leading singer for nearly fifteen years. She was mortally bored, a condition that explains her increasingly willful extravagance and her costly passion for gambling.

In 1830, Rossini was thirty-eight, Isabella forty-five. They were not to meet again for nearly four years. In Bologna, Giuseppe Rossini was left behind to take care of his son's affairs, watch over Isabella, try to pacify her, attempt to lead her to economies—and turn over to her, mostly on a monthly basis (a procedure that irritated her extremely), the income that Rossini had fixed on her. A letter that Giuseppe wrote his son on December 31, 1830, foretold many similar messages that were to travel from Bologna to Paris over the next three years—and often were to remain unanswered. In it, he said: "On Wednesday the 20th both I and your wife were made a little less upset, and that because of having received your words, it having been a long time that we had not received any, and for that reason we have spent the Holy Christmas Holidays better, but like two lost souls, and on Christmas Day our table was made up of your wife, me, and her two maidservants. You can imagine with what happiness that was."

On April 18, 1833, Giuseppe was to write his son: "You know much better than me your wife's character, she is all grandeur in her thinking, and I am tiny in mine. It pleases her to squander and to give pleasure to her idolators, and it pleases me to enjoy my tranquillity and peace, and I don't give a damn for them all . . ." Five days later, he wrote: "Your wife has left for her Grand Villa; may God give her peace and quiet and also leave all the rest of us in quiet. She has become so fine now that she has to have her hair done by a hairdresser, and that because of her good humor and because of those most accursed dogs, which have ruined sofas, rugs, and everything beautiful that we have in the city." Giuseppe constantly fulminated against Isabella's extravagances.

Liking and not liking Isabella, Giuseppe Rossini found fault with most of her ways and actions. In the letters to Paris, he referred to her first as "the dear Isabella," then as "your wife," then as "your lady"— and at one point as "my lady, the Duchess of Castenaso." In a sad letter concerning her which he wrote to Rossini on August 4, 1833, Giuseppe said: "When your wife left for the country, she had everything locked up, so that I had to buy plates, glasses, and bottles, a thing that they don't do even in Turkey. And how one has to behave to love and get along with a proud and disgraceful woman, a spendthrift who looks only for ways to show spite, and that because one doesn't want to kowtow to her grandeurs and insanities; and she does not remember her birth, that she too was the daughter of a poor trumpet player like me and that she has a sister in Midrit [*sic*] who bombards her with letters; she does not remember when Crescentini[n] gave her lessons out of charity at the time when they were in Madrit [*sic*], or so many other things that I could say but do not say. And I do say only: *Evviva* the Venetians for the time when they hissed her to death,[n] it would have been better if they had done with her as they intended, and then my poor wife would not have died of distress, and if things go on in this way, I too shall go crazy. You are lucky to be far away, and may God always keep you thus so that you can always be tranquil and enjoy your peace, which you probably could not enjoy near her; and she thanks the Heavens a thousand times for having taken you as a husband; for if she had married a man who thought as she thinks, by now both of them would have been in the poorhouse."

Romain Rolland well said: "The old Giuseppe Rossini has in this correspondence much less the tone of a father than that of an upright steward, of an old domestic, devoted and grumbling."[n] His letters are written in a bold hand on paper that he ruled in lines so as to keep the words and their components marching straight across the pages. His spelling, syntax, and grammar are uncertain. But one can only come from a reading of Giuseppe Rossini's letters with respect and warm liking for the hard-pressed man who wrote them. His frequent detailed accountings of the financial situation in Bologna—with their full attention to the smallest amounts of income and outlay—are fascinating documents of Italian daily life in the early 1830's.

Whether Giuseppe Rossini's belief that his daughter-in-law's behavior had contributed to his wife's fatal illness was justified or unjustified, he can scarcely be censured for not always sympathizing with Isabella—who had declined into the pitiable state of a once-feted woman who was now unwell, past the days of her public glory, and left behind in what must have seemed to her a sluggish backwater by a husband who continued to be active and famous. And yet, Giuseppe Rossini was human: at times he even pled Isabella's case with his son, trying hard to picture a happy future when the three of them might live together contentedly. But what he sent to Rossini as a picture of Isabella's behavior in Bologna and Castenaso cannot have made her disaffected husband eager to return to her, or even to keep in regular communication with her. By the time of Rossini's return to Bologna in November 1836 to stay, she would be fifty-one and he would have become attached to Olympe Pélissier, the peculiar, admirable, infuriating younger woman who would become his second wife after Isabella's death in 1845. Rossini's constantly prolonged stay in Paris from September 1830 on marked the fraying-out of his first marriage, which did not survive Isabella's forced retirement from the stage and the end of his own career as an operatic composer.

A letter (Bologna, April 8, no year) from Isabella to Lorenzo Bartolini presents her view of the life of a retired *prima donna* and abandoned wife:[n]

"When fortune is remote from you, everything conspires against you, I must tell you that my health is always bad, that my affairs go from bad to worse, and in order to distract myself I have turned to gambling, with such disaster that I cannot take a card that doesn't become a victim. The idea that it would change has driven me too far and got me into difficulties, I have a magnificent portrait in miniature (a remnant of past grandeurs), which aroused wonderment in Paris and which at Naples, done by M. Le Comte, cost me three thousand francs, at Florence there are so many English people who make collections of beautiful things, couldn't you undertake to sell it? Dear Bartolini, believe that my situation is one of the most horrible and you, who have demonstrated such friendship for me in all circumstances, don't abandon me, this cannot compromise you, seeing that no one could recognize the original and it could be said to be an ideal; tell me what I should do to send it to you and write me your address so that I don't have to send it by post. I await a prompt reply and, full of gratitude, I am always your ISABELLA.

"The daphnes have come to a sad end, the rain has ruined them all, the gardener, having been very ill, left them in the ground and everything went wrong."

Rossini had intended to remain in Paris only the month that he had supposed would be enough for straightening out his financial affairs there. By September 12, 1830, however, he was back at Petit-Bourg as Aguado's guest. Then, having no apartment in Paris, he went to stay near Severini in rooms up many narrow stairs under the roof of the Théâtre-Italien (Salle Favart). Among the numerous guests whom he received in that tiny apartment was Pedro I, ex-Emperor of Brazil— who in March 1830 had created Rossini a Knight of the Order of the Southern Cross. But Rossini mostly lived in an operatic milieu, associating chiefly with Italians and singers of Italian: Giuditta Pasta, Giulia Grisi, Maria Malibran, Luigi Lablache, Giovanni Battista Rubini, Antonio Tamburini, and many lesser lights. On November 8, 1830, however, he was writing to his Bologna friend and financial adviser the Swiss Emilio [Émile?] Loup: "The sadness here is great and the excitement immense; but I hope to embrace you again quickly and to take pleasure in the blessed Bolognese tranquillity, which I prefer to everything else." His determination to retire, or at least to enjoy a prolonged holiday, was steady.

Paris was much changed from the city that Rossini and Isabella had left in mid-August 1829. Louis-Philippe, much less interested in opera than Charles X had seemed to be (the Citizen King had small feeling for any art), was held to a thin civil list; he was far too busy trying to establish his regime and dynasty to devote care or time to musical matters. Administration of the Opéra had been taken from the Civil List and assigned to the Ministry of the Interior, which had delegated it to a private group. All agreements between the former Royal Household and individuals had been annulled. These included Rossini's revised contract of 1829 (if it was still in effect), but he strongly—and in a legal sense correctly—maintained that a change of regime had no bearing upon Charles X's promise to him of a lifetime annuity of 6,000 francs, a claim that it would take him five years to validate. Very soon, Rossini's agents were involved in a double struggle, legal and administrative, as they tried to establish his continuing right to the annuity. That struggle, dragging on until December 1835, kept Rossini in France, one short visit to Spain and one to Italy excepted, until his victory was won.

Cut off from the Opéra, Rossini turned his attention to the Italien, which he continued to enrich by recruiting to it not only the finest Italian singers of the epoch, but also such of his younger contemporaries among Italian composers as Donizetti, Mercadante, and Bellini, thus helping the Italien to rise to the acme of its glory.

On February 4, 1831, Rossini left Paris with Aguado on a pleasure trip to Spain. They reached Madrid on February 13. That night, Rossini conducted a performance of *Il Barbiere di Siviglia* put on in his honor and attended by King Ferdinand VII. The Madrid correspondent of *Il Redattore del Reno* reported: "It is impossible to describe the welcome given to this idol of Europe by the audience. At the end of the opera, two hundred artists of the theater and the Royal Chapel gathered under the celebrated composer's window to offer him a magnificent serenade." Rossini was received at court. In 1855, he told Hiller about his reception, saying of Ferdinand VII: "He smoked all day long. I had the honor of being presented to him when Aguado and I made a short excursion to Madrid. He received me smoking in the presence of the Queen.[*] His appearance was not very attractive or even clean. After we had exchanged a few pleasantries, he most kindly offered me a half-smoked cigar; I bowed and thanked him, but did not accept it. 'You are wrong to refuse it,' Maria Cristina said to me softly in good Neapolitan, 'this is a favor not extended to many.' 'Your Majesty,' I answered in the same way (I knew her from earlier days in Naples), 'first of all, I don't smoke; secondly, under these circumstances, I could not guarantee the consequences.' The Queen laughed, and my impudence had no further consequences. . . .

"The graciousness bestowed upon me by the King's brother Francisco was much less dangerous. Maria Cristina already had given me to understand that in him I should find a great admirer. She advised my going to him immediately after my audience with the King. I found him alone with his wife,[*] making music, and I believe that a score of one of my operas stood open on the pianoforte. After a brief conversation, Don

Francisco turned to me with great kindness and told me that he had a great favor to ask of me. 'Permit me to perform Assur's aria [from *Semiramide*] for you—but dramatically.' Somewhat astonished and not knowing the meaning of all this, I sat down at the piano to accompany him. The Prince meanwhile went to the other end of the salon, assumed a theatrical pose, and then, to his wife's supreme pleasure, proceeded to perform the aria with all sorts of motions and gestures. I must say that I had never experienced anything like it."

Aguado introduced Rossini to his eminent priestly friend Manuel Fernández Varela, a state counselor who was burning to possess an autograph composition of his own by Rossini. He asked Aguado to persuade the composer to set the *Stabat Mater* exclusively for him. Rossini, who admired Pergolesi's setting of the medieval poem, had no wish to compete with it. But Varela was so insistent that at last, not wishing to offend a friend of his Maecenas, he accepted the commission. He insisted, however, upon Varela's promising that he would never let the music out of his hands or permit its publication. Whether he began to compose the setting in Madrid or waited until his return to Paris is unclear; but he did complete the six most important sections. Then, suffering from a lumbago that kept him in bed for weeks, he found himself unequal to satisfying the persistent demand from Madrid for instant delivery of the *Stabat Mater*. Thereupon he entrusted composition of the less important sections to his friend Giovanni Tadolini," who completed the work.

The autograph of the Rossini-Tadolini *Stabat Mater* was sent to Varela in Madrid with this legend on its title-page: "*Stabat Mater*, composed expressly for His Excellency Don Francisco [*sic*] Fernández Varella [*sic*], Grand Cross of the Order of Carlos III, Archdeacon of Madrid, Commissioner-General of the [Santa] Cruzada, dedicated to him by Gioachino Rossini—Paris, March 26, 1832." Varela remained unaware that his prized score was only in part a composition by Rossini, whom he rewarded with a gold snuffbox studded with eight large diamonds which later was found to be worth between 10,000 and 12,000 francs. The Rossini-Tadolini *Stabat Mater* appears to have been sung only once: on Holy Saturday 1833, it was heard in the Chapel of San Felipe el Real, Madrid, as performed by more than one hundred singers. Thereafter, it was left idle until after Varela's death in 1837. Then his testamentary executors—he willed his large fortune to the poor—sold the manuscript for 5,000 francs to one Oller Chetard, who in turn sold it to the Paris music publisher Antoine Aulagnier, thus setting in motion the interlinked, agitated events that eventually produced the all-Rossini *Stabat Mater* (see page 212).

More than a painful lumbago afflicted Rossini after his return from Madrid to Paris toward the end of March 1831. He had begun to show signs of nervous exhaustion and was suffering painfully from what almost certainly was a gonorrheal infection. Whether or not he was well enough to go to the Opéra on November 21, 1831, and thus be present at the triumph of Louis-Désiré Véron's new regime in the *première* of Meyerbeer's *Robert le Diable*, he quickly understood the significance of the event. His attitude toward the vocal style required by Meyerbeer probably was reflected in what Azevedo wrote of *Robert*: "We do not have to estimate it here except in its relations to Rossini's life; and so we limit ourselves to saying that, by the way in which the voices in it are treated, all the results of the long and patient effort of the composer of *Guillaume Tell* to lead the artists of our foremost opera house to the state of veritable singers were, if not completely destroyed, at least singularly diminished and compromised."

Rossini, that is, now was witnessing further movement away from the light, sensuous agility of early romantic *bel canto*—a movement in which, in Paris, his own operas to French texts had played an introductory role. Although *fioriture* and the other determining elements of that earlier manner remained integral to Meyerbeer's conception of operatic vocalism, the demands that he made on singers in stamina and volume already were nearer to those of *Das Liebesverbot*, *Rienzi*, and *Der fliegende Holländer* than to those of Cimarosa and Paisiello—most notably because of his increasing demand (of which Rossini himself had been accused exaggeratedly) that they sing against a big, importantly dramatic orchestra.

On December 12, 1831, Frédéric Chopin wrote a letter from Paris to his friend Tytus Woyciechowski, reporting to him on the chief excitements of Parisian life: "Through Paër, who is court conductor here, I have met Rossini, Cherubini, [Pierre-Marie-François de Sales] Baillot, etc.—also Kalkbrenner. . . . The hardest thing is to get women singers [Chopin wanted to give a concert]. Rossini would have let me have one from the [Italian] opera if he could have arranged it without M. Robert, the assistant conductor [*sic*], whose feelings he did not want to hurt with 200 or 300 such requests. But I have told you nothing up to now about the opera. I had never really heard *Il Barbiere* until last week, with Lablache Rubini, and Malibran (Garcia). Nor had I heard *Otello* until I heard it with Rubini, Pasta, and Lablache, nor

L'Italiana until with Rubini, Lablache, and Mme Raimbeaux [Raimbaux]."

Some of Chopin's news was startling: "Malibran played Otello and she [Schröder-Devrient] Desdemona. Malibran is small, and the German woman is huge; it looked as if Desdemona would smother Otello. . . . [*Robert le Diable*] is a masterpiece of the new school, in which devils (huge choruses) sing through speaking-trumpets and souls arise from graves . . . in which there is a diorama in the theater in which at the end you see the interior of a church, the whole church, at Christmas or Easter, lighted up, with monks, with all the congregation on benches, with censers—even with the organ, the sound of which on the stage is enchanting and amazing and nearly drowns out the orchestra; nothing of the sort could be put on anywhere else."

From February—and especially from May—to September 1832, Paris was pervaded by a cholera epidemic. Soon after the February performances of Bellini's *Il Pirata*, the theaters began to be deserted. Rossini, still ailing, escaped the threat of the disease by going with Aguado to Bayonne, where he was desperately bored." He found southern France more attractive when, in the summer, the Aguado family and he moved along the French side of the Pyrenees. Édouard Robert, eager to lure him back to Paris, wrote him on September 12 that the epidemic was dying out and that he could safely come back." On that same day, Boieldieu wrote in a letter: "I count on finding Rossini in Toulouse, where he is with the Aguado family, who take him everywhere without its costing him anything. He is very happy!" But Rossini was not happy; his health was deteriorating alarmingly. He was back at Petit-Bourg with the Aguados early in October."

By then, Rossini needed a sympathetic constant nurse and attendant. He found that (and possibly but not certainly a mistress as well) in Olympe Pélissier, a thirty-three-year-old woman whom he probably had met for the first time at Aix-les-bains." Daughter of an unmarried woman, Olympe was born in 1797. She was known at first as Olympe-Louise-Aléxandrine Descuilliers, but after her mother married a man named Joseph Pélissier, who adopted her, she was styled Olympe Pélissier. The late Franco Schlitzer wrote that her mother "forsaw for her adolescent daughter 'no better destiny . . . than that of being protected' in the sense that the word, a synonym for *cocotte*, had in the old gallant nomenclature. And while the girl was still a child, she brought her 'protectors,' whom the girl always accepted in an adverse spirit and without any throb of love, without amorous assent, but only so as to profit from their money and make herself a 'position.' In that she succeeded thoroughly, being by nature neither extravagant nor a lover of luxury nor given to caprices; different from other women of her sort, she was economical and a good manager." Édouard Robert, who had enjoyed associating with Rossini on a man-to-man basis in the absence of Isabella, was not pleased when Rossini acquired a protective new female companion: he called Olympe "Madame Rabatjoie No. 2" —the Second Mrs. Spoilsport.

Olympe had recently been the mistress of Horace Vernet, later noted for his genre and battle paintings and then as director of the French Academy at Rome, where one of his most famous charges was the young Hector Berlioz (he also painted a familiar portrait of Mendelssohn). The painter exhibited no pique when Olympe transferred her attentions to the musician: he later painted Olympe's face as that of Judith in his *Judith et Holopherne*." That she had been the mistress of several other men is certain.

Associating with Rossini and his friends, Olympe developed her instinctive taste for music. She was to meet most of the leading figures in most walks of Parisian life for the next four decades. She was on friendly terms with Balzac: on January 2, 1832, she wrote him: "Can I depend upon you for next Monday at nine o'clock? Rossini is coming to dinner, and it will provide a good beginning for the New Year. You must be your most charming self; a period of rest should have made you more brilliant than ever." On October 24, 1834, Bellini, writing from Paris to Francesco Florimo at Naples, said in his usual egocentric tone: "Among other things, the other day I met in the office of the management [of the Théâtre-Italien] his [Rossini's] inamorata, Madame Pélissier, and I acted enchanted to see her and asked her permission to call on her at home. Yesterday evening I saw that my attention had produced its effect, as both she and those who were in her loge applauded [*La Sonnambula*, with Grisi and Rubini] in transports."

A manuscript survives at Pesaro of a solo cantata with piano accompaniment dated "Parigi, 1832," and entitled *Grande scena—Giovanna d'Arco*. Beneath the title, Rossini wrote: "Cantata for solo voice with piano accompaniment composed expressly for Mademoiselle Olympe Pélissier by Rossini." In 1852, Rossini provided *Giovanna d'Arco* with string accompaniment, also revising the text with the help of Luigi Crisostomo Ferrucci and Barone Eugenio Lebon. When, on April 1, 1859, Marietta Alboni sang a version of the cantata at one of the Rossini musicales, the guests were enraptured, much to the delight of Olympe, who justly regarded it as "her" piece (see page 304)."

Of Rossini in the early 1830's, Zanolini wrote: "He fell ill in 1832, and Olympe wanted to be his nurse. He needed, above all, that someone should take care of his health: he overindulged himself like most of those not restrained by family ties. With an apparently robust appearance, of an attractive and smiling aspect, of a happy and joking nature, he often found himself indisposed; being very sensitive, he could very easily change by a sudden angry impetus, but could more easily be moved by great joy, by tenderness of affection, by compassion; and any serious misfortune or bitterness of spirit could upset his nerves so sharply that he would become exhausted and worn out as though from a long illness. Olympe not only took care of him diligently in illness, but also knew how to induce him to avoid causes for it, to lead a better-regulated life."

Rossini, in fact, was to exhibit more and more the determining characteristics and symptoms of the so-called manic-depressive personality. Bruno Riboli, in a very suggestive if not wholly convincing "Medico-Psychological Profile of Gioacchino Rossini," argues for a determinable relationship among Rossini's physical constitution, his psychological nature and development, and his withdrawal from operatic composition after 1829. In the jargon of psychoanalytic anthropology, Riboli classifies Rossini as having had a physical makeup "*al tipo picnico*" ("of the pyknic type"). Then he gives the medical evidence that before Rossini was forty, he suffered from persistent blennorrhoeal urethritis that necessitated his making sometimes daily use of a catheter out of fear that his urethral canal might become blocked. This painful procedure was an intermittent part of Rossini's daily life for seven or eight years. Having examined the surviving report by a physician, Riboli writes: "At the age of 44, he mitigated his passion for women and abandoned the use of liquors and overheating foods. But already, long before this period, hemorrhoids had manifested themselves, and during the losses of blood from them, his health was much improved. . . ."

Riboli continues: "In reality, the chronic urethritis in itself . . . though in a grave and painful form, does not alone suffice to explain the strong physical and psychic prostration into which Rossini fell. Indeed, 'la Pélissier,' a good observer, repeatedly notes that Rossini appears 'changed even more morally than physically.' In Rossini at this period, then, there was manifested an emotional hypersensitivity with a depressive state which, through mechanisms of psychosomatic dynamics familiar today, as well as with a psychic symptomatology of melancholy, anguish, inhibition of psychic activity, determined profound physical disturbances such as loss of weight, diarrhea, and strong general debility. If one keeps in mind that he was seized by other depressive episodes, still more evidently pathological, at Florence after 1848, with manifestations of desperate anguish, auditory illusions, and ideas of suicide, one can understand why psychiatry must consider Rossini as a cyclothymic[n] temperament who in depressive crises reaches typical expressions of the manic-depressive psychoses."

Whether so detailed a diagnosis as Riboli's can be accepted whole or not, it is addressed to facts about Rossini. It also makes certain that the post-*Guillaume Tell* Rossini could no longer have found a satisfactory mate in Isabelle Colbran, but would have found something like perfection in the untiringly attentive, protective, even worshipful Olympe—and that his desertion of Isabella for Olympe cannot be ascribed to preference for a new sexual companion twelve years younger than his wife. Whatever satisfactions he may have found in his life with Isabella during their early years together at Naples, she had exercised upon his career as a composer, especially in causing him to devote himself to *opera seria* rather than to *opera buffa*, a strong influence that many have regarded as harmful. Olympe, on the other hand, entering his life after his retirement from opera, was to be an unfailingly good influence for nearly forty years, both because of the peculiarities of his physical and mental conditions and because of her own singularly protective, self-effacing attitude.

Early in 1834, Rossini wrote to Gaetano Donizetti, inviting him to come to Paris to compose an opera for the Théâtre-Italien, an action that caused the nervous, jealous Bellini considerable anguish. From Florence, on February 22, five days before the *première* of his *Rosmonda d'Inghilterra* there, the flattered Donizetti replied:[n]

"Most Honored Maestro: The flattering expressions in your letter would invite me to do everything, or rather, I shall say, to abandon everything and free myself from everything in order to be in Paris with you.

"However, a previous obligation that I have with La Scala for Carnival would prevent me from being able to be with you in the autumn, as I must do the first opera. If this good fortune that I owe to the Honored Rossini, and for which I shall be eternally grateful, could

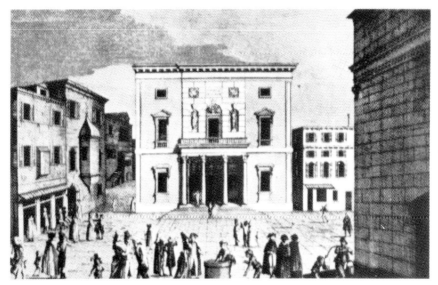

THE TEATRO LA FENICE, VENICE, ABOUT 1813

THE TEATRO ALLA SCALA, MILAN, ABOUT 1812

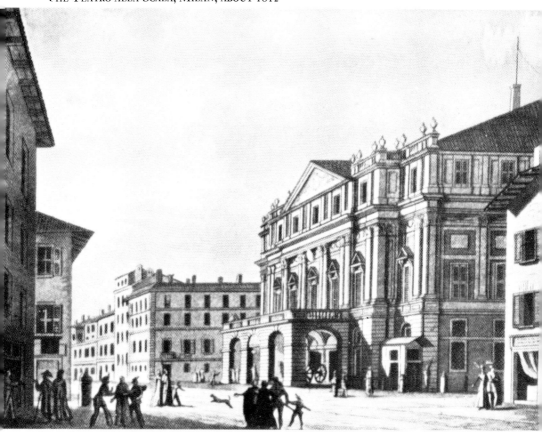

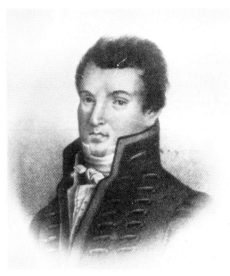

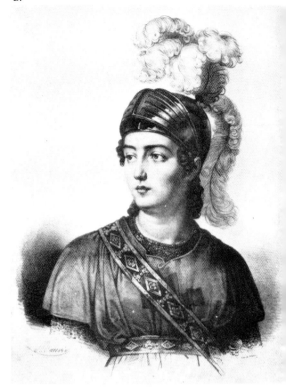

A. Domenico Donzelli

B. Giuditta Pasta
   as Tancredi

C. Geltrude Righetti-Giorgi

D. Gilbert-Louis Duprez as
   Arnold in *Guillaume Tell*

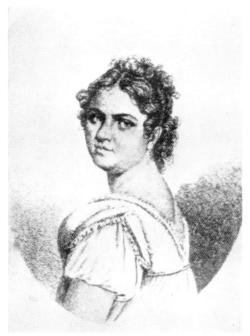

C.

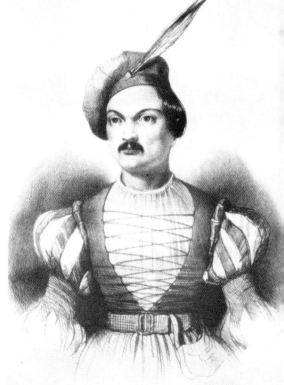

D.

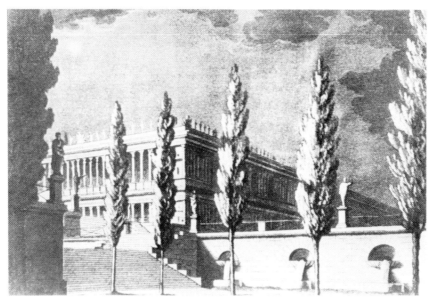

ORIGINAL STAGE-SET PAINTING FOR *Aureliano in Palmira*,
BY CAMILLO LANDRIANI, LA SCALA, 1813

ORIGINAL STAGE-SET DESIGN FOR *La Gazza ladra*,
BY ALESSANDRO SANQUIRICO, LA SCALA, 1817

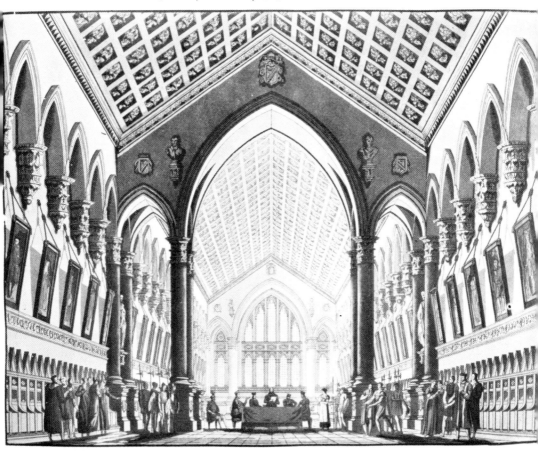

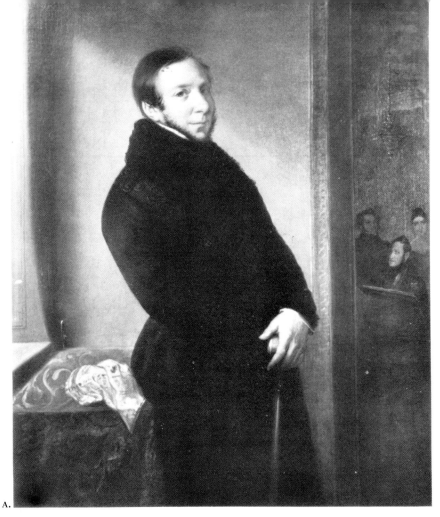

A.

A. Domenico Barbaja

B. Olympe Pélissier

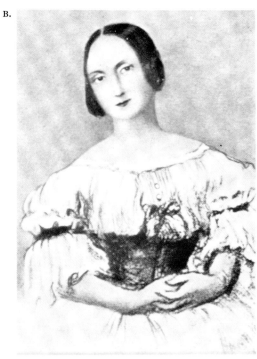

B.

be deferred, for example to another year, or at least if I could know how long the theater season lasts in Paris, and thus see if it would be possible for me to divide time between Milan and Paris, then I should be most content; as for the financial arrangements, everything is fine, as I should be paid completely by the pleasure of being at Rossini's side and protected by him. I beg you, then, to arrange that I shall not have to miss such good fortune, and on my side I shall not spare myself fatigue or labor, as my gratitude for so great a favor will be eternally lively.

"I have so much wanted to come to Paris . . .

"Shall I perhaps lose so beautiful an occasion because of another contract? No, Rossini, no, for Heaven's sake.

"Believe me to be the last among your servants but the first among your admirers.

"Answer me, or have someone answer me, to Naples, as I shall leave here Saturday after going on stage on Thursday. Yours completely, GAETANO DONIZETTI."

Rossini's high regard for Donizetti as a musician was to be demonstrated even more clearly four years later at Bologna, where Donizetti was to conduct the first performances in Italy of Rossini's *Stabat Mater*. In 1834, Rossini found a way to adjust the Italien's schedule to Donizetti's: after Donizetti fulfilled his contract with La Scala (*Gemma di Vergy*, December 26, 1834), he did go to Paris, where his *Marino Faliero* was staged with mild success at the Italien on March 12, 1835, six weeks after the very successful *première* there of Bellini's last opera, *I Puritani di Scozia*.

Echoes from old operatic battles still reached Rossini. On April 24, 1834, Eugenia Tadolini wrote him about sharp criticisms that had been directed against her by a writer (almost certainly G. Battaglia) in a Milanese periodical called *Il Barbiere di Siviglia*.ⁿ They concerned *fioriture* that she had used in "*Una voce poco fa*" during a singing of *Il Barbiere* at the Teatro Carcano. The writer had called them arbitrary additions. Tadolini wrote that she had been taught the ornaments by Giulia Grisi, who in turn had had them from Rossini in Paris. "Authorized by you, I also said that these embellishments were demonstrated to me by Rossini, for which reason, as I now want to persuade someone, I shall beg you to answer me, confirming in writing what you kindly said to me *viva voce*."

Rossini's reply to Tadolini appears not to have survived. But another *Milanese* periodical, *L'Eco* (No. 100), quickly printed a letter to its

"Signori Editori" signed "Your Associate R. S." which clearly indicates that Rossini supported the singer's position:

"One of your colleagues, the editor of *Il Barbiere di Siviglia*, hurls excommunications against anyone who dares to add any ornaments to their singing roles in the operas of Rossini. Although among the culprits whom he would like punished could be found the greatest artists and the leading talents, I do not want to restrain his wrath, but only to ask him why he wants to place all the onus on Madama Tadolini, who did not add to her cavatina a single appoggiatura, a single note that had not been inserted by Rossini himself. When the role of Rosina, originally composed at Rome for a contralto, was performed at Paris, under Rossini's supervision, by a soprano voice, he thought it opportune to add to the cavatina some *fioriture* suited to the sort of voice that was to sing it, and among the artists whom Rossini rehearsed in it with the *fioriture* added was to be found precisely Madama Tadolini, whose talents he always has admired and whose abilities he had always appreciated, and who, in the opera *Il Barbiere* at the Carcano, did nothing but perform in the presence of the great Maestro [*sic*] what he himself had taught her, and certainly in such a way as to obtain the audience's applause.

"*Authorized by Rossini* [italics in original] himself at the moment when he left Milan to defend Madama Tadolini against an accusation as false in the basis of the accusation as it was immoderate, considering the terminology of which your colleague made use, I beg you to insert these few lines in your estimable pages and to gratify, etc. *Your Associate* R. S."

The editor of *Il Barbiere di Siviglia* reacted quickly. In the issue of August 23, a "Reply of the critic of this journal to the letter inserted in Number 100 of *L'Eco*" was signed G. Battaglia:

"In one of my recent articles I asserted, as I assert and always shall assert—not only in one journal, but even in a hundred journals, if I had a hundred journals—that Signora Eugenia Tadolini *altered* the characteristic original *fioriture* of the role of Rosina in *Il Barbiere di Siviglia*, alas! performed recently at the Carcano for A SINGLE EVENING." In a flurry of picturesque invective, the writer went on to question his opponent's veracity, to attack him for his anonymity, and finally to demand to see a written authorization from Rossini for the added and altered *fioriture*. Not very convincingly, he argued that if Rossini had in fact given oral sanction to them, he had done so out of the merest politeness. And there, as far as available documents show, the polemic

rested. Needless to say, both soprano and contralto Rosinas, even supposing that they posses faithful copies of Rossini's original, have gone
on dealing with Rosina's *fioriture* as they have seen fit.

In Paris, Rossini again was much occupied with his fight to establish his continuing right to the lifetime annuity." He also was involved
in profitable financial speculation. Azevedo wrote: "The author of the
present book saw Rossini at the Paris Bourse in 1833 and 1834. He was
as assiduous as the brokers; he gave orders, received replies, in a word,
did everything done by people who conduct their own affairs." But
Rossini soon became so weak that his physicians urged him to go to
Italy "to breathe the air of his native land." Early in November 1833,
Bologna heard rumors that he had taken a vinegar cure to lose weight.
In June 1834, after the seasonal closing of the Italien, he left for Italy
in the company of Robert and Severini, who went in search of new
operas and of new singers. They were in Milan on June 11, when Rossini
was welcomed like a homecoming conqueror: on June 15, he reached
Bologna. He had been away two years and nine months.

Rossini spent about two months recuperating at Castenaso. On
July 20, 1834, he wrote to a friend named Vanotti in Milan: "I stay
in the country. The pastoral life suits me: oh, how beautiful plants
are; how much the moon delights me, the song of the birds, the murmuring of water. Everything enchants me . . ." In Paris, meanwhile,
word that Rossini had died was being passed about excitedly. On July
19, Édouard Robert wrote to his brother Joseph in Paris that he would
return there about August 25 with Severini and Rossini, whom they
would pick up in Milan. "Rossini is feeling very well," he noted, "and
by his presence necessarily will formally give the lie to the good souls
who kill him off with such assurance and ease."

Late in August, in fact, Rossini returned to Paris very much alive,
his health temporarily so much improved that he was ready to lead a
social life again: on September 1, for example, he and Olympe were
honored guests at one of Balzac's dinner parties. Early in 1834 (March
21), the Tribunal de Première Instance de la Seine had ordered his annuity paid him in perpetuity. The government had appealed that ruling
on May 23; the appeal had inched along through other courts. Finally,
on December 24, 1835, an opinion of the Committee on Finance found
Rossini's claim payable. On the basis of that ruling, the Ministry of
Finance decided that the pension thenceforth would be paid from
Treasury funds, and that payment would be retroactive to July 1, 1830,

since which date Rossini had received no payments. By his persistence, he had won a victory that would make the rest of his long life financially easier.

On September 4, 1834, Vincenzo Bellini, writing from Puteaux, outside Paris, to Francesco Florimo in Naples, said: "He [Rossini] has arrived here: he received me very well; I hear that he speaks well of me. . . . He has told [Conte Carlo] Pepoli that my frank nature pleases him and that my music tells him that I must have deep feelings. Pepoli answered that my greatest gift is to speak well of all musicians, without exception . . . and then said other things that Rossini agreed with. Then I asked him to advise me (we were alone) like a brother to a brother and begged him to love me well: 'But I do love you well' (he answered). 'Yes, you love me well' (I added), 'but you must love me better.' He laughed and embraced me."

Bellini's next phrase was as characteristic as his false picture of his attitudes toward other musicians: "Let's wait for circumstances to let us decide whether or not he speaks truthfully!" Intensely jealous of both Pacini and Donizetti, Bellini was at work on the score of *I Puritani di Scozia*, and therefore naturally was doing everything possible to secure and maintain Rossini's interest and support. On November 24, 1834, he wrote to his and Rossini's friend Filippo Santocanale at Palermo: "I don't want to fail on this occasion to implore you to attend to Rossini's affairs" and to tell you and beg you to interest yourself greatly in them, as he wants once and for all to see them taken care of so that he will not merit the bad humor of his wife, who is the owner. I now receive continuous politeness from Rossini, as now he protects me and wishes me well, and I can repay him at this moment only by giving you this plea, about which he doesn't know. But in the meantime, sure that you will grant this prayer from me, I can feel the satisfaction of being able to repay with interest the friendship that this immense man demonsrates for me; do you understand? If his protection becomes stronger, my glory will profit very much, as in Paris he is the musical oracle." And, with almost pathological insistence, in letter after letter, Bellini described his conquest of Rossini, upon whose favorable attitude he seemed willing to design the future of his own career.

The *première* of *I Puritani*, at the Théâtre-Italien on January 24, 1835," was entirely successful. This delighted Rossini, who wrote to Santocanale on January 26: "Knowing how much affection you feel for our mutual friend Bellini, I give myself the pleasure of informing you that the opera he composed for Paris, *I Puritani in Iscozia* [*sic*], was received most happily. The singers and the composer were called out twice onto the stage, and I should tell you that these demonstrations are rare in Paris and that only merit obtains them. You will see that my prophecies have been realized and with a sincerity beyond our greatest hopes. This score shows notable progress in orchestration, but I urge Bellini daily not to let himself be seduced too much by German harmonies, but always to rely for his structure on simple melodies full of real effect. I beg you to tell my good Caserano [?] about Bellini's success and to say that I assure him that Bellini's score for *I Puritani* is the most finished that he has composed up to now."[n]

For some years, Rossini had been composing occasional songs and duets for concerts and other occasions. Troupenas had been pestering him for permission to publish a collection of them. Rossini finally consented, and in 1835 the *Soirées musicales* appeared. They were subtitled *Collection de 8 Ariettes et 4 Duos italiens avec accompagnement de Piano.* Besides their long life as salon entertainments, the pieces also became familiar in transcriptions. Richard Wagner orchestrated the last of them, "*I Marinai,*" and conducted it at Riga in March 1838. Radiciotti wrote: "Rossini's composition, highly expressive but formally very simple, gains much in color and efficacy with the new instrumental dress; but if Wagner gave a little something of his own to the work of the Pesarese, it is not improbable that the latter, in his turn, exercised a certain influence upon the composition of *Der fliegende Holländer* with his work, for it seems that one hears something like it in a scene of that opera."[n]

More enduring than Wagner's transcription of a single duet from the *Soirées musicales* was the publication by Ricordi, also in 1838 (in *La Strenna musicale*), of a sort of preview of Liszt's *Soirées musicales de Rossini transcrites pour piano*, some of which were to enjoy long, widespread popularity with virtuoso pianists and accomplished dilettantes.[n] In March 1835, too, Rossini presented to the young daughter of a Parisian impresario, Louise Carlier (later Mme Benazet), a collection of manuscript vocal pieces with piano accompaniment by eighteen composers, himself included.[n] It was inscribed "*Album de Musique, offert par G. Rossini à Mademoiselle Louise Carlier/Mars 1835.*"

By 1835, the Théâtre-Italien, in the direction of which Rossini was collaborating in earnest with Robert and Severini, had begun to offer some of its most brilliant nights. In 1832, its season had opened with *Matilde di Shabran* (Rubini as Corradino, Luigia Boccabadati as Matilde). That season also had offered *La Cenerentola* (Fanny Eckerlin, Tamburini); *Semiramide* (Giulia Grisi, Rosmunda Pisaroni, Marco

Bordogni, Filippo Galli, Tamburini); Bellini's *La Straniera* (Giuditta Grisi, Rubini, Tamburini); *Mosè*; *Otello*; Donizetti's *Anna Bolena* (Giuditta Pasta, Eugenia Tadolini, Rubini, Lablache). The three years later (January 24, 1835), the Italien's audience heard the *première* of Bellini's *I Puritani di Scozia;* on March 12, it received its own Donizetti opera, *Marino Faliero* (Giulia Grisi, Rubini, Tamburini, Lablache—the four singers by then coming to be called "the *Puritani* Quartet"). At the Opéra, on the other hand, Rossini's influence had practically vanished; further, his French operas had all but left the repertoire by the night when Duprez's sensational appearance as Arnold provided a reason for keeping *Guillaume Tell* active there. Many French opera lovers expressed resentment of the treatment being accorded Rossini's operas by the Opéra directorship."

On September 23, 1835, Bellini died at Puteaux in circumstances so incomprehensible that they at once led to unfounded statements that he had been poisoned. On October 3, Rossini—who had become fondly protective of the vain, arrogant young Sicilian genius, and who was to devote considerable effort to helping settle Bellini's estate in Paris—wrote to their friend Filippo Santocanale in Palermo: "I have the sad satisfaction of telling you that the exequies of our deceased friend were carried out with general love, with extraordinary solicitude on the part of all the artists, and with pomp that would have sufficed for a king too; two hundred voices performed the funeral Mass, the leading artists in this capital joined in competing to sing in the choruses; after the Mass, they took the road to the cemetery (where poor Bellini's body will rest until other arrangements are made); a military band of one hundred and twenty musicians escorted the cortège; every ten minutes, a blow on the tamtam resounded, and I assure you that the mass of people and the sorrow that one saw reflected on all the faces produced an inexpressible effect; I cannot tell you how great the affection was which this poor friend of ours had inspired. I am in bed, half dead, for I won't hide from you that I wanted to be present when the last word was pronounced over Bellini's grave; and as the weather was awful, it having rained all day—but that didn't discourage anyone, not even me, though I had been unwell for several days—my having stayed for three hours in the mud and drenched with water has been bad for me . . ."

The ceremony at the Invalides had exceeded Rossini's decription of it: Habeneck had conducted a chorus of 350 singers; the soloists had been Nicholas Ivanoff, Lablache, Rubini, and Tamburini; and the honorary pallbearers had included not only Carafa, Paër, and Rossini, but also the seventy-five-year-old Cherubini. Bellini was buried in Père-Lachaise, where a monument was erected the next year. Not until 1876 were his remains transported to his birthplace, Catania, where the principal public park now bears his name and the house in which he was born has become a museum devoted to his life and music.

In Vienna on April 9, 1836, the new co-impresario of the Kärnthnertortheater, Carlo Balocchino, handed Felice Quinterio, a Milanese banker, a letter to deliver to Rossini in Paris. In part it said: "I do not fail to beg you please to tell me if you would be disposed to compose the music of a new opera, which would be used for the spring season of the year 1837 at this Imperial Royal Court Theater of the Kärnthnertor. The librettist and subject of this opera would be selected with your approval, and the singers to be signed on would be of the first quality. Above all, I shall not omit saying that the good Viennese of the First Nobility would receive you with open arms and that my associate Signor [Bartolomeo] Merelli [would be] in an ecstasy of joy if he were to have the good fortune of foretelling in our theatrical announcements that the First Maestro of Music, that unique talent, would come to crown our efforts for this, our arduous enterprise. I omit speaking to you of the price for your masterwork, being very sure that you would be willing to establish an equitable one, by which I mean one suitable to the present conditions of the theaters." Rossini's certainly negative answer appears not to have survived. Nearly seven years had elapsed since the *première* of *Guillaume Tell*, but opera-composing and its inescapable concomitants did not attract him.

The question of his annuity having been answered to Rossini's satisfaction, he had no reason to linger in Paris: he could keep his hand in at the Théâtre-Italien by post; he had nothing further to expect or desire from the Opéra. He was planning his return to Bologna when his friend the banker Lionel de Rothschild took him on a trip to Belgium and the Rhineland in June 1836. In a letter of June 26 to Emilio Loup, Rossini said: "I have made a trip to Frankfurt, passing through Brussels, Antwerp, Aix-la-Chapelle, Cologne, Coblenz, Mainz, etc., and I assure you that nothing in the world is more beautiful than the banks of the Rhine. What richness, what vegetation, what cathedrals, what objects from olden times! I do not speak of the pictures by Rubens and Wandik [Vandyke], as I should want to have twenty pages to describe their beauties and number to you. I am truly satisfied with this little trip, the entire purpose of which was to attend at Frankfurt the marriage of Lionel Rotschildt [sic], my very dear friend."[n]

Stopping first at Brussels, Rossini had been honored by the local opera orchestra, which had given a concert outside his hotel; that had been followed by a concert by members of the local Académie Phil-harmonique, who also named him an honorary member. He visited Antwerp and returned to Brussels by train—an experience that so un-nerved him that he never again could be persuaded to travel by railroad; he is said to have suffered from frazzled nerves for several days.[n] Back in Brussels, he was presented to Leopold I, King of the Belgians (whom he had met in London in 1824), who created him a *chevalier* of the Belgian Order. At Liège, his welcome was even more effusive than at Brussels: a local paper stated that the whole city had turned out and that serenades to Rossini had been offered by the orchestra, the military band, and singers from the opera.

At Frankfurt, Rossini again was lavishly feted. A large banquet in his honor was given at the Main-Lust, where he heard the prayer of the pretended pilgrims from *Le Comte Ory* sung as a vocal quartet to verses praising him; at the end of the repast, among toasts and cheers, an embarrassingly overwrought speech was pronounced. Ferdinand Ries interpreted for Rossini. Toasts were drunk to German composers, including Hiller, Mendelssohn, Ries, Jacob Rosenhain, and Aloys Schmitt. Through Ries, Rossini said: "I shall preserve this affecting wel-come in my memory my whole life, but it is above all in my heart that I shall carry it." He stayed in Frankfurt a week. Hiller later told of a supper at his home during which everyone present praised Rossini to his face and virtuoso followed virtuoso in performing sonata movments, nocturnes, and variations on motives from *Guillaume Tell*, all the while sweating from the intense heat then settled upon the city. Only Rossini, Hiller said, remained impassive, smiling at everyone, saying something polite to each.

At Hiller's, too, Rossini met Mendelssohn, who had just reached Frankfurt after a night in a diligence, for which reason Rossini, who was eager to hear him play the piano, suggested that the pleasure be postponed until the next day. "I was stupefied," Hiller wrote,[n] "to see Felix submit to Rossini's amiable demands as, sitting near the piano, [Rossini] made observations and criticisms in such terms as to make one understand that the heart, and not only the intellect, spoke in him." The forty-four-year-old Rossini and the twenty-seven-year-old Mendelssohn met several times more during the succeeding days, and Rossini's assumption of the role of a world-famous elder composer slightly ruffled the younger man. One day when Mendelssohn was swimming in the Main with Hiller, he said:

"If your Rossini makes another remark to me like the one that he made to me this morning, I'm not going to play for him again."

"What did he say to you?" Hiller asked.

"You heard him too."

"No, truly. Furthermore, he was sitting closer to you."

"Do you mean to say, then, that you don't understand French?"

"But, yes, I do understand it," Hiller answered.

"Well, when I played my étude, he mumbled between his teeth: 'That smells of Scarlatti's sonatas.' "

"I don't really see that there is anything offensive in that remark."

"Nevertheless . . ." Mendelssohn sputtered.

As the two young men were about to part, Mendelssohn asked: "And so you think that I should see Rossini again?"

"Certainly."

"Well, so be it! Until tomorrow, then, for the love of Rossini."

Writing from Frankfurt on July 14, 1836, Mendelssohn told his mother and his sister Rebecka: "Yesterday morning I went to Hiller's, and can you guess whom I found there? Rossini, big and fat, in his most amiable and festive mood! Truly, I know few men who can be as spirited and amusing as Rossini when he wants to be. And we did nothing but laugh. I promised to have the Society of S. Cecilia sing the B-minor Mass and other things by Bach for him; it would be beautiful for Rossini to become an admirer of Bach. But he is of the opinion that each country has its customs, and that when one is with the wolves one should learn to howl. He says that he is enthusiastic about Germany and that if in the evening he finds himself on the Rhine and the wine list is given to him, [the result is that later] the waiter has to accompany him to his room, as otherwise he'd never find it again. About Paris and all the musicians there, about himself and his compositions, he tells the funniest and most amusing things, and he shows almost unbounded respect for everyone present, so that one would actually believe him if one didn't have eyes to watch his sly face. But intelligence, vivacity, and polish at all times and in every word; and whoever doesn't think him a genius must hear him hold forth only once, and he'll change his mind immediately."

Hiller wrote that at Trouville in 1855, Rossini "described a good performance of his [Mendelssohn's] Octet which he had heard in Florence, and Mme Pfeifer, the very able pianist from Paris who was in Trouville at the time, and I had to play the A-minor Symphony four-handed. 'Mendelssohn knew how to treat the smallest motif with so much sensitivity and with such spirit,' he said afterward. 'How does it happen that he never wrote operas?[n] Didn't all the theaters ask him to?' " When Hiller explained that no German theatrical manager would think of commissioning an opera, Rossini remarked: " 'But if young talents are not encouraged, if they aren't given an opportunity to acquire experience, nothing will ever come of them.' " Hiller replied that German composers retained a strong preference for instrumental music. " 'They usually begin with instrumental music,' " Rossini agreed, " 'and that may make it difficult for them later on to subject themselves to the restrictions imposed by vocal music. It is hard for them to become simple, whereas it is hard for Italians not to be trivial.' "

On August 16, 1836, Rossini was at Kissingen in Bavaria, perhaps for a brief cure.[n] Returned to France, he completed arrangements for the handling of his affairs there during a prolonged absence. Then, on October 24, he left for Bologna, traveling via Turin, Milan, and (November 9) Mantua. He sent reports of his journey back to Severini at the Théâtre-Italien. *La Revue musicale* remarked: "The illustrious Swan of Pesaro has left for Italy: he wants again to see his father, too advanced in age to undertake the trip thither. May the beautiful Italian sky inspire him again; may the great composer swiftly bring back another masterpiece for the Opéra or for the Théâtre-Italien!"

That writer clearly had no notion of Rossini's resentment of the fate of his French operas at the Opéra—where the Rossinian fare had come to consist of Act II of *Guillaume Tell* and Act III of *Moïse*, but where no expense had been spared to guarantee the extraordinary success of Meyerbeer's *Robert le Diable* (November 21, 1831) and *Les Huguenots* (first performed on February 29, 1836, Rossini's forty-fourth birthday). Rossini appeared to have no intention of composing another opera. In September 1885, however, the poet-librettist Achille de Lauzières wrote[n] that Rossini had told him that he would have taken up opera-composing again only if he had been offered a good libretto dealing with either Joan of Arc or Rebecca (*Ivanhoe*); Rossini well may have been referring to the years just after 1829.

Rossini returned to Bologna on November 23, 1836. Then, writing from Castenaso, he told Severini of being "feted in Milan and Bologna;

sonnets, odes, etc., on my return. At Milan, I bought carriages and horses, and I am blissful here in the country." On November 28, he wrote Severini: "Here I have found my father in good health and delighted, as you can easily believe, to see me. My wife is well and very reasonable [evidently Rossini already had discussed with Isabella the arranging of a formal separation]. Both of them send you a million tender things . . . I thank you for your friendliness toward Olympe; she writes me many things regarding it, and I am and always shall be obliged to you for anything you care to do for her . . . I assure you that up to now I feel the greatest indifference over having abandoned the capital of the world . . . The only privation I feel is that of you and of Olympe; but I hope that time will restore everything to me . . . Embrace Olympe . . ."

Olympe was on Rossini's mind constantly. In one letter to Severini, it would be: "If you see Olympe, say many tender things to her for me." In another: "Signor Severini is requested to give Olympe some tickets each time that extracts from Rossinian operas are performed." Or: "If you see Olympe, embrace her for me, and if she needs advice or help, I beg you to give it to her." The presence of Isabella was not making up for the absence of the affectionate, undemanding, protective Olympe. Not many months would pass before Rossini would consummate a formal separation from Isabella and invite Olympe to come to Bologna to live.

On February 26, 1837, Alessandro Lanari, then impresario of the Teatro La Fenice, Venice, wrote Rossini from Florence to suggest that the opera to be given for the reopening of La Fenice—which had been destroyed by fire on December 13, 1836—should be *Guglielmo Tell*. From Bologna, Rossini replied in part: "I answer your letter, in which you proposed that I travel to Venice to stage *Guglielmo Tell*. . . . I am most flattered by the gracious invitation, but, not knowing where I shall be at that time, it would be hard for me now to take on an arrangement with you for that reason; further, I shall tell you frankly that I do not think the choice of *Guglielmo Tell* a happy one for the opening of a new theater; music of a melancholy tint, peasants, mountains, miseries, etc., etc., are badly associated, in my view, with the solemnity of the opening of La Fenice . . ."[n] What Rossini really desired was to remain at his ease in Bologna, doing nothing—or at least nothing that would involve him with impresarios, librettists, singers, all the exhausting paraphernalia of the operatic stage.

CHAPTER XII

1837-1842

B Y JANUARY 1837, plans were nearly complete in both Paris and
Bologna for Olympe Pélissier's removal from her home city to
Rossini's. On January 26, giving her legal name as Olympe-Louise-
Aléxandrine Descuilliers, she dated her will, which she left with her
friend Hector Couvert. She had put Couvert in charge of her assets,
instructing him to turn over her annual income from them to Rossini,
her *"légataire universel."* The will provided for her mother ("Madame
Pélissier, née Descuilliers"), who was to receive 5,000 francs annually;
for her sister, Augustine Clurel, and her children; and for her sister-in-
law ("Madame Pélissier") and her children. Olympe also had planned
her own burial: "Rossini will decide if by my conduct I have merited
reposing near him one day. My last wish will be to be buried near his
mother; if Rossini does not judge that to be fitting, a plot will be
bought in perpetuity so that my mother can repose near me." Her
definite ideas about where her body should lie were to cause curious
difficulties more than forty years later, when plans were being formu-
lated for removing Rossini's remains from Père-Lachaise Cemetery in
Paris to Santa Croce in Florence.

In Bologna, meanwhile, Rossini was completing his legal separation
from Isabella. On February 5, 1837, writing to Severini, he explained
that his tardiness as a correspondent had been caused by the negotiations
over the formal pact: ". . . she will establish a household apart from
me; I have done things nobly, so that now everyone is against her for
her unending insanities." Intending to go on living in the Strada Maggiore
palazzo, in January 1837 he had bought a contiguous building in another street; in February, he acquired from his friend the Marchese

Sampieri a coach house above which there were rooms." His decision to dispose of this complex of buildings in May 1839 may have been occasioned, as Corrado Ricci suggested, by his feeling uncomfortable in quarters originally bought, redesigned, and redecorated for a sumptuous existence with Isabella. Or, as others have supposed, after his father's death in April 1839 he may simply have felt too melancholy and alone there.

Édouard Robert reported to Rossini by letter that Olympe had left Paris in her "old hovel of a carriage," weighed down by an enormous collection of cases and bundles containing "above all, table linen, the heaviest thing in the world." En route to Bologna, Olympe wrote to Couvert from Turin to describe the extreme discomfort of the Chambéry-Turin stage of her wintry trip (she had been alarmed by a blizzard in the Cenis Pass). On March 8, 1837, she wrote Couvert from Bologna, which she had reached ten days before. The letter, largely concerned with financial details, also erupts into these characteristic pell-mell sentences:

"Rossini has not wanted to let me be placed, in Bologna, in the position of an equivocally situated woman. He has wanted me on a level equal with his wife, and without precisely [imposing me] upon Mme Rossini and the world, he has posed the problem so well that Mme's friends have persuaded her that it would be better for her to keep her husband near her than to drive him away forever. She has understood that she could not break off our liaison even if she wanted to; so, Rossini never having ceased to deserve her esteem and recognition, she must now learn how to make for her husband the sacrifices that all women resign themselves to making, she must receive me in her home as an accepted fact. On my arrival, then, things have been put in that manner. I had to go to Mme Rossini, whom I found pretty and unaffected; she was pleased with me at a moment, my good Couvert, when I would have fled Bologna had I dared. I know Rossini; if his wife is even a little good to me, I shall sacrifice myself to the proprieties." By these last words, Olympe probably meant that she was reconciled to living alone. Rossini did not consider it possible for her to share quarters with him openly in Bologna, and during the nine years before their marriage, she lived at three successive addresses."

The next words in Olympe's letter of March 8, 1837—"God gave me strength a long time ago to see only a friend in Rossini"—probably meant either that she was not then physically Rossini's mistress (which seems altogether likely in view of his illness) or that she understood that she could not become the second Signora Rossini in a country where divorce did not exist. Plunging on after that clause, Olympe told Couvert: ". . . . and as nothing can alter the nature of our present relationship, I hope that I shall find compensation in the new position that Rossini assures me; his friendship and protection will console me for some sacrifices of self-esteem which I make for his personal tranquillity. Today, my dear Couvert, I have no *arrière-pensée* about Rossini, who conducts himself toward me so nobly . . ."

On March 12, Rossini wrote to Carlo Severini, saying: "Olympe is invited to lunch with Mad. Rossini tomorrow; tell [Édouard] Robert, who will be enchanted." Five days after that, he reported to Severini: "Olympe lunched the other day with Mme Rossini, who, furthermore, was friendly with her, and everything goes well." And on March 29, still keeping Severini informed, he wrote: "Isabella, *papà*, and Olympe send you a thousand regards; this last has been very well received everywhere, and Isabella is behaving herself very well in this delicate situation."

Regarding the Isabella-Olympe confrontation, Zanolini (who, as Corrado Ricci wrote, "knew matters thoroughly" but "says too little") wrote: "After Olympe's arrival, Isabella's insistence was such that Rossini had to accompany her [Olympe] to Castenaso [actually, the meeting almost certainly occurred at Isabella's winter residence in Bologna]. Isabella and Olympe became acquainted, sounded each other out, and for a brief period frequented each other as though united in sincere friendship; later, this *ignis fatuus* went out from lack of air; one day they separated in a rage, and they never saw each other again."

Olympe eventually accepted her new life in Italy calmly and even with pleasure, telling Couvert to liquidate her Paris interests, rent her apartment, sell whatever she would not need, and relieve himself of further responsibility for her by transferring her funds to Rossini. But before she reached that state, she went through painful days of adjustment. In April 1837, for example, she wrote Couvert in her usual breathless way:

"[Rossini] defers to all my caprices, but [says] that if I leave Bologna, I shall never hear from him again and that even if I were to weep he would not give me a thought, as then he would see that I was not made for the honorable position that he has created for me. When I have been unable [*sic*] to reply, I have begged him to spare me his anger, I have enumerated the promises that he made me in Paris: that if I should not be happy in Bologna, he would establish me in Milan or Florence [and have said] that the sacrifices I must make to create an honorable position are beyond my moral strength, so that he has no right to criticize me because I seek happiness according to my own tastes . . ." Can this last have meant that Olympe, accustomed to regular sexual satisfaction, but not receiving it from Rossini, had been dallying with other men?

Olympe went on: ". . . that I was bored with his world in Paris, and that something that I need to buy is also useful to me in [relieving] the sufferings of my self-esteem. [I said] that I would have sacrificed the Eternal Father Himself to give up my whole life for him, that I wanted to leave, I should say with a profound feeling of gratitude for the Maestro, who, after a little reflection, has come back to better feelings toward me, and I think that he has understood that my bad spiritual state deserves a little more indulgence. Now he has been good to me as never before in his life. He has promised me that if in a year I am not perfectly happy, we will establish ourselves in whatever part of Italy suits me best [and has said] that I must give in to him so as to let him make me happy in my way . . ."

In a city the size of Bologna, the triangular situation cannot have been a pleasant one for Rossini, Isabella, or Olympe—and must have been very difficult for the elderly Giuseppe Rossini. In September 1837, however, the act confirming Rossini's legal separation from Isabella was signed. By their 1822 marriage contract, she had assigned to him the entire income from her patrimony and half of its ownership: she had held property and credits in Sicily as well as the land and villa at Castenaso, with an estimated cash value of 40,000 Roman scudi (about $126,000). In turn, Rossini now assigned to her from the income a monthly sum of 150 scudi (a little more than $470), the entire use of Castenaso, and an amount to cover the rent of winter quarters in Bologna.

When that necessary arrangement had been made, Rossini took Olympe to Milan early in November for a stay of about five months. Reaching there on November 9, they moved into rooms in the Palazzo Cantù at the Ponte San Damiano. On November 28, Rossini wrote to Severini: "I am here in Milan enjoying a rather brilliant life; I give musicales or musical gatherings at my home each Friday. I have a handsome apartment, and everyone wants to attend these reunions; one passes the time, eats well, and speaks of you often. I shall spend the whole winter here and return to Bologna at the end of March . . ." In a postscript he added: "The Teatro alla Scala is unbearable; I foresee that I shan't go to two performances during the winter season."[n]

On December 26, 1837, Rossini wrote to Antonio Zoboli in Bologna: "Milan is a city of many resources, and life here is rather agreeable. My musical evenings make something of a sensation . . . Dilettantes, singers, *maestri*, all sing in the choruses; I have about forty choral voices, not counting all the solo parts. Madame Pasta[n] will sing next Friday. As you can imagine, this will be counted an extraordinary novelty, as she doesn't want to sing in any other home. I have all the artists from the theaters, who compete to sing and feel driven to struggle all day long to prevent the admission of any new satellites. The most distinguished people are admitted to my soirées; Olympe does the honors successfully, and we carry things off well." These Milan evenings in the winter of 1837–8 were first rehearsals for the later Rossini *samedi soirs* in Paris.

During the night of January 14–15, 1838, two hours after a performance of *Don Giovanni*, fire destroyed the Salle Favart, then the home of the Théâtre-Italien in Paris. Flames surged up in a scenery storeroom; in an hour, the whole building was gutted (and a large collection of music which Rossini had left there was destroyed). Carlo Severini, who lived in the building (in which Rossini too had stayed when last in Paris), escaped the flames by leaping fifteen feet to the ground. Landing on a pile of stones, he broke his spine and died almost instantly. Learning this news from the papers, Rossini was grief-stricken. His friend had visited Italy less than a year before, and had acquired not far from Bologna a property (Rossini referred to it as "La Severiniana") on which to build a home for his retirement. He had not then, in fact, intended to go back to Paris, but his co-manager, Édouard Robert, had persuaded him to return, after which he had corresponded intimately with Rossini, sending him news and gossip: Rubini was well again; Fanny Tacchinardi-Persiani, received coldly at her Paris debut, had begun greatly to please the Italien's audiences; he had seen Olympe's mother, who was well. Rossini mourned not only the loss of a close friend, but also the disappearance of his closest remaining contact in France.

Robert, now sole director of the Théâtre-Italien, not only had been placed in intense difficulty by the destruction of the Salle Favart and the death of Severini, but also himself had received painful burns in the fire. Rossini, whose business affairs in Paris Severini had been handling, and who had owed him a large sum of money, at once arranged to have it paid to Robert, whose funds were tied up because the Italien's account in the Banque de France had been in Severini's name and could not now be drawn upon, his estate not having been settled. Rossini wrote Robert at length,[n] making suggestions, discussing financial and other problems, and reporting that he had written two letters to important people in Paris regarding the future of the Italien. On February 24, Robert (who had succeeded in transferring the Italien to the Salle Ventadour) wrote Rossini to say that the repertoire of four operas being offered was continuingly successful. It included *Lucia di Lammermoor*, with Fanny Tacchinardi-Persiani and Rubini; on the day when Robert was writing, the first new production of the season, that of Donizetti's *Parisina*, was to be presented.

"In sum, everything goes well," Robert added, "except myself, who am forced again to remain in bed. I had wanted to get out too soon; the wounds on my legs reopened; now I had to stay in bed for fifteen days. . . . Ah, dear Maestro, that you are not here! How precious your good advice, your wisdom, would be to me! If you are not coming, at least write me, then, I implore you. I await your answers with great impatience." Rossini did not go to Paris. Robert's troubles multiplied. He had to move the Italien again, this time from the Salle Ventadour to the Odéon. At the end of the 1839 season there, he gave up the directorship and was very temporarily succeeded by Louis Viardot (who the next year would marry Malibran's sister, Pauline Garcia).

At the Teatro Re, Milan, on February 17, 1838, a curious entertainment called *I Rossiniani in Parigi* was staged. Its verses were by Giambattista Savon; its music had been adapted by Antonio Ronzi, a tenor, from several operas by Rossini.[n] Whether or not Rossini and Olympe attended this imitation of *Rossini à Paris*, Scribe's 1835 *vaudeville*, is not known. On March 10, Franz Liszt dated at Milan a chronicle for the *Revue et Gazette musicale*, Maurice Schlésinger's persistently anti-Rossinian Paris periodical: "Rossini, returned to Milan, the scene of his early youth [*sic*]—that youth so exuberant, amorous, abandoned to the breezes of mad joys—Rossini become rich, idle, illustrious, has opened his home to his compatriots, and during the entire winter a numerous society has filled his salons, hastening to render homage to

one of Italy's greatest glories. Surrounded by a swarm of young dilettantes, the Maestro has taken pleasure in making them study his most
beautiful compositions; amateurs and artists all consider it an honor
to mingle amicably at his concerts. There are few cities in Europe in
which music can be cultivated as much as it is in Milanese society;
Rossini justly said that we artists would be bested completely in the
competition here. Alongside Madame Pasta, you could have seen the
two young Branca girls,[n] their voices as fresh as their faces: beside
Nourrit, Count Pompeo Belgiojoso and his cousin Tonino,[n] of whom
Tamburini and Ivanoff might be jealous."

In 1882, Emilia Branca Romani published a biography[n] of her
husband, Felice Romani, who had died in 1877. She was a passionate
defender of Romani against all charges (several of them fully justified).
Her book is far from dependable, but her pictures of Milanese musical
life in 1837–8 (when she had been one of Liszt's "two young Branca
girls") and of Rossini's role in it describe events at which she had been
present. "That was a memorable year for the *bell'arte* in Milan," she
wrote. "Rossini was lively, gay, and had great zest for making music.
The most elegant society disputed for him turn by turn: everyone
wanted . . . to entertain him, to hear his voice, to drink in one of his
words, to receive his advice. Foremost among them all was the Branca
family, which on the night of December 19 [1837] gave a musicale in
honor of the living genius of harmony, with the guests selected from
among the most eminent artists, writers, and notables. The most perfect
taste, the finest criteria, ruled the choice of the music both sung and
played; and the celebrated Rossini ceded to the first excitement of the
ladies of the place and seated himself at the piano as regulator of those
inspired melodies to which he himself had given spirit; at the conclusion,
there was even a concerted piece that the great master had composed
at the age of only fourteen years, and that piece was heard with such
delight, was found to have such an abundance of beauties, that it seemed
to be the first time that one heard that famous quartet from *Demetrio
e Polibio*."

That not everything ran smoothly for Rossini and Olympe in that
Milanese winter is suggested by the memoirs of Liszt's mistress, the
Comtesse d'Agoult—though, like Emilia Branca, she is not always a
witness to be trusted. She said that Rossini attempted to introduce
Olympe into good Milanese society by means of the musical evenings
over which he had her preside, but that not a single woman of respecta-

ble standing attended them. From Milan, however, Liszt had written to the Comtesse (then at Como): "I am on the best terms with Rossini and Mlle Pélissier—she pleases me as you know"—could the Comtesse have been jealous of Olympe? On her return from Como, the Comtesse thought that Rossini would present Olympe to her, but noted that "instead of that, they both have kept silent and peaceful, and after a first visit of ten minutes, Rossini never has called on me again." Perhaps Rossini or Olympe did not like the Comtesse d'Agoult—many people did not—and it is curious to note that her legal and social position was little different from Olympe's: she was not married to Liszt, by whom she had had two daughters (one of them the future Cosima Wagner) and would have a son in 1839.

Rossini was tempted to linger among the cosmopolitan, musical, flattering attractions of Milan beyond the date originally named for his return to Bologna. But his seventy-nine-year-old father began insistently to call him home. He and Olympe returned to Bologna after March 30, 1838, but Rossini would be in Milan again by the following September to appear with Pasta as an honored guest at a large musical party given by Metternich.

In January 1839,[n] the commissioners charged with studying ways to restore the decadent fortunes and quality of Bologna's Liceo Musicale suggested the appointment of the alumnus Rossini as their perpetual consultant. Having been approved unanimously, the proposal was transmitted to Rossini. He did not accept immediately: he was very unwell, and the alarming condition of his aged father's health was seriously aggravating his increasing depression. Many letters written by Olympe during the years from 1839 to 1843 testify to his nervous hypersensitivity and physical suffering. They justify the belief that the report on him by a physician, probably written out in or just before February 1842[n] for Olympe to forward to Paris, refers particularly to the period beginning in the early months of 1839. The urethritis with which it largely deals was to torment Rossini for a long time; in itself, it would be almost enough to explain the moods of black despair, at times so unreasoning as to resemble incipient madness, into which he now began frequently to fall.

Giuseppe Rossini, who had celebrated his eightieth birthday on November 3, 1838, died on April 29, 1839. His son suffered deeply over the loss of this man, with whom he had been on close, warm terms for more than forty years. When his friend Aguado learned of the state of prostration into which Rossini had collapsed immediately after Giuseppe's death, he wrote to offer the luxurious hospitality of his Paris mansion. The *Revue et Gazette musicale* No. 23 of 1839 announced Rossini's imminent return to Paris. But the physicians attending him in Bologna forbade a journey to France—which, in any case, Rossini probably had little desire to undertake. At about this time, Rossini wrote to an unidentifiable friend:"

"I have lost everything most precious that I had on earth, without illusions, with no future, imagine how I pass the time! My physician wants me to go to Naples to take the mud baths, sea baths, and another cure of decoctions. I spent such a cruel winter that I must decide to make this trip, a trip that under other circumstances would have been delicious for me, but which in the sorrow in which I live will be of complete indifference to me. May I at least be cured of my glandular troubles and articulation pains, which transfixed me throughout the past winter."

On April 28, as his father lay dying, Rossini, too overwrought to write, dictated a letter" accepting the position of permanent honorary consultant to the Bologna Liceo Musicale:

"Excellency: If by long study and assiduous exercise in music I have succeeded in being worth something in it and in acquiring a not inglorious (if unmerited) fame, I must be grateful chiefly to this Liceo. It was there that I learned the first rudiments of this beautiful and difficult art, which, moreover, is not the least glory of our Italy. It was there that I received my first encouragements, which made me more daring in launching myself on the risky profession that I practiced for so many years. It is, therefore, in payment of a just debt that I should labor for the Liceo itself with all my strength in every activity that might be able to preserve and increase its luster. And I will do so with a very happy spirit and with faith that I shall be able to show, by works more than by words, how dear this city is to me and how much gratitude I feel for these schools, which nourished my talent and my heart.

"Therefore I accept with real exultation of spirit the honorable office of perpetual honorary consultant of the Special Commission for the Re-formation of the Liceo Musicale and express my lively thanks to Your Excellency, to the Honored Commission, and to the respected representatives of the community who thus have honored me. Further, may Heaven grant me the favor of being able to be of some use to the Liceo itself in some matter, as I now can wish for nothing other than to render myself useful by my example and my words to my sweet adopted city and to end my life honorably here, where I took up my most divine art under such favorable auspices.

"I have the honor to call myself, with much respect, Obedient, devoted, GIOACHINO ROSSINI."

Despite his unhappy condition, Rossini then paid one visit to the Liceo, with which he later was to work seriously and long. Then, on June 20, he and Olympe set out for Naples, which he had not visited since leaving there with Isabella ten years before. They were in Rome on June 23. Then they went on to Posillipo, where they were guests at Barbaja's fine villa. Two days after their arrival, Rossini went into Naples to visit San Pietro a Maiella, where he was greeted enthusiastically by professors and students and had to sit through a concert arranged to honor him. The Neapolitan correspondent of the *Revue et Gazette musicale* thereupon reported, certainly without foundation, that Rossini had been commissioned to compose for the Teatro San Carlo a four-act *opera seria* to be called *Giovanni di Monferrato*, to a text by the Neapolitan writer Luigi Guarniccioli.

On August 11, 1839, writing in French to Antonio Zoboli in Bologna, Olympe said: "Oh, my dear Zoboli, do you know, Barbaja is a man of unexampled originality. He has an excellent heart, but no sort of education. At Bologna I shall entertain you by telling how this King of Impresarios stupefied me." Rossini too may have been entertained by his old friend, but the stay beside the Bay of Naples did not improve his state of mind or physical health. He and Olympe remained at Posillipo until early September. On September 11, they were in Rome, where for two days he again refused all invitations. The impresario of the Teatro Valle insisted that he attend a performance of *Semiramide*; Rossini stayed away. The Società Filarmonica wanted to regale their honorary president at an extraordinary sitting; Rossini regretted his inability to attend. On September 13, after dining with the Duca di Bracciano (Torlonia), Rossini and Olympe left by coach for Bologna, which they reached on September 17. He mightily wanted to devote his attention to the Liceo, of which he now was in effect acting director, but his health continued to be so bad that he was unable to do so until January 1840.

Having sold his *palazzo* in the Strada Maggiore, Rossini spent his first Bologna winter therafter in another in the same street. Thence he moved to a house in the Via Santo Stefano, where he remained a short time before moving to the Degli Antonj family's *palazzo* in that street. Not until 1846 would he once again return to the Strada Maggiore, then to occupy quarters in a *palazzo* belonging to his old friend the tenor Domenico Donzelli. Olympe's letters dated just before and just after the stay in Naples clearly indicate a gradual worsening of Rossini's condition. She describes him as suffering from extreme nervous oversensitivity leading to crises of emotional depression. She told Hector Couvert that Rossini could not free himself from the effects of his father's death, that he went about saying that his father had died too young and should have lived at least two years more. If he accidentally picked up some object that had been his father's, she wrote, he often wept for whole hours. "He is with friends of his," she wrote on May 13, 1839, "who do not know how to explain a sorrow that, despite his superiority, resists even his self-love; he is sick, he can neither sleep nor eat." On October 1, 1839, she wrote that a treatment of baths at Bagnoli had done him no good and that he could scarcely stand.

In mid-January 1840, Rossini was able to attend the admission examinations at the Liceo—and apparently to conduct its orchestra in the attendant exercises (a local paper noted this as his first performance of the duties conferred upon him). This meant no more than that he was enjoying temporary respite from his sufferings. In February and March, his physicians found it necessary to insert drops of oil of sweet almond, mallow, and gum into his urethra. A month later, his condition was much worse. He reported a sensation of heaviness in the perineum; the urethral secretions had become more abundant and included striations of blood. Leeches were applied to his perineum—after which he suffered complete blocking of the urethral canal, which caused him such pain that a surgeon inserted a catheter for twenty-four hours. For a time, Rossini also suffered from pruritis of the scrotum. He was bled; he was given warm baths; he was dosed with mild decoctions. Nothing helped.

Olympe did not lose her sense of balance or her ability to see matters sometimes in a better light. On March 3, 1840, she wrote to Couvert: "We are unwell ... it is from eating too much ... the Maestro and I live to eat ... and we acquit ourselves of this duty religiously." Rossini had given her a "very elegant small carriage" and a brace of horses, and she reported that she gave herself "Parisian airs" when out driving. After eight years of sharing Rossini's life, she was to say: "I am neither proud nor gracious, I am a fat woman who is occupied from morning to evening with digesting."

In September 1840, Olympe reported to Couvert that though the general state of Rossini's health then seemed good, his malady was chronic. Later that year, she again was anxious about him, and into the summer of 1841 she wrote few letters that did not dilate upon Rossini's physical suffering and mental depression. It is to be doubted that he was able to derive much satisfaction from the Bologna staging of *Guillaume Tell* as *Rudolfo di Sterlinga* during the second half of 1840.ⁿ Nor can he have been much cheered by word that the bust of himself (along with one of Conte Giulio Perticari) finally had been installed in the lobby of the Teatro Nuovo at Pesaro, which in 1818 had taken the place of the Sole, demolished shortly before.

Some of Rossini's characteristic humor flashes out from a letter that he wrote on September 13, 1840, to his Venetian pharmacist friend Giuseppe Ancillo. "For you alone, my dearest friend," it begins—and continues: "You will know that to please my friend [Nicholas] Ivanoff, I have been corresponding with Signor Caresana, Secretary to the Presidency of the Teatro La Fenice, over the matter of choosing the first score in which Ivanoff should make his first appearance. This choice will not be easy, as Ivanoff is a delicious singer, but special. With reservation, being the composer, I have proposed *Guglielmo Tell* under the name *Rodolfo di Sterlinga*, as it was presented by Ivanoff himself early in October at the Teatro Comunale in Bologna. Signor Caresana, to whom I had offered my cooperation for this score, told me that Signor Mocinigo [Mocenigo] did not like to have scores given except under their original titles (first f——), that the part of the *donna* was too small for Madame Devancourt [Derancourt] (second f——), and that means for performing this score did not exist in Venice (third f——), and that, finally, the government would not give its approval to this score (fourth and final f——). I have not mentioned this opera again or replied to those miserable observations because I don't want them to suppose that I have the usual weakness of composers, which is that of wanting to see only their own works performed. You know that in my simplicity I f—— my works, the public, presidencies, etc., etc., but in the interests of your Theater and for the company already formed, it is impossible to find a better score. Sebastiano Ronconi does the part of Tell perfectly. In this part, and in company with Ivanoff, he had a very brilliant success in Florence during the past spring. La

Devancourt, *who is very far from being a star for the Fenice*, would be well placed in the role of Matilde. [Jenny] Olivier would be delicious in that of the son, [Paolo] Ambrosini excellent as Valter, and Ivanoff divine as Arnoldo. The Bologna libretto (which your government could not forbid under any pretext) has been adjusted by me, and I assure you that it goes well—few secondary parts—I guarantee the success. You, *mediating associate*, move yourself, speak, intrigue, see Mocenigo, listen to Caresana, revolutionize Venice, succeed, and preserve for yourself, by bringing about the adoption of *Rodolfo di Sterlinga*, the esteem and love of G. ROSSINI.

"There's not a minute to lose. Understand? How many autographs! ! ! !"[n]

Although nothing came of these negotiations, in mid-February 1841—Rossini's continuing ailments apparently seeming somewhat less alarming—Rossini and Olympe went to Venice, taking two servants with them and putting up at the Locanda dell'Europa. The chief, and perhaps only, reason for this trip was Rossini's wish to help his friend Vincenzo Gabussi (1800–46), a Bolognese composer, whose opera *Clemenza di Valois* was to be given its *première* at La Fenice during that Carnival season. Perhaps because of Rossini's presence as a Gabussi supporter, the opera was disapproved of only mildly at its first performance. Nor was Venice more beneficial for Rossini than for Gabussi. Before leaving Bologna, he had begun to suffer from violent diarrhea, and it continued throughout his Venetian sojourn. When he returned to Bologna, the condition—which oddly was then attributed to water drunk in Venice—worsened for three or four months despite desperate attempts to end it.

Rossini was back in Bologna by March 4. He apparently remained unaware for some time that on March 21, the Pontifical Academy of Bologna sat in solemn session to make him an honorary associate for his efforts with the Liceo Comunale.[n] For he was naggingly, continuously unwell. In April, Carl Gustav Carus, a famous Dresden physician, stopped off in Bologna. Rossini consulted him. Carus judged that the chronic urethral inflammation was related to painful hemorrhoids from which Rossini also suffered. He prescribed a long dosage of "flower of sulphur" mixed with cream of tartar and ordered periodic application of leeches to the hemorrhoids; more immediately, he prescribed castor oil rather than salts and told Rossini that a cure at Marienbad had been effective in like cases.

Rossini did not go to Marienbad. On May 9, 1841, strong enough to devote time and consecutive thought to the Liceo's affairs, he wrote to Domenico Donzelli in Vienna to purchase much-needed music: "I have need to ask you to waste a little time for me. This is the matter: ask some *maestro* with good musical taste to select for you pieces for solo clarinet, clarinet and piano, trios, quartets, quintets, septets, etc., for several wind and stringed instruments. I am told that there are many brilliant pieces of this sort by Maestro Mendelssohn; the whole problem is to have good advice, both in the matter of choice and in that of cost, seeing that these pieces are to be used by the Liceo Comunale. If there exist songs in Italian or French by the aforementioned Mendelssohn for soprano or tenor, with piano accompaniment, acquire them. The general costs will be repaid you by me, and I'll remit the amount to your agent [Andrea] Peruzzi, from whom I've often had news of you. You take care of the costs of the pieces you buy; thus you too will have contributed to the good of the hometown establishment. Understand well that I do not intend them to be exclusively by Maestro Mendelssohn; all the *maestri* will be good. Weber, for example, has done good pieces, and many others. Make me a good collection, worthy of us all."

In June, Rossini's Bologna physicians decided that he must take a water cure at Porretta, down the Reno Valley toward Pistoia. He and Olympe stayed at Porretta for between three weeks and a month, but to no avail: his urethritis remained unchanged, the secretions increased, he lost so much weight that he soon was complaining of weakness after the slightest exercise. Olympe wrote Couvert that the diarrhea had been aggravated and that the doctors did not know what to do. Rossini, she said, was "even more changed morally than physically, he feels profoundly sick, his general weakness is such that he hasn't in him the energy to move." By June 21, he was again in Bologna, a very sick man. There, during the summer, he was visited by the Beligan musicologist François-Joseph Fétis, then fifty-seven and at work on the second edition of his eight-volume *Biographie universelle des musiciens et bibliographie générale de la musique*,[n] which was to include almost ten two-column pages on Rossini's life and works. The first result of Fétis's visit to Bologna was an article published in Paris by the *Revue et Gazette musicale* (No. 61, 1841), which in part read:

"Rossini has put his hand to the regeneration of the Bologna Liceo Musicale. Those who saw his flabby negligence in the administration of the Paris Théâtre-Italien in 1824, and who recall his jests about the

grotesque position of Inspector General of Singing in France, attached
to him by the Vicomte La Rochefoucauld, will balk at believing that
he can bring help to a school that needs help of every sort; but Rossini,
very different from what he once was, now is a serious man. He has
wanted only the title of honorary director because he has accepted no
stipend, but he goes to the Liceo almost every day, he pays attention
to the condition of the students and the studies, he occupies himself
with improvement of the teaching, and himself presides over the rehearsals for the concerts, the performances at which improve constantly,
thanks to his salutary advice.

"Unhappily, the poor state of his health is not one of the least
obstacles to the activity that he would like to display. I confess that
I was sorrowfully struck when, upon entering his house, I saw his
body so emaciated, his features aged, and I do not know what feebleness in his motions. A malady of the urinary tract, contracted many
years ago, is the principal cause of this depression; the death of his
father, plunging him into the most intense sorrow, finally has struck
him down completely. For one of the characteristic features of this
artist's nature is filial piety.

"This man whose *boasted* egoism and *boasted* indifference have
become proverbial in Paris, this man always was an affectionate son.
On hearing the first word of his father's illness, he rushed from Milan
to Bologna. When the old man died, Rossini did not want to re-enter
the *palazzo* in which he had lost him. So that *palazzo*, which he had
beautified at great expense, was sold. The consequence of this misfortune
for Rossini was a long and painful illness that put his life in danger
fifteen months ago, and the traces of which still are visible.

"Despite the bad condition of his health, Rossini is much more
active today than he was when he was well. During the summer, he
lives in a country house that he has rented, a short distance from
Bologna [the Villa Cornetti, beyond the Porta Castiglione]; but he
goes into the city almost every morning, borne there swiftly by his
good, handsome horses. After a short rest in the apartment that he
occupies during the winter, he goes to the Liceo, visits some friends,
and deals with affairs: then he returns to the country, where he unites
around the table two or three times each week the foreigners who visit
him and some of his devoted friends. . . .

"When I reached his country house near Bologna, he called my
attention to the pianoforte in his salon and said: 'You must be aston-

ished to see this instrument here.' 'And why?' I asked him. Without answering the question, he added: 'This instrument is not here for me; they use it when I'm not here, and I never hear it.' The next day, I asked him if he does not sometimes feel the need to compose, not for the theater, from which his position and his health keep him remote, but at least for the Church, in which I think that he could do new things; smiling, he answered me with a certain bitterness: 'For the Church! Am I then, perhaps, a learned musician? I? Thank God, I no longer occupy myself with music.' 'I am sure that the desire will return to you.' 'How can it return to me, seeing that it never has come to me? . . .'

"Furthermore, I have reason to believe that it would not be difficult to make him forget his vexations. The conversation referred to above took place before witnesses, at the table; but when, just before I left Bologna, finding myself alone with him, I returned to the discussion, he proceeded to give me serious attention. He again spoke of the in-sufficiency of his scholastic training as rendering him unable to write for the Church and declared that he no longer had the spirit to return to the study of the elements of fugue and counterpoint. 'Listen to me!' I replied, 'in order to make good use of that theory, one must have absorbed it when young and have it ready under one's pen. Those forms, foreign to your way of feeling, would impede the free flow of your imagination. Further, what can be done with them has been done. Your mission is not to follow paths traced by others, but to open new ones. Although I am of the opinion that today we are far removed from the character favorable to church music because we are introducing the dramatic genre into it. For this very reason I think that you could take the lead in it; because no one better than you could render it expressive and pathetic. There you have what you still could do for the art; there you have a noble aim for the autumn of your career.'*

"I don't know, but I believe that I converted a convert despite the apparent objections that he raised; for at the very moment when our conversation touched upon this subject, he was coming to an agreement with a publisher for the publication of his *Stabat.* . . .*

"A neglected education, a natural tendency to jest about everything, the wandering life of an Italian composer—which led him to meet a multitude of people without leaving him time for forming true friend-ships—the agitation, I might almost say the delirium, of a life entirely in the grip of different sorts of sensations: all those causes combined

have given him that appearance of indifference to everything which
has been mistaken for egoism. Now, however, concentrated in the
repose that for a long time has been forced upon him, he has become
reflective and everything in him has been awakened. Thus, when the
poor relatives of Bellini, living in Catania, turned to him, asking him to
collect together whatever the young composer had possessed at the
moment of his untimely end, the composer of *Guillaume Tell*, ignoring
the offensive comparisons that were being made in Italy at that time
between his own talent and that of the Catanese, took pains to verify
the estate, about 40,000 francs, which he then had transferred to [Bel-
lini's] family. . . .

"I must confess it, and I never concealed it during my talks in his
house: if the true character of Rossini has not been known, the fault
is his own, as he seems to have delighted in calumniating himself, expressing feelings that are not his, and in fact taking no trouble to deny the
false stories that are in circulation about him . . .

"May the time come quickly in which he will dare to show himself
as he really is, and then the world will be stupefied to realize that a
great man can have gone to such lengths to make himself small."

On July 25, 1841, *Le Temps* (Paris) had run a report that the Duca
di Modena had wanted to commission Rossini to compose an opera
for the inauguration of the new Modena opera house, but that Rossini had declined the commission. But events were culminating which
would lead him to the completion of one of his major works. Their
beginnings dated back to 1831 and, more immediately, to 1837. Varela,
the Spanish prelate to whom Aguado had introduced Rossini in Madrid
in 1831, and upon whose insistence he had composed a *Stabat Mater*
with Tadolini, had died in 1837. On December 1 of that year, his heirs
had sold the Rossini-Tadolini manuscript (which they believed to be
Rossini throughout) to Oller Chetard for 5,000 reales (approximately
$720 in today's buying power). At Paris on September 1, 1841, in
turn, Chetard signed the following bill of sale:

"I, the undersigned, declare that I sell, cede, and alienate to M.
Antoine Aulagnier, music publisher, rue de Valois, Palais-Royal, number
9, at Paris, the original score of the *Stabat Mater* of G. Rossini, as having
acquired it by an authentic deed and with rights for all places and all
times, from the testamentary executors of the Reverend Father Don
Francisco Fernández Varela, who himself had ordered this work from
Rossini and paid him for it, as is set forth in the Spanish deed herewith
and annexed to the present deed. I further declare that I cede to M.

Aulagnier all the rights that were given me by that deed dated December 1, 1837. The present sale is made by means of the sum of two thousand francs of quittance."

Having acquired the *Stabat Mater*, Aulagnier wisely wrote to Rossini to inquire if he had made any secret formal reservations about its publication when sending the manuscript to Varela. Rossini's reply was definite: "On returning from the country, I find your letter, which has been awaiting me for four days; this is what explains my delay. You inform me that you have been sold a property that I merely dedicated to the Reverend Father Varela, reserving to myself to have it published when I considered it convenient. Without entering into the sort of swindle that someone has wanted to perpetrate to the detriment of my interests, I declare to you, *monsieur*, that if my *Stabat Mater* should be published without my authorization, whether in France or abroad, my very firm intention is to pursue the publisher to death. What is more, *monsieur*, I must tell you that in the copy that I sent to the Reverend Father, there are to be found only six numbers of my composing, I having charged a friend to complete what I could not complete because I was gravely indisposed; and as I do not doubt that you are a good musician, it will be easy for you, by examining that copy, to perceive the difference in style existing between one number and another. A little while later, restored to health, I completed my work, and the autograph of the new numbers exists only in my possession. I very much regret, *monsieur*, not to be able to allow publication of my *Stabat Mater*. Hoping for a more favorable occasion in order to demonstrate the distinguished consideration with which I call myself your devoted Gioachino Rossini."

The letter, possibly disingenuous, is difficult to evaluate. It is possible that in fact Rossini had composed the additional numbers for the *Stabat Mater* "a little while" after dispatching the patchwork score to Varela; it is more likely that he had composed them much later, and perhaps after first learning of what had happened to the Varela score. He had known of the sale of the manuscript by Varela's heirs before receiving Aulagnier's letter: on September 22, 1841, he had signed at Bologna the following contract with Eugène Troupenas:

"I, the undersigned Gioacchino Rossini, composer of music, presently residing at Bologna in Italy, declare by the present deed that I cede full proprietary rights, and without reservation, to MM. Troupenas et Cie, music publishers at Paris, in the music of a *Stabat Mater* that I composed in that city in 1832. This cession, the aim of which is publication of this work in the form that the purchaser may deem most proper, whether with orchestral accompaniment or with only piano accompaniment, in France and in all other countries, without exception; that sale, I say, is made in return for a payment of 6,000 French francs, payable next February 15 at the office of MM. Rothschild *frères* at Paris.

"I undertake to recognize as needed all sales that MM. Troupenas et Cie may make of the present composition, and I declare that up to now I never have given anyone the right to publish it.

"Made in duplicate between the parties.
"Bologna, September 22, 1841.
"Approved, what is written above.
"Gioachino Rossini."

Having acquired the manuscript of the *Stabat Mater*, in good faith, Aulagnier fought back. What he did is explained by a letter that Rossini wrote to Troupenas from Bologna on September 24, 1841: "I have received your letter of the 16th of this month, and I am going to busy myself right away with putting metronome markings into my *Stabat*, as you wish. In the last letter that I received from M. Aulagnier, he uses the copy that he possesses to menace me with a lawsuit, asserting that the gift that I received from the Reverend Spaniard is, for him, a contract of sale on my part. This amuses me greatly. He also threatens to have the said *Stabat* performed in what he calls a monster concert. If such a thing really is being planned, I mean by this letter to give you full and complete authority to have the tribunals and the police prevent him from having a work performed in which only six numbers of my composing are to be found.

"By this same courier, I send you three numbers that I have scored; all that remains for me to do further is to send you the last final chorus," which you will receive the coming week. Try not to boast of the merit of my *Stabat* too much in the newspapers, as we must prevent them from making fools of you and me. I send you two letters from M. Aulagnier so that you may be informed of his intentions, and this, be it understood, for you alone. It would also be good that you should know that I have answered, telling him that I never signed a contract of sale with the Reverend Varela; that I merely dedicated the *Stabat* to him; and that, for the rest, most of the numbers are not of my composing; that I am ready to pursue to death, whether in France or abroad, any publisher who desires to perpetrate a swindle."

Zanolini wrote that when Rossini was completing the new numbers of the *Stabat Mater* in Bologna, friends who had been with him at a meal the preceding day called upon him. They asked him what he was doing. Rubbing his forehead, Rossini answered: "I am searching for motives, and all that comes into my mind is pastries, truffles, and such things." The "discreet friends," Zanolini added, thereupon left him in peace.

Antoine Aulagnier was already in motion. Working in collaboration with Maurice Schlésinger, music publisher and proprietor of the *Revue et Gazette musicale*,[n] he secretly had ordered plates of the Rossini-Tadolini *Stabat Mater* made by the Hamburg firm of Cranz. Troupenas learned of this action, had the plates sequestered legally, and brought suit against Schlésinger and Aulagnier for falsification and theft—an action that was to earn Rossini the continued dislike of the *Revue et Gazette musicale*. The trial was long and bitter: at one juncture, a Troupenas aide named Masset encountered Schlésinger in a court ante-chamber, denounced him in scarifying terms, and even began to punch him. The court decided that Rossini's having dedicated the *Stabat Mater* to Varela and having accepted a valuable gift from him did not con-stitute a sale. It therefore affirmed Rossini's right to dispose of his property as he wished—and also threw out Troupenas's rash suit against Schlésinger and Aulagnier.[n] In the end, Troupenas would publish the all-Rossini *Stabat Mater*, Aulagnier the six numbers which did not appear in Troupenas's edition because they had been composed not by Rossini but by Tadolini.

In late October 1841, sections of the *Stabat Mater* were sung in Paris privately at the home of Pierre-Joseph-Guillaume Zimmerman, a prominent pianist-composer. On Sunday, October 31, leading journalists and critics attended a more formal performance of six numbers—very probably including some or all of those newly composed or completed —which Troupenas held in the private salons of the Austrian pianist Henri Herz. The solos were sung by Pauline Viardot-Garcia, Mme Théodore Labarre, Alexis (Alexis Dupont), and Jean-Antoine-Just Géraldy. Théodore Labarre supplied the piano accompaniment; Auguste-Mathieu Panseron led the chorus, Narcisse Girard the double quartet. Adolphe Adam attended for *La France musicale*, for which he wrote a report that was the first, though only partial, critical analysis of the *Stabat Mater* and at the same time the first hymn in its praise.

What happened thereafter was told by the Escudiers:[n]

"After the first private audition, we had had no doubt of success with the public; we had become fanatics of that music and, strong in our conviction, we went to see M. Troupenas to ask him if he would cede to us for three months the exclusive right to perform the *Stabat Mater* in Paris.

" 'What amount do you offer me?' M. Troupenas replied to us.

" 'Eight thousand francs.'

" 'The work cost me only six thousand; the offer delights me. In an hour, M. Masset, my associate, will be with you, and he will bring you the answer.'

"M. Masset was on time. The answer was an agreement. Then and there, we counted out eight thousand francs for him, and in exchange he handed us a copy of the manuscript.

"If M. Troupenas had fulfilled our desires readily, that was because he had been alarmed excessively by the difficulties of a public perform-ance. And there we were, in our turn, knocking on the doors of theaters and meeting only disappointments. M. Léon Pillet, then director of the Opéra, answered us by saying that his theater was not made for church music and that we must take the *Stabat* to the Madeleine or Saint-Roch. M. Dormoy, who was directing the Théâtre-Italien, refused to associate himself with us, and was not persuaded of success. Only one means remained to us, and that was to rent the auditorium of the Italien, to take on at our own expense the soloists, the chorus, and the orchestra. We did not hesitate.

"It was necessary, above everything, to assure ourselves of the collaboration of leading artists. Mme Giulia Grisi and M. Mario did not immediately appreciate the scope of the work, and greeted our project coldly. Tamburini alone understood us; after having read the *Pro peccatis* twice and having cast his eye over the whole of the work, he exclaimed: 'It is beautiful, it is admirable; I will see Mmes Grisi and Albertazzi and M. Mario; in the meantime, you can absolutely count upon me.' That same evening, M. Dormoy told us that those artists would sing the *Stabat*. We deposited the sum of six thousand francs to guarantee the chief expenses—which finally rose to eight thousand francs. The only stipulation that we made was that no person not attached to the theater should be admitted to the rehearsals.

"The next day, the *Stabat* shone in huge letters on the *affiche* of the Théâtre-Italien. Two days later, the chorus and orchestra were convoked for the first rehearsal. More than six hundred orders for admission to it were sent to M. Dormoy, who had to respond negatively, as per our agreements. Only ourselves and the director of the theater were in the auditorium on the day of the first rehearsal. After the Introduction, the artists were stupefied and did not know how to express their amazement, and as we proceeded with the reading—for it was nothing more than a reading—the interpreters of the *Stabat* were more and more dominated by emotion. The unaccompanied quartet [*Quando corpus morietur*], the tenor aria, the *Inflammatus*, the *Pro peccatis*, led to the peak of enthusiasm; at the end, all bows were struck against their instruments, and from the heart of the orchestra and the choral mass rose a unanimous shout of admiration.

"The effect of that rehearsal rapidly spread outside. All the seats for the first performance were taken in one day. From all sides came demands to know the day on which the second rehearsal would take place; it would have required a hall four times the size of that of the Italien to contain the curious who wanted to attend.

"But that time again the auditorium remained completely empty; that was our wish. We forebear to depict the fanaticism that took hold of the performers at that second rehearsal; it was a kind of delirium.

"Finally the solemn moment arrived. Rossini's *Stabat* was sung before an immense throng on January 7, 1842, in the Salle Ventadour at two o'clock in the afternoon.

"Rossini's name was shouted out amid the applause. The entire work transported the audience; the triumph was complete. Three numbers had to be repeated: the *Inflammatus*, the unaccompanied quartet, the *Pro peccatis*, and the audience left the theater moved and seized by an admiration that quickly won all Paris.

"Up to that night, the Théâtre-Italien had been dragging along pitiably under M. Dormoy's direction. The *Stabat* could bring it a new life; the director understood that and regretted having refused the association we had offered him. The next day, very early in the morning, he came to us, despair in his soul, begging and supplicating us to cede to him the *Stabat*, which could re-establish his tottering fortunes. He was in a position to refuse us the auditorium for further performances. The feeling of friendship that linked us to M. Dormoy swept away selfish preoccupations; we could have earned one hundred thousand francs by exploiting the new masterpiece, but we ceded our rights to M. Dormoy for a net profit of twelve thousand francs. The

Stabat was sung fourteen times during the season and earned the direction more than one hundred and fifty thousand francs.

"Two months later, on April 10, 1842, Rossini—who was not so insensitive as some would have one believe—wrote us this letter:

" 'My dear sirs,

" 'I have learned of all that you have done for the performance of my little *Stabat Mater* at the Théâtre-Italien. I did not know that M. Troupenas had ceded to you the rights that I had conferred upon him. I am doubly enchanted, seeing that the affair has been good for you and that, thanks to your excellent friendship for me, the work has had interpreters who have assured its success. Accept my very sincere thanks, which I hope to be able to renew to you in person at Bologna, as from what M. Troupenas has written me, you should be coming here soon. G. Rossini.' "

That the *Stabat Mater* would strike Protestant and other non-Latin ears as "theatrical" and not truly religious in tone was forecast by the reactions to it of North German musicians referred to by Heinrich Heine (a convert to Christianity in his youth), writing in the year of its first performance:[*]

"It [the *Stabat Mater*] is still the topic of the day, and the very criticisms leveled against the great master from North German sources testify most clearly to the originality and depth of his genius. The approach is said to be too worldly, too sensuous, too playful for the religious subject, too light, too pleasant, too entertaining; these are the groaning complaints of a few heavy, boring critics. Although these gentlemen do not pretend to exaggerated spirituality, they surely are plagued by very limited and erroneous conceptions of sacred music. Musicians as well as painters have completely wrong views on the treatment of Christian subjects. The latter feel that the true essence of Christianity must be rendered in thin, emaciated contours and should be represented in as weak and colorless a manner as possible; in this respect, [Johann Friedrich] Overbeck's drawings are their ideal. So as to contradict this misconception with a fact, I point to the paintings of saints by the Spanish school; there, fullness of contour and richness of color predominate. Yet nobody would deny that these Spanish paintings exhale the most intense Christianity and that their creators were no less believing than the famous masters who were converted to Catholicism in Rome in order to be able to paint with more immediate fervor. The sign of the truly Christian element in art is not external thinness and pallor, but a certain inner profusion to which one cannot be converted and which cannot be learned in either music or painting. Consequently, I find Rossini's *Stabat* much more truly Christian than Felix Mendelssohn-Bartholdy's oratorio *St. Paul*, which Rossini's enemies praise as a model of the Christian approach.

"Heaven forbid that because I speak this way I should be thought of as in any manner wishing to criticize a master as distinguished as the composer of *St. Paul*. Furthermore, the author of these lines never, never would find fault with the type of Christianity in the aforementioned oratorio because Felix Mendelssohn-Bartholdy was born a Jew. However, I cannot refrain from pointing out that when Herr Mendelssohn embraced Christianity at Berlin (he was converted only at the age of thirteen), Rossini already had given it up and had submerged himself completely in the worldliness of operatic music. Now that he has left the latter again and is dreaming back to his Catholic youth, to the times when he was a choir boy in the Pesaro Cathedral or when, as an acolyte, he assisted at Mass—now, when organ sounds of yore again emerge from his memory and he reaches for his pen in order to write a Stabat, now he certainly does not have to construct the spirit of Christianity for himself scientifically or, even less, to copy slavishly Handel or Sebastian Bach. He needs only to recall the marvelous sounds of his youth! However serious, however profound the grief in this music, however powerfully it sighs and bleeds the sublime, it always retained something childlike and naïve, reminding me of the performance of the Passion by children which I had witnessed at Cette. Yes, when I first heard a performance of Rossini's *Stabat*, I suddenly found myself thinking of that pious little pantomime. It represents the terrible, sublime martyrdom, but in the most naïve accents of youth; the awful wails of the Mater Dolorosa are to be heard, but as if from the lips of an innocent little girl; alongside the bleakest mourning weeds, the wings of graceful *putti* rustle. The terror of the Crucifixion was mitigated as if by a pastoral play, and awareness of the infinite surrounded and enclosed the whole just as the blue sky had shone on the procession at Cette and the blue sea on the beach along which it had moved. This is Rossini's eternal grace, his indestructible tenderness, which no impresario, no music merchant can destroy or even dim! However much meanness and crafty intrigue he may have met with in the course of his life, his music shows no trace of bitterness. Like the Fountain of Arethusa, which preserved its original sweetness despite the bitter currents that flowed through its waters, so Rossini's heart has preserved its melodic charm and sweetness though it received more than its share from all of this world's cups of bitterness.

"As I have said, the *Stabat* by the great Maestro was the outstanding musical event of the year. I report nothing about the first performance; suffice it to say that Italians sang. The auditorium of the Italian Opera seemed like the vestibule of Heaven; holy nightingales sobbed and fashionable tears flowed. *La France* musicale also produced most of the *Stabat* during its concerts and, of course, to the greatest acclaim. It was during those concerts that we also heard Herr Felix Mendelssohn-Bartholdy's *St. Paul*, attracting attention by its proximity, so that he himself invited comparison with Rossini. With the general public, this comparison was not at all advantageous to our young compatriot; after all, isn't it as though one were to compare Italy's Apennines and Berlin's Templow Mountain? Not that this diminishes the merits of Templow Mountain, which already deserves the respect of the large masses because it has a cross on its summit. 'In this sign thou shalt conquer.' But, of course, not in France, the land of unbelievers, where Herr Mendelssohn always had been a failure. He was the sacrificial lamb of the season, whereas Rossini was its musical lion, whose sweet roars are still reverberating.'"ⁿ

CHAPTER XIII

1842-1846

D URING 1842, Rossini was working to restore the Liceo Comunale to its onetime glory. He had assigned the school of violin to the severe Giuseppe Manetti; that of piano to Stefano Golinelli, whom Hiller called the best pianist in Italy; that of clarinet to his friend Domenico Liverani. His major problem remained unsolved: the school lacked a suitable professor of counterpoint and composition, a post that involved acting as director. Rossini first had offered this post to Mercadante, who had accepted. Then rumors had been heard that Mercadante also had been offered the directorship of San Pietro a Maiella at Naples, a much more imposing position. And on the day on which Mercadante had promised to take up his duties in Bologna (October 1, 1840), a letter from him had announced that "unforeseen and commanding family circumstances and private interests" obliged him to return to Naples. Outraged, the *Gazzetta di Bologna* had published an attack on Mercadante, accusing him of dishonesty and lack of forthrightness. To the Marchese Carlo Bevilacqua," Rossini had written: "Your Excellency can judge of my stupefaction and my indignation!"

Next Rossini tried Giovanni Pacini, who replied that he did not feel equal to such large responsibilities. In October 1841, at about the time of the first partial singing of the *Stabat Mater* in Paris, Rossini had held out to Donizetti both the directorship of the Liceo and a position as *maestro di cappella* at San Petronio. Perhaps as much because of pride hurt at having been the third choice as because of not wanting to be tied to Bologna, Donizetti had rejected the offer. He would hear much more about it in March 1842.

Although audiences' reactions to Rossini's *Stabat Mater* were being repeated over and over, guaranteeing the international fame of this unprepared-for music, Rossini himself had not yet heard a performance of it. When a Bologna singing was suggested, he not only took a very active part in the arrangements for it, but also requested that everyone participating should contribute his services gratis so that all income from the sale of tickets could be put into a fund for erecting a home for superannuated musicians." A committee of prominent Bolognese assisted him. The first plan was to have the *Stabat* sung at the Liceo; the final decision was to hold only rehearsals there and to have the performances in the Archiginnasio, a handsome large building with a suitable auditorium. On March 2, 1842, Donizetti wrote to his Bergamo friend Antonio Dolci: "Rossini has written me to go to Bologna to conduct his *Stabat*, putting at my disposal his house, his wealth, and his life. Think well how honorific a matter this is. There will be a hundred singers and more . . . The Stabat will be on the 17th or 18th [of March] . . ."

Of the four vocal soloists, two were to be professionals—Clara Novello, a young English soprano of Italian descent, and the Russian tenor Nicholas Ivanoff—and two talented dilettantes—Clementina Degli Antonj and Rossini's close friend Count Pompeo Belgiojoso, whose brother Ludovico came from Milan with him and sang among the tenors in the chorus. The chorus included several well-known singers, most notably the bass Carlo Zucchelli and a young girl from Città di Castello who was to become renowned as Marietta Alboni. Members of the accompanying orchestra included the bassoonist Giovanni André; the doublebass player Luigi Bortolotti; the trumpeter Gaetano Brizzi, of whom Donizetti said that on the Day of Judgment the Eternal Father would summon him to wake the dead; the oboist Baldassare Centroni; the flutist Domenico Gilli; the violinist Giuseppe Manetti; the cellist Carlo Parisini; the cellist Carlo Savini, a dilettante whom Rossini had recruited after failing to lure Giovanni Vitali from Ascoli Piceno to act as first cellist; the violinist Francesco Schiassi; and the clarinettist Serafino Veggetti. When Rossini asked Stefano Golinelli to serve as rehearsal pianist, Golinelli refused. Thereupon Rossini wrote him: "My very dear friend: I don't believe in your ailments, I don't accept your refusal, and I demand that you come to this morning's rehearsal, where I shall be better able than the physician to judge the state of things. In this situation I need talents and good friends; you combine the two specialties, and therefore, even at the cost of your life, cannot abandon me.

The very great claims that I press upon you are because of the very great love that I bear you . . ." Golinelli served.

More than seventy instrumentalists made up the orchestra; the chorus numbered between eighty and ninety-five singers. Rossini asked that the final rehearsal (March 17) be reserved for members of the Liceo faculty and relatives of the performers. But when he was told that others were very eager to be present, he agreed to let them buy admissions, thus increasing the fund for the rest home; when the three singings were over, the total for that cause had risen to 1,306.31 scudi (about $4,125), the price of ticket having been set at one scudo.

Donizetti went to Bologna from Milan, where he just had attended the *première*, at La Scala, of Verdi's *Nabucodonosor*. He found the rehearsals of the *Stabat Mater* very well advanced. The reliable Annibale Gabrielli (a grandson of Donizetti's brother-in-law) wrote[n] that on the day of the final rehearsal, the ailing and thitherto invisible Rossini appeared, grasped Donizetti's hand, and said in a high, emotional voice: "Signori, I present Gaetano Donizetti to you: I confide the performance of the *Stabat* to him as the only person capable of conducting and interpreting it as I created it."

The *Stabat Mater* was sung at the Archiginnasio under Donizetti's direction on March 18, 19, and 20. The first performance had been scheduled for eight-thirty in the evening. The throng outside the Archiginnasio was huge; inside, more than 650 ticket holders burst into waves of applause upon Donizetti's appearance, then settled back in total silence to hear Rossini's music. The evening was an unmarred triumph for everyone involved. On March 20, Donizetti wrote to his Neapolitan friend Tommaso Persico: "We are up to the third and final performance today. The enthusiasm is impossible to describe. After the last rehearsal, which Rossini attended in full daylight, he was accompanied to his house amid the shouting of more than five hundred people. The same thing the first night under his windows, though he was not in the room. And yesterday the same. And *la Novello* and Ivanoff and the dilettantes Degli Antonj and Conte Pompeo Belgiojoso of Milan and I have been *écrasés* by the applause and shouting, poems, etc."

Of the final singing, Zanolini, noting that Rossini had become hypersensitive and could be upset by the smallest things, wrote: ". . . on the evening of the 20th, while the *Stabat* was being performed, he was staying—so as to avoid the intense heat in the hall—with some of his most intimate friends in a fresh, well-ventilated adjacent room, when one of them produced a newspaper and read a passage in which the music that at that very moment was being raised to the sky by extraordinary applause was spoken of abusively. Everyone, Rossini included, laughed; then, stirred by conflicting emotions, he fell victim to a trembling and a copious sweat that diminished little by little, so that when the final number had been repeated, he was able to respond to the summons of those applauding, enter the hall, and go out onto the platform, where he embraced and kissed Donizetti, to whom, if he could, he meant to attribute a large part of the good success of the *Stabat*. In the meantime, the people in the *piazza* were shouting for Rossini. From a window of the Archiginnasio, it was announced that the great Maestro was indisposed, and the applauding throng dispersed. . . .

"Recovered completely from the sudden faintness, fully satisfied by the great success of the *Stabat*, Rossini gladly accepted an invitation from his friends, and that same evening went to the house to which he had given his name while [re]constructing it, and where a supper in his honor had been prepared. The news having spread, the gay and festive banquet was accompanied by the town band and the applause of a large crowd that wanted to force the great Maestro to appear. Rossini went out onto the balcony to thank the musicians and the applauders, who raised still noiser *vivas* and then, satisfied and content, drifted away. He also was satisfied and content, and with words that came from the heart, he showed himself touched by gratitude for such proofs of esteem and cordial affection: no illness, he said, could induce him to leave Bologna, the Bolognese were his townsfellows, brothers, and good and beloved friends from whom he wanted never to separate himself again, and whom, in his old age, as in the first years of his adolescence, he wanted to have as his companions."[n]

Donizetti's brother-in-law, Antonio Vasselli, evidently had predicted that Donizetti would earn little by his conductorial work at Bologna. For on April 4, 1842, writing to him from Vienna, Donizetti said: "Do you know that Rossini gave me four [diamond] studs for having conducted the *Stabat*? If one considers their value, you have won; but if one thinks of their donor, I am right. Do you understand? If you could see how he really wept on leaving me!" Rossini had called Donizetti "the only *maestro* in Italy who knows how to conduct my *Stabat* as I wish it"; and on April 24, 1842, he wrote to Angelo Lambertini, director of *La Gazzetta privilegiata di Milano*, that he was very grateful "to the excellent performers, and in particular to Donizetti, who has done me an immense service with his vigor and his intelligence. The condition of my health did not permit me to conduct the *Stabat;* in that case, who better than he?"

Nor did Rossini intend to let Donizetti out of his grasp: his vigor and intelligence could be very useful to the Bologna Liceo. In the letter to Persico quoted above, Donizetti had written: "Rossini besieges me and seduces me to accept the direction of the Liceo and the *cappella* [San Petronio] here. If it does not prove to my liking, I can quit whenever I wish. Leaves of absence: twice yearly. What shall I say?" Some negotiations took place before Donizetti's departure from Bologna, for on April 12, Rossini sent this letter to him in Vienna:

"My well-loved Donizetti: I send you some emendations made by the Marchese Bevilacqua on the page that was left with me, and I beg you to consider them, but without regarding this as an ultimatum. Because you indicated that you would give harmony lessons, it occurred to the aforementioned Marchese that you would want to give the lessons in counterpoint, high dramatic composition, ecclesiastics, etc., etc. But I recall clearly that you do not want to have the boredom of the scholastic part, but want to occupy yourself only with the most interesting part, and we are in perfect accord about that. If the commune must take on the expense of a *maestro* for harmony and counterpoint, you will have to be satisfied with fifty zecchini [a little more than $332] per month; [but] I would like you to reflect that during your leaves of absence, your remuneration, however small, will not be suspended or diminished, which means that for your months of service, you will have about seventy-seven zecchini monthly. These are miserable pittances, it's true—but we are in Bologna!

"Six months of leave as a contractual condition are excessive; it seems to me that four and a half months would be enough. Your presence at Bologna is indispensable in mid-September, the period during which admissions to the Liceo are made and they prepare to open the school, which happens early in October; the time at which they prepare the *festa* for the patron saint at San Petronio; the period, finally, of the big fall performance. Once you are established here, I guarantee you all the leaves that you will want. I will take this up verbally with the Senator, and in that, as in anything else, I will be the intermediary, certain that I can succeed in satisfying you. Don't abandon me, Donizetti! The feelings of gratitude and affection which I hold for you merit some sacrifice on your part. If you wish to bring funds to Bologna, I will make good, safe investments for you; doing that, you will find yourself handsomely compensated for your current sacrifices. The Marchese [Camillo] Pizzardi[n] is delighted to offer you his delicious apartment, which I mentioned to you, and you will be lodged as you deserve. . . . Remember that you are idolized in Bologna. Think that here one lives in lordly fashion on a few scudi; reflect, decide, and console him who is blessed to call himself your affectionate friend. GIOACHINO ROSSINI."[n]

Donizetti's answer to that cry from the heart appears not to have survived.[n] On May 10, 1842, however, he wrote to Giuseppina Appiani, a friend of both Rossini and himself, that his letter, in turn, had elicited no reply from Rossini, who probably was *"vexé, contrarié."* Four days before that, he had written Vasselli that he hoped that the Bologna question might be settled within a few days. "I am still waiting for his [Rossini's] letters. Bologna is sad, I shall be bored, but at least I'll have a place to rest myself. The distraction and satisfaction of shaping pupils will serve to prepare me for a less sorrowful decrepitude, if I ever reach it. By every courier I expect news of the yes or the no." Donizetti soon accepted appointment at Vienna as *Maestro di Cappella e di Camera di Corte* and *Maestro Diretorre de' Concerti Privati di Sua Maestà Imperiale Reale Austriaca.* When Vasselli scolded him by letter for having thus removed himself from Italy instead of accepting the Bolognese positions, Donizetti replied (July 25, 1842): "To let pass a thousand Austrian lire [about $475] per month for doing nothing, and many months of freedom, in order to earn fifty scudi, give lessons at a conservatory, direct it and conduct, and compose pieces for the chapel, with two or three months of leave! This is how one lives at court, and I prefer . . . the courtly!"

Having failed in his attempts to lure Mercadante, Pacini, and Donizetti to the Liceo, Rossini allowed the communal authorities to appoint Antonio Fabbri as its professor of counterpoint and, *ipso facto*, its director. He did not, however, permit his own interest in the Liceo to slacken. On the contrary, his failure to attract an outstanding musician to its directorship seemed to increase the close attention that he continued thereafter to give to it. At the scholastic exercises on June 15, 1842, the compositions performed included Beethoven's *Egmont* overture and a chorus from Hadyn's *Die Schöpfung*, music still feared as advanced and somewhat exotic in Italy, but insisted upon by Rossini.

In April 1842, meanwhile, Rossini had been grieved by news that his friend Aguado was dead. Then fifty-eight, Aguado had set out from

Paris to visit his native Spain. Traveling by carriage the sixteen miles from Oviedo to the Biscayan port of Gijón, in part over a road that he himself had had built, he was overtaken by a storm that blocked his way. He set out to cover the rest of the distance on foot. Reaching Gijón weary and all but frozen, he suffered a stroke and died a few hours later." Rossini had Olympe write to Hector Couvert in Paris to inform Aguado's family that he now owed to them 50,000 francs that he had borrowed from Aguado—and which he wanted them to obtain by retiring the amount from his Rothschild bank account. Couvert took this opportunity to transfer to the Rothschilds the responsibility for Olympe's Paris holdings; all of Rossini's own financial dealings in France thereafter were handled by the Rothschild bank.

In June 1842, Rossini was made a knight of the recently instituted Order of Merit in the Sciences and Arts by Friedrich Wilhelm IV of Prussia. And his name-day in 1842 was made a civic festival in Bologna. Outside the house in which he lived, a gigantic balloon was sent aloft that afternoon. When darkness fell, magnificent fireworks were set off and the *Stabat Mater* was played in a transcription for fourteen wind instruments by Giovanni André." Antoine Aulagnier's attempt to publish and perform the Rossini-Tadolini *Stabat Mater* had set off a train of events which had burnished Rossini's worldly reputation and brought him back to participation in events beyond the walls of his home and those of the Liceo Musicale. For him, in fact, that train of occurrences had served to improve everything but his health. It was scarcely to be wondered at that during 1842 the twenty-nine-year-old Verdi should have written to his friend the Contessa Emilia Morosini: "I have been in Bologna for five or six days. I went to visit Rossini, who greeted me very politely, and the welcome seemed to me sincere. However that may be, I was very pleased. When I think that the reputation alive throughout the world is Rossini, I could kill myself, and with me all the imbeciles. Oh, it's a great thing to be Rossini!"

Among the nearly fifty surviving letters from Rossini to Michele (Sir Michael) Costa, one written from Bologna on September 12, 1842, to London, reflects brightly the euphoric state of mind (if not of body) in which the Bolognese acclaim for his *Stabat Mater* had left its composer:

"MOST ESTEEMED FRIEND: It is [Domenico] Liverani, my charming friend, who will deliver the present letter to you. He has fulfilled his duty by coming *to serve you* in the Greatest Capital. Now you have another duty to fulfil, and that is to help him to earn some of the *Ghinee* [guineas] of which he has great need! ! ! I demand from your omnipotence and friendship that you obtain for him all the means needed to give a Magnificent Concert in the High Season. I demand further that you impose him upon those Noble Milords in their private musical Entertainments, called Concerts, the sort in which Puzzi and Dragonetti take part. He will give out some sound on the clarinet or stroke of the tongue foreign to the harmony or the measure. Nothing can be done about that. Let the money come in, and I'll think of the rest . . . You will find my manner of writing to you strange and, to tell the truth, a little Imperious; what could you expect? The success of the *Stabat Mater* (unforeseen) has gone so completely to my head that I have become a Nero. You have a feeling heart, you are arbitrary of character, you command everybody, how can I not have hopes for my good Liverani? I also recommend him to Mr. [Benjamin] Lumley, whom I saw in Bologna. Be happy, grant my prayers, and believe me wholly your affectionate G. ROSSINI."[n]

On December 15, 1841, Olympe had written to Hector Couvert to ask him to arrange a consultation of the most celebrated Parisian specialists in diseases of the urinary tract. She had told him that Rossini's physician in Bologna was preparing a summary description of his condition over five years, beginning with 1836. On February 6, 1842, she sent the report[n] to Couvert, evidently hoping that she could take Rossini to Paris in the near future. For more than a year, however, Rossini felt too unwell, weak, and depressed to take the hopeful journey. Meanwhile, honors continued to be paid him. On January 24, 1843, the Bologna Consiglio Comunale concluded a sitting by approving a motion that a bust of Rossini be installed in the Liceo. On February 4, the city of Pesaro placed an incised plaque on the house in which Rossini had been born and struck a medal to celebrate two performances (February 16 and 17) of his *Stabat Mater* at the Teatro Nuovo. And on March 15, King Otto of Greece conferred upon him the Cross of Knight of the Royal Order of the Saviour.

Rossini meanwhile was proposing methods for increasing the Liceo's meager funds. His friends Domenico Liverani and Carlo Parisini were joined on March 19, 1843, at the Liceo by Donzelli, Zucchelli, the Modenese violinist Sighicelli, and an orchestra in a benefit concert of music by Mozart. Much more was earned for the school by a semi-amateur performance of Rossini's *Otello* at the Teatro Contavalli on

May 4: Rossini, though planning to leave for Paris and possible surgery ten days later, conducted. Three members of the Poniatowski family" sang leading roles: Prince Giuseppe (Otello), Prince Carlo (Elmiro), and Princess Elisa, Carlo's wife (Desdemona). The *canzone* of the off-stage gondolier was sung by Donzelli. The audience included Mme Isabella Colbran-Rossini and such other renowned singers as Nicholas Ivanoff; Antonio Poggi and his wife, Erminia Frezzolini; Francesco Pedrazzi; Zucchelli; Domenico Cosselli; Cesare Badiali; and Desiderata Derancourt. Rossini and the principal protagonists had to appear many times at the end of the opera to acknowledge long, loud applause.

Not satisfied with the prolonged, ineffective ministrations of Bologna physicians—and probably as the direct consequence of word received from Hector Couvert that he had arranged a consultation with Paris doctors—Rossini and Olympe finally decided to risk the trip to France so that he might be treated by the very renowned surgeon Jean Civiale." On May 11, 1843, Rossini paid a farewell visit to the Liceo. It was Friday, the day of the weekly student exercises. When they had concluded, he formally entrusted care of the institution to Alessandro Mombelli," Giuseppe Manetti, Gaetano Gasparri, and Antonio Fabbri during his absence. Then, in a highly emotional state, he said: "The day when I shall be able to return to this place will be for me the most beautiful of my life. . . ." The next day, the professors from the Liceo went to his quarters to return his call and bid him a sad, uncertain farewell.

At seven-fifteen on the morning of May 14, Rossini and Olympe set out for Paris. Four days later, Giuseppe Verdi wrote from Parma to Luigi Toccagni: "For the rest, there is no news. Ah, Rossini passed through Parma the other evening on his way to Paris. I went to call on him; naturally, that's understood." At about the same time, Verdi said in a letter to Isidoro Cambiasi: "I have seen the Supreme Maestro, who is leaving shortly for Paris, and on his return will stop in Milan." The Rossinis were in Turin on May 16; thence they traversed the Cenis Pass during a storm that must have recalled to Olympe a similar storm that had frightened her when she had gone through the Cenis in the opposite direction six years before. They reached Lyon on May 20.

Arriving in Paris on May 27, Rossini and Olympe settled into lodgings at No. 6, place de la Madeleine; they were to remain in Paris until September 20. Immediately, eager visitors began to pour in to see Rossini. Léon Escudier wrote: "His house had the look of a theater entrance. There was a persevering queue. All the callers could not penetrate into the illustrious composer's apartment." During the four months of Rossini's Paris sojourn, more than 2,000 people—musicians, writers, diplomats, painters, and other prominent Parisians and foreigners—made a path to that door. Antoine Étex prepared to carve a statue of Rossini by sketching him from life; Ary Scheffer painted a large oil portrait of him. All of this activity, however, occurred at the beginning and end of the visit: shortly after Rossini's arrival, Dr. Civiale forbade him almost all activity, even including writing or any extended conversation.

For about three months, Rossini was kept in almost total isolation. When Duprez succeeded in seeing him and begged for a new Rossini opera in which to sing, Rossini's answer was: "I came upon the scene too early and you too late." Because Spontini, Meyerbeer, and Donizetti[n] also were in Paris, a periodical remarked that though the city lacked new operas, it could not be said to lack composers. The director of the Opéra wanted to honor the visitor with a gala evening of selections from *Il Barbiere di Siviglia*, *Otello*, *Le Siège de Corinthe*, and *Guillaume Tell*, but Rossini could not attend. The Schlésinger *Revue et Gazette musicale*, still smarting from the lost struggle over the *Stabat Mater*, vituperated him for not wanting to compose more operas for the Paris stages.

On June 20, Rossini wrote to Antonio Zoboli in Bologna: "I am progressing slowly in my cure; I live by privations. Civiale tells me pretty words; we shall see!" On August 20, he reported to Zoboli: "Better late than never. I didn't want to write to you before being well advanced on my cure, so as to be able to inform you about the state of my health. I found a treacherous situation in Paris which worked against the complete medical-surgical treatment that was prescribed for me; a thousand incidents and constant irritations impeded the progress of my treatment. For about three weeks, things have changed, and only now can I tell you that I am fully content about having come here to have myself re-established, a thing that I now believe certain. At the end of September, I'll be in Bologna, and we'll be able to take our daily walks and eat good *tortellini*."

Léon Pillet, about to become director of the Opéra, begged Rossini for a new work, probably in August. "I am too unwell to risk myself by composing something new," Rossini told him. "If you absolutely want to perform one of my works at the Opéra, I'll tell you one with which I wanted to make my debut in this theater when I took its direction: *La Donna del lago*, which never has been performed at the Théâtre-Italien in satisfactory style despite the merits of some of the singers. It was, of all my operas, the one that I thought most suitable to the French stage, the one that, more than the others, had need of your big choruses, your magnificent orchestra, your beautiful staging. In that sense, I preferred it to *Le Siège de Corinthe.* I even had the libretto touched up in that direction by Emmanuel Dupaty,[n] but then I had to give up the notion of having it performed because I lacked a singer who could sustain the role of Malcolm. Now that you have [Rosine] Stoltz at your disposition, you would do well to profit by it." Circumstances balked Pillet's attempt to carry out Rossini's suggestion, but by a roundabout course the abortive negotiations would lead, in December 1846, to the staging at the Opéra of a curious *pastiche* of Rossini excerpts called *Robert Bruce.*[n]

The necessity of remaining much alone and of devoting all of each morning to his cure had depressed Rossini, who for a time had suffered intensely from thoughts and fantasies of death. Nonetheless, his physical condition improved so markedly that he and Olympe set out for Bologna from Paris on September 20, 1843.[n] In Turin a week later, he called at the Accademia Filarmonica. Leaving Turin on September 28, he reached Bologna on October 4—and began at once to minister to the Liceo Musicale. He also started attending a few operatic performances, particularly when the work offered was new or by one of his friends. One of the first performances that he heard in Bologna in October was the local *première* of Verdi's *Nabucodonosor*, already being referred to as *Nabucco*. During that month, he received, in a letter from Meyerbeer, official notification that in June he had been elected an Honorary Member of the Berlin Royal Academy of Fine Arts.

Rossini was briefly stirred from creative lethargy early in 1844 when he was asked to contribute to the celebration by the city of Turin of the third centenary of Tasso's birth. Taking up the "*Coro dei bardi*" from *La Donna del lago*, he enlarged it into a kind of cantata built upon occasional verses by Conte Giovanni Marchetti, a littérateur from Sinigaglia then living in Bologna. He composed a new introduction for it, modified its accompaniment, and added a closing section that was judged especially effective when the new "*Coro*" was sung in the grand salon of the Palazzo Carignano at Turin on March 10, 1844.

Half unwilling, Rossini was again to be lured into composition when Troupenas, his Paris publisher, traveled to Bologna to call upon him in the spring of 1844. In Paris in 1843, Rossini had learned that his friend the Bolognese composer Vincenzo Gabussi had turned up the score of incidental music that Rossini had composed (probably in 1813–16) for a staging of Giambattista Giusti's Italian translation of Sophocles's *Œdipus at Colonos*.[n] Gabussi had taken his find to the music publisher Masset (Troupenas's former aide?), who obtained this quittance from Rossini: "I, the undersigned G. Rossini, composer of music, authorize M. Masset to publish in whatever form he wishes my manuscript of *Œdipus at Colonos*, which he has acquired from Signor Gabussi, and I bind myself to recognize arrangements that he may make abroad. Gioachino Rossini, Paris, June 28, 1843." Thus Rossini tried to guarantee that Gabussi should profit from Masset's publication of the score.

Azevedo said that the Rossini incidental music for *Œdipus at Colonos* had been played at the time of its composition as part of a private amateur performance of Giusti's translation. But when the heirs of Giambattista Bodoni published the translation at Parma in 1817, Giusti said in a note to it: "A celebrated *maestro di cappella* set my choruses to music and was generously recompensed by me. A little later, I discovered that the accompaniments were lacking on many pages. I turned to him, and he took back the pages; and despite the several demands that I have made upon him year after year, I have been unable to recover them. . . ."

Many details of this incident remain unrecoverable: why Rossini never delivered to Giusti the accompaniments that the poet expected; why neither Masset nor his successor, Brandus,[n] ever published the complete score; how Troupenas came into possession of two of its choruses. For what Troupenas had in mind in going to Bologna in the spring of 1844 was to obtain Rossini's permission to have two choruses from *Œdipus at Colonos*, plus a third chorus to be composed for the purpose, published to new texts in French. At first, Rossini demurred, telling Troupenas to keep the choruses hidden in his strongbox. But the publisher produced a double motive for his doing something more. The trip from Paris to Bologna had been costly and time-consuming; Gabussi might still reap some financial reward for his original rediscovery of the score. Rossini let himself be convinced. He thought poorly of his youthful choruses, even calling them "too inferior" to be issued. But he finally agreed to Troupenas's repeated suggestion that he compose a "passport" for them in the form of a new, third chorus; thereupon he set an anonymous doggerel prayer to the Virgin.

Troupenas having returned to Paris, on June 22, 1844, Rossini signed and posted to him a copy of the score of the third chorus, which he had completed at the Villa Cornetti.[n] Troupenas then had the three choruses supplied with French texts: *"La Foi,"* by Prosper Goubaux, *"L'Espérance,"* by Hippolyte Lucas, and *"La Charité"* (the new music) by Louise Colet. As published by Troupenas,ⁿ the tripartite work was sung for the first time at the Salle Troupenas on November 20, 1844. Auguste Panseron conducted; Henri Herz accompanied at the piano; the chorus of twelve Conservatoire graduates was joined, in the solos, by a recent prize winner. Many music critics were in the audience, as were Adolphe Adam, Auber, and Fromental Halévy. Adam reviewed the performance for *La France musicale*, saying that *"La Foi"* would suffice to establish a lesser composer's title to glory; that *"L'Espérance"* earned praise by its "majestic opening, happy development, and the beautiful simplicity of its epilogue"; and that *"La Charité"* gave proof of compositional genius. In the *Journal des débats* of December 6, 1844, however, Berlioz slashed ironically at the choruses: *"La Foi* will not move mountains; *L'Espérance* lulled us sweetly; as for *La Charité*, which M. Rossini just has prepared for us, it must be conceded that it cannot have interfered greatly with the growth of his musical fortune, and that his alms-giving will not ruin him.'"ⁿ

In May 1844, Rossini was feeling strong enough to go to Ferrara to hear Domenico Donzelli sing in Saverio Mercadante's 1839 opera *Il Bravo*. His presence in the opera house touched off prolonged applause. The orchestra honored him between acts by playing the overture to *Semiramide*—and would have gone to serenade him outside his lodgings if a storm had not broken over the city. In Bologna, too, his popularity continued: on August 19, 1844, Costanza Tibaldi, daughter of the tenor Carlo Tibaldi, wrote to a friend about the gala celebration of Rossini's name-day: "The band played five pieces, four of them from the *Stabat* and one from *Guglielmo* [*Tell*], and the *evvivas* for Rossini were general, as you understand. When the music was over, the table was laid for the forty performers, all of whom, seated at the table, were served by waiters joined by [Vincenzo] Rasori, Gaetanino, Liverani (an eminent composer of music and professor at the Liceo), and Rossini himself; and there the *evvivas* were repeated."

On January 28, 1845, Rossini wrote from Bologna to Verdi, then in Milan preparing for the *première* at La Scala (February 15) of his *Giovanna d'Arco*. The chief purpose of the letter was to pay Verdi for an *aria di bravura* that he had composed, evidently on Rossini's order, for Nicholas Ivanoff:

"MOST ESTEEMED MAESTRO AND FRIEND: What will you ever say

of my long silence? A boil *or nail in the flesh* spread over my legs and arms, and without telling you of the pain that I have suffered, I will tell you only in my justification that it has been impossible for me to write you before today to thank you exceedingly for what you have done for my friend Ivanoff, who feels himself blessed to have possession of one of your delicious compositions, which has earned him a brilliant success at Parma.

"Herewith you will find a draft for 1,500 Austrian lire [about $712] which you will accept not as payment for your work, which deserves much more, but as a simple gesture of thanks on the part of Ivanoff, there resting on me alone all the obligation to you, whom I esteem and love.

"*I Due Foscari* made a furor at Florence; thus it will be with your *Giovanna d'Arco*. That is desired for you with all his heart by he who is completely your affectionate and admiring G. ROSSINI."

Rossini's continuing interest in musical occurrences is demonstrated again by a letter that he wrote from Bologna on March 10, 1845, to Elena Viganò, then in Paris. To this singing daughter of the famous choreographer Salvatore Viganò, he commented—clearly in reply to word from her about the enormous popular success of Félicien David's symphonic ode *Le Désert*ⁿ—"I thank you for the news that you gave me regarding Signor David. I am not pleased for him that they place him in the line of Beethoven, Mozart, etc. That is the way to do damage to his future."

The even tenor of Rossini's days was jangled late in August 1845 by receipt of word that Isabella lay gravely ill at Castenaso. Apparently he had not seen her except on public occasions since the disagreement between her and Olympe eight years before. But on September 7, 1845, he and Olympe drove out to Castenaso, having learned that Isabella (by then sixty) was dying. Of this meeting, Zanolini wrote: "Olympe was present and said nothing; if she felt any painful effect, she knew how to hide it." Rossini talked with Isabella alone for about half an hour and emerged from her bedroom with his cheeks bathed in tears. He instructed her servants to take the most assiduous care of her. For the succeeding month, he received daily reports on her condition—and on October 7 was told that she had died after having spoken his name several times. Almost exactly thirty years had elapsed since the dazzling Colbran had created the role of Elisabetta at the San Carlo in Naples. Rossini's thoughts well may have roved back to the era that had ended for her, as for him, when she had sung the title role of *Semiramide* at Venice in 1823, thus closing his career as a composer of operas for Italy. He was now free to marry Olympe; but he did not do so for more than ten months. Nor did he ever live at Castenaso after Isabella's death. He rented out the property for several years and then, in March 1851, sold it.

At about the time of Isabella's final illness, Giovanni Ricordi decided to install a bust of Rossini in his Milanese establishment; he ordered the sculpture from Cincinnato Baruzzi. On May 17, 1846, its unveiling took place in the foyer of La Scala. The musical program for that event was made up of chronologically ordered excerpts from Rossini's operas and an *Inno a G. Rossini* that Donizetti's friend the Sicilian composer Placido Mandanici had composed to appropriate lines by Felice Romani.ⁿ Rossini was also to be memorialized in marble at the Paris Opéra during 1846, the statue being dedicated on June 9. During Rossini's 1843 stay in Paris for medical treatment, Antoine Étex had sketched him. A committee had been formed to raise among Rossini's admirers a subscription with which to pay Étex to complete the statue: it had included Auber, Donizetti, Duprez, Luigi Lablache, Meyerbeer, Léon Pillet, and Ary Scheffer. The doggedly unfriendly *Revue et Gazette musicale* (Nos. 51 and 53, 1843) had slashed at the committee's purpose and deliberations. In May 1845, Étex went to Bologna for the special purpose of sketching Rossini's hands for the sculpture. A friend who made the trip with him published an anonymous account of the visit in *Iberia Musical;* in part, it reads:

"As our carriage proceeded toward the great composer's home, we encountered him along the way where he was walking with some friends; he seemed an antique philosopher surrounded by disciples hanging on his words. Presented to him, we received a truly friendly and affectionate welcome; he took us under the arms and led us to his house, speaking familiarly of France and of the present state of music. He errs who believes that Rossini is indifferent to what is going on in the artistic world. . . . I having said frankly that I had found the Italian theaters in a deplorable state, he added: 'You are correct. Now it is not a question of who sings better, but of who shouts most. In a few years we won't have a voice in Italy.' And he cited the tenor Donzelli, saying: 'Look! That is a singer!'

"When we reached the doorway to his house, he told us of his displeasure at not being able, because of his legs, to act as cicerone for

our excursions in Bologna and its surroundings; but he indicated to us
the way to see in a short time everything in Bologna and the countryside
which is most interesting for a foreigner. . . .

"Rossini constantly laments the condition of his health, and particularly the weakness of his legs; but I believe that his illness resides
more in his spirit than in his body. His face shows no suffering; he walks
with the agility of a man of thirty; his conversation is animated, his
glance penetrating.

"My friend Étex had come to seek out the Maestro for a purpose
. . . to model the hands of the illustrious composer for the marble statue
that he is to carve for the Paris Opéra.

" 'My hands are those of any other man,' the Maestro said with
his usual smile, showing them to Étex. Then he added: 'Do you know
the Bolognese sculptor Baruzzi? Tomorrow we'll go to him together;
in his studio you will find the needed instruments for working, and
there you'll be able to dispose of my hands.'

"In Baruzzi's studio, Étex saw the colossal bust of Rossini which
this sculptor had then completed. There, having the Maestro sit in an
armchair, he was able to shape the hands. That evening, we spent five
happy hours in the house of the great composer, whom we found in a
large circle of friends, including many artistic celebrities."

Étex's statue—which was destroyed in the fire that burned the
Opéra (Salle Le Peletier) to the ground on October 29, 1873—showed
Rossini seated, his legs crossed. Pen in hand and with music paper on his
knees, he was portrayed in a meditative mood. The statue was unveiled
during a concert of Rossinian music in which the Opéra's orchestra
was joined by Laure Cinti-Damoreau, Duprez, Tamburini, Paul Barroilhet, Italo Gardoni, and other soloists. The Paris press was very harsh
in describing Étex's statue. Admitting that it supplied a good likeness
in detail, they said almost unanimously that it failed to capture Rossini's
personality or character. In *Lutèce*, Heine had a good time with it, writing: "Whenever M. Spontini passed near it, he always bumped himself
against it. Our Meyerbeer is much more wary: when he goes to the
Opéra of an evening, he always takes the precaution to avoid encountering this statue, or tries to avert his eyes, just as the Jews of Rome, even
if they are in a hurry, always take a long detour so as not to pass near
the Arch of Titus, erected in memory of the destruction of Jerusalem."

On March 18, 1846, the Belgian Académie Royale des Sciences, des
Lettres, et des Beaux-Arts issued at Brussels a diploma naming Rossini

one of its foreign associates. During his protracted operatic inactivity, Rossini was coming to be regarded as something of a conservative, and was therefore amassing official honors. In fact, he was not much interested in social or political matters except as they directly affected his own person and life. But when a group of distinguished Bolognese dated, on June 10, 1846, a petition for governmental reforms addressed "To His Eminence the Very Reverend Signor Cardinal Tommaso Riario Sforza, Camerlengo of the Holy Church, and to the Sacred College of the Most Eminent Signori Cardinals convened in Conclave," Rossini signed it. The stimulus for the drawing-up of this daring petition had been the death of Gregory XVI and the election as Pope of Giovanni Maria Mastai-Ferretti, who was to take the name Pius IX on June 16.

Around Rossini's signature at the foot of the document can be seen, among many other names, the signatures of Conte Giovanni Marchetti, Marco Minghetti, and other noble and otherwise prominent Bolognese. Like thousands of other Italians elsewhere, they were placing illusory hopes on the newly elected Pope's reputation as a liberal. In no sense revolutionary, this windy petition nevertheless—given the reactionary tenor of pontifical rule at the time—marked its signatories as dangerous malcontents. But after the coronation of Pius IX on June 16, 1846, Rossini was invited to compose a ceremonial piece to honor the occasion and the new Pope. Again taking up the *"Coro dei bardi"* from *La Donna del lago*, he fitted it to a text attributed to a Canonico Golfieri, calling the resulting chorus *Grido di Esultazione Riconoscente alla Paterna Clemenza di PIO*. What had been a female chorus had become male; the instrumentation had been altered; a new terminal cadence was necessary. The resulting piece was sung in Bologna on July 23, 1846, on the level space at the foot of the stairs leading up to San Petronio from the Piazza Maggiore. Rossini conducted. The enthusiasm was tremendous. Then, news of the *Grido* having been spread, it was repeated at the Teatro Carcano, Milan, on June 8, 1847.

Meanwhile, on June 12, 1846, Léon Pillet had set out from Paris to visit Rossini in Bologna; he was accompanied by the composer Louis-Abraham Niedermeyer and the librettist known as Gustave Vaëz (pseudonym of Jean-Nicolas-Gustave van Nieuvenhuysen). Their purpose was to make the final arrangements for staging at the Opéra, as Rossini had suggested, *La Donna del lago* as fitted to a French text. Pillet did not linger in Bologna, but Niedermeyer and Vaëz (who was later to summon Alphonse Royer to his assistance) found the task before them finicking and long. The new French text dealt with Robert Bruce, and thus preserved the Scottish locale of Tottola's original 1819 libretto. The collaborators soon were shaping not a French version of *La Donna del lago*, but a pastiche of numbers from it, *Armida*, *Zelmira*, *Bianca e Falliero*, *Torvaldo e Dorliska*, and *Moïse*.[n]

On July 15, when Niedermeyer and Vaëz prepared to leave for Paris, Rossini gave them this letter for Pillet:[n]

"MY DEAR MONS. PILLET: These two words will be brought to you by Mess.rs Niedermeyer and Vaëz. For their characters, for their personal amiability, and for their talent, you could not have given me collaborators who could simplify my task better. Our work is finished. Your latest plans did not fit in with the pieces that I have chosen for our noble *pasticcio*. Therefore I beg you to hew to the letter of everything that has been settled. I understand that no change will be made in my work; that is the only recompense that I expect from you.

"Receive, I beg you, my dear Mons.r Pillet, the expression of my devoted feelings. GIOACHINO ROSSINI."

Robert Bruce was staged at the Opéra on December 30, 1846, having been postponed from mid-December to December 23—the date on the printed libretto—and then to the later day because of the illness of Rosine Stoltz.[n] The first audience was too excited over attending what is half believed to be a genuine Rossini *première*, too divided in reaction to what it was seeing and hearing, to notice that for the first time the Opéra's orchestra included a recently invented instrument, later to be known as the saxophone. Many of its members, however, realized that several of the singers were not at their best. Stoltz became so enraged when one faction in the audience tried to suppress another faction's applause for her that she shouted imprecations from the stage —including, many said, "*le mot de Cambronne*."

Robert Bruce, which was to pile up thirty performances and to be revived in the summer of 1848, aroused violent controversy. Pillet found it necessary to rush to the defense of this mélange against attacks by Charles Duponchel, who was striving to become his successor at the Opéra. Some critics attacked the very idea of such a pastiche. Louis Desnoyers, who published a 136-page book on the controversy, tried to dodge the aesthetic-ethical issue by asserting that *Robert Bruce* was in fact not a pastiche or a new opera, but an arrangement or "completion" of *La Donna del lago*. The *Revue et Gazette musicale*, perdurably anti-Rossinian, attacked *Robert Bruce*, Rossini, his librettists, and Pillet for having perpetrated a profanation. In the *Journal des débats*, Berlioz reproached Rossini for "lack of respect for the artistic details that create the true expressiveness and fidelity of his characters."

Most reasoned and vigorous of the attacks upon *Robert Bruce* was that published by the Hungarian pianist Stephen Heller in the form of a letter to *The Musical World* (London). Describing Rossini as the "great corrupter of music," Heller denounced his "effeminate cavatinas . . . passions without truth . . . hypocritical phraseology . . . lack of taste . . . trivial and vulgar ideas." As translated into French and published in *La Critique musicale*, Heller's diatribe came to the attention of Olympe Pélissier. Probably without consulting the impassive Rossini, on January 17, 1847, she snatched up a pen and addressed Pillet as follows:

"Reading in *La Critique musicale* of January 17 a letter addressed to the director of *The Musical World* by Mr. Stephen Heller, what can I say to you? As, stupefied, I perused that mass of insults, of stupid circumlocutions, pronounced with as much triviality as ignorance, impudence, and bad taste, my blood congealed in my veins, my cheeks turned purple with indignation. How could I, a woman—that is to say, a mere atom—revenge an insult that passes beyond all human imagining? I set to work. I have sent the director of the [*Journal des*] *Débats* a box containing two magnificent ass's ears; the first as a gift for M. Bertin, editor in chief of the *Débats*; the second for M. Hector Berlioz, the renowned composer of music, to send to his illustrious friend, the modern Midas otherwise called Stephen Heller. The ears were wrapped in fodder. All this took me infinite time: the ears never satisfied me; what I wanted was to create an imitation that, on the opening of the box, would provoke fresh hilarity and an appearance of the real thing. I hope that the said box will be opened in front of the director or the employees of the *Débats*; it is quite impossible that this gift will not reach the addressee, as I attached to the two ears, as a frontispiece, the article of January 17, being persuaded that M. Bertin will be charmed to forward the said decoration to whoever deserves it. Rossini knows nothing about all this; his *sang-froid* is so directly opposed to my nature that I have upset myself to the point of being unwell. He makes happy fun of Mr. Stephen Heller, not knowing this miserable fellow even by name; he asserts that this gentleman has full right to have his opinion, and that it should be respected. *Così sia per la mia.*"

We do not know whether or not Olympe's remarkable package

reached its destination. We do know that—perhaps helped along by the beginning of this exchange of insults—*Robert Bruce* earned Niedermeyer 15,000 francs (500 francs per performance for thirty performances). Rossini, who had accommodated Pillet with a "new" Rossini opera, but who had not earned one franc thereby, felt able to smile at the high moral tone of indignation struck by Duponchel, Heller, and others. Having begun its career at the Opéra on the last day but one of 1846, *Robert Bruce* was to be heard the following October at Brussels and in November at The Hague before returning to the Opéra in the summer of 1848.

In Bologna, meanwhile, the accession of Pius IX had had a further effect upon Rossini the *pasticheur*. The Roman historian Giuseppe Spada had invited him to set occasional verses by Conte Giovanni Marchetti as a cantata honoring the new pope. Offhandedly, Rossini agreed; he well may have been plotting still another avatar for the *"Coro dei bardi."* Then he changed his mind, writing to Spada on August 6, 1846: "I am very late in answering your most valued letter; I have been and still am unwell; there you have my justification. As soon as I received your letter, I informed Conte Marchetti that I had a chorus to which new verses could be put, and that I was at his disposition; up to now I have had no answer. As far as my composing a cantata, you should not forget, my excellent friend, that I laid down my lyre in 1828 and that it will be impossible for me to take it up again. If this magnificent occasion had presented itself when I was able, I should have embraced it with enthusiasm; now I am among the invalids and must be musically mute. If Marchetti decides for the chorus, I shall send if off quickly . . ."

Spada did not surrender. Through two of Rossini's Bolognese friends—the Marchese Camillo Pizzardi and V. Cristini—he brought to bear so much pressure that Rossini finally agreed to prepare a cantata-*pasticcio*. When someone later wanted to publish the resulting *Cantata ad Onore del Sommo Pontefice Pio IX*, he replied that publication was impossible because the music belonged to other publishers, who had paid him for it. What Marchetti had to do, then, was prepare verses for music already existing. On October 25, 1846, Rossini wrote Spada: "I have delivered to the Marchese Pizzardi my composition to the poetry of Conte Marchetti, so that it can be sent to you quickly; if this work ever should be performed, what is required is a beautiful and fluent soprano voice for the character of *La Speranza* and another for the tenor *L'Amore pubblico*. The part of the *Corifeo* is not much;

for it, only an accurate voice is needed. The bass *Genio cristiano* should have strength and courage. You will find the two *Corifee* in the chorus of maidens, followers of *La Speranza*; have them be pretty and possibly possessed of ingenuous voices. The military band must be placed opposite the orchestra, this to bring out certain echo effects. The chorus numerous, the listeners patient, etc., etc. My good friend, these are the few instructions that I believe necessary; if the music were to be conducted by the Marchese [Raffaele] Muti [-Papazzurri], I should be completely at peace and [feel] blessed."[n]

The true first performance of this *Cantata* (introduction, soprano solo, tenor solo, quartet, choruses) was given in the auditorium of the Accademia Filarmonica at Bologna on August 16, 1846, seemingly as a run-through for Rossini on his name-day; the Roman performance for which it had been prepared took place in the Senate on the Campidoglio on January 1, 1847.[n] The press noted that the audience numbered more than 1,500, including thirteen cardinals; the Duke of Devonshire; a brother of the King of the Two Sicilies; and a Princess of Saxony. The walls of the Senate had been hung with mottoes written by Giuseppe Spada's brother Francesco. At the back, on a star-sprinkled hanging, this appeared:

TO PIUS IX

EXCELLENT PONTIFEX MAXIMUS

CANTICLE OF GRATITUDE AND OF PRAISE

JOYFUL ROME CONSECRATES

IN ITS IMMORTAL AND VENERATED NAME

SOLEMNLY INAUGURATING

ON THE CAMPIDOGLIO

THE BEGINNING OF THE NEW YEAR

CHAPTER XIV

1846-1855

O N AUGUST 16, 1846, the day of the first run-through of Rossini's cantata for Pius IX, he and Olympe Pélissier were married. Shortly before, Rossini had rented from the Marchese Annibale Banzi a villa just outside Bologna's Porta Santo Stefano. In a chapel adjacent to that property, his friends the bassoonist Antonio Zoboli and the tenor Domenico Donzelli acted as witnesses to his second marriage. Rossini was fifty-four, his bride forty-nine. The marriage act in the parish church of San Giovanni in Monte reads: "Year 1846, August 16. Publication [of the banns] having been omitted by the usual license, the M.R.S. Parish Abbot of San Giuliano has joined in matrimony, according to the prescription of the Council of Trent, the Most Illustrious Cavalier Gioachino Rossini, widower of the late Signora Isabella Collina [*sic*] Cobrand [*sic*], son of the late Giuseppe and the late Anna Guidarini, of the Parish of Saints Vitale and Agricola, and the Signora Olimpia Alessandrina, daughter of the late Joseph and the late Adelaide Descuillier [*sic*], of this parish of San Giovanni in Monte. Witnesses, the Signor Antonio Zoboli and the Signor Domenico Donzelli." Rossini's second marriage was to endure without serious disagreements until his death twenty-two years later; Olympe would survive him, earnestly and loquaciously enacting the role of a great man's widow, until her own death, in her eighty-first year, on March 22, 1878.

The Rossinis were not to enjoy their placid Bolognese life very long: the year soon was 1848. Whether because Rossini had been alarmed by the civil disturbances reported from many quarters or because of some other reason, on April 26, 1848, he deposited his will with the Bolognese notary Cesare Stagni. In it he named the Liceo Musicale as his chief heir. The next day, a band of military volunteers about to leave for Lombardy to take part in the struggle for independence gathered outside the Palazzo Donzelli to honor him. When he stepped out onto a balcony to thank them, he was greeted by applause—but also by catcalls and hostile shouting. Voices were heard to call out: "Down with the rich reactionary!"

Word had been spread that Rossini's sympathy for the liberal (nationalist) cause, evidenced by his having signed the petition to Cardinal Riario Sforza, had cooled considerably at news of excesses being committed by the patriots. Distrust and dislike of Rossini by liberals and radicals had intensified after he had contributed only 500 scudi and a pair of horses, nothing more, when solicited by a Bolognese commission raising funds to support the struggle for independence. The surly attitude of several men in the throng below his windows terrified the always timorous Rossini. He later asserted that his apparently untoward reaction had resulted from knowledge that people had been killed in Bologna that day without anyone's raising a hand to arrest their assailants. Also, Olympe, who happened to be unwell, was as frightened as Rossini. In a panic, they decided to leave Bologna immediately. The next morning (April 28, 1848), they set out by early post for Florence.

What had lain behind the demonstration against Rossini is made clear, as Radiciotti first pointed out, by a manuscript chronicle left by one Bottrigari, regarded as one of the most fanatic and hotheaded of the Bolognese radical patriots. In it he called Rossini "a cold egoist, a despiser of anything but money" and remarked that the performance of the chorus *"La Carità"*—that is, *"La Charité"*—had been "the more effective and not a little surprising because everyone knew that charity never had found a place in the celebrated Maestro's heart." That Bottrigari entertained a distorted picture of Rossini is indicated by his statement that "he took no interest in the Liceo, the direction of which had been confided to him." Significantly, this libel is dated April 29, 1848, two days after the demonstration outside the Palazzo Donzelli. The true cause of the trouble was that Rossini had declined to take any active part in the revolutionary struggle.

A large proportion of the Bolognese evidently did not share Bottrigari's attitude toward their most renowned fellow townsmen. Some of them asserted that the demonstration against him had been the work of Sicilian troops passing through the city—but did not explain how Sicilians would have acquired detailed knowledge about Rossini or his attitudes. Others of them went to Padre Ugo Bassi, an ardent patriot who even had played some part in inciting the anti-Rossini feelings that had got out of hand, and asked him to persuade the composer to return from Florence. On April 29, at the suggestion of the pontifical legate, Bassi preached in San Petronio, urging the populace to remain calm. After sundown that day, he invited the people to follow him to the Palazzo Donzelli when the military volunteers would have returned to their barracks. There he stood between torches on a balcony and ardently defended Rossini, saying that they did not love Italy who did not respect the Italians who had honored her most, that "the fact that Italy was not yet inclined to German music was owing to Rossini's genius," and that the composer of *Guglielmo Tell* could only be a partisan of freedom. Bassi demanded that the Bolognese demonstrate their esteem and affection for Rossini, their gratitude to him, and their sorrow over his departure.

The *Gazzetta di Bologna* of May 2 called the sermon "the handsomest of all the triumphs of the celebrated Padre Ugo Bassi's fervid eloquence" and ended its comment by joining its voice to Bassi's invitation to Rossini to come back to Bologna. Bassi sent an account of the evening of April 29 to Rossini in Florence, almost begging him to return. Rossini replied on May 1:

"Very Illustrious and Reverend Sir: The Bolognese people, whose esteem is so dear to me, could not choose a better interpreter than you, oh *signore*, to make its feelings of affection more gratifying to me. Please, then, oh *signore*, have the kindness also to be the interpreter of my feelings of gratitude to them. Bologna always was the center of my sympathies. There, from my earliest years on, as I recall with pleasure, I learned the art of music—and be it permitted me to say with the poet—*Lo bello stile che m'ha fatto onore.*"

"To Bologna, even amid the attractions and plaudits of Europe's greatest metropolises, my thoughts, my affections, my heart always returned. In Bologna, retiring from the tumults of the world, I established my tranquil residence and my modest—and not, as others now believe, my immense—fortune. In Bologna I have found hospitality, friendship, the best of all good things, the tranquillity of the last years of my life. Bologna is my second home, and I glory in being its son, if not by birth, by adoption.

"From the sincerity of these feelings, you, oh *signore*, will easily gather the sweet impression that has been brought me by the honorable invitation that the city of Bologna has sent me through you, and how much I desire to return within its walls. If the present indisposition afflicting the health of my wife had not prevented me, I should, on the arrival of your letter, have flown to thank all those good friends, brothers, and compatriots who so love me and are so loved by me in return. But the state in which she is at present does not permit the repetition for the time being of so tiring a trip, and the affection that I bear her does not allow me to leave her at this hour. I cherish the hope, for her and for myself, that she will be restored to good health promptly and that, in reply to the Bolognese public's cordiality, I shall be able very soon to renew in person, in company with her, those thanks which I now must express to you by letter, and which, oh *signore*, I beg you to present to them by the organ of your eloquent and powerful voice.

"I am also most deeply moved and satisfied to learn that you, oh *signore*, have suggested, and that the Bolognese public has adopted, the idea of offering me the occasion to try my hand again at my abandoned profession on an Italian Hymn written by you, and which I, a true and enthusiastic Italian, shall make every effort to adapt to song and to the enthusiasm of all Italy as it applauds our great and beneficent Sovereign, Pope Pius IX.

"Receive, oh *signore*, the assurance of the high esteem and consideration with which I have the honor to be your most devoted servant. GIOACHINO ROSSINI."

Before Bassi could send Rossini the verses for the projected Italian Hymn, he himself had to leave Bologna. Near Treviso, he was wounded seriously. The text therefore was supplied by Filippo Martinelli. In mid-May at Florence, Rossini contrived a harmonized melody in march rhythm to which it could be sung. On May 19, he sent the sketch to Domenico Liverani in Bologna, asking him to provide the instrumentation: "In the accompaniments I have indicated the melodies and the essential harmonies, as well, too, as the rhythms of the accompaniment; it will be up to you to fill out all this with the greatest vigor and adopt the key best suited to the instruments available. It hurts me to give you this bother, but I know that your heart will find pleasure in helping me."

Liverani did as he had been asked, sending the result to Florence, whence Rossini wrote him on June 3: "I have received the chorus, with which, as regards the accompaniments, I am entirely satisfied: your heart could not help entering into all my ideas, my thoughts. Bravo, Menghino; your labor is complete and perfect. I do not write phrases of gratitude because you, feeling as you do, find enough recompense in doing things to please me." Liverani thereafter wrote him that this *Coro dedicato alla guardia civica di Bologna* would be sung in the Piazza Maggiore between two other pieces, the first of them the overture to *L'Assedio di Corinto*. To this piece of news, Rossini replied on June 11: "I don't find it unsuitable that the chorus should be performed in the Piazza Maggiore. Considering the brevity of the chorus, to play it between two other pieces is good; only, I do not approve of making the overture to *L'Assedio di Corinto* [*Le Siège de Corinthe*] the first piece. That piece is too brilliant to have it precede the chorus. Instead, I'd have the overture as the third and final piece, and for the first I'd love a majestic piece like, for example, the prelude to [Meyerbeer's] *Robert le Diable*, or perhaps another in the manner of that for the *Stabat* which exists at San Petronio. Thus the program would be:

"No. 1. Majestic piece. 2. Chorus. 3. Overture to *L'Assedio di Corinto* . . ."

On May 24, Senator Gaetano Zucchini was handed the score of the *Coro*, which Rossini had dedicated to the city of Bologna and its Civil Guard. Two days later, Zucchini and an officer of the Guard wrote to thank Rossini. Their flowery letter included this passage: "The Hymn, which you have had the courtesy to dedicate to the Municipality and to the Bologna Civil Guard, has transformed our sorrow into purest joy. You have added a gem to your immortal crown, and Italy is beautified by a new musical glory." Radiciotti's comment on that last sentence was just: "To tell the truth, the music of this hymn adds nothing to the composer's deserts or to the glory of Italian art. We have seen that every time Rossini turned his hand to occasional compositions, his vein failed him. This happens also to other great masters (Verdi, for example), and the reason is understandable."

"Menghino" Liverani conducted the first singing of the *Coro* on the evening of June 21, 1848 (the anniversary of Pius IX's coronation), in the festively illuminated Piazza Maggiore. The instrumental and vocal performers numbered more than 400." The vast audience reacted with the most intense enthusiasm (certainly in part stimulated by Martinelli's inflamed, flatulent text) and demanded that the *Coro* be repeated. Although their reaction confirmed the admiring attitude of a sizable proportion of the Bolognese toward Rossini, no more than Bassi's summons did news of it persuade Rossini and Olympe to abandon the relative security of Tuscany."

Rossini may have been sincere in protesting his continuing love for Bologna, and even in making repeated statements that he longed to return there. Nevertheless, he was to discover that (musical matters excepted) Florentine life was culturally on a higher, more varied, and more entertaining level than life in Bologna. That attractiveness, combined with his wavering and often desperate health, would keep him in the grand-ducal capital until September 1850. During more than two years, in fact, he did not even visit Bologna, which was connected with Florence by a road that, though difficult and bumpy, stretched through the Apennines for no more than sixty-five miles.

Rossini's hypersensitive nature and deteriorating physical state had been disturbed intensely by the event that had led to his taking refuge in Florence. There is no doubt that he suffered at this time from what Bruno Riboli called "always graver symptoms of desperate anxiety." Much of the time, in fact, he now showed the stigmata of a manic-depressive personality sunk to its nadir. Only the untiring, affectionate ministrations of Olympe led him through this darkening labyrinth. The worst was not constant: Rossini's moods fluctuated unpredictably and seemingly without cause. At some times he was all but completely prostrated; at others, he joined tentatively in the socio-musical gatherings that formerly had delighted him.

Republican Paris, recovering slowly from the revolution that had driven Louis-Philippe into exile in February 1848, had not forgotten Rossini. Taking up the score and libretto of *Il Viaggio a Reims*, the odd almost-opera with which Rossini had saluted the coronation of the last of the Bourbon kings twenty-three years before, Jean-Henri Dupin refashioned Luigi Balocchi's text into a two-act *opera comica* called *Andremo a Parigi?* ("Shall We Go to Paris?"). What had been a meeting at the Inn of the Golden Lily and a decision to attend Charles X's coronation at Reims now became a group at Plombières discussing the streetfighting of 1848 and its decision to go to Paris to see what had happened. The lines that had referred to fighting at the Trocadéro now referred to fighting in the place du Palais-Royal. This exceedingly strange *pasticcio* was given the first of its few performances at the Théâtre-Italien on October 26, 1848."

Rossini had taken no part in arranging this farrago of music that he had used in *Il Viaggio a Reims* and, in part, in *Le Comte Ory*. The critic of the *Revue et Gazette musicale* contented himself with saying: "The performance was cold and boring. The great Maestro's strokes of genius could not break the ice. The charming introduction, which is the same as that to *Le Comte Ory*, the duet of the cavalier and Corinna, which is the same as that of Comte Ory and the Comtesse, the great unaccompanied number, and the admirable finale were listened to without enthusiasm. Nothing is simpler: one has heard all this too often, and much better done." *Andremo a Parigi?* soon died a natural death.

Of the very numerous surviving Rossini letters, an amazing proportion dates from 1848, 1849, and the first nine months of 1850 and was written from Florence. These are mostly to his financial, legal, and musical agents in Bologna, particularly Gaetano Fabi, Domenico Liverani, and Angelo Mignani, whom he bombarded with sometimes daily requests for information, financial accountings, exact details of what they had done for him, and insistences that they pay close attention to all his instructions. When, for example, he learned from Fabi that an Austrian officer had been billeted in his Bologna apartment, he replied: "You must see that the Colonel doesn't tear the linen too much and that it is handed over to him and accepted back from him with all due care. For the rest, the honor is great, and one must be satisfied." Many of the 1848 letters signed by Rossini were written out by someone else: the suggestion that he was too unwell to write them himself is strengthened by the wavering lines of the signatures.

The Rossinis led a generally quiet life in Florence. News that heavy fighting had taken place in Bologna certainly increased their determination to remain away. During an encounter at Bologna on May 8, 1849, Conte Marco Aurelio Marliani, who had studied briefly with Rossini and who had seen his operas staged at the Théâtre-Italien in Paris,[n] was killed. A liberal, Marliani had become a fervent, active partisan of independence. In Florence, Rossini occasionally was seen in public: on January 20, 1850, he acted as an honorary pallbearer at the funeral of the sculptor Lorenzo Bartolini, holding one of the ribbons attached to the catafalque car; on May 20, 1850, he wrote out a page of music[n] inscribed to the sculptor's widow. A more ponderable return to music was occasioned late in 1850 when the painter Vincenzo Rasori gave Rossini a canvas representing, as symbolic of sacred music, David playing a harp. Wanting to show his gratitude, Rossini chose a translation by Giuseppe Arcangeli of a poem by Bacchilides, set it as *Inno alla Pace*, and sent it off to Giovanni Pacini for orchestration. No record of its having been performed at the time has come to light, but a critique of it was published in *Teatri, Arti e Letteratura* (Bologna) in January 1851. The score, long lost, was turned up late in the 1950's at Imola, in the home of a descendant of the Marchese Daniele Zappi, who had married a Poniatowski.[n] The music, certainly showing influences of then-recent operatic styles (it sounds as though Rossini had been listening attentively to both Bellini and Donizetti), is lyric and serene: nothing about it suggests a composer in abject depression.

In mid-September 1850, Rossini finally decided to venture a visit to Bologna. He almost certainly wanted to see for himself whether the hundreds of complex instructions that he had sent to Fabi, Liverani, and Mignani had been carried out. Before leaving Florence, however, he began negotiating to rent the second floor of the Palazzo Pianciatici there, thus certifying his intention to remain in Tuscany.[n] For the trip to Bologna, he offered to pay for an escort of four mounted *carabinieri* from Loiano into the city, and asked for permission to display protective weapons while at his Bolognese residence. He found the Bolognese authorities vigilant, Bologna "more classical than usual"; its inhabitants, he said, went about with long faces. No sooner was he in Bologna than he was longing for the attractions of Florence, for the attentions of Olympe, for the Friday social gatherings, and for the enjoyable visits with his friend Laudadio Della Ripa at the Villa Loretino.

The unsettled conditions in Bologna did not reassure Rossini. By January 1, 1851, he was writing from there to his Florentine friend Giulio Carboni that he expected to be able to "embrace him tenderly" early in May; on February 24, he wrote to Prince Carlo Poniatowski that he definitely would be back in Florence early in May. The jewelry, silver, paintings, and statuary from his Bologna *palazzo* had been crated. On February 12, he had waited upon the Austrian governor of Bologna, Count Nobili, asking him for permission to have the crates conveyed to Florence under military escort. Even if he had nursed any faint intention of staying longer in Bologna, an incident on May 1 would have killed it. He was at home with friends that day when Count Nobili unexpectedly called to see him. As soon as the Austrian official entered the room, Rossini's companions ostentatiously left. He had to receive the governor alone. He considered his friends' defection not so much an affront to Nobili and Austria as a criticism of himself and an insult to his position as host. He left for Florence four days later and never visited Bologna again.

Gaetano Gaspari was to say of Rossini: "He could no longer bear to hear Bologna spoken of. The name that he always gave the people from there was *assassins*." When the Cremonese musician Ruggero Manna asked Rossini to suggest a director for his formerly beloved Bologna Liceo, Rossini referred to the city as "the noble homeland of aggressions and *mortadelle*." In November 1852, he sent his servant Vincenzo from Florence to Bologna to assist Fabi in selling off furniture and other domestic impedimenta remaining in the Palazzo Donzelli apartment. "I authorize you, then," he wrote Fabi on November 9, "to make whatever changes in price you may deem necessary so that the matter can be ended and I shall hear no further talk about this ill-fated story."[n]

On October 30, 1852, replying to a request from Donzelli that he compose a piece for the tenor's daughter Rosmunda and another to be interpolated into *Il Barbiere di Siviglia*, Rossini told his friend: "Have you forgotten then, my good friend, the state of constantly increasing mental impotence in which I live? Please believe that it was a sense of delicacy rather than of vanity which led me to renounce glory and profit, making me hang up the key to my lyre so early; music needs freshness of ideas; I have only languor and hydrophobia." While keeping Florence as his official residence for the next four years, Rossini spent up to eight months of each year taking ineffective cures at Montecatini and Bagni di Lucca. During those four Florentine years, he lived in several rented places in and near the city—including a house in the Via Larga (now Via Cavour); the Pinzauti family's Villa Normanby; and the Villa Pellegrino, just outside the Porta San Gallo.

On July 2, 1853, Rossini bought three contiguous buildings that had belonged to the Medici family. Adjacent to what is now known as the Palazzo Medici-Riccardi, these were the Palazzo Pucci and an adjoining *palazzina*, both in the Via Larga, and a house on the Via dei Ginori, behind them.[n] Although he spent considerable sums on their improvement, he never settled in them, despite which a stone of the principal *palazzo* was incised to read: *"In questa casa che fu sua— dimorò alcun tempo—Giovacchino Rossini"* ("In this house, which was his, Giovacchino Rossini lived for some time").[n]

When feeling sufficiently well, Rossini fraternized with many of Florence's other distinguished residents, including Laudadio Della Ripa; the noted surgeon Giorgio Regnoli; the lawyer-politician Vincenzo Salvagnoli; the renowned Latinist and librarian of the Laurentian

Library, Luigi Crisostomo Ferrucci (also a close friend of Donizetti); two political exiles from pontifical Rome, Filippo Mordani and Giuseppe Barilli; the composer-conductor of the Società Filarmonica, Teodulo Mabellini; and the very popular composer of *stornelli* Luigi Gordigiani. Ferdinando Martini (1841–1928), a prominent writer-politician, recalled in his *Firenze granducale* (1902) events that he had witnessed as a boy in Florence. He had seen Rossini at the palazzo of Monsignor Minucci, Archbishop of Florence, on the day in 1854 when word reached the city of the death of the liberal patriot Silvio Pellico. Martini wrote that Rossini thereupon went to the piano and improvised a brief funeral composition in Pellico's memory while the other guests clustered about him.[n] He reported that Nicholas Ivanoff often sang at Minucci's and that there he heard the trio from *L'Italiana in Algeri* sung by the Archbishop, Donzelli ("who was past sixty and had the very freshest of voices"), and Rossini—who also had played the piano accompaniment. That same day at lunch, Martini noted, Rossini ate only a single slice off the roast. "I did not understand the reason for such abstinence then; now I understand that the Archbishop's abundant but plain fare could not delight the *papillae* of that palate, accustomed to all the refinements of gastronomy."

One passage in Martini's memoirs is especially vivid: "There were the Maestro, three or four of his friends, and a long-haired dog—a moth-eaten, nauseating, pestilential dog, the delight and care of the mistress of the house; she would have sacrificed her husband's fame to it without even thinking. That stinking, dried-up beast shuffled from one person's knees to another's, and this one and that one, with glances shooting forth hatred and invoking the municipal dogcatcher, but with caressing manner so that the Signora should not take offense, got rid of it by passing it to one another in such a way that the pain of having it on one's lap, though profound, was short and shared. Finally the fetid carcass got to me; I was near the Signora, and naturally could not tell it to go away. I did not have the courage to set it back on the floor so that it could take up its rounds again; it squatted on my lap, yawning with the beatitude of that unhoped-for repose, and went to sleep! Who could describe the tenderness of the amorous glances that Signora Rossini threw my way? If I had not been twelve years old and she very close to sixty, who knows how it would have ended? It is true that her glances were only half for me; they began in my direction, but ended up on the very hairy dog. And, after the glances, the words of praise for my poise

(I did not dare to move), for my ingeniousness, for my height; there was nothing about me that she did not praise."

Next, Olympe turned to Rossini and, pointing out the twelve-year-old Martini, said: "You ought to make him into a musician." Rossini accepted the command, asking the boy to sing. "An inner voice," Martini wrote, "told me that I was not going to do myself honor, but nonetheless I was very happy for that summons, which freed me from the miasma, which would have cut me off in the flower of my youth if it had continued. I handed the sweet burden to the Signora; she took it back, caressed it, apologized to it for having disturbed its slumber, and perhaps at heart reproved herself for not having foreseen that in order to launch an artist she would have to disturb that mound of hair." Martini's attempt to sing evoked from Rossini the comment: "My boy, I hope that you are going to become a fine man! But you will never strike a right note if you live a hundred years!"

From Florence, Rossini still was keeping track of the career of his beloved friend Nicholas Ivanoff. On April 15, 1852, he wrote to Ivanoff at Bologna:

"DEAR NICOLINO: I hear with pleasure that you have been negotiating with several people about the Fair of Sinigaglia, and I also hear that they want to put on the *Rigoletto* of our friend Verdi. I should like, before you accept the engagement to sing this opera, for you to consult Verdi so that he can tell you with that frankness which is native to his proved goodwill toward you, whether you can discharge this obligation comfortably and whether, to further this end, he would be willing to open the box of his happy inspiration to compose something for you to assure your success." When writing to him or calling upon him, give him my cordial greetings and tell him that, for what value they may have, I add my own to your prayers that he should keep the Ivanoffian vessel on its course.

"Farewell, Nicolino. Believe me Your Affectionate G. ROSSINI."

Few Rossini compositions, and they negligible, survive from his Florentine years. They include a *Canzonetta* dated April 5, 1852 (another setting of the Metastasian lines beginning *"Mi lagnerò tacendo"*), probably for an autograph album; a *Bolero* presented to Contessa Antonietta Orloff-Orsini, dating from the summer of 1852; and an adaptation, to a translation by Ferrucci, of the solo cantata on Joan of Arc which he had presented to Olympe in 1832. A letter that Rossini sent to Ferrucci, very probably in 1852, regarding the "vulgarization" of the

Joan of Arc text is of special interest because it includes thoughts and theorizing derived from his long experience in writing for voices."

"Do you feel in the vein to put some strophes on Joan of Arc into the vulgate for me? Come, and we'll do it together. Eugenio [Lebon] will help too.

"You ask me how it is that the contralto almost never figures among the principal parts in composing. That is not, certainly, because it has lost its natural attractions. Go to a sung Mass and you will understand this. Anyone gifted with a good ear waits for the *Sanctus* to judge the organist's ability. It is there, with the *vox humana* stop, with pathetic development, most often in an andante, that he makes his way into the hearts of the devoted. The organist is the first teacher of logic, which he measures out beat by beat.

"The contralto is the norm to which voices and instruments should be subordinated in a fully harmonized musical composition. If one wanted to downgrade the contralto, one could drive the *prima donna assoluta* to the moon and the *basso profondo* into a well. And that is to see the moon in a well. What is best is to work on the middle strings, which always manage to be in tune. On the extreme strings, one loses as much in grace as one gains in force; and from abuse they tend toward paralysis of the throat, turning as an expedient to declaimed—that is, forced and toneless—singing.

"Then the need is born to give more body to the instrumentation, to cover the excess of the voices, to the detriment of the musical coloring. That is the way it is done now, and it will be worse after me. The head will conquer the heart: science will lead to the ruin of art; and under a deluge of notes, what is called *instrumental* will be the tomb of the voices and of feeling. May it not come to pass! ! ! !"

When *Moïse* was revived successfully at the Paris Opéra in 1852, Nestor Roqueplan, director of the theater, discovered that Rossini was only a *chevalier* of the Légion d'honneur. He approached the government of Napoleon III with the proposal that Rossini be promoted to *commandeur* without passing through the grade of *officier*. The official decree naming Rossini a *commandeur*, dated April 12, 1853, was sent with a letter in which Achille Fould, Minister of State, urged Rossini to compose a new masterpiece. A more exotic honor also was awarded Rossini when, in 1853, Abdul Medjid, Sultan of Turkey, sent him the Order of Nicham-Iftihar" in appreciation for a *Marcia militare* that Rossini had dedicated to him in 1852.

Early in April 1853, the Grand Duke of Tuscany ordered that *Guglielmo Tell* be staged in the Palazzo Pitti in the composer's honor. Rossini "presided" at the performance, but did not conduct, that task being assigned to Jefté Sbolci. The Florence correspondent of the *Revue et Gazette musicale* (Paris) reported the event fully; he concluded his account with the comment: "This magnificent musical solemnity, ordered by the Grand Duke, having succeeded in making Rossini reappear at the head of a body of musicians all glorying in performing under his eyes one of the most beautiful dramatic operas ever written, gives hope that, after a repose of twenty-five years, the man of genius will understand that, as he still preserves his intellectual faculties intact, no pretext any longer exists for the drying-up of that marvelous source from which so many inspired works emerged to delight the world."

Only Olympe and a few of Rossini's closest friends seem to have understood that he had become a despairingly sick man—and that his nervous, physical, and moral illness was intensifying as he entered his early sixties. On January 17, 1853, Giuseppina Strepponi, writing to Verdi from Leghorn, said: "Ivanoff, who came to see me, spoke to me of you with the greatest pleasure and esteem. Rossini is not, as he might have been, happy. That man thought that he could annihilate his heart by means of his intelligence; now his heart is avenging its rights, searching for those feelings of affection which it cannot find. The heart in its turn is defeating the mind!"

Rossini's wit, however, had not deserted him. Receiving a package of sausages and stuffed *pasta* from Giuseppe Bellentani of Modena, he wrote a letter of thanks on December 28, 1853, "To the Very Illustrious Signor Giuseppe Bellentani, Very Famous Sausage Dealer, Modena." It is headed: "From the so-called Swan of Pesaro to the Eagle of Estensian Sausage Men," and reads: "You have wanted to impress me by soaring very high, by bestowing upon me specially prepared *zamponi* and *cappelletti*; and it is entirely proper that I, as though from the marshy homelands of the ancient Padusa [Po], should raise a loud cry of special gratitude to you. I found your collected works complete in every way; and I am as pleased by the internal mastery as by the joy of delighting in the finesse of your renowned compositions.

"I do not set your praises to music because, as I told you in another letter, I live in the world of harmony as an ex-composer. Good for me, better for you! You know how to touch certain keys that satisfy the palate, a surer judge than the ear because it depends upon delicacy of touch at its most sensitive point, the source of all energy; to please you,

I touch only one of these keys, and it is that of my deeply felt thanks for your numerous attentions. I should like it to serve to stimulate you to higher flights, so that you might wear a laurel wreath, one with which your very much indebted servant would gladly crown you. Your much-obliged servant, Gioachino Rossini. Florence 28 December 1853."

Bellentani, a very excitable man, gathered a crowd of Modenese together in their Piazza Grande, reading and rereading the letter to them. Then he had it framed, placed lights around it, and worked himself up into a such a state of agitation that his never certain control of his emotions gave way; after four days of super-excitation, he was removed to an asylum at Reggio Emilia for a cure. That he recovered his self-possession quickly appears proved, however: Rossini would be writing to him, again with thanks for delicatessen produce, on February 27, 1854—a letter in which he sadly said: "Tormented by a persistent nervous ailment, I cannot for the time being enjoy the exquisite tastes you have prepared. I limit myself to reading the historical notes on gastronomy which you have sent me . . ."[n]

In January 1854, Rossini received a letter from Count Stephen Fay, a Hungarian Knight of Malta who had some renown as a pianist. Fay besought him to supply his Hungarian admirers with a new opera or, lacking that, a large new religious piece. Fay's letter, which seems not to have survived, probably was written in Latin because he lacked any common living language with Rossini. We know it only from versions of its contents published in the *Post* (Pest), the *Niederrheinische Musikzeitung*, and *La France musicale*, and from a summary printed in *La Gazzetta musicale* (Florence). Rossini's reply, dated "*XIV Kal. februarias*"—January 19—was sent in a Latin translation by Ferrucci. It set forth Rossini's artistic, as opposed to his personal, reasons for refusing to compose more for the stage. He expressed himself as out of sympathy with contemporary manners of composition, especially those tending toward "excessive knowledge," which "diminishes the heart's pleasure while making strength of intelligence dominate." Further, he said, he disliked librettos that "magnify unworthy subjects, even horrible crimes."

Perhaps having forgotten some of the texts that he himself had set —such as that for *Semiramide*—Rossini probably intended that comment as criticism of Scribe's sanguinary texts for Halévy and Meyerbeer, notably in *La Juive*, *Les Huguenots*, and *Le Prophète*, though he may equally have been thinking of such a blood bath as Salvatore Cammarano's *Il Trovatore* (1853) for Verdi. The old Rossini glimmered toward the end of the communication to Fay: "I always have had a predilection for Hungary. While it is true that Tokay wine never is missing from my table, yet from now on, Hungary will be doubly dear to me, most amiable Knight, because it shelters you."

At the time of the letter to Fay, Rossini was at the lowest point of his ill health. Eyewitness testimony to his pitiable condition survives in the memoirs of Filippo Mordani[n] and in Emilia Branca's biography of Felice Romani, quoted from earlier. Mordani saw Rossini often in Florence between May 1854 and April 1855. On May 7, 1854, having been introduced to Rossini by Ferrucci, Mordani noted: "This is the first time that I have spoken with this very famous—but oh, so unhappy—man! And of what use is his very great fame to him? The light of his high intelligence seems on the verge of darkening . . . some of those who frequent his house have told me how he gives vent to heavy laments and sighs, unexpectedly breaks into violent sobbing, and often, looking into a mirror, accuses himself of cowardice and says: 'To what have I come, and what was I in this world? And what will people say when they see me reduced to having to be led about by a woman, like a small boy?' "

Rossini told Mordani that he suffered from a species of "hydrophobia" which prevented him from sleeping enough or enjoying the flavors of food. As explanation of this condition, Rossini said: "I exercised my fantasy too much, and this, my nervous sensibility . . ." and added: "But my trouble began in 1847 . . ."[n] On January 8, 1855, Rossini and Mordani met in the Piazza del Duomo. During their ensuing stroll together, Rossini remarked: "I have all of woman's ills. All that I lack is the uterus." A little later, he referred to himself as "the father of those who suffer from nervous trouble." Two days later, when he was again talking about Bologna, he told Mordani "how in 1848 people were killed, and, though many soldiers were about, no one lifted a hand to arrest the cutthroats. 'And don't you know that if what happened hadn't happened, they had a list of more than a thousand people to kill?' And when uttering these words, he became terribly disturbed and flushed. Then: 'They asked me to do things that I couldn't do. Did they want money? I'd have given it to them, and I had it. But they wanted me to become chief of all the bands in Italy and to wear military clothes like a youth of eighteen . . .' "

On February 13, 1855, Rossini told Mordani that for fourteen months he had slept only in snatches of five minutes at a time, that he envied beings who felt nothing, and especially animals. "Death is better than living this way," he said. "All illusions about life have fled me. I always thought little of human glory, knowing how easy both the ascent and the descent are." When Mordani met Rossini again more than two months later, just before the Rossinis' departure for Paris, Rossini said: "Nobody knows the pain that our nervous disease brings. Look—I can't raise my arms more than this." That is, Mordani explained, he could lift them only to his head. "But never believe that when the nervous trouble lays hold of me, my intelligence becomes clouded or ever loses any of its lucidity. Oh, no, that never happens . . ."

Neither quiet summer life in the Tuscan countryside near Florence nor the baths of Montecatini[n] and Bagni di Lucca (where Rossini had passed the summer of 1854 from June 28 on) had helped him at all. Mordani reports a singular "magnetic" cure performed on Rossini early in October 1854 by a "Conte Ginnasi," who "magnetized the nightcap, blowing into it and caressing it on the outside. Poor Rossini!" His nerves were constantly jangled; he often cursed himself; at least once, he held a knife to his throat and begged friends to end his suffering. "A truly miserable life!" Mordani exclaimed after looking at Rossini's "pallid face, the eyes languid and deep-sunk, the cheeks hollow, the head drooping . . ."

Emilia Branca Romani's description of a visit to Florence which she made in 1854 with her husband, her sister Matilde, and Matilde's husband, Juva, confirms Mordani's reports. Rossini, she wrote, was suffering from a "neurosis which, altering all his fibers, rendered him almost monomaniac. . . . Rossini truly was sick, disturbed, nervous, very much weakened and depressed in spirit. According to him, the world had forgotten him, and he would have liked to forget the world, by removing himself from it. . . . The conversation turned on nothing but the discomforts that he suffered or imagined that he suffered, and on the details of the cure that his physician, Professore [Maurizio] Buffalini, ordered him to undergo, but which he had no desire to submit to docilely. Sometimes the altered Maestro moved around the room with agitated steps, struck his head, and, fulminating against his adverse fate, exclaimed: 'Someone else in my state would kill himself, but I . . . I am a coward and haven't the courage to do it!'[n] Nothing could calm that changed mind. Decidedly, his fervid imagination, his powerful fantasy, had rebelled to his detriment, degenerating into mania."

After the Romanis and the Juvas had dined with the Rossinis, Olympe, "when the opportune moment seemed to her to have arrived

. . . opened the door into the salon where the pianoforte was, prepared it, but was careful not to take in the lamps. Night had fallen.

"Signora Matilde Juva, a most intelligent woman, beautiful and with an exquisitely insinuating manner, knew so well what to do that little by little, assisted by Romani, she induced the *Papà-Maestro*, as she called him, to enter the salon, seat himself at the pianoforte, and accompany her in the *romanza* from *Otello*, which he once had taught her lovingly.

". . . The Maestro allowed himself to be carried along, so to speak, but on the condition of remaining in darkness. To the little party were added the usual friends for the evening, who were: Prince Poniatowski, Counts Zappa [Zappi] and Ricci, the painter Vincenzo Rasori, Ferrucci —a famous Latinist—a young foreign gentleman, a pianist who was staying in Florence to study counterpoint, and a few other intimates. All moved into the salon, in which the only light was that reflected through the door from the dining room, where a lamp burned on the table.

"Rossini was seated at the pianoforte, with his Matildina standing beside him, ready to sing, and with Romani on his left. The great Maestro, his agile fingers running arpeggios on the keys, trilling, capriciously indulging his fancy in the prelude to the famous *Otello romanza*, quadruplicated, centuplicated it, producing a *fantasia alla Thalberg*, magnificent, astonishing, dumbfounding. One would have said that, far from being sluggish, he did nothing but practice on the pianoforte keyboard.

"The admiration felt by those privileged listeners was immense, but no one dared to show it, for Signora Pélissier, her finger to her lips in sign of silence, had passed in front of them all; she was afraid of disturbing the Maestro. When the prelude was finished, Rossini said to Signora Juva: 'Now it's your turn, dear Desdemona.' She, moved almost to tears, produced singing so expressive, so impassioned, so correct, that she scarcely had finished when Rossini, seized by a very strange access of sensibility, began to weep violently and sob deeply like a small boy. He was shaking (*storico*). . . . Those present were embarrassed . . . but then Romani joined his wife in saying comforting words to the Maestro, who remained seated at the pianoforte, kissing and rekissing the talented singer's hands.

"Calm was re-established; and Rossini, letting his fingers run along the keyboard again, drawing forth magical sounds, proposed to the woman beside him, who still had not moved, that she sing the cavatina from *Semiramide*. Signora Juva agreed jubilantly, but feared that she might not remember it well. 'But still, dear Matildina, you must sing without music, for I don't want lights . . . I'll act as your prompter,' he added. And with him playing with the brilliance of a great pianist and varying the prelude and preceding chorus with new passages in good taste, as in the *Otello romanza*, the cavatina was performed from beginning to end without any sort of hitch, evoking great admiration from everyone, especially from the Maestro, who this time, in a satis-fying state of mind, wanted to embrace and kiss his SEMIRAMIDE, as he said, and paid her a world of compliments. 'Behold, Rossini reconciled with music!' the friends exclaimed in unison, and each in turn con-gratulated the other. Madame Pélissier, with expansive gratitude, pressed the hands of Romani and Juva and embraced the Branca sisters, her friends, for the good that they had done her. . . .

"From that evening on, a little music always was made in the Rossini house—Rossinian music, be it well understood, or very old classics—that is, as long as the two families, Romani and Juva, remained in Florence, which was for about one month. The lucid interval for Rossini's mind was not of much longer duration; the hypochondriac-nervous accesses again seized him, with greater or lesser intensity, but persistently."

Word was diffused, in fact, that Rossini had lost his mind. There-upon, Olympe felt it necessary to deny the gossip publicly. On October 22, 1854, *La Revue et Gazette musicale*, Paris, said: "We are happy to be able to give our readers news that contradicts what has been published in the papers recently about the state of Rossini's health. In a letter sent to us, a letter written under his dictation by his wife and signed by him, the illustrious composer congratulates himself on the fact that, despite the suffering that he has undergone, he has preserved the full and complete use of his faculties."

Everything else having failed, Olympe again decided to take Rossini to Paris, believing both that French medical science might accomplish what Italian physicians had been unable to do and that complete change of ambiance might of itself benefit him. After the most careful planning and long delays, the decision was carried into action. On April 26, 1855, accompanied by the two servants Tonino and Ninetta, Rossini and Olympe left Florence for Paris. Their friend Masetti rode out as far as Lucca with them. They spent several days in Nice, where local musicians serenaded them in the garden of the Hôtel des Étrangers. They reached Paris about May 25. Rossini was never to see Italy again. But after some further delay, occasioned by continuing bad health, the nearly fourteen years of his final apotheosis were about to begin.

CHAPTER XV

1855-1860

T HE JOURNEY from Florence to Paris, lasting nearly a month with stopovers, did nothing to improve Rossini's condition. At the first of the homes that he and Olympe occupied in Second Empire Paris, No. 32, rue Basse-du-Rempart,[n] he was not able to receive most of the very numerous people who called. When a very few of them—Auber, Carafa, Joseph Méry, Panseron, Comte Frédéric Pillet-Will, Baron Lionel de Rothschild, Sampieri—were admitted, those who had not seen Rossini for some years found him, at sixty-three, frighteningly emaciated, pallid, and weak, his mind altogether lacking its former vivacity. Eating without pleasure, digesting with difficulty, he quickly became exhausted. It was said that the many barrel organs heard in the neighborhood of his lodgings pained him so intensely (especially when, in a manifestation of his disturbed mental state, he heard each tone accompanied by the third above it) that Olympe gave the concierge a small fund with which to bribe them to go away.

Slowly, however, Rossini began to improve. He saw Verdi, who was in Paris for the *première* of *Les Vêpres siciliennes* at the Opéra on June 13, 1855.[n] *La France musicale* reported him as saying to the younger man: "You don't know in what a prison I've been confined!" One of the first signs of a revival of Rossini's humor was noted when, speaking to Carafa of his friend's ancient riding nag, he said: "Eh, Don Michele, I didn't see you go by on horseback today. You must realize that your Rosinante is beginning to canter with appoggiature." Talked into visiting the studio of the photographer Mayer to view a picture of Bologna, he sat quietly, staring at it. Covertly, Mayer took a photograph of him and, when Rossini prepared to leave, handed him the fixed negative. Rossini's comment after looking at the likeness of himself was: "You have played an ugly joke on me."

Generally, however, Rossini remained quietly at home—where, he later said, Olympe surrounded him with a triple defense, the concierge, the servant Tonino, and herself: "The first is a small fortress, the second a formidable bastion; as for the third, to get past it, one needs to be invincible."[n] A young German composer, a protégé of Comte Charles-Robert de Nesselrode, managed to squeeze past the three defenses. Then, all atremble, he placed before Rossini a *Melody* that he had composed for violin. Rossini scanned the manuscript page after page. "The Devil!" he said. "Eighteen pages! What a robust melody! I never saw anything like it. But there must be something good here. Leave it with me so that I can look at it. Come back, and I'll show you which sixteen pages should be suppressed; if you want to save them all, put in sixteen pages of *pizzicati!*" Definitely, Rossini's mental weather and physical resilience were improving. His cheeks began to take on a natural flush, his eyes to brighten, his speech to sound more flavorsome and firm. Out walking with Panseron, he was irritated by passersby who stared at him, moved past, and then returned for a closer, longer look. "See those movements," he said. "They're like ascending and descending scales." Delighted to hear his old friend joking, Panseron replied: "Of which you are the tonic."

Castil-Blaze stated in his somewhat unreliable history of the Théâtre-Italien[n] that Rossini's *Stabat Mater* was sung in Paris at least six times per year from 1842 on, and that some ecclesiastics who greatly prized it remarked to him that they ought to have a Mass by the same composer. Had Rossini composed one? "No," Castil-Blaze reported himself as replying, "and here is how I know it. One evening [in 1837] at the Théâtre-Favart, when the admirable A-flat quintet 'Crudele sospetto'[n] from *La Donna del lago* had been performed on the stage, that vocal ensemble seemed to me to fit so well the words '*Qui tollis peccata mundi*' from the Mass that I sang them in Rossini's presence in the little foyer, saying to him: 'Doubtless you borrowed this fragment from some Mass of your composition.' 'Not at all. It is an accidental effect. I never have written anything for the Church.' 'With twenty of these accidents, one could complete an admirable Mass.' 'Complete it. That's up to you. . . .'

"Seventeen years later, in 1854, I again went on a pilgrimage to Mormoiron, a village in the Vaucluse department where I have an infinity of offspring, *miei rampolli* [my offshoots or descendants]. In that blessed place, I rediscovered the choral society of which M. l'abbé Peytié, rector of the canton, the Choron[n] of our time, was the founder and chief. . . . I was attending one of the society's rehearsals when the famous '*Qui tollis peccata mundi*' came into my mind and I sang it at the keyboard, naming its composer. 'What? A Mass by Rossini?' the elderly *maître de chapelle* exclaimed. 'Yes, the Mass from *La Donna del lago*.' 'What does it matter? This song—isn't it solemn, religious to a supreme degree? Let us see, let us see. Go on, continue!' 'Impossible. I don't know any more.' 'Repeat for us ten, twenty times this admirable fragment, this delicious "*Qui tollis*" to which you are going to give a head and a tail so as to make a blazing, solemn, ravishing Mass, a worthy sister of the *Stabat Mater*! . . .'

"To parody an aria is a difficult matter in itself, even though one is permitted to turn the new words around at pleasure in order to adjust them to the given music. But to adapt the unchangeable text of the Mass to melodies that one must preserve in all their purity; to maintain perfect accord of feeling, color, expression among the disparate elements that you are uniting; to maintain that accord to the point of making people believe that the expatriated songs were composed for their new words, *hoc opus, hic labor est*. That was the way that Gluck arranged his French operas. Nevertheless, I attained the goal; it was not done without both pain and pleasure. I had completed the Rossini Mass by the time I had to return to Paris. I was not able to attend the performance [of it] that was given on Christmas Day [at Mormoiron], but I had word of that solemnity and of the second [performance], even more satisfactory than the first. . . .

"The other day, March 14, 1856, during a long walk with Rossini on the boulevard, I recalled to him that '*Qui tollis peccata mundi*' and said: 'Our Mass is finished. Even better! It has been sung twice!' And then, at once, behold the famous *maître de chapelle* calling off the names of all the sections, which I sang to him *sotto voce*.

" '*Credo in unum Deum*?'

" '*Ecco ridente in cielo*.'

" 'At least you treated it chorally?'

" 'Certainly—wasn't that its original form in *Aureliano in Palmira*?'

" 'Bravo! Perfect! I doubted that I had made a Credo that majestic and that well accented. The Kyrie?'

" '*Santo imen!* A religious chorus from *Otello*.'

" 'Christe eleison?'

" 'The canon quintet from *Mosè*.'

" 'Incarnatus?'

" 'Ninetta's prayer [from *La Gazza ladra*].'

" 'Crucifixus?'

" 'The chorus of shades from *Mosè*.'

" 'Let's pass from the solemn, the sad, to the gay. *Cum Sancto-Spirito, Et vitam venturi saeculi*—that's where the masters place their fugues full of vivacity, sometimes of brilliant madness.'

" 'I took the animated strettas from the *Cenerentola* quintet, the finale of *Semiramide*.'

" 'Good hunting!'

" 'Allow me to submit to you the manuscript of your Mass.'

" 'No. I'll see it when it has been engraved and printed. It is a real tour de force, happily carried out. I answer to you for its success . . .'

"Three gentlemen stopped us, and Rossini introduced me to their lordships by saying: 'This venerable and sainted patriarch [Castil-Blaze was seventy-two in 1856] is my second father. It is he who has translated me into French, Provençal, Latin, and has given me possession of a new empire. That isn't all: the fellow now wants to lead me into Paradise. I'm not much alarmed: I don't think that he's in a great hurry to start leading the way.' "

Early in July 1855, Rossini went to Trouville on the advice of his physicians. There he enjoyed the companionship of Ferdinand Hiller, carrying on long conversations with him. Hiller set down the gist of those talks in the second volume[n] of his *Aus dem Tonleben unsere Zeit*, published at Leipzig in the year of Rossini's death. In part, he wrote:

"I had been introduced to Rossini when I reached Paris as a very young man [about 1828]. There, as well as later on in Milan, I saw him very often; always and everywhere he was most gracious and sympathetic. During the two or three weeks that I spent in Trouville, I passed the greater part of my time in his company. . . .

"Rossini is now sixty-three years old. His features are but little changed. It would be difficult to find a more intelligent face than his: a well-chiseled nose, an eloquent mouth, expressive eyes, and a marvelous forehead. His physiognomy is of Southern vivacity, truly eloquent whether being humorous or serious, irresistible in expressing irony, a mood, or roguishness. His voice is as pleasant as it is flexible; no South German can sound more pleasant to the ear of a well-educated North

German than Rossini—when he chooses to. His is the most sociable nature imaginable. I do not think that he ever tires of having people around him, of conversing, of telling stories, and—what is rarer—of listening. With this, he has the even disposition to be found only among people from the South: for children as well as for the aged, for the mighty as well as for the lowly, he always finds the right words without altering his manner. He is, then, one of those happy creatures born with everything, and in whom all modifications occur naturally and most organically. Nothing in either his music or his personality is violent—and for that reason both have won so many hearts."

Rossini told Hiller how much he had enjoyed the younger man's performances of Bach, and then added: "What a colossal creature Bach was! To write such a quantity of works in such a style! It's inconceivable. What is difficult or impossible for others was child's play for him. What about that beautiful edition of his works [the *Bach Gesellschaft*]? I first heard of it from a Leipzig family who visited me in Florence; it was probably owing to them that the first two volumes were sent to me, but I'd like to have the subsequent volumes too." When Hiller said that all he need do was subscribe to them, Rossini was delighted. Then he said: "Bach's portrait in the first volume is marvelous. It shows such extraordinary intellectual force. Bach must also have been an eminent virtuoso." He then asked Hiller if many of Bach's works were performed in Germany. When Hiller replied that many, but still not enough, were heard, Rossini's comment was: "Unfortunately that is not possible in Italy, and now less than ever. Unlike you Germans, we cannot organize huge choruses of amateurs. Formerly we used to have good voices in church choirs—but that is all gone. And since the death of [Giuseppe] Baini," even the Sistine [Chapel choir] is getting poorer all the time. . . ."

The conversation turned to singers and singing, and Rossini said: "Most of the important singers of the present owe their talent more to fortunate natural endowment than to their training. This is true of Rubini, of Pasta, and of many others. The true art of *bel canto* ended with the disappearance of *castrati*; one must agree to that, even if one cannot wish to have them back. Their artistry was all that those people could have, and so they devoted the most assiduous diligence and untiring care to their training. They always turned into able musicians, and when their voices faltered, they were at least excellent teachers."

On another occasion, the conversation veered to Italian composers of the past. Hiller asked Rossini whether or not he had heard many of Paisiello's operas. "They already had more or less vanished from Italian stages during my youth," Rossini told him. "Generali, Fioravanti, Paër, and especially Simone Mayr were popular then." When Hiller asked his opinion of Paisiello, Rossini replied: "His music moves past the ear pleasantly, but neither its harmony nor its melody is anything special, and I never was particularly interested in it. His principle was to compose a whole piece around a small motive—which makes for little vitality and even less dramatic expressiveness." Hiller wanted to know if Rossini had met Paisiello. "I saw him in Naples after his return from Paris, where he had made a considerable fortune. Napoleon liked to hear his music, and Paisiello boasted about that rather naïvely by telling the whole world that the great emperor especially loved his music because he could listen to it while thinking about other matters. What strange praise! But at that time his gentle music was generally preferred—after all, each era has its own taste."

"Was Paisiello an interesting person?" Hiller asked. And Rossini said: "His appearance was pleasant, strong, almost imposing, but he was terribly uneducated and immeasurably insignificant. You should have read one of his letters! I don't even want to mention his handwriting, or his spelling—I'll let that go—but the clumsiness of his expressions, the shallowness of his ideas, cannot be imagined! Now, Cimarosa was a quite different person—a fine, educated mind." Hiller remarked that all he knew of Cimarosa was *Il Matrimonio segreto* and (from reading the score) *Gli Orazii e Curiazii*. Rossini said: "There isn't much to the latter. On the other hand, an *opera buffa* by him exists, *Le Trame deluse*, which is really excellent." "Better than *Il Matrimonio segreto*?" Hiller inquired. "Incomparably more significant. The second-act finale (it's almost too large for a last finale) is a real masterpiece. Unfortunately, the libretto is insufferable." I can also recall an aria from his oratorio *Isacco*[n] which has a passage in which the harmony is extremely dramatic and striking. Pure inspiration—for, as you know, he was not a great harmonist."

Hiller asked where the manuscripts of Rossini's operas were: "I believe that you don't have many of them." "Not a note," Rossini told him, adding: "I was entitled to demand them from the copyist after a year, but I never took advantage of that. A few may be in Naples, a few are in Paris—I don't know the fate of the others." Hiller interjected: "Perhaps you don't even own the engraved scores and piano scores of your operas, Maestro?" "What for?" Rossini asked. "No music has been played in my home for years. Should I study them, perhaps?" Hiller persisted: "And the opera *Ermione*, which your biographers say you are secretly saving for posterity—what about it?" "It's with the others," Rossini told him. Hiller went on: "You once told me about that opera that you had made it too dramatic—and that it had been a failure." "Quite justifiably," Rossini replied, amused. "It was terribly boring."

During September, another musician visited Trouville: Sigismund, Ritter von Neukomm (then seventy-seven), who had studied with Michael Haydn and from 1816 to 1821 had been in Rio de Janeiro as court music director to the Emperor Pedro I. Hiller presented Neukomm to Rossini, and the talk turned to Dom Pedro, of whom Rossini said: "He was nice enough to send me a decoration. I thanked him for it later, when he came to Paris somewhat against his will. And as I had heard about his compositions, I offered to have something by him played at the Théâtre-Italien. He gladly accepted." Here Neukomm interrupted: "He would have conducted it himself if you had asked him." "Not really!" Rossini said. "He sent me a cavatina, which I had copied out after adding only a few trombones. It was well played at one of the Théâtre-Italien concerts and received very decent applause. In his loge, Dom Pedro seemed very pleased about it—at least, he thanked me very warmly." Hiller continued: "Here I should like to add something to complete this little anecdote. I mentioned it at the salon of the Comtess B. 'I recall that evening very well,' the Comtesse said. 'Dom Pedro came to the Tuileries after the concert, and he seemed completely transported with joy. He maintained that it was the greatest happiness of his entire life. Coming from a man who had just lost a kingdom, those expressions of enthusiasm struck us as rather strange.' "

Rossini returned to Paris from Trouville toward the end of September 1855. Early the next month, the Théâtre-Italien began a season during which his operas occupied a large place. It started with *Mosè*, conducted by Giovanni Bòttesini. The manager's hope that Rossini would attend at least one performance was not realized. Nor does Rossini seem to have gone to the Italien on the evening of March 20 and 21, 1856, when it housed singings of his *Stabat Mater* and his choruses *La Fede, La Speranza, La Carità* (the Italian translation of *La Foi, L'Es-*

pérance, La Charité). His physical condition, however, continued to improve. His physicians suggested that he complete his cure by taking the waters at Wildblad in Württemberg. En route there in June 1856, he stopped off at Strasbourg, where in the evening the local orchestra, the chorus from the opera, and a number of fervent dilettantes joined to perform under the windows of his hotel room the overture to *Il Barbiere di Siviglia*, choruses from *Le Comte Ory*, and the overture to *Guillaume Tell*.

Somewhat later, the *Theater-Journal* (Munich) reported: "Among the guests at Wildblad, one person has the privilege of attracting the attention of all the bathers; he is an elderly man, a little tremulous in his motions, but with an open physiognomy and a lively eye who is inscribed on the hotel register under the name *Rossini, composer of music*. He behaves very politely toward all who pay attention to him. A young man a, great admirer of the celebrated musician, introduced himself, telling him that he could not make up his mind to leave Wildblad without having seen him. '*Eh, bien!*' the Maestro answered him in French, '*Monsieur, regardez-moi! Vous voyez ça un vieux rococo!* ["Well, then, sir, look at me! Here you see a rococo old man!"].'"

Early in August, Rossini went on to Kissingen, where he was sought out by Maximilian II, King of Bavaria. Then, after a stay at Baden for further mineral-water treatment, he went back to Paris with the noted horn player Eugène Vivier in late September. Soon after reaching Paris, he was serenaded again, this time by the popular Alfred Musard, whose dance orchestra of twenty players performed from memory "*La Pastorella delle Alpi*" from the *Soirées musicales* and the overture to *La Gazza ladra*.

Having found the Paris summer oppressive, in May 1856, the Rossinis had rented a small Passy villa from the music publisher Jacques-Léopold Heugel.ⁿ When the Paris municipal authorities learned that Rossini would like to have a permanent villa of his own in the Beauséjour quarter of Passy, near the Bois de Boulogne, they offered him free lifetime use of a property to be selected by him, the understanding to be that it would revert to the city after his death. Rossini replied that, though he appreciated the offer, he was not so poor as to have to accept it or so rich as to be able to leave to the city of Paris the handsome villa that he planned to build. On September 18, 1858, therefore, the city sold him at a favorable price (90,000 francs) a parcel of land adjacent to the Bois, just to the left of the Porte de Passy. Rossini half-jokingly explained that he had chosen the land because it was in the shape of a grand piano; that this remark was not wholly facetious is suggested by the fact that the elaborate flowerbeds that were to surround the villa would be laid out in the shapes of musical instruments, including cellos and doublebasses.

Rossini's agreement with the city of Paris stipulated that after his death and that of Olympe, the city would be able to buy back the property by paying to their heirs the purchase price of the land plus that of the building to be erected upon it, that price to be determined by an expert appraiser. The cornerstone of the later famous Villa Rossini was not to be laid until March 10, 1859, by which time the sixty-seven-year-old composer evidently believed that he and Olympe still had years of good life ahead."

In the autumn of 1856, the Frankfurt music publisher Karl August André, intending to ingratiate himself with Rossini, sent him a portrait of Mozart—and in the accompanying letter compared Rossini to Mozart. On October 13, Rossini wrote him in French: "Allow me to thank you for the flattering way in which you offer me the portrait of the immortal Mozart, the master of us all ! ! ! but whom one cannot imitate, and to whom is so justly due the admiration upon which Germany prides itself. I do thank you for the esteem that you have for me, nothing could be said that could be more pleasing to me than the point of comparison that you establish between him and me, but here I must assert to you that the intention cannot be accepted as a fact." Rossini always enjoyed honest praise, but he knew, and always had known, that he was no Mozart, and the terseness of his comment shows that he was fully conscious that André knew it too."

By the spring of 1857, Rossini had begun to compose again. On Olympe's name-day (April 5) of that year, he handed her a manuscript headed *Musique anodine*. It consisted of a prelude for piano and six different settings of the Metastasio lines beginning "*Mi lagnerò tacendo della mia sorte amara.*" The first page carried this inscription:

MUSIQUE ANODINE
Prélude for the Piano
Followed by Six Little Songs composed
on the same words, of which Two for soprano, one for
mezzo-soprano, one for Contralto, and two
for Baritone
with Piano accompaniment

I offer these modest songs to my dear wife Olympe
as a simple testimonial of gratitude for the
affectionate, intelligent care of which she was prodigal
during my overlong and terrible illness
(Shame of the [medical] faculty)

GIOACHINO ROSSINI
Words by METASTASIO
Paris, this April 15, 1857.[n]

Rossini became constantly more gregarious as his spirits rose. The rented city quarters in the rue Basse-du-Rempart soon became too constricted for the social activity that he increasingly required and enjoyed. Friends located ampler quarters for the Rossinis on the *premier étage* (second floor) of a large building at No. 2, rue de la Chaussée d'Antin, at the northeast corner of that street and the boulevard des Italiens, a building in which the fashionable portrait painter Franz Xaver Winterhalter also lived. Rossini at once set about furnishing his new home, buying finically selected pieces of furniture and ordering many of his possessions to be sent on from Italy. The apartment consisted of a reception hall; a large bedroom with adjacent bathroom; a small sitting room reserved for Olympe; a very spacious grand salon with three windows on each street; a dining room; a master bedroom for Rossini; a den; and an ample kitchen (the servants' quarters were not specified).

The reception hall soon was decorated with engravings by Rossini's friend Luigi Calamatta of paintings by Correggio at Parma. The grand salon held a Pleyel grand piano, some large urns, and the 1815 portrait of Rossini by the Viennese artist Mayer, showing him in a green mantle and red beret; on either side of it hung copies of paintings by Rembrandt. In the dining room, glass-doored armoires held silver; between the two windows, which gave on the boulevard des Italiens, stood an inlaid mechanical organ surmounted by a group of monkey musicians carved in wood.[n] A wall rack running around the room held pieces of fine porcelain; the pictures on the walls were hunting and fishing scenes.

Rossini's bedroom—which he gradually came to use both as a study and as the place for receiving callers—contained a canopied, curtained bed. With time, this room swallowed an astonishing miscellany of objects. On the mantelpiece ticked a clock topped by a bronze bust of Mozart. On a small Pleyel piano stood photographs of the Queen of Spain and the King of Portugal, both inscribed to Rossini. The walls were covered with photographs and landscape paintings. Between the two windows stood a large mahogany armoire in which slowly piled up the brief pieces—the *Péchés de vieillesse* ("Sins of Old Age") and others—which Rossini composed after *Musique anodine*. In the center of the room, near the piano, a table was littered with periodicals, books, music, and letters: Rossini used it for composing, reading, and writing letters and often sat behind it when receiving visitors. Here, too, when the mood was upon him (which was increasingly often), he sat to listen to music that others wanted him to judge and to singers eager for his opinion, by which they meant his approbation. Olympe, it was said, upon hearing the strange sounds that often drifted from this room, would say: "Rossini is at the fair again!"

Rossini's den housed a cabinet crammed with small *objets d'art*, including a Madonna that he believed to be an original Leonardo da Vinci and a supposed Benvenuto Cellini silver piece of which he was inordinately proud. Its furnishings also included a trophy cabinet displaying halberds and small firearms; musical instruments—among them violins, flutes, clarinets, trumpets, and a large ivory syrinx that he had bought from the tenor Mario—and busts of Rossini[n] and Napoleon I signed by Lorenzo Bartolini. Between the two windows stood a desk; in its drawers were spread out jewels that had been Isabella's, brooches, rings, and snuffboxes, as well as the nearly thirty decorations that had been conferred upon Rossini. During the final years of his life, the miscellany in this den was completed by a gift presented to him on his seventieth birthday by Mario: a tobacco jar from Scotland, made from a goat's head of which the horns had been silvered.

Rossini's daily regimen came to be all but invariable. He rose at about eight o'clock and breakfasted on a roll and a large glass of coffee (sometimes replaced in later years by two *oeufs à la cocque* and a glass of Bordeaux wine) while Olympe opened and rapidly summarized for him the newly arrived mail.[n] Then Rossini received callers until about ten-thirty, when he put on a long cloak, fastened his cravat with a favorite pin bearing a portrait of Handel, and sallied forth. Weather permitting, he strolled the boulevards for an hour or climbed into a fiacre to pay calls on such of his friends as the Rothschilds and Comte Pillet-Will. Often, too, he dropped in at various shops to carry out commissions for Olympe and to buy food.

One day the young Edmond Michotte accompanied Rossini on a foray into the Marais district, their objective being a *pasta* shop run by an Italian named Canaveri. When they had climbed the stairs to the third floor, Rossini addressed the shopkeeper: "Are you Canaveri? I have been told that you have Neapolitan macaroni; show them to me." Then, staring coldly at what the man had put before him, he said: "These? But these are Genoese macaroni!"

"Signore, I assure you . . ." the man began to protest.

"So, that's it?" Rossini answered. "If you don't have Neapolitan macaroni, I don't want to know anything else. Good day!" And he started back down the stairs.

Left behind, Michotte said to Canaveri: "Do you know who that gentleman is? Rossini, the great composer."

"Rossini?" the merchant answered. "Don't know him. But if he knows as much about music as he does about macaroni, he must write beautiful stuff!"

At the bottom of the stairs, Michotte reported this exchange to Rossini, whose comment was: "A good thing! Not one of my panegyrists ever has risen to such a hyperbole of praise!"

In warmer weather, Rossini might ride of a morning to the Bois de Boulogne, stroll up and down the avenue des Acacias for a while, and then climb back into a fiacre so as to reach home about an hour after noon. There he sipped a glass of wine or cordial, but usually ate nothing until six o'clock, when the table was set with a simple but well-prepared mixture of Italian and French dishes. On Saturday, the Rossinis came to have up to sixteen, but commonly no more than twelve, dinner guests; many others were asked to arrive after dinner to participate in music or listen to it.

Rossini seldom dined out more than twice a year: before the annual move to Passy for the summer, with his friend Bigottini (a son of the ballerina Emilia Bigottini); and, upon returning to Paris for the winter, with Comte Pillet-Will. Otherwise, Saturdays excepted, he went to his bedroom alone after dinner, slept briefly, and then smoked a light cigar. Later, in the evening, he returned to the dining room, where Olympe read aloud from the newspapers. Intimate friends often dropped in after eight-thirty to discuss current happenings and to gossip. Once, it was said, Tonino entered to announce the arrival of Enrico Tamberlik, whose high C-sharp chest tone then was a subject of animated discussion and the object of almost hysterical audience acclamation. Rossini's reaction was: "Have him come in. But tell him to leave his C-sharp on the coatrack. He can pick it up again when he leaves."[n]

Panseron was present on one such evening when Rossini played pieces by Haydn and Mozart on the piano. Wondering aloud why

Haydn's cantata *Arianna a Naxos* (1789), which he preferred among Haydn's vocal compositions after *Die Schöpfung* and *Die Jahreszeiten*, never was sung at the Conservatoire, he began, after some preluding chords, to sing it *sotto voce*. Then, letting his voice swell out, he continued from memory through the twenty-five minutes of the cantata. On that same evening, he demonstrated the way that Giuseppe Prinetti had taught him to play scales with thumb and index finger, performing in that awkward way a phrase for violins in the first finale of *Il Barbiere di Siviglia*. These evenings were not allowed to last too late. Rossini stole occasional glances at a clock, and when, at exactly ten, he said: "Behold the canonical hour," everyone departed.

Saturday evenings were more formal. Engraved invitations, with the guests' names and the date filled in by pen, were sent out. One of these surviving in the Bibliothèque Nationale, Paris, reads: "*Monsieur & Madame Rossini prient* Monsieur *de queux de St. Hilaire de leur faire l'honneur de venir passer la Soirée chez eux, le 29 fevrier. On est prié de remettre en entrant son invitation. 2, rue de la Chaussée d'Antin R.S.V.P.*" At about nine o'clock, Olympe stood in the large salon—opened only for these occasions—to receive the arriving guests. The first of these famous *samedi soirs* occurred on December 18, 1858; the last took place on September 26, 1868. During those ten years, one guest was there almost always: Michele Enrico Carafa, Principe di Colobrano, Rossini's old friend who had collaborated with him on *Adelaide di Borgogna* and *Mosè in Egitto*. And eventually almost every French and foreign musician and other artist of note, as well as many well-known political, social, and commercial people, attended one or more of the Rossini Saturday nights.[n]

The Rossini cuisine was praised more often for its lavishness than for its peculiarly combined foods, which often included delicacies sent to Rossini as gifts: macaroni made by nuns at L'Aquila and forwarded by Francesco Florimo,[n] Seville hams, Modenese *zamponi*, olives from Ascoli Piceno,[n] Bolognese *mortadelle*, cheeses from Gorgonzola, and special wines. Some hungry people seem to have sought invitation to the Chaussée d'Antin to eat, but the real *clou* of the Rossini *samedi soirs*—which provided dinner only on occasion, and then for only a small percentage of the guests—was the conversation, the music (particularly when it meant new music by the host), the skits prepared and performed by such talented entertainers as Gustave Doré and Eugène Vivier, and Rossini's acidulous comments.

Rossini himself pre-selected the musical program, which often was printed in advance (many of the printed programs survive in Michotte's collection at the Brussels Royal Conservatory). He did not usually dress formally; he did not appear in the grand salon except to accompany a singer or instrumentalist, but preferred to remain in the less crowded adjoining dining room. The Rossini soirées became so famous that an invitation to one of them was very highly valued and sometimes doggedly fought for. Those who wanted to receive a second invitation had to pay open court to Olympe. Radiciotti wrote: "I know of one person of high standing among my acquaintances who, on visiting Rossini, failed to render particular homage to Madame Olympe, and she never forgave him for this oversight."

Fortunately, not everyone understood Rossini's commentaries. One evening, a *diva* sang badly and then went to the dining room to receive Rossini's opinion of her performance. "Oh, my dear friend!" he said. "What do you want me to tell you? No, no. I cannot say anything to you!" The lady told the other guests that the Maestro had been unable to find words to express his admiration. Obliged to say something to Gabrielle Krauss, whose artistry went far toward compensating for her flawed vocal production, he remarked: "You sing with your soul, and your soul is beautiful," a sentence that her admirers solemnly reported to the newspapers. When a society lady had succeeded in all but destroying an aria, she excused herself to Rossini by saying: "Pardon me, *cher maître*, I am a little frightened." Rossini's reply was: "And so am I."

Sigismond Thalberg, returning to Paris after an absence of ten years, participated in a program at one of the *samedi soirs*. Among the other guests that night were Alboni, Grisi, Frezzolini, and Fodor-Mainvielle. When Thalberg had finished playing, Rossini hastened up to him, embraced him, and said to the entire assemblage: "Grant that Thalberg just now has given you a lesson in singing such as you never have had before." On a few occasions, compositions by others especially prepared for the musicale were heard. At the first of them (December 18, 1858), for example, Maria Mira and the tenor Biéval sang a chamber opera called *La Laitière de Trianon*, with libretto by Galoppe d'Onquaire and music by Jean-Baptiste Weckerlin, librarian of the Conservatoire. After it had been applauded warmly, Mira and Biéval sang as an encore a short piece, also especially written for the occasion, honoring Rossini.

In 1858, Rossini accepted the presidency of a twelve-man commission set up by the French government to establish a standard musical pitch (Auber, Berlioz, Fromental Halévy, Meyerbeer, and Ambroise Thomas were the other composer-members of the commission, which also included two physicists—one of them Jules Lissajous—and four bureaucrats). Regarding this appointment as purely honorary, Rossini never attended a sitting of the commission, thus infuriating Verdi, who disapproved of the commission's recommendation, made in 1859, that the musical A be stabilized at 435 vibrations per second. Writing to Ricordi from Madrid early in 1863, Verdi noted that the Ricordi *Gazzetta* had reported him as approving completely of the new "*diapason normale*," and complained: "On the contrary, last year I told Rossini that a standard diapason was useful and desirable, but that the commission had been wrong in lowering it too much. By way of complete reply, Rossini told me that he could not discuss the matter because he had never attended a sitting of the commission. And he was its president!"

Rossini had begun to devote some time each day to composition. When Max Maria von Weber visited him in 1865, he was awkward enough to ask why his host had decided never to compose for the theater again. "Quiet!" Rossini replied, gesturing. "Don't talk to me about that! Moreover, I compose constantly. Do you see that cabinet full of music? All of it has been written since *Guillaume Tell*. But I don't publish anything; and I compose because I can't help myself." As he produced these little pieces, some of them serious, more of them farcically or satirically intended and sardonically or nonsensically entitled in a manner later repeated by Erik Satie, a copyist carefully made clean copies of them. One day, Rossini pointed out to the copyist that he had changed a natural to a sharp. The man replied that he had done so to make the chord sweeter. "Right," Rossini said. "The chord is sweeter; but it would be *your* chord and not *mine*. Now correct it, and in the future do me the favor of writing *my* chords. If, then, they make too disagreeable an impression upon you, tell me so frankly; I'll compensate you when you have completed your task." Telling Filippo Filippi about this incident. Rossini added: "Do you know, the copyist goes on correcting me, and perhaps he's right, but I'm an obstinate boy, a stubborn pupil, and here and there I restore the chords that upset him."

Olympe lovingly gathered up these compositions and put them under double lock in her husband's bedroom. She guarded them so fiercely that when a caller wanted to hear one of them, she grumbled and demurred until Rossini quietly ordered her to fetch the desired manuscript. The ease with which he always had composed had not lessened: if he was writing when a friend dropped in, he simply put down his pen for the duration of the visit; when the guest had departed, he picked it up again and went on from the notes at which he had been interrupted.

Although Rossini often referred to himself deprecatingly as a "pianist of the fourth class," he had lost none of his remarkable pianistic ability. On April 8, 1864, writing to Giovanni Pacini, who had invited him to compose a piece for the Società del Quartetto at Florence, he said: "I abandoned my musical career in 1829; this long silence has lost me the power to compose and awareness of the instruments. Now I am simply a pianist of the fourth class, and though I thus classify myself modestly enough, as you see, the pianists of all nations (who entertain me at my home) wage secret, bitter war against me (behind my back), so that I cannot find pupils despite the modest charge—twenty soldi—for my lessons; nor am I allowed to perform, for I am not asked to; and I therefore live (as a pianist) under a public scourge. . . . *Giovanni mio!* . . . 'If you don't weep now, for what are you wont to weep?' . . . "[n]

Le Ménestrel (Paris) published on July 30, 1920, some informal memoirs that had been found among Louis Diémer's papers after his death in 1919. Diémer recalled: "I was presented to Rossini by M. Heugel. The Maestro asked me to play his new compositions for him, and I gladly accepted. Thus I became the habitual pianist of his weekly soirées, interpreting his manuscripts each Saturday—I had to study them at his house because he did not want to entrust them to anyone. After two or three times [readings], I succeeded in committing to memory the pieces to be played in the evening. He had composed many, including a most diverting parody of Offenbach's music, to be played with one finger; a tarantella in which one heard the passing of a parade (I played it once during a big benefit concert with choruses conducted by Jules Cohen); certain preludes; *Profound Sleep with Startled Awakening*; and finally a series of little pieces that he called '*Les Petits Riens*,' to which he gave such curious titles as *The Hors d'œuvres, The Anchovies, The Radishes, A Caress for My Wife*, etc. . . ."[n]

"At one of these suppers, which were always intensely interesting, there were present the *maestri* Auber, then director of the Conservatoire, and Verdi, who was passing through Paris: Auber, a very spirited conversationalist; Verdi, taciturn . . .

"At Rossini's home I had occasion to hear the most famous singers:

Alboni, Tamberlick, Duprez, Faure, Delle Sedie, Conneau, Mira (who sang splendidly a delicious song by the host, 'L'Orpheline du Tyrol'),[n] Adelina Patti, whom we had the unexpected pleasure of admiring there for the first time. She was then seventeen years old, and a few days earlier had made her debut at the Théâtre-Italien in *La Sonnambula* . . .[n] Among the instrumentalists, Sivori, Sarasate, the violoncellist Braga, our great and dear Maître Saint-Saëns, Mathias, the excellent Italian pianist Stanzieri, and finally Rubinstein and Liszt—who gave the first audition of his noted *Légendes—Saint François d'Assise prédicant aux oiseaux* and *Saint François de Paule marchant sur les flots*— at Rossini's home.

"Rossini himself also played the pianoforte deliciously, without using the pedals, and with a silvery touch. One day it entered his head to have me sing a song that he had composed on only one note, the interest of which was entirely in the accompaniment; I did not agree, so then Alboni sang it—to the greater satisfaction of everyone. Instead, I played a four-hand march with him and accompanied another of his beautiful pieces, entitled 'Un Mot à Paganini,' which Sivori often delighted to play.[n]

"The close of these evenings often was enlivened by the gay *chansons* of the celebrated Variétés actor Levasseur. Once we also had the surprise of seeing Taglioni, the creator of *La Sylphide*, dance a gavotte and a minuet. Although she was no longer young (she was then the wife of Comte Gilbert des [de] Voisins), she still delighted us by her great art."

The first time that Adelina Patti attended one of the Rossini musicales, she sang "Una voce poco fa." Saint-Saëns wrote:[n] "Unhappily, I was not present at the soirée during which Patti was heard at Rossini's for the first time. It is known that when she had performed the aria from *Il Barbiere*, he said to her, after many compliments: 'By whom is this aria that you just have let us hear?' I saw him a few days later: he still had not calmed down. 'I know perfectly well,' he told me, 'that my arias must be embroidered; they were made for that. But not to leave a note of what I composed, even in the recitatives—really, that is too much!' And in his irritation, he complained because sopranos insisted upon singing this aria, which was composed for a contralto, and did not sing so much that he had composed for soprano."

Patti had been presented to Rossini by Maurice Strakosch, her brother-in-law and mentor. It was said that Rossini, commenting upon her overdecorated rendition of "*Una voce poco fa*," remarked to her: " . . . I did not recognize the finale: probably it was altered by your teacher, who has Strakoschonized it."[n] Saint-Saëns reported: "The *diva*, for her part, was much annoyed. But she reflected: to have Rossini as an enemy, that would be a serious matter. Some days later, she went repentantly to ask for his advice. It was wise of her, for at that time her astonishing, fascinating talent was not yet perfected.

"Two months after this encounter, Patti, with the Maître accompanying, sang arias from *La Gazza ladra* and *Semiramide*, coupling with her brilliant qualities the absolute correctness that she has always displayed since then."[n]

On March 10, 1859, Rossini, Olympe, and a few of their friends presided ceremoniously over the initiation of work on the Passy villa. Rossini buried a small casket containing a medal that had been struck off for the *Stabat Mater*. Then, officiating with trowel and mortar, he laid the first stone, striking it symbolically three times. Olympe, who was to be in charge of the gardens to surround the villa, planted a rosebush. Rossini told Doussault, architect of the villa, that he had considered burying a recently discovered coin of Caracalla for the joy of anticipating the disputes that its rediscovery one day might provoke.

As work on the villa went forward, Rossini fell into the habit of visiting its site every day. At about seven o'clock each morning, he could be seen walking toward Passy—often in the company of his friend Conte Pompeo Belgiojoso—his long greatcoat fluttering about his nankeen pantaloons as he politely acknowledged the greetings of passersby. At the building site, he paid the strictest attention to each detail of the construction of the villa, the floor plan of which he himself had suggested to Doussault. The wall and ceiling decorations were the joint work of a Ravennese academician named Bisteghi and a specialist in chiaroscuro, Samoggia. The villa included a comfortably spacious salon, a dining room, a first-floor master bedroom and adjacent study, a bedroom for Olympe, a kitchen, and smaller dependencies. The salon ceiling was decorated with cartouches containing portraits of Palestrina, Mozart, Cimarosa, and Haydn; it also included a likeness of Padre Mattei. The dining-room ceiling had similar portraits of Beethoven, Grétry, and Boieldieu. The furnishings were much less heavy and cluttered than those in the Chaussée d'Antin apartment: one of the Rossinis' chief desires, there in the country, was for light and air. His bedroom had simple mahogany furniture; the adjoining study contained a small Pleyel piano and a desk. Its windows gave on Olympe's garden, which displayed a large urn topped by a representation of the Three Graces carved by Germain Pilon.

In the spring of 1861, the Rossinis made the first of their annual moves from the Chaussée d'Antin to the Beauséjour villa. That the Maestro was in residence in Passy always was announced by the mounting of a gilt lyre on the entrance gate. Weckerlin reported[n] that one day Rossini and a friend walked past the Passy villa of Lamartine, then reputed to be in financial straits. When the friend called Rossini's attention to a gilt *"lyre"* that Lamartine too had had placed above his gateway, Rossini remarked: "He should have put a *tirelire* [in effect a coin bank] there." Beyond the Rossinis' own lyre-topped entrance, passersby could see into the gardens, their flowerbeds laid out in the shapes of musical instruments.

Rossini had begun to make an occasional appearance at public musical events. In 1858, he went to the Opéra-Comique for a rehearsal of Carafa's 1823 success, *Le Valet de chambre*. That year he also was at the Salle Ventadour for the dress rehearsal of Prince Giuseppe Poniatowski's 1840 opera *Don Desiderio*. Poniatowski, addressing the orchestra, had said: "Messieurs, Maestro Rossini has done us the honor of attending the rehearsal!" A prolonged burst of applause followed. Rossini sat through the rehearsal, listening intently and often praising the composer. After a first-act sextet, he took Poniatowski's hands and said: "One sees very clearly that you have studied the great masters seriously. Cimarosa must have been content!" Like many of his similar remarks, this one combined courtesy and criticism.

In January 1859, the Société des Concerts du Conservatoire celebrated its thirty-first anniversary: its first concert (which had included a Rossini aria and the big duet from *Semiramide*) had been given under Habeneck's direction on March 9, 1828. Rossini had promised Auber, now director of the Conservatoire, that in good weather he would attend one of the concerts. The Empress Eugénie was present when, on April 17, 1859, Rossini heard a program that included part of his *Stabat Mater* and the finale of *Moïse*. At the end of the Inflammatus, the audience hailed him vociferously; after the *Moïse* excerpt, the concert was interrupted for fifteen minutes of applause that made Rossini weep. Leaving the hall on Auber's arm, he was cheered by the audience.

In 1861, Rossini went to the Opéra for a rehearsal of *La Stella di Messina*, a ballet composed by his Neapolitan friend Conte Nicolò

Gabrielli. *La Revue et Gazette musicale*, become less anti-Rossinian with the passing years, reported: "One piece of good fortune which touched this new ballet was that of having received, before its birth, the visit of Rossini, who deigned to attend its dress rehearsal. The orchestra saluted the illustrious *maestro,* playing the overture to *Guillaume Tell*; the cry of *Viva Rossini!* echoed from all parts of the hall. He was so moved that he besought Alphonse Royer to speak for him and to thank the performers." Radiciotti reported that during this visit to the Opéra, Rossini discovered an error in the published score of the *Tell* overture"— and that when he pointed it out, the publisher ordered it corrected; unfortunately, the error persists in many editions, thus depriving Rossini of a very effective dissonance.

Late in 1859, Torribio Calzado, the Cuban who had become director of the languishing Italien, staged an unhappy Rossinian performance. He already (1855) had revived *Mosè in Egitto* by putting on a balletless Italian version of *Moïse*. In 1856, he had staged *La Cenerentola*. In 1857, he had announced the intention of producing a "new Rossini opera" entitled *Un Curioso Accidente*, but had not staged it then or in 1858. This appalling *pasticcio*, to a two-act libretto by Arcangelo Berettoni, contained ill-used music from *La Cambiale di matrimonio*, *La Pietra del paragone*, *L'Occasione fa il ladro*, and *Aureliano in Palmira*. Hearing that it was finally about to reach the stage of the Italien, on November 11, 1859, Rossini sent the overeager Calzado a letter in French:

"MONSIEUR: I am told that the *affiche* of your theater has announced a new opera by me under this title: *Un Curioso Accidente*. I do not know whether I should have the right to prevent the performance of a composite in two acts (more or less) of old pieces of mine; I never become involved in questions of these sorts related to my works (none of which, by the way, bears this title: *Un Curioso Accidente*). In any case, I am not opposed . . . to the performance of this *curious accident*. But I cannot let the public called to your theater and your subscribers believe that it is, to start with, a new opera of mine or even that I have had anything to do with the arrangement to be produced. I approach you, then, to beg you to remove from your *affiche* the word *new* and my name as the composer, and to replace them with the following: Opera arranged on pieces by M. Rossini by M. Berrettoni [sic]. I demand that this change appear on tomorrow's *affiche*; if it does not, I shall be obliged to claim from the law what I now claim from your loyalty."

Calzado removed the offending announcement, but did not replace it with one reading as Rossini had specified. He went ahead with the production, even enlisting such excellent singers as Alboni and Cesare Badiali. The *première* of *Un Curioso Accidente*—which proved to be its only performance—occurred at the Italien on November 27, 1859. "One still had time to note a graceful comic trio for male voices," Pierre Scudo wrote," "taken from *La Pietra del paragone*, and a very beautiful duet belonging to *Aureliano in Palmira.*"

Fortunately, Rossini's position among opera lovers, in Paris as well as in Italy, was to be influenced by the appearance of a phenomenon that he and others long had supposed extinct: genuine Rossini singers of great brilliance in the older manner. Had the Turinese sisters Barbara and Carlotta Marchisio been born at the turn of the century rather than, respectively, in 1833 and 1835, Rossini might even have been wooed back to the composition of opera after *Guillaume Tell.* They appeared too late for that, but they were to give a new generation the opportunity to hear several of Rossini's operas sung as though the new manners of singing required by Halévy, Meyerbeer, and the middle-aged Verdi had not intervened—and were to be one chief reason for the creation of his last large composition, the *Petite Messe solennelle.*

Barbara Marchisio, a contralto–mezzo-soprano who had sung in concert in Turin when only sixteen, had been discovered by the impresario Bartolomeo Merelli. After further training, she had made her operatic debut in Madrid in 1856 as Rosina in *Il Barbiere di Siviglia.* Thereafter, she had successfully sung Azucena in *Il Trovatore*, the title role of *La Cenerentola*, and parts in Donizetti's *Linda di Chamounix* and *Lucrezia Borgia.* Her sister Carlotta, a soprano, had made her first operatic appearance in the title role of *Norma.* During the 1856–7 season, the sisters had also initiated their double career by appearing together in three Rossini operas: *Matilde di Shabran*, *Semiramide*—the work in which they were to be most celebrated—and *Guglielmo Tell* (in which Barbara sang the small role of Jemmy). Thereafter, they had continued to sing both separately and together; as a greatly admired duo, they added appearances in Rossini's *Otello* (Barbara as Desdemona, Carlotta as Emilia). Reaching La Scala, Milan, in the season of 1858–9, they evoked extraordinary excitement in *Semiramide* (thirty-three perform- ances), *Norma*, and Enrico Petrella's *Il Duca di Scilla*; in addition to appearances in other operas, they added at La Scala the next season *Il Trovatore* and *La Cenerentola.*

News of the Marchisios, and especially of their remarkable restora- tion of *Semiramide*, reached Paris quickly. The playwright Charles-

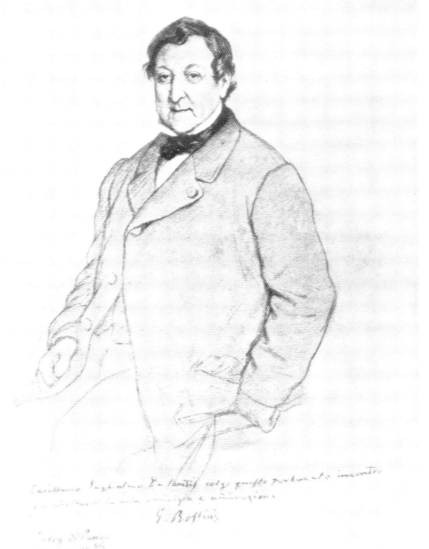

Carissimo Guglielmo De Sanctis colgo questo motivo tanto incontro
per dichiararle la mia amicizia e ammirazione

G. Rossini

Parigi d'Passoi

A.

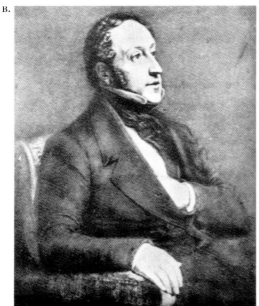

B.

A. Rossini in 1862,
    by Guglielmo De Sanctis

B. Rossini in 1843,
    by Ary Scheffer

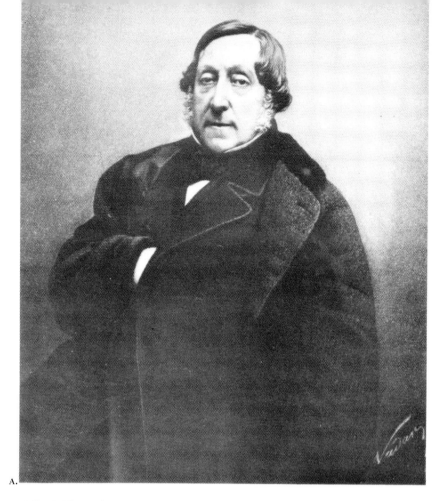

A. ROSSINI ABOUT 1858,
PHOTOGRAPH BY NADAR

B. THE CONSERVATORIO
ROSSINI, PESARO, WITH
DEATHBED SKETCH OF
ROSSINI BY GUSTAVE DORÉ

C. ROSSINI ABOUT 1860

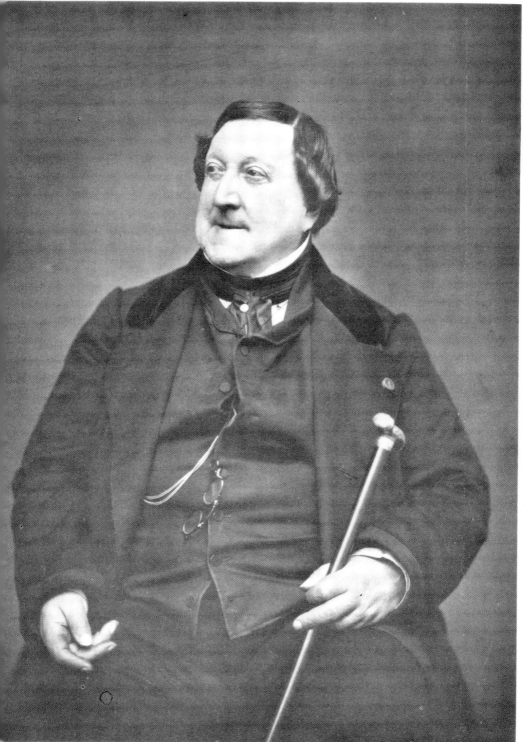

C.

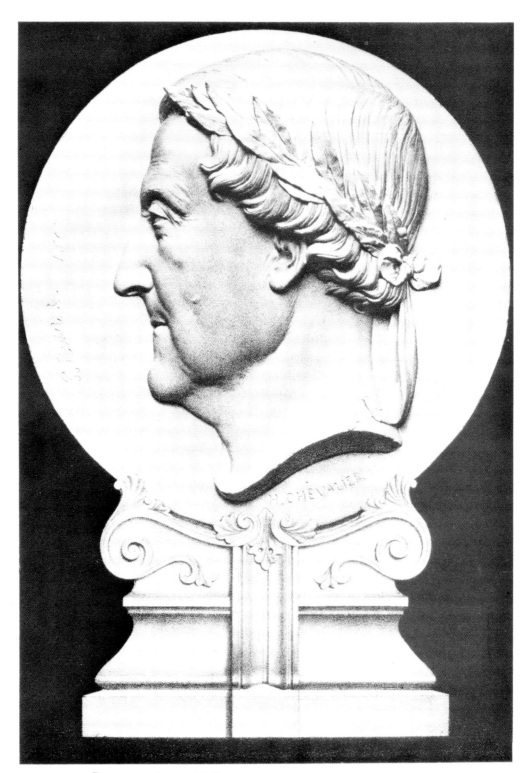

ROSSINI IN 1864, BY H. CHEVALIER

Camille Doucet had heard them as Semiramide and Arsace at the Teatro San Benedetto, Venice, where they had gone in the summer of 1858, and had spread word about them after his return to Paris. As Turinese, the sister sang French as well as Italian, and the management of the Opéra therefore became interested in them, sending Pierre-Louis Dietsch to Italy to bring back a full report on their qualities. He later said that not since the days of Malibran and Sontag had he heard the renowned second-act duet in *Semiramide* sung with such perfection. The Opéra management acted with eager swiftness, signing up the sisters for the summer season of 1860 and deciding to have them make their first Paris appearance in a French translation of *Semiramide*.

The translation of Rossi's libretto for *Semiramide* was entrusted to François-Joseph Méry, later to be one of the librettists of Verdi's *Don Carlos*. The Opéra directorship and Rossini gave Carafa the considerable task of reshaping to the French text in four acts the originally two-act score and of composing the music for the ballet that was mandatory at the Opéra. By a three-sided arrangement, Rossini assigned to Carafa, then seventy-two and not in a flourishing financial state, all author's rights in the French version of the thirty-seven-year-old score: "My dear Carafa: As it is proposed to stage my opera *Semiramide*, and as I take, as you know, no part in anything of this sort, I beg you to take charge, giving you the most complete latitude for all the arrangements that you will consider it necessary to make. Because the result will be your work, it will also be your property, and all author's rights, in the theater and outsde it, will belong to you. Your most affectionate G. Rossini."[n]

The Marchisio sisters, who had been singing at the Teatro Regio in Parma during the 1859–60 season, were in Paris rehearsing in *Semiramide* by early April 1860. Rossini, who evidently had heard them during a rehearsal, greeted them when they called at the Chaussée d'Antin with the words: "My dear babies, you have brought a dead man back to life!" The first performance of the extravagantly staged opera was given on Monday, July 9, in positively Ninevesque gorgeousness; the effect upon the audience was so overwhelming that twenty-nine repetitions were called for by mid-December. As the composer's royalty for each performance was about 500 francs, Carafa earned in a little over five months about 15,000 francs (more than $8,500).

In the second volume of his *L'Année musicale*, Scudo published a long review of the Marchisio *Semiramide*. He described Carlotta as "a dark young girl, somewhat plump, with a narrow forehead and a vivacious physiognomy, more intelligent than beautiful. Lacking elegance and plastic beauty, Carlotta owes her favorable reception to an extended, equal, soprano voice of sweet timbre, which is projected effortlessly and enters the ear moderately and caressingly. Her vocalizing is easy and brilliant . . . In the singing of this girl one notes an impetuosity of temperament which should, however, not be mistaken for the *élan* of passion. She is an Italian singer of the old school, caring more for the quality of the sound than for feeling, more for the musical phrase than for dramatic expression, desiring more to please than to move. Carlotta is excellently seconded throughout the opera by her sister Barbara, no better favored by nature as regards her physical appearance. She has a contralto voice which, though it does not have the depth or roundness of Alboni's, nonetheless is more even and does not present, running its range (of almost two octaves), that break in continuity from the chest tones to the others which usually is noticeable in contraltos. She vocalizes with the same ease as her sister, but her taste seems more secure and of higher quality . . . In the duet . . . between Semiramide and Arsace, the two singers fulfill themselves turn by turn; the fusion of these two voices, brought together by nature and by art, forms a combination perfect enough to recall the best days of the Théâtre-Italien. It is not grandiose art producing strong dramatic emotions; it is a delicate pleasure, a sensuality of the ear tempered by a light moral emotion that sweetly penetrates the heart: *per aures pectus irrigat*, as a Latin poet happily said. . . . But, in any case, the Rossinian *Semiramide*, interpreted by two such excellent singers and by M. [Louis-Henry] Obin,[n] constitutes a spectacle worthy of the Théâtre de l'Opéra and of the capital of the civilized world."

The Marchisios also sang at the Opéra in *Guillaume Tell* and at the Théâtre-Lyrique in a French version of *Il Trovatore*. When the Rossini-Carafa *Semiramide* was published in a handsome edition, Rossini presented a copy of it to them with this inscription: "To my beloved friends and incomparable interpreters, Carlotta and Barbara Marchisio, possessors of that song which is sensed in the soul." He was to make use of their special talents again in 1864. Carlotta died, aged only thirty-six, in 1872, but Barbara—who survived until 1919, dying at eighty-five[n]— would be heard at the Palazzo Vecchio, Florence, in May 1887 in the performance of the *Stabat Mater* sung in celebration of Rossini's re-burial in Santa Croce.

CHAPTER XVI

1860

DURING THE PREPARATIONS for *Semiramide* at the Opéra with the Marchisio sisters, Richard Wagner called on Rossini in the Chaussée d'Antin. It was March 1860. Wagner, who had completed *Tristan und Isolde* in his Swiss exile in August 1859, had come to Paris the next month, largely in the vain hope of achieving production of the new music drama there. In January 1860, he had conducted at the Théâtre-Italien (Salle Ventadour) three concerts consisting of excerpts from *Der fliegende Holländer*, *Tannhäuser*, and *Lohengrin* and the prelude to *Tristan*. He and his wife, Minna, were living at No. 16, rue Newton, near the Barrière de l'Étoile, when Edmond Michotte" took him to meet Rossini, of whom he had said in Michotte's presence: "Rossini—it's true that I haven't seen him yet; but he is caricatured as a great epicurean, stuffed not with music—of which he was emptied long ago—but with *mortadella*!"

Wagner had a personal motive beyond that of protocol for wanting to call upon Rossini. As Michotte interpreted it, Wagner "had no illusions, as goes without saying, about the welcome that a setting-forth of his doctrines would receive. . . . Also, it was not with the intention of being understood that Wagner had asked for the interview; but above all in the hope of being able to study psychologically at close range this strange musician, miraculously endowed, who, after so astonishingly swift a rise in the development of his creative faculties—from which *Guillaume Tell* finally emerged—then, at the age of thirty-seven, had had nothing more urgent [to do] than to separate himself from his genie as one disembarrasses oneself of an encumbering burden, in order to bury himself in the bourgeois *farniente* of a colorless life without worrying more about his art than if he never had practiced it. That was the phenomenon that attracted Wagner's curiosity, and which he wanted to be able to analyze."

That Wagner should have felt some bitterness toward Rossini was easily understandable. As Michotte wrote: "It was asserted that during one of the weekly dinners for which the composer of *Il Barbiere* brought together some noted guests, at the point at which the menu mentioned '*Turbot à l'allemande*,' the servants placed before the guests a very appetizing sauce, of which each of them then took his portion. Then nothing else was served. The turbot did not appear. The guests, perplexed, asked one another: What does one do with this sauce? Then Rossini, maliciously enjoying their embarrassment, and himself gulping down the same sauce: 'And so,' he exclaimed, 'you are still waiting for something? Enjoy this sauce; believe me, it's excellent. As for the turbot—alas! the principal dish . . . It is just . . . the fishman forgot at the last moment to bring it; don't be astonished. Isn't it the same with Wagner's music? . . . Good sauce, but no turbot! . . . no melody.'

"It also was said that another time a visitor entered Rossini's study and surprised the Maestro, all attention, turning the pages of an enormous score . . . That of *Tannhäuser.* After further efforts, he stopped: 'At last, this isn't bad!'—and he sighed. 'For half an hour I've been searching . . . now I'm beginning to understand some of it!'—The score was upside down and backwards! And behold, at exactly that moment, a loud fracas was heard from the adjoining room: 'Oh! oh! what's this,' Rossini went on, 'that polyphony: *Corpo di Dio!* but it strongly resembles the orchestra of the Venusberg.' Whereupon the door was opened brusquely and the valet entered to inform the Maestro that the maid had dropped a whole platter of cutlery!

"Impressed by these stories, which he believed to be true, Wagner, as is understandable, hesitated to present himself at Rossini's home. I took pains to reassure him. I made him understand that all those nonsensical stories were pure inventions that a hostile press amused itself by spreading to the public. I added that Rossini—whose character I was in a position to know through and through better than anyone else, as the result of long intimacy and daily contacts—had too lofty a mind to belittle himself by sillinesses that did not even have the merit of being intellectual, and against which he himself never stopped protesting vehemently. [Michotte adds here in a footnote: "In fact, Rossini just had published in the newspapers a denial on the subject of 'these malicious hoaxes.' He used to say that he feared two things in this world: *catarrhs* and journalists; that the former engendered *humeurs mauvaises* [distempers] in his body and the latter a *mauvaise humeur* [bad mood] in his mind."]

"I succeeded in undeceiving Wagner, assuring him that he could present himself at Rossini's without fear, that he would be received in the most cordial way. That decided him. He expressed the wish that I accompany and introduce him. The meeting was set for the morning two days later.

"Nevertheless, I forewarned Rossini, who replied at once: 'But that goes without saying; I'll receive M. Wagner with the greatest pleasure. You know my hours; come with him when you wish.' Then he added: 'Have you at least made him understand that I am an utter stranger to all the stupidities about him which have been attributed to me?' "" And so Michotte and Wagner presented themselves in the Chaussée d'Antin."

"When we were announced," Michotte's account reads, "the Maestro was just finishing his lunch. We waited for several minutes in the grand salon.

"There Wagner's glance fixed immediately upon a portrait of Rossini in which he was depicted half-length, life-size, wrapped in a long green mantle and with his head covered by a red cap—a portrait that has been reproduced in gravure and later became well known.

" 'That intellectual physiognomy, that ironic mouth—it was surely the composer of *Il Barbiere*,' Wagner said to me. 'This portrait must date from the era in which that opera was composed?'

" 'Four years later,' I told him. 'This portrait, painted at Naples by Mayer, dates from 1820.'

" 'He was a good-looking youth, and in that land of Vesuvius, where women take fire easily, he must have caused lots of ravages,' Wagner answered, smiling.

" 'Who knows?' I said. 'If he had had a valet as devoted to bookkeeping as Don Giovanni's Leporello, might he perhaps have surpassed the number *mil e tre* set down in the notebook?'

" 'Oh, you exaggerate,' Wagner answered, '*mil* I'll agree to, but *tre* more, that's really too many!'

"At this moment, the *valet de chambre* came to tell us that Rossini was awaiting us.

"As soon as we entered: 'Ah! Monsieur Wagner'—he said—'like a new Orpheus, you don't fear to enter this redoubtable precinct . . . '

(And without giving Wagner time to answer): 'I know that they have thoroughly blackened me in your mind . . .' [Michotte's footnote: "In reporting the conversation between the two masters, I have tried as much as possible to reproduce it in its integral form. It is quasi-textual, in particular as far as Rossini is concerned, he having married as his second wife Olympe Pélissier, a Parisian, and being used to speaking the French language, of which he knew all the fine points, argot included. As for Wagner, less familiar with this idiom, he frequently multiplied circumlocutions in the attempt to express his thought precisely.—I have thought it my duty at times to sum up in more concise and literary language what he said."]

" 'With regard to you, they load me with many quips that, furthermore, nothing on my part could justify. And why do I suffer from this fate? I am neither Mozart nor Beethoven. Nor do I pretend to be a wise man; but I do hold to that of being a polite one and of refraining from insulting a musician who, as you do—according to what I have been told—tries to extend the limits of our art. Those great devils who take pleasure in busying themselves about me should at least grant me, lacking other merits, that of having some common sense.'

" 'As for slighting your music, first I should have to know it; to know it, I should have to hear it in the theater, as it is only in the theater, and not by the simple reading of a score, that it is possible to bring equitable judgment to bear on music meant for the stage. The only composition of yours that I know is the march from *Tannhäuser*. I heard it often at Kissingen when I was taking a cure there three years ago. It produced a great effect and—I assure you sincerely—for my part, I found it very beautiful.'

" 'And now that all misunderstanding between us is, I hope, dissipated, tell me how you are finding your stay in Paris? I know that you are in discussions about staging your opera *Tannhäuser*? . . .' "

Wagner, after thanking Rossini for this friendly welcome, said: " 'Believe above all, I beg you, that even if you criticize me sharply, I shall take no offense. I know that my writings are of a nature to give birth to wrong interpretations. Faced with expounding a large system of new ideas, the best-intentioned judges can mistake their significance. This is because I am late in being able to make the logical and complete demonstration of my tendencies by performances of my operas as nearly complete and perfect as possible.'

"ROSSINI: 'That is fair; for deeds are worth more than words!' "

When Wagner, telling of his struggle to get *Tannhäuser* performed, mentioned the word "cabal," Rossini interrupted animatedly: " 'What composer has not felt them, to begin with the great Gluck himself? As for me, I have not been spared—far from it. On the evening of the *première* of *Il Barbiere*, when, as then was customary in Italy for *opera buffa*, I played the clavicembalo in the orchestra to accompany the recitatives, I had to save myself from a really riotous attitude on the part of the audience. I thought that they were going to assassinate me.'

" 'Here in Paris, where I came for the first time in 1824, having been summoned by the direction of the Théâtre-Italien, I was greeted with the sobriquet "Monsieur Vacarmini" ["Mr. Uproar"], which I still have. And it's not a thing of the past, I assure you, for me to be abused in the camp of some musicians and press critics leagued in a common accord—an *accord* as perfect as it is major!'

" 'It was no different in Vienna when I reached there in 1822 to mount my opera *Zelmira*. Weber himself, who furthermore had been fulminating against me in articles for a long time, pursued me relentlessly after the performances of my operas at the Italian court theater . . .' "[n]

" '. . . But we were talking about cabals,' Rossini continued. 'This is my opinion on the subject: there is nothing to be done about them except fight them with silence and inertia; that is more effective, believe me, than answers and anger. Ill will is legion; anyone who only wants to argue or, if you like this better, to fight against that sow will never strike the last blow. For my part, I spat on such attacks—the more they buffeted me, the more I replied with *roulades*; I fought sobriquets with my *triplets*, satires with my *pizzicati*; and all the hurly-burly stirred up by those who didn't like them never, I swear to you, was able to force me to give them one less blow on the big drum in my *crescendos* or to prevent me, when it suited me, from horrifying them with one more *felicità* in my finales. The fact that you see me with a wig, believe me, does not mean that those *b...utors* succeeded in making me lose a single hair from my head.' " [Michotte's footnote: "When, during the course of the conversation, his mind brought up some memory or some natural difficulty that excited him, he thought little of academic language to frame his thought, but gave free voice to vocables of which it is enough, I think, to underline the first letter for the rest to be divined."]

The conversation next turned to *Tannhäuser*. When Wagner spoke of the difficulty of completing the translation of the text into French,

Rossini said: "But why, in the manner of Gluck, Spontini, Meyerbeer, don't you start from the beginning by writing an opera with all the numbers adapted to a French libretto? Wouldn't you then be in a position to take into consideration the taste that predominates here and the special atmosphere of theatrical matters inherent in the French spirit?'

"WAGNER: 'In my case, Maestro, I don't think that that could be done. After *Tannhäuser*, I wrote *Lohengrin*, then *Tristan und Isolde*. These three operas, from both the literary point of view and the musical, represent a logical development of my conception of the definitive and absolute form of the lyric drama. My style has undergone the inevitable effects of that gradation. And if it is true that today I sense the possibility of writing other works in the style of *Tristan*, I swear that I am incapable of taking up my *Tannhäuser* manner again. Well, then, if I were in the position of having to compose an opera to a French text for Paris, I could not and should not follow any other road than the one that has led me to the writing of *Tristan*.'

" 'Further, a work like that, comprising such a disturbance of the traditional forms of opera, certainly would remain unappreciated and would have no chance, under the present conditions, of being accepted by the French.'

"ROSSINI: 'And tell me, what in your mind has been the point of departure for these reforms?'

"WAGNER: 'Their system was not developed all at once. My doubts go back to my first attempts, which did not satisfy me; and it was rather in the poetic conception than in the musical conception that the germ of these reforms suddenly entered my mind. My first works, in fact, had a literary objective above all. Later, preoccupied with the means to use in enlarging the meaning by the very penetrating addition of musical expression, I deplored the way in which the independence with which my thought was moving in the visionary realm was decreased by the demands imposed by routine in the form of the musical drama.' [Michotte's footnote: "One should not lose sight of the fact that Wagner was born in 1813."]

" 'Those *bravura arias*, those insipid duets manufactured fatally on the same model, and how many other hors d'œuvres that interrupt the stage action without reason! Then the *septets*! For in every opera that was to be respected, it was necessary to have a solemn septet in which the drama's characters, setting aside the meaning of their roles, formed a line across the front of the stage—all reconciled!—to come to a common accord (of often what accords, good Lord!) in order to supply the public with one of those stale banalities . . .'

"ROSSINI (interrupting): 'And do you know what we called that in my time in Italy? *The row of artichokes*. I assure you that I was perfectly aware of the silliness of the thing. It always gave me the impression of a line of porters come to sing in order to earn a tip. But what could you hope for? It was the custom; a concession that one had to make to the public, which otherwise would have thrown sliced potatoes at us . . . or even some that hadn't been sliced!'

"WAGNER (continuing without paying much attention to Rossini's interruption): 'And as for the orchestra, those routine accompaniments . . . colorless . . . obstinately repeating the same formulas without taking into account the diversity of the characters and situations . . . in a word, all that concert music, foreign to the action, with no reason for being there except the *convention*—music that in many places obstructs the most famous operas . . . all that seemed to me something contrary to good sense and incompatible with the high mission of an art noble and worthy of that name.'

"ROSSINI: 'Among other things, you just referred to the *bravura arias*. Well, what do you think? That was my nightmare. To satisfy at the same time the *prima donna*, the first tenor, the first bass! . . . there were those jolly fellows—without forgetting, above all, those of the terrible feminine gender—who thought it sensible to count the number of measures in one of their arias, then come to me to declare that they would not sing because another of their colleagues had an aria containing several measures more, not to mention a larger number of trills, or ornaments . . .'

"WAGNER (gaily): 'It was measured by a ruler! Nothing was left for the composer to do but take a musical *meter* as collaborator for his insiprations.'

"ROSSINI: 'Let's simply make it an aria-meter! Really, when I think of those people, they were wild animals. There you have the very people who, by making my head sweat, soon made me bald. But let's leave that and go on with your reasoning . . .

" 'In effect, and without replying, it seems to deal with the rational, rapid, and regular development of the dramatic action. Only—that independence claimed by the literary conception, how to maintain it in alliance with that of musical form, which is nothing but *convention*? You yourself used the word! For if one must obey the sense of absolute logic, it goes without saying that when speaking, one does not sing; an angry man, a conspirator, a jealous man does not sing!' (Humorously): 'An exception, perhaps, for lovers, whom, in a strict sense, one can have *coo* . . . But, even more forceful: does one go singing to one's death? *Convention* in the opera, then, from beginning to end. And the instrumentation itself? . . . Who, then, when an orchestra is unleashed, could pinpoint the difference of description for a storm, a riot, a fire? . . . always *convention*!'

"WAGNER: 'Clearly, Maestro, *convention*—and in very large amount —is imposed upon one, for otherwise one would have to do away completely with the lyric drama and even the comedy in music. It is none the less indisputable, however, that this convention, having been raised to the level of a form of art, must be understood in a way to avoid excesses leading to the absurd, the ridiculous. And there you have the abuse against which I am reacting. But they have wanted to muddy my thought. Don't they represent me as an arrogant man . . . denigrating Mozart?'

"ROSSINI (somewhat humorously): 'Mozart, *l'angelo della musica* . . . But who, short of sacrilege, would dare to touch him?'

"WAGNER: 'They have accused me, as if it were a mere trifle, of repudiating all existing operatic music—with rare exceptions, such as Gluck and Weber. They refuse, clearly with closed minds, to want to understand my writings. And in what a way! But far from denying the charm—*as pure music*—of lots of admirable pages in justly famous operas, or not myself feeling it, and in the highest degree, it is against the *role* of that music when it is condemned to be used as a purely diverting hors d'œuvre, or where, a slave to routine and foreign to the stage action, it is not systematically addressed to anything but the ear's sensuality—it is against that role that I want to rise up and react.

" 'An opera, in my view, being destined by its complex nature to have as its objective that of forming an organism concentrating the perfect union of all the arts that contribute to making it—the poetic art, the musical art, the decorative and plastic art—isn't this a disparagement of the musician's mission, this wish to confine him to being the simple instrumental illustrator of just any libretto, which imposes upon him in advance a summary number of arias, duets, scenes, ensembles . . . in a word, of *pieces* (pieces—that is to say, things cut up in the true sense of the word) which he must translate into notes, almost like a colorist filling in proofs printed in black? Certainly there are many examples of composers inspired by a moving dramatic situation who have written immortal pages. But how many other pages of their scores are diminished or nullified because of the vicious system that I am discussing! Well, as long as these follies persist, as long as one does not feel prevailing a complete reciprocal penetration by music and poem, or that *double conception,* based, from the start, on a single thought, the true music drama does not exist.'

"ROSSINI: 'That is to say, if I understand you correctly, that to realize your ideal, the composer must be his own librettist? That seems to me, for many reasons, to be an insurmountable condition.'

"WAGNER (very animated): 'And why? What reason is there against having composers, while they are learning counterpoint, study literature at the same time, search history, read legends? Which would lead them instinctively thereafter to become attached to a subject, poetic or tragic, related to their own temperament? . . . And then, if they lack ability or experience to arrange the dramatic intrigue, wouldn't they still be in a position to go to some practiced dramatist with whom they could associate themselves in a steadily maintained collaboration?

" 'Furthermore, among dramatic composers, there have been few, I think, who have not at times instinctively displayed remarkable literary and poetic aptitudes: rearranging or refashioning to their own taste either the text or the arrangement of a given scene which they have felt differently and understood better than their librettist. Not to go farther afield, you yourself, Maestro—let us take for example the scene of the oath-swearing in *Guillaume Tell*—would you tell me that you followed servilely, word by word, the text given you by your collaborators? I don't believe it. It is not difficult, when one looks at it closely, to discover in many places effects of declamation and of gradation which bear such an imprint of *musicality* (if I may say it that way), of *spontaneous inspiration,* that I refuse to attribute their genesis exclusively to the intervention of the textual scheme that was before your eyes. A librettist, whatever his ability, cannot know—above all, in scenes complicated by ensembles—how to conceive the arrangement that will suit the composer when creating the musical fresco as his imagination will suggest it.'

"ROSSINI: 'What you say is true. That scene, in fact, was drastically altered to my specifications, and not without trouble. I composed *Guillaume Tell* at the country house of my friend Aguado, where I was spending the summer. Out there, my librettists were not at hand. But

Armand Marrast and [Adolphe] Crémieux (parenthetically, *two future conspirators* against the government of Louis-Philippe), who also were staying at Aguado's country place, came to my assistance with changes in the text and versification which I needed in order to work out, as I had to, the plan of *my own conspirators* against Gessler.'

"WAGNER: 'There you have an implicit confession, Maestro, which already partly confirms what I have just been saying; it would be enough to enlarge that principle to establish that my ideas are not so contradictory, so impossible of realization, as they may appear at first.

" 'I assert that it is logically inevitable that, by an entirely natural evolution—perhaps a slow one—there will be born, not that *music of the future* which they insist upon attributing to me the pretension of wanting to give birth to all alone, but the *future of the music drama*, in which the general movement will play a part and from which will arise an orientation—as fecund as it will be new—in the concept of composers, singers, and public.'

"ROSSINI: 'In short, it is a radical revolution! And do you think that the *singers*—let's talk about them right away—habituated to displaying their talent in virtuoso singing, which is to be replaced, if I divine clearly, by a sort of *declamatory recitative*; do you think that the *public*, habituated to, let's use the word, the *vieux jeu*, will finally submit to changes so destructive of the entire past? I doubt it strongly.'

"WAGNER: 'There certainly will be a slow education to achieve, but it will be achieved. As for the public, does it form the masters, or do the masters form the public? Another situation in which I see an illustrious demonstration in you.

" 'Wasn't it, in fact, your very personal manner that made people in Italy forget all your predecessors; that won you, with unheard-of rapidity, an unexampled popularity? Well, Maestro, your influence, once having passed the frontier, didn't it become universal?

" 'As for the singers, whose resistance you cited to me as an objection, they will have to submit, to accept a situation that, furthermore, will improve their position. When they have perceived that the lyric drama in its new form will not furnish them, it is true, with the elements of easy success owing either to the strength of their lungs or to the advantages of a charming vocal organ, they will understand that nonetheless the art demands a much higher mission of them. Forced to give up isolating themselves in the personal limitations of their role, they will identify themselves with both the philosophic and the aesthetic spirit dominating the work. They will live, if I may express myself this way, in an atmosphere in which—*everything forming part of the whole*—nothing should remain secondary. Further, broken of the habit of ephemeral successes won by fleeting virtuosity, delivered from the torment of having to expend their voices on insipid words aligned in banal rhymes, they will perceive the new possibility of surrounding their names with a more glorious and durable aureole by incarnating the characters that they represent—incarnating them by complete penetration of their psychological and human *raisons d'être* in the drama; by basing themselves on deepened studies of the ideas, customs, character of the period in which the action takes place; by joining irreproachable diction to the prestige of masterly declamation, full of truth and nobility.'

"ROSSINI: 'From the point of view of *pure art*, those unquestionably are long views, seductive perspectives. But from the point of view of musical form in particular, this is, as I said, the fatal blow to declamatory melody—*the funeral oration of melody!* Otherwise, how ally expressive notation, to say it that way, of each syllable of the language to the melodic form, in which precise rhythms and symmetrical concord among the constituent elements must establish the physiognomy?'

"WAGNER: 'Certainly, Maestro, if applied and pushed with such rigor, such a system would be intolerable. But if you want to understand me correctly, note that far from brushing melody aside, on the contrary I demand it, and *copiously*. Isn't melody the vitality of every musical organism? Without melody, nothing is or could be. Only, let us understand one another: I demand that it not be the sort of melody which, shut up inside the narrow limitations of conventional procedures, submits to the yoke of symmetrical periods, persistent rhymes, foreseeable harmonic progressions, obligatory cadences. I want melody *free, independent,* unfettered. A melody particularizing by its own characteristic contour not only *each character* in such a way that he cannot be confused with another, but also *each event, each episode* inherent in the context of the drama. A melody of very precise form which, while conforming to the sense of the poetic text in its multiple inflections, can extend itself, contract itself, prolong itself [Michotte's footnote: " 'A melody in the struggle [*mélodie de combat*],' Rossini added quickly. But Wagner, carried along in what he was saying, paid no attention to that really droll interruption. I pointed it out to him later. 'For a *charge*,' he exclaimed, 'and, behold, at least one that is galloped into in a good corner of the mind. Ah! I'll remember that: *mélodie de combat* . . . A lucky hit!' "] according to the conditions required by the musical effect that the composer wants to obtain. And as for that sort of melody, Maestro, you stereotyped a sublime specimen in the scene of *Guillaume Tell*, "*Sois immobile*," where the very free song, accentuating each word and sustained by the breathing strokes of the violoncellos, reached the highest summits of lyric expression.'

"ROSSINI: 'So I made *music of the future* without knowing it?'

"WAGNER: 'There, Maestro, you made music for all times, and that is the best.'

"ROSSINI: 'I'll tell you that the sentiment that moved me most during my life was the love I had for my mother and my father, and which they repaid at usurious rates, I'm happy to tell you. It was there, I think, that I found the note that I needed for the scene of the *apple*—in *Guillaume Tell*.

" 'But one more question, Monsieur Wagner, if you'll permit me: how to fit into this system the simultaneous employment of two, of several, voices, as well as that of choruses? Should one, in order to be logical, forbid them? . . .'

"WAGNER: 'In fact, it would be rigorously logical to model musical dialogue on spoken dialogue, assigning the word to the characters one after the other. But, on the other hand, too, one admits that, for example, two distinct people can, at a given moment, find themselves in the same spiritual state—sharing a common feeling, and as a result joining their voices to identify themselves in a single thought. In the same way, several assembled characters, if there is a discussion involving the diverse feelings animating them, can sensibly use the faculty of expressing them simultaneously while each one individually determines what is his own.

" 'And do you understand now, Maestro, what immense, what infinite resources are offered to composers by this system of applying to each personage of the drama, to each situation, a typical melodic formula, susceptible in the course of action—while preserving its original character—of lending itself to the most varying, the most extended, developments? . . .

" 'Further, these ensembles in which each character exists in his individuality, but in which these elements are combined in a polyphony appropriate to the action, these ensembles no longer will present the spectacle, I repeat, of those absurd ensembles in which the characters, animated by the most contradictory passions, find themselves at a given moment condemned without rhyme or reason to unite their voices in a sort of *largo d'apothéose* in which the patriarchal harmonies only make one think "that one cannot be better than in the bosom of his family." [Michotte's footnote: "An allusion to the very popular finale [*"On ne saurait être mieux qu'au sein de sa famille"*] of *Lucile*, an opera by Grétry."]

" 'As to choruses,' Wagner continued, 'it is a psychological truth that the collective masses obey a determined sensation more energetically than the isolated man; such as dread, fury, pity . . . Then it is logical to admit that the crowd can express such a state collectively in the sound-language of the opera without a shock to good sense. Furthermore, the intervention of choruses, granted that it is logically required by situations in the drama, is a power without equal and one of the most precious agents of theatrical effect. Among a hundred examples, shall I recall the impression of anguish in the vivid chorus in *Idomeneo*—*"Corriamo, fuggiamo!"*—not to forget either, Maestro, your admirable fresco in *Moïse*—the very desolate chorus of the shades!? . . .'

"ROSSINI: 'Again!'—striking his forehead, and very amusingly— 'decidedly, then, I had—me too—some disposition for the *music of the future*? . . . You are salving my wounds! If I were not too old, I'd start over, and then . . . let the *ancien régime* beware!'

" 'Ah, Maestro,' WAGNER replied immediately, 'if you had not laid down your pen after *Guillaume Tell* at thirty-seven years—a crime!— you yourself don't know everything that you could have pulled from that brain there! At that time, you had done no more than begin . . .'

"ROSSINI: (returning to a serious tone): 'What would you have? I had no children. Had I had some, I doubtless should have continued to work. But, to tell you the truth, after having labored for fifteen years during that so-called very *lazy* period and having composed forty operas, I felt the need of rest and returned to Bologna to live in peace."

" 'Also, the state of the theaters in Italy, which during my career already left much to be desired, then was in full decay; the art of singing had darkened. That was to be foreseen.'

"WAGNER: 'To what do you attribute such an unexpected phenomenon in a country in which beautiful voices are superabundant?"

"ROSSINI: 'To the disappearance of the *castrati*. One can form no notion of the charm of their vocal organ and consummate virtuosity— which those best of the best possessed in default of something else, and by a charitable compensation. They also were incomparable teachers. To them generally was confided the teaching of singing in the master schools attached to the churches and supported at the churches' expense. Some of those schools were famous. They were real academies of singing. Pupils flocked to them, and a number of them frequently abandoned the choir lofts to devote themselves to a theatrical career. But after a new political regime was installed throughout Italy by my restless contemporaries, the master schools were suppressed and replaced with some *conservatories* in which, though good traditions existed, absolutely nothing of *bel canto* was *conserved*.

" 'As to the *castrati*, they vanished, and the usage vanished in the creation of new customs. That was the cause of the irremediable decay of the art of singing. It having disappeared, *opera buffa* (the best of what we had) was adrift. And *opera seria*? Audiences, who even in my time had showed themselves not very likely to raise themselves to the height of that great art, now showed no interest whatever in that sort of spectacle. The announcement of an *opera seria* on the posters usually had the result of attracting some plethoric spectators wanting to breathe in a cooling aria [a pun on the word air] remote from the crowd. There you have the reasons, and there were also others, why I judged that I had something better to do, which was to keep silent. I committed suicide, and *così finita la comedia* [*sic*].'

"Rossini rose, clasped Wagner's hands affectionately, adding: 'My dear Monsieur Wagner, I don't know how to thank you enough for your call, and particularly for the exposition, so clear and so interesting, that you have been kind enough to give me of your ideas. I who no longer compose, being at the age at which, rather, one *decomposes* while waiting to be truly *undecomposed*—I am too old to begin looking toward new horizons; but your ideas—whatever your detractors may say—are of a sort to make the young reflect. Of all the arts, music is the one which, because of its unsubstantial nature [*essence idéale*], is most exposed to transformations. They are unlimited. After Mozart, could one have foreseen Beethoven? After Gluck, Weber? And the end certainly is not after them. Each one must strive, if not to advance, at least to discover the new without worrying about the legend of a certain Hercules, a great traveler toward the visible, who, having reached a certain place beyond which things were no longer very visible, is said to have set up a column and then retraced his steps.'

"WAGNER: 'Was it perhaps a private hunting stake, to prevent others from going on farther?'

"ROSSINI: '*Chi lo sa?* Doubtless you are right, for one is assured that he displayed a brave predilection for hunting lions. Let us hope, however, that our art never will be limited by a placer of that sort of columns. For my part, I belonged to my time. To others, to you in particular, whom I see vigorous and impregnated with such masterly impulses, it falls to create the new and to succeed—which I wish you with all my heart.'

"Thus ended that memorable interview, in which, during the long half-hour that it lasted, these two men—in whom the intellectual verve of one aroused the humorous repartee of the other—never, as I can attest, had the air of being bored. . . .

"While going down the stairs, Wagner said to me: 'I swear to you that I didn't expect to find in Rossini the man who appeared before me. He is simple, natural, serious, and shows himself quick to be interested in all the points that I touched upon during this short talk. I couldn't set forth in a few words all the ideas that I develop in my writing about the conception that I have formed of the essential evolution of the lyric drama toward other destinies. I have had to restrict myself to some general views, citing practical details only when that could make the point immediately. But be that as it may, it was to be expected that my declarations would seem excessive to him, given the systematic spirit that prevailed when he made his career, and with which he necessarily remains deeply imbued today. Like Mozart, he possessed melodic inventiveness to the highest degree. Further, that inventiveness was marvelously seconded by his instinct for the stage and for dramatic expression. What might he not have produced if he had received a forceful and complete musical education? Especially if, less Italian and less skeptical, he had felt within him the religion of his art? There can be no doubt that he would have taken off on a flight that would have raised him to the highest peaks. In a word, he is a genius who was led astray by not having been well prepared and not having encountered the milieu for which his high creative abilities had marked him. But I must declare this: of all the musicians whom I have met in Paris, *he alone is truly great.* . . .'

"So I put my notes in order, and that same evening, as usual, went to Rossini's, where one always was sure to meet some real personalities. There I found, among others, Azevedo, a music critic attached to the journal of the *Opinion Nationale*, a fanatic Rossinian and one of the most violent persecutors of Wagner.

"Rossini, seeing him, addressed him banteringly: 'Eh, Azevedo, well! I saw him, he came . . . the monster . . . your *bête noire* . . . Wagner!'

"While the Maestro then moved on to talk with Carafa, Azevedo took me aside to ask for some details about that interview. But an instant later, Rossini came to interrupt us: 'You talked in vain,' he went on, addressing Azevedo. 'This Wagner—I must confess—seems to me to be endowed with first-class faculties. His entire physique—his chin most of all—reveals an iron-willed temperament. It's a great thing to know how to *will*. If he has to the same degree, as I believe he has, the gift of *being able*, he will get himself talked about.'

"Azevedo fell silent; but then he whispered in my ear: 'Why is Rossini addressing the *future*? This animal, zounds! now does nothing but talk too much about him in the *present*. . . .'

"I have said above that the two masters never met again.

"After the failure of *Tannhäuser* at the Paris Opéra, the French and some German journalists published at Wagner's expense new stories to which Rossini's name again was attached. Then some maladroit friends intervened—one asks with what aim—to present the Italian Maestro's attitude to Wagner's eyes in a disadvantageous light. They picture him as neither more nor less than a false good fellow. I tried to enlighten Wagner on this subject and tell him the exact truth. [Michotte's footnote: "I insisted above all that he should decide—with the aim of ending the persistence of these false rumors—to publish, *in extenso*, the account of all that had taken place during his interview with Rossini. . . . He refused. 'What good would it do?' he answered. 'With regard to what concerns his art and the way in which he practiced it, Rossini didn't tell me anything more than his works demonstrate. On the other hand, if I report the exposition of my theories as I sketched them for him, that will be, for the public, a repetition as brief as it would be useless, they being sufficiently divulged by my writings. Then there remains my appreciation of the man. Here, I confess to you, I was very much surprised to discover—if only in the way in which he talked to me about Bach and Beethoven—how much his intellect, nourished much more than I had thought on German art, showed itself to be superior. He grew swiftly in my estimation. Historically, the moment for judging him has not yet arrived. He is still in too good health and is too much in view as he strolls the length of the Champs-Élysées (I hear, from those who meet him, all the way from the place de la Concorde to the Barrière de l'Étoile) for it to be possible to assign him now the place that he will take up among the masters, his predecessors and contemporaries who walk now and forever in the Elysian Fields of the other world.' Wagner persisted in this view; one can detect it in the obituary article that he devoted to Rossini in 1868. There he held himself to a very summary account of the 1860 interview."]

"Rossini, no less annoyed, charged Liszt, among others, to invite Wagner to return to see him so that he might furnish indisputable proofs of his entire innocence. Wagner declined that invitation, giving as pretext that these pullulating tales would only increase more from the moment when the journals learned that he had paid another call on Rossini—that these men had not as yet, in this respect, overlarded their tittle-tattle with *Pater, peccavi*—that all this put him in a false position . . . that, furthermore, he kept himself from further discussion of Rossini, never having varied from the impression of profound sympathy for the nobility of his character which he [Wagner] had had since the first visit that he [Wagner] had paid him . . .

"That was the end of the matter. He remained obdurate, though I once again unsuccessfully renewed a final invitation on the part of Rossini when he charged me with returning to Wagner's house the score of the 'Graner' Mass, which Liszt had lent to the Maestro.

"I believe that the real reason for Wagner's refusal resided rather in the conviction that undertaking a second interview with the Italian master would profit him little. The purpose that he had proposed to himself in soliciting a first interview had, as I have explained, been achieved. He desired nothing further.

"The two masters, then, never saw one another again; but I can certify that whenever Rossini's name came from Wagner's lips or pen, the latter never departed from the deference and profound esteem that he had conceived for him. It was the same with Rossini, who later on often asked me about the success that Wagner's operas were meeting with in Germany, and regarding which he often charged me to transmit to the latter his congratulations and remembrances."

CHAPTER XVII

1860-1863

SIX MONTHS after receiving Wagner in the Chaussée d'Antin, Rossini welcomed to his Passy villa the man who came to be regarded as the foremost anti-Wagnerian: Eduard Hanslick. The Austrian writer published in the *Neue freie Presse*, Vienna, an extended account of his visit to Rossini. In part, it reads:[n]

"I found Rossini in his small study on the first floor of his Passy villa. He was in the midst of writing out a score, and the friendly expression on his face, as well as the welcoming, outstretched hand, seemed to apologize for the awkwardness with which he got up when I entered. Rossini's head, so different from the well-known portraits of him when he was at the height of his glory, still impresses one as that of a great and charming person. Beneath the philistine brown wig, there still is a cheerful, clear brow. The sparkle of his brown eyes is intelligent and friendly. The rather long though beautifully shaped nose, the fine, sensuous mouth, the round chin, testify to the old Italian's former good looks. From portraits, one would imagine Rossini taller than he actually is; and it is true that his massive head seems to suggest a taller body. Although handicapped by corpulence and increasing difficulty with his legs, Rossini insisted upon taking me to his downstairs parlor. Supported by a cane, he descended the stairs slowly and did the honors of his home with obvious pleasure. 'The whole villa,' he said, 'was built completely and furnished in fifteen months. A year and a half ago, the whole site was bare.' The walls and ceiling of the room are embellished with pleasant frescoes. Rossini himself chose their wholly musical subjects and then had them executed by Italian artists. One painting shows us Mozart summoned to the imperial box at the Opera by the Emperor

Joseph II after the performance of *Le Nozze di Figaro*. Another shows us Palestrina surrounded by his pupils, and so forth. The spaces between the larger pictures are occupied by portrait medallions of Haydn, Cimarosa, Paisiello, Weber, and Boieldieu—'*Mon très bon ami Boieldieu!*' my host repeatedly exclaimed. . . .

"The Maestro was in extremely high spirits, and was very talkative. I did not even feel the ugly temptation of so many tourists, who, for their own benefit, squeeze every famous person like a lemon. Memories of Vienna, which he had not seen since 1822, seemed to animate the old Maestro happily. At one point, he mentioned one of his own operas, *Zelmira*, which he composed for Vienna at that time. 'It was in Vienna,' he said in praise, 'that for the first time I found an audience that knew how to listen. I was quite overwhelmed by that attentive interest: in Italy, the audience chatters away during the music and becomes quiet only when the ballet begins.'

"An authentic description of Rossini's feelings about his enthusiastic biographer Stendhal (Henri Beyle) seemed too important for me to avoid a modest question about it. Rossini answered that he had seen this most charming of his admirers only once, but never had spoken to him. He had seen him in Italy at the home of the singer Pasta. Someone had told Rossini (probably in a spiteful, exaggerated way) that Stendhal had boasted of a close acquaintance with him, and he 'didn't want to have anything to do with such a liar.' I scarcely need mention that I pitied that scorned lover, now in his grave, and did not leave untried a well-intended rehabilitation of him.

"We sat down on a sofa from which we had a view of the sun-drenched flowerbeds in the garden. In front of us was a table covered with sheets of music; they were almost exclusively new arrangements from *Semiramide*, potpourris, impromptus, quadrilles, and similar stuff that the publishers dutifully had sent to the pillaged composer. A few months earlier, a French version of *Semiramide* had been performed at the Opéra, and so it had come back into vogue. . . . Rossini himself knew about the performance only from hearsay. He had not been to a theater in sixteen years, 'and it is at least that long,' he added, 'since anyone has known how to sing. They scream, they bellow, they wrestle!'

"He was much more interested in the latest political drama of the world itself than in 'the stage, which represents that world.' Despite his admiration for and confidence in Garibaldi, Rossini refused to give a favorable prognosis for the future of the Italian movement. 'I know my compatriots,' he said, shaking his head. 'They want more and more, and are never satisfied. Italy is too small for its many large cities; their mutual jealousies will never end, never will give way to voluntary subordination.'

"While Rossini went on talking in this pleasantly animated way, I was delighted to observe in his features the lively interplay between intelligence and kindly sincerity. His words and his appearance displayed that same childlike quality and naïvete which we notice to some degree in all men of genius. Having surrendered to the soft, smooth tides of secure leisure, never having aged beyond his joy in nature, art, or goodfellowship, incapable of any ambition, the old Maestro thus has lived the life of an epicurean sage for the past thirty years. As he no longer thinks about his own art or expects that others should do so, one can understand the pleasant objectivity with which Rossini surveys the contemporary musical scene; he is the disinterested spectator who watches without envy or bitterness, though not always without irony. . . .

"Great musical controversies and turning points, as, for example, *Zukunftsmusik* [music of the future], have no interest beyond curiosity for the composer of *Il Barbiere*. A year ago, Rossini took the baths at Kissingen. As soon as he appeared in the pump room, the band played selections from his operas. 'You can scarcely imagine how boring that was for me. I thanked the leader and told him that I'd much rather hear something that I didn't know, by Richard Wagner, for example.' He then heard the march from *Tannhäuser*, which he quite liked, and another piece that he no longer could recall. That's all he knew of Wagner. Rossini wanted to know a little something about the subject of *Lohengrin*. After I had explained it as briefly and clearly as possible, he exclaimed gaily in his funny accent: '*Ah, je comprends! C'est un Garibaldi qui s'en va aux nues!* ["Ah, I understand! It's a Garibaldi who ascends to the sky!"].' Richard Wagner had visited the old gentleman recently, and 'didn't seem at all like a revolutionary,' a description with which anyone who knows that dainty little man, that untiring and witty conversationalist, would gladly agree. Wagner, Rossini went on, introduced himself at once with the quieting assurance that he had not the slightest intention of overthrowing existing music, as people said he had. 'My dear sir,' Rossini interrupts him, 'that doesn't matter at all. If your revolution succeeds, then you were absolutely right; if you are unsuccessful, then you have miscalculated in any case, revolution or no revolution.' Rossini did not want to admit knowing about the malicious joke, currently being circulated in Paris, which compares Wagner's music to 'fish sauce without fish.' I would have believed him completely if he had not added in his droll, solemn manner: *'Je ne dis jamais de telles choses* ["I never say such things"].' Well, one knows so many and such certain *'de telles choses'* fathered by Rossini that his tendency to irony is completely beyond doubt. In that vein, he is credited with having exclaimed recently, after looking through a Berlioz score: 'How fortunate that this is not music!'

"The kindly gentleman was so untiring as both conversationalist and listener that I myself had to think of returning him to his quiet occupation. I therefore accompanied him back upstairs to his study, where he bade me a very cordial farewell. Because the famous master had become precious and dear to me as a person, I did not leave him without emotion. Along stately avenues and past gleaming villas, I ambled toward Saint-Cloud. Through open windows, like the perfume of roses, came the sweetest melodies of *Guillaume Tell.* Instinctively I touched my hat and saluted back toward the villa, its golden lyre sparkling like a little star."

At about the time of Wagner's and Hanslick's calls, Rossini also was visited by an impresario named Achille Montuoro, through whom he sent warm greetings to Giuseppe and Giuseppina Verdi. Under date of *"Primo aprile"* 1860 in the letter copybooks kept by Giuseppina (the renowned *"Coppialettere"*), this appears as part of a reply to Montuoro: "Does Rossini really love us? He is the eternal father of composers, past and present, but we had thought that the verb to love did not exist in his dictionary. [Crossed out is an alternative ending to the sentence: "that he does not love anyone."] For the rest, nobody more than us wishes that sovereign genius a long and happy life."

Many of the small compositions that Rossini was producing at this time were to be heard first at his Saturday-night musicales. In the beginning, he often gave copies of them to friends, but when he learned that two of them[n] had been published without his permission, he dispensed with presentation copies except on the rarest occasions. The music of the *samedi soirs* was by no means confined to Rossini's own. From information supplied him by Edmond Michotte from his collection of printed and handwritten musicale programs, now in the Library of the Royal Conservatory of Music, Brussels, Radiciotti compiled a partial list of the music heard at the musicales. Some of the performances and performers deserve to be recalled.

On January 22, 1859, for example, Adelaide Borghi-Mamo joined Giulia Grisi in the big duet from *Semiramide*; then Borghi-Mamo sang a number that Rossini had composed for and dedicated to her—and concluded with a Neapolitan song. Two weeks later, the program included *Le Paradis perdu*, a dramatic scene by Liszt's seventeen-year-old pupil Théodore Ritter (Bennett). The evening of February 26, 1859, included a new chamber opera by Galoppe d'Onquaire and Weckerlin, whose *La Laitière de Trianon* had been sung at the first *samedi soir*; called *Le Mariage en poste*, it was sung by Marie Mira, Biéval, and Bussine. Marie Taglioni and another ballerina danced the gavotte and Tyrolienne from *Guillaume Tell* while the singers present half-improvised from memory the chorus that accompanies these dances in the opera.

The program for April 1, 1859 (unusually, a Friday) was printed:

1. PRÉLUDE DE L'AVENIR, *for piano* . . . . ROSSINI
   Performed by Mme Tardieu [de Malleville]
2. *Duet from* L'ITALIANA IN ALGERI . . . . ROSSINI
   Sung by Messieurs Badiali and Bélart
3. *Cavatina from* IL BARBIERE DI SIVIGLIA . . . . . . ROSSINI
   Sung by Mme Alboni

---

1. *Caprice, for violin and piano, on* OTELLO . . . . . ROSSINI
   *Composed and performed by Messieurs Accursi
   and Stanzieri*
2. *Aria from the* STABAT, "PRO PECCATIS" . . . . . . ROSSINI
   Sung by M. Badiali
3. CHANSON ESPAGNOLE . . . . ROSSINI
   Sung by M. [Buenaventura] Bélart
4. GIOVANNA D'ARCO, *cantata* . . . . ROSSINI
   Sung by Mme Alboni

M. Schimon will be at the piano.

Radiciotti quotes from a published report on this program, but does not name the publication. The section of it referring to *Giovanna d'Arco* (the cantata that Rossini had presented to Olympe in 1832) in part reads: "What was awaited impatiently was *Giovanna d'Arco*; *tout Paris* was already discussing the promised performance of this unpublished cantata at least two weeks ago. When Rossini, giving his arm to Alboni, approached the pianoforte to accompany this composition himself, all those present felt a shudder of emotion; the eyes of the ladies were bedewed with tears. One thought involuntarily of all the masterpieces developed in that vast brain, of *Tancredi, L'Italiana in*

Algeri, Il Barbiere di Siviglia, Otello, La Cenerentola, La Gazza ladra,
Semiramide, Moïse, Le Siège de Corinthe, Le Comte Ory, Guillaume
Tell, and other admirable conceptions, and one felt I do not know what
sublime sensation at the thought that one was about to hear a still-
unknown work by that brilliant genius.

"At the moment for her to interpret her part, Mme Alboni was
unable to control her own agitation . . .

"Mme Alboni, after the first measures, had been able to overcome
her panic; she never had seemed so beautiful, so dramatic. At the end
of the piece, she threw herself into the arms of Rossini, who pressed
her emotionally to his heart. The success of this beautiful work was
enormous: Auber, Scudo, Poniatowski, Rothschild, Carafa, etc., surrounded the composer and loaded him with congratulations."

On Good Friday, March 29, 1861, the *Stabat Mater* was sung at
the Rossinis'. Barbara and Carlotta Marchisio, Cesare Badiali, and the
tenor Soleri were accompanied by a double string quartet, the members
of which included Antonio Bazzini and Gaetano Braga. On the Good
Friday of 1863, a long program included numbers from Pergolesi's
Stabat Mater and Rossini's; among the singers were Giulia Grisi,
Alessandro Bettini, Zelia Trebelli-Bettini, and Badiali. Three pieces
from the *Album de château* under the temporary titles of "*Prélude de
l'avenir*," "*Prélude de mon temps*," and "*Prélude de l'ancien régime*"[n]
were played by, respectively, Albert Lavignac, Louis Diémer, and
Jacob Rosenhain.

The program for the evening of March 31, 1865, again was printed.
It shows selections from *La Gazza ladra, Le Comte Ory, Le Siège de
Corinthe, La Cenerentola,* and *Guillaume Tell* sung by, among others,
Marie Battu, Jean-Baptiste Faure, and Louis-Henri Obin. Several
smaller Rossini pieces completed the musicale. Adelina Patti was one
of the performers on March 9, 1866 (there was a printed program),
taking part in ensemble numbers from *Moïse* and *Il Barbiere di Siviglia*
and singing Desdemona's romance from *Otello.* That program also included an aria from Verdi's *Un Ballo in maschera,* sung by Enrico Delle
Sedie, and the trio from *Crispino e la comare* by the Brothers Ricci;
among the other singers were Italo Gardoni and Antonio Tamburini.
On Holy Saturday 1866, the Rossinis' dinner guests included Liszt and
Camillo Sivori; a promised singing of the *Stabat Mater* had to be canceled because of a singer's indisposition, and the substitute program
included the tenor song "*Il Fanciullo smarrito*" and a baritone *cabaret*

chansonette" entitled "*Le Lazzarone*," with text by Émilien Pacini, a satire on gluttony which includes the indication "Spoken while smacking the lips."

A miscellaneous program heard on April 17, 1866, provided music by Rossini, Jean-Baptiste Faure, Mozart, and Gounod.[n] A note states that the pianist will be M. Maton, the harmonium player M. Savignac (*sic*), the violinist M. Sarazate (*sic*); the singers included Faure and three Maries—Battu, Miolan-Carvalho, and Sass-Castelmary;[n] the chorus of

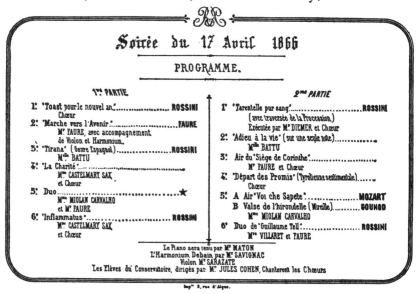

Conservatoire pupils was directed by Jules Cohen. *Le Ménestrel* thus reported the evening of April 18, 1868 (Rossini was then seventy-six): "The only evening *de rigueur* given this year in Rossini's home took place last Saturday: heard were, among the singers, Mmes Alboni and Battu, Mm. Delle Sedie and Gardoni; among the instrumentalists, the pianists Diémer and Lavignac, and the violinist Sivori. As usual, the Maestro's unpublished works made up the chief offerings of the concert; and they left no one discontented. Mme Alboni sang a song on the Chinese scale,[n] which is both a real masterwork and a tour de force of composition: it is a scale made up of six tones without semitones: C, D, E, F-sharp, G-sharp, A-sharp, C.[n] This daring and curious manner of singing the scale produces very odd harmonic combinations; and nonetheless one would believe them very natural. In short: it is a discovery by the Maestro (and he is fully capable of them).

"Then Mme Battu sang the cantilena on a single note and the tenor Gardoni '*Il Fanciullo smarrito*,' a veritable jewel. M. Lavignac played '*Un Rien*,' the '*Barcarolle vénitienne*,' the '*Valse de boudoir*'; M. Diémer '*Un Profond Sommeil*'; and, finally, Sivori '*Un Mot à Paganini*,' an admirable elegy written for the violin with the ability with which *Il Barbiere* was written for the voice, and performed . . . as Sivori knows how to do it. The accompanying piano was in the hands of the excellent Peruzzi."[n]

R

Soirée du 1 Mars 1867.

PROGRAMME.

1ʳᵉ PARTIE.	2ᵐᵉ PARTIE.
1ᵉ Petite Fanfare à 4 mains..............ROSSINI Exécutée par l'Auteur et M. DIEMER	1ᵉ Romance del 'Ballo in Masquera'............VERDI M. DELLE-SEDIE.
2ᵉ Duo du 'Mariage secret'..............CIMAROSA M. AGNESI et ZUCCHINI.	2ᵉ Terzetto da 'Camera......................COSTA M. A. PATTI, M. GARDONI et GALVANI.
3ᵉ Duo de 'la Traviata'..................VERDI M. A. PATTI, M. GARDONI.	3ᵉ Le 'Lazzarone' (Paroles de M. PACINI).......ROSSINI M. BARRÉ.
4ᵉ Spécimen de mon temps............ROSSINI Exécuté par M. PLANTÉ.	4ᵉ Ouverture de 'Semiramide'..............ROSSINI M. PLANTE.
5ᵉ Cavatina 'Semiramide'............ROSSINI M. A. PATTI.	5ᵉ 'Il Fanciullo Smarrito'..............ROSSINI M. GARDONI.
6ᵉ Terzetto 'Italiana in Algeri'............ROSSINI M. GARDONI, AGNESI et ZUCCHINI.	6ᵉ Quartetto 'Rigoletto'..................VERDI M. A. PATTI et LLIANNES, M. GARDONI et DELLE-SEDIE.

PIANO : M. PERUZZI

Lith. Carbuck, 3, r. d'Alger.

The last of the Rossini musicales was held on September 26, 1868. *Le Ménestrel* said: "The Saturday evening at the Rossini home must be included among the most brilliant of the season: Mme Alboni, Mme [Christine] Nilsson, and M. Faure, no less; Mme Nilsson murmured her *Swedish airs* with moving grace; M. Faure sang like a great artist a poetic sonnet of Maître Duprat; Mme Alboni repeated for at least the twentieth time an adorable song by Rossini composed on the tonal base of what he called the *Chinese scale*. At the close, M. Lavignac performed on the piano some unpublished works by the Maestro." With that evening, the *samedi soirs* came to an end: Rossini lived only fifty days more.

In the summer of 1860—between the visits of Wagner and Hanslick —the renowned pianist, teacher, and composer Ignaz Moscheles visited his son Felix in Paris. The boy had seen Rossini several times after meeting him during an earlier visit from his father. They went to call upon Rossini in Passy. Moscheles and his wife later wrote:[n]

"Felix has been made quite at home in the Villa on former occasions. To me the 'Parterre Salon,' with its rich furniture, was new, and before the Maestro himself appeared, we looked at his photograph in a circular porcelain frame, on the sides of which were inscribed the names of his works.[n] The ceiling is covered with pictures illustrating scenes out of Palestrina's and Mozart's lives; in the middle of the room stands a Pleyel piano. When Rossini came in he gave me the orthodox Italian kiss, and was effusive in expressions of delight at my re-appearance, and very complimentary on the subject of Felix. In the course of our conversation, he was full of hard-hitting truths, and brilliant satire on the present study and method of vocalization. 'I don't want to hear anything more of it,' he said, 'they scream! And all that I want is a resonant full-tone, not a screeching voice. I care not whether it be for speaking or singing; everything ought to sound melodious.' He then spoke of the pleasure he felt in studying the piano; and 'if it were not presumption' (he added), 'in composing for that instrument; in playing, however, his fourth and fifth fingers would not do their duty properly.' He complains that the piano is, now-a-days, only maltreated. 'They not only thump the piano, but the armchair, and even the floor.'"

Rossini told an anecdote of his early years. Visiting a small Italian town, he had been routed out of bed by the resident *maestro di cappella* and borne off to hear one of his own operas—in the performance of which he had to substitute for a missing doublebass player. "This reminded me," Moscheles goes on, "of what I once experienced to my cost at York, when the parts of the of the tenor and the lowest bassoon for Mozart's symphony in D major were missing. On the piano I showed Rossini what the effect was. He laughed heartily, and then asked for a little real music; after I had extemporized, he said: 'Is that printed? It is music that flows from the fountain head. There is reservoir water and spring water; the former only runs when you turn the cock, and is always redolent of the vase, the latter always gushes forth fresh and limpid. Now-a-days people confound the simple and the trivial; a motif of Mozart they would call trivial if they dared.' When we talked of the Leipzig 'Conservatoire,' he was delighted to hear that encouragement was given to the serious study of organ-playing, and he complained of the decay of Church music in Italy. He was quite enthusiastic on the subject of Marcello's and Palestrina's sublime creations. . . . When

I next came, Rossini, yielding to my request, but not without modestly expressing diffidence in his own powers, played an Andante in B flat, beginning somewhat in this style:

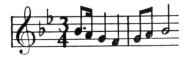

in which, after the first eight bars, the following interesting modulation was introduced:

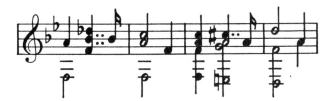

The piece is what we Germans would call tame. He then showed me two manuscript compositions, an Introduction and Fugue in C major, and a sort of pastoral Fantasia, with a brilliant Rondo in A major, which I had to play to him. When I added a ♮ to the manuscript, he declared 'it was worth gold to him.' Clara, who was with me, and had already mustered up courage sufficient to sing my *'Frühlingslied'* and *'Botschaft,'* to Rossini's satisfaction, was obliged to repeat both songs before the singers Ponchard[n] and [Nicholas-Prosper] Levasseur, who had just stopped in. I accompanied, and in answer to Rossini's observation that I had enough flow of melody to write an opera, rejoined, 'What a pity that I am not young enough to become your pupil!' I then had to play from his manuscripts, and that raised me 'to the kingship of pianists.' 'Whatever I am,' I replied, 'is due to the old school, the old master Clementi,' and on my mentioning that name, Rossini goes to the piano, and plays by heart fragments out of his Sonatas."

Shortly after Moscheles left Paris, his son Felix wrote to him about other meetings with Rossini. "The conversation turning upon German music," he reported, "I asked him 'which was his favourite amongst the great masters.' Of Beethoven he said: 'I take him twice a week, Haydn four times, and Mozart every day. You will tell me that Beethoven is a Colossus who often gives you a dig in the ribs, whilst Mozart is always adorable; it is that the latter had the chance of going very young to Italy, at a time when they still sang well. . . .' I asked him if he had met Byron in Venice? 'Only in a Restaurant,' was the answer, 'where I was introduced to him; our acquaintance, therefore, was very slight; it seems he has spoken of me, but I don't know what he says.' I translated for him, in a somewhat milder form, Byron's words, which happened to be fresh in my memory: 'They have been crucifying Othello into an Opera, the music good but lugubrious, but, as for the words, all the real scenes with Iago cut out, and the greatest nonsense instead, the handkerchief turned into a billet-doux, and the first singer would not black his face—singing, dresses, and music very good.' The Maestro regretted his ignorance of the English language, and said, 'In my day, I gave much time to the study of our Italian literature. Dante is the man I owe most to; he taught me more music than all my music-masters put together, and when I wrote my "Otello" I would introduce those lines of Dante—you know—the song of the Gondolier. My librettist would have it that gondoliers never sing Dante, and but rarely Tasso, but I answered him, 'I know all about that better than you, for I have lived in Venice, and you haven't. Dante I must have and will have. . . .'

"Rossini has in the kindest way composed a piece expressly for my imitation of the French horn, and written it into my album; it is exactly adapted to my voice, or rather to my blowing powers. Above is this inscription:

" 'Thème of Rossini, followed by two variations and Coda by Moscheles père,' offered to my young friend Felix Moscheles.

G. Rossini, Passy 20th August 1860.'

"On receipt of a copy of this piece, which was forwarded to Moscheles, he at once carried out Rossini's suggestion, and after writing the 'Two Variations and Coda,' asked the Maestro's permission to dedicate to him the work in the amended form. The following answer was received:

" 'Paris, Passy, 1861.

" 'MON MAITRE (DE PIANO) ET AMI,—

" 'Allow me to thank you for your friendly letter. Nothing could or should be more agreeable to me, more flattering, than a dedication from you. This testimony of your affection is an inestimable prize in my eyes. I thank you with all the warmth I have and which has not yet frozen my old heart.

" 'You asked me for authorization to have engraved the little theme that I noted down for your dear son;—it is granted you. Nothing more of an honor, dear friend, than to associate my name with yours in this little publication, but alas! what is the role that you are making me play in so glorious a marriage? That of the composer granting you, the great patriarch, exclusivity as a pianist. Why don't you want to admit into the great family one more, what! although I have put myself very modestly (but not without lively suffering) in the category of pianist of the fourth class? Do you want, then, dear Moscheles, to make me die of chagrin?

"'You will succeed, you great pianists, in treating me as a Pariah, yes, you will be responsible, before God and before men, for my death.

"'Please remember me to Madame and the dear children while accepting for yourself the sincere affection of your heartfelt friend.

G. ROSSINI.'"

On January 22, 1860, Rossini composed, signed, and dated a page of music that his friend the Sienese inventor Giovanni Caselli[n] wanted to telegraph from Paris to Amiens as a demonstration of his new *pantele-grafo*. In 1887, at the time of the removal of Rossini's body from Paris to Florence, the exhibition of Rossini autographs displayed at the Circolo Filologico in Florence included that page, together with the pantele-graphic reproduction of it. During the late 1850's and early 1860's, too, Rossini occasionally attended daytime informal musicales at the homes of musicians and other friends, including the Vicomtesse Grandval, the composer-violinist Adolphe Blanc, and Comte and Comtesse Frédéric Pillet-Will.

Rossini's residences in the Chaussée d'Antin and Passy continued to be waystations through which musicians passed en route from Italy to other parts of Europe. Often they elicited from him one of his very numerous letters of introduction and recommendation. In June 1859, he gave Mme Miolan-Carvalho such a letter to Costa in London, heading it: "One of the High Priests of the Musical Temple of Paris to the Supreme Pontiff of the Musical Temple of London." On May 30, 1861, again writing to Costa—this time to introduce Joseph Wieniawski— he told his "Dearest Son": "Here again is one of my paternal autographs for you. In France, they bring twenty sous; in England, given the im- mense wealth of the Country, they ought to sell for at least Two *Scel- lini* [shillings]. Let the buyer beware! ! !" The jocular, self-depreca- tory tone persist through most of the letters to Costa, whatever their real subject.[n]

In June 1861, a commission making arrangements for the London Exhibition of 1862 addressed Auber, Meyerbeer, and Rossini, asking each composer to provide a new piece to be performed during the opening-day ceremonies. Declining to compose such a piece, Rossini wrote: "If I were still of this musical world, I should feel it a duty and pleasure to prove on this occasion that I am not at all forgetful of England's noble hospitality."[n] He reacted differently, however, when invited to provide a composition for a concert to be given by the Société des Concerts du Conservatoire to raise funds for the Florentine committee charged with erecting a monument to Cherubini (who had died in Paris on March 15, 1842). The result was to be one of his most extraordinary compositions.

Earlier, Rossini had composed for Conte Pompeo Belgiojoso *Le Chant des Titans*, a piece for four bass voices in unison, to a text in French by Émilien Pacini dealing with a furious assault on Mount Olympus by Titans. An incomplete autograph score of it at Pesaro (it has only vocal, harmonium, and bassoon parts) bears the following description after the title: "(*Encélande, Hypérion, Coelus, Polyphème, 4 fils de Titan, le frère de Saturne). Avec accompagnement de piano et d'harmonium, pour quatre voix de basses—de haute Taille—Soli à l'unisson. Paroles de E. Pacini*"; at the bottom of the last page, Rossini wrote: "*Laus Deo—G. Rossini, Passy September 15, 1861*" The sanguinary text begins: "*Guerre! Massacre! Mort! Carnage!/Fils de Titan, que votre rage / Venge enfin un trop long outrage / Par le glaive exterminateur!*" Now Rossini arranged the accompaniment for large orchestra, calling for at least eighty-four performers, preferably more —plus the original four bass voices. And on October 5, 1861,[n] he wrote to Alphonse Royer, then director of the Opéra, where the Cherubini memorial concert was to be held:

"Monsieur et ami. In view of a request sent me by the Committee of the Société des Concerts du Conservatoire de Musique, I just have obtained the favor of the performance of a little vocal piece of my composing, which should be given by the aforementioned society for the raising of a monument to the honor and memory of the learned and celebrated Cherubini. I have composed my piece for four bass voices (of the highest quality) *in unison*. It is entitled *Le Chant des Titans*, and for that performance I need four gallant fellows. I request them from you, who are the happy director. Here are the names: Belval, Cazaux, Faure, Obin *a perfetta vicenda* [in perfect order]! As you see, I note them in alphabetic order to prove to you that I have not at all forgotten the theatrical conventions! ! ! Would you, my dear

Monsieur Royer, give me a new mark of your sympathy by making yourself my interpreter to these *messieurs*, asking them in my name to lend me their presence for the performance of my *Chant des Titans*, in which, *be reassured*, there is not the smallest roulade, chromatic scale, trill, or arpeggio; it is a simple chant in a rhythm that is titanic and ever so little violent. One small rehearsal with me, and everything will be said! If my health permitted, I should very gladly go (as would be my duty) to see your valiant artists, to ask the favor I aspire to: alas! my friend, my legs bend just as much as my heart leaps, and this heart comes to you in advance to testify to all its lively gratitude. It guides my hand in reiterating to you feelings of the greatest esteem and the sincere friendship of your affectionate GIOACHINO ROSSINI, pianist of the fourth order."

Le Chant des Titans was sung for the first time at the Opéra on December 22, 1861. It was to be sung again in Vienna on April 15, 1866, during a concert given to raise funds for a monument to Mozart; on that occasion, the program would include another Rossini piece, *La Notte del Santo Natale*, a pastorale for bass and eight-voice chorus which he had composed in 1863 (when it had been sung at one of the *samedi soirs*). On June 6, 1863, Rossini had written to someone in Vienna, evidently in the belief that the performance was to occur soon:[n]

"Illustrious Sir,

"Instructions and prayers that I permit myself to address to the organizer of the Mozart concert and its program. I write in Italian, my native tongue, because I know that it is very familiar in Vienna.

"I have sent two of my unpublished compositions to the illustrious Austrian consul to be forwarded to Vienna and performed during the aforementioned concert:

"I.—*La Nuit de Noël* (pastorale in the Italian style)[n]

"II.—*Le Chant des Titans*.

"These two pieces should be performed in the order indicated above: I and II. For the first, in addition to the solo bass, there is needed a piano, or two pianos in unison if the place is large, with the harmonium (or the old philharmonicon). Twelve voices will suffice for the chorus. Of this piece, I send the score and some vocal parts.

"For the second piece, *Les Titans*, four first basses of vigorous and extended voice are required, men of warm spirit so that they can emphasize the rhythms of this composition strongly, they being its chief foundation. For it, I send the score, the orchestral and tam-tam parts, and the vocal parts.

"I should wish these two numbers (one after the other, be it understood) to be performed at the beginning of one of the sections of the concert (the opening number excluded).

"I declare myself proud and happy to be able, by a small homage, to contribute to honoring the memory of the veritable Titan of music, Mozart, whom I began to admire in my adolescence and who always was my idol and my master. May the Viennese—who were so courteous to me during my stay among them in 1822—accept the homage that I am happy to offer to their great and immortal fellow townsman and be indulgent *once more* toward my two compositions, which are the work of an old adorer of Mozart.

G. Rossini.

"P.S.—In the supposition that my compositions must be translated into the German language, I beg the poet-translator to preserve well the prosody and the musical rhythms. It remains clearly understood that, once the performance at the concert has taken place, my compositions (scores and parts) will be sent to their composer in Paris by the agency of the aforementioned Austrian consul, and that it remains forbidden to make any copy *under penalty of the law*, the proprietary right being reserved exclusively by the composer."[n]

One week after the singing of *Le Chant des Titans* at the Opéra, *La Revue et Gazette musicale* said of the piece that it "had greatly astonished the listeners: Rossini never has showed himself in this formidable aspect, and something different was expected from him. A repetition was demanded, as if by one voice. The orchestra began again, and then the composition was understood a little better; but in order for it to have been understood completely, it would have been necessary for the words to be printed and distributed to the listeners: which doubtless will be done another time." The critic then remarked on the savage accents and explosions of sound adapted to the text. The real Rossinian vocal line was not in it, he wrote, the vocal part being only a series of savage vociferations. He found the orchestral effects unprecedented, though the composer had not employed extraordinary means: trumpets and trombones entered only at intervals; percussion appeared only at the end.[n] The effect, he concluded, was produced by wise disposition of the parts and by the grouping of the instruments, by the choice of chords and modulations, and by the vigorous nature of the reiterated instrumental pattern that formed the texture of this highly original composition.

Rossini, meanwhile, was not being forgotten by Italy. On August 19, 1861, he addressed Conte Costantino Nigra, the notable diplomat-poet-philologist who was then Italian ambassador to France: "Excellency, if my uncertain health did not prevent me, I should be at your residence the coming Thursday before noon to present my gratitude and take the oath according to the Statute of the Order of Knights of the Order of Civil Merit of Savoy, which His Majesty Vittorio Emanuele II, in his sovereign benevolence, has deigned to confer upon me. May it please Your Excellency to believe me, with profound esteem, your most devoted servant." The sovereign of newly united Italy was honoring one of his most famous subjects.

During 1862, the Italians visiting Paris who flocked to the Rossinis' included Franco Faccio and Arrigo Boito,[*] who arrived together with a warm introduction to Rossini from Tito Ricordi. The two young men were at the Opéra on December 22 for *Le Chant des Titans*, which they admired intensely, seeing in it a promise that their own music—which they judged to be the new and future music—might eventually make its way. Boito reported that a female admirer had told Rossini that she found *Le Chant des Titans* "*très gracieux*," and that Rossini, astonished by the inapplicability of the adjective, had replied: "Oh, Madame, it's nothing but a jest!" Boito and Faccio were allowed to show their host the score of their collaborative patriotic cantata *Le Sorelle d'Italia*. He appears to have praised it, for on April 1, 1863, Boito's brother Camillo wrote to him: "I am glad that Rossini has liked your music; he is not much of man for understanding every forward step." The young visitors returned several times to see Rossini; as early as December 19, 1862, Camillo had written to Arrigo: "I am glad that Rossini has taken you under his wing—he can be a great help to the young; and that wherever; a word from him, venerated as the God of Music—could put you both on solid ground."

When, in April 1863, Boito and Faccio were about to leave Paris, they went to bid farewell to Rossini. He gave each of them a signed photograph of himself, using the word "colleague" in both inscriptions and calling Boito "*mio caldo collega*" (roughly, "my ardent colleague"). Then he handed each of them a small packet, saying: "Everything can be useful to the young." Descending the stairs, the two men could not restrain their curiosity. To their hilarious amazement, the packets contained all of the calling cards that they had left at the Rossinis' during their stay in Paris.

When Tito and Giulio Ricordi saw Rossini in Paris in 1867,[n] he remarked: "Speaking of music, I met two attractive young men from your Conservatory: Faccio and . . . Goito." Giulio Ricordi corrected him: "Boito." And Rossini went on: "That's right, Boito; but what a Devil of a name! . . . it's always difficult for me to pronounce, and I start out with a G to get to the B. What is your Boito doing? . . . I liked him very much: I think that he has the stuff in him for something out of the ordinary! What pleasure I'd feel for Italy. Giulio, who surely must be Boito's friend, will send me word of that young fellow's doings, as he ought to get himself talked about soon." A few weeks after the failure of the first version of Boito's *Mefistofele* (La Scala, March 5, 1868), Rossini wrote to Tito Ricordi: "I want to be remembered to Boito, whose fine talent I appreciate infinitely. He sent me his *Mefistofele* libretto, from which I see that he wants too precociously to be an innovator. Don't believe that I war on innovators! I only wish that what might be attained in a few years not be done in a day. Let dear Giulio read *Demetrio e Polibio*, my first work, *benignly*, and *Guglielmo Tell*; he'll see I wasn't a crawfish."

In the spring of 1862, the Roman painter Guglielmo De Sanctis (1829–1911), who had met Rossini in Florence in 1851, was in Paris. Sixteen years later, he published[n] an account of his May–June 1862 meetings with the seventy-year-old composer. At Florence, he had thought Rossini sarcastic and bitter; when he had remarked that to have one's name universally known must be a satisfaction, Rossini had answered: "That's all very well, but glory is no compensation for the trials of living." In Paris, De Sanctis found a much less acerb and embittered man, though one still without illusions. During his first call at the Chaussée d'Antin, two Frenchmen who also stopped in fawned on Rossini, murmuring fulsome compliments. After they left, Rossini said to De Sanctis: "We've been going through the usual. I'm condemned always to listen to the same things, which drive me to take a dislike to the human species." He invited the painter to come to Passy the next Friday and bring some of his sketches.

Taken into Rossini's bedroom-study at the villa on May 10, De Sanctis found his host writing. The old man glanced up, noticed that the caller was carrying a portfolio, and said very brusquely: "Have you perhaps come to make a portrait of me? Never, because I haven't the patience to sit still, and being a model agitates my nerves and keeps me from sleeping. Well, believe me, maybe you'd have more success working from a photograph." De Sanctis reminded him of the invitation to bring samples of his work. "If that's it," Rossini said, calming down, "then come in." He pushed aside the pages on which he had been working, had De Sanctis place the portfolio on the table, and carefully examined the sketches, which included portraits from life. Then, preparing to leave, De Sanctis said: "For ten years a page has been reserved for Rossini, but now that he has refused, I must resign myself to his decision." Completely mollified, Rossini said: "Listen, if you'd be satisfied to sketch me while I'm writing, so that I wouldn't be forced to remain still, then come whenever you like and stay here as long as you think necessary and as pleases you." This about-face so elated De Sanctis that he walked some distance from the villa before realizing that a fine drizzle was falling.

On May 14, De Sanctis was at the villa while Rossini downed his usual large cup of *café au lait*, into which he dipped pieces of bread. Then, as they walked toward the bedroom-study, Rossini stopped to strum a few chords on the piano. Taking courage, De Sanctis asked to hear him play. Rossini hesitated, he wrote, letting "his pudgy hands run along the keyboard with a light touch, eliciting very sweet chords with so little effort that one scarcely could perceive the motion of his fingers." Then Rossini said: "If you want to hear me play, I warn you that I'm a second-class pianist. The pieces that you'll hear are among my recent compositions, and I have called them '*Une Caresse à ma femme*' and '*Memento.*' "[n] De Sanctis wallowed in the consciousness that the man whom he regarded as the greatest living Italian was playing just for him.

"Rossini takes the very greatest pains when copying out his writings," De Sanctis wrote, "never wearying of perfecting them, often going back to read them over and alter notes, which he is in the habit of erasing with a scraper with truly singular patience. One never would say that a man of such fervent imagination could lend himself to such minutiae. Another thing that I observed about him was the regularity of his habits, not to mention the symmetrical order in which he placed the furniture and objects around him. The room that he habitually occupied for many hours each day, both for receiving and for working, was his bedroom. There, the writing table was in the center, and on it set out in perfect order were the papers, his indispensable scrapers, the pens, the inkstand, and whatever else he needed for his writing. Three or four wigs were placed in a row on the mantel, evenly spaced. On the white walls hung some Japanese miniatures on rice paper, and some Oriental objects had been placed like a trophy on the chest of drawers; the bed, against the wall, always neat; a few simple chairs around the room. It all had the look of neatness and order, which it is a pleasure to see, but which did not give the notion of a room lived in by an artist, whom we more easily imagine inclined to disorder. When, struck by that perfect orderliness, I showed my surprise to the Maestro, he said to me: 'Eh, my dear fellow, order is wealth.' "

Remarking equally the regular schedule of Rossini's daily life, De Sanctis wrote that each morning, after returning from his stroll in the Bois de Boulogne, Rossini "changed his clothes, and if he was perspiring, took off his wig and put a towel, folded double, on his head, and in that guise walked up and down the room until he was completely free of sweat. He never let anyone see him during those moments, but none-theless, one day when we returned together from the walk, I was per-mitted to be in the room as a sign of special favor, and was able to see him in that odd get-up, which gave me time to observe Rossini's beautifully shaped and compeltely bald cranium, which reminded me of the head of Cicero or Scipio Africanus."

De Sanctis describes Rossini's appearance this way: "I see him still, round-shouldered, his paunch protruding, as he moved about the salon with short steps, doing with much simplicity the honors of the house. From his looks, one would not have judged him to be an artist and one of the greatest geniuses of our time. The reddish-blond wig that crudely outlined his forehead and temples contrasted strangely with his rather pallid and meticulously shaved face. His powerful imagination was evidenced only by his vivacious and penetrating eyes, just as one divined from his lips, thin and shaped slightly toward the sardonic, that he was a man of uncommon intelligence. There was not a trace of arrogance in him, or of that heavy manner which people of great fame not rarely take on."

By May 16, De Sanctis had finished sketching Rossini. The very lifelike drawing bears across the bottom this inscription in Rossini's handwriting: "Very dear Guglielmo De Sanctis. I take this oppor-tunity to attest to you my friendship and admiration. G. Rossini, Passy, Paris, 15 May 1862." The painter continued to be a welcome guest during the rest of his stay in Paris. Commenting on Rossini's tendency to discuss the past, De Sanctis wrote: "He could be thought of as like a beautiful woman in her declining years who is pleased to recall her good days, when she was courted and praised by all." But Rossini also discussed current events, notably on the Italian political scene, of which he said: "The only benefit that I can foresee from national unification is that of a new intellectual awakening among the Italians; for the rest, I have small faith, for however men may align themselves, they always are the same as far as their passions go. In 1848, I was accused of being a reactionary because I didn't agree with those who believed that they could get rid of the Austrians by means of hymns and shouts of '*Evviva l'Italia!*' Time proved me right. But I can't fail to see that those childishnesses succeeded in some manner too; just as I must render justice to Mazzini, though I was opposed to his doctrines, for having, by his continuous agitation, upheld and always kept alive among the Italians the spirit of liberty and independence, thus making the present unity of Italy possible."

When De Sanctis asked Rossini if composing tired him, the old man answered: "My dear fellow, if that were the case, I should never have written anything, for I am lazy by nature. I wrote *Il Barbiere di Siviglia* in thirteen days, working constantly amid the babblings of my friends. Being alone never has pleased me. When I was in a mood for composing and had no company, I sought out some." Then the painter asked him why he had introduced so many roulades and other ornaments into his music. "The motive was simple," Rossini averred. "Singers formerly did it on their own, in the worst taste. In order to forestall such indecencies, I decided to write them out myself in a form more suitable to my music; but it was never because I believed ornamentation essential for beautiful singing."

On June 3, De Sanctis was the Rossinis' dinner guest. The young Italian spoke of the loneliness he felt at being so far from his beloved mother. Moved, Rossini said: "I too loved my mother very much, the greatest affection I have felt in my life. It was to please her that I was induced to take a wife, whereas I should have preferred to remain single." De Sanctis asked him why he had abandoned his career so early. And this time Rossini's explanation was: "If I had had children, I'd have gone on writing [operas] despite my natural inclination to laziness. But being alone and having enough to live on comfortably, I never have gone back on my decision, neither for offers of profit nor for the flattery of honors. Impresarios, kings, emperors often have tempted me in every way. Well," he added, here slapping De Sanctis on the back and smiling, "retiring in time requires genius too."

When De Sanctis asked Rossini his opinions of the great Italian composers, his host began by saying: "The greatest of them all, in my view, though a foreigner, is Mozart. He knew how to make himself Italian in song and to be, at the same time, very skilled in composing, and thus to deal admirably with the serious as well as the facetious. A thing that's not given to everyone." He called Donizetti "one of the most productive and versatile talents of our time," adding: "Being his close friend, I reproved him many times for following the rhythm of my music too closely, and thus making himself less original. When, on the other hand, he followed his inspiration without preconceived ideas, he was very original, as is demonstrated by *Anna Bolena*, by *Lucia*, and by *L'Elisir d'amore*."

Of Bellini, Rossini told De Sanctis that he was "great above all in *Norma* and *I Puritani*. He had a very beautiful spirit, exquisitely delicate; but he lacked abundance of ideas when writing. It was true, however, that he had not had time to display himself in full, having died while still young and at the most beautiful moment of his artistic life." Of Mercadante: "I can't say more than that he makes good music; but I don't at all care for his very rough character or his manners, which are almost boorish at times." Of Verdi: "I like very much his almost savage nature, not to mention his great power for expressing the passions." Possibly he was alluding to Wagner when he remarked that non-Italian composers seemed to him "to lack sun"—by which De Sanctis understood him to mean that they lacked Italian warmth and spontaneity. Rossini added that in his opinion, music was made to delight the spirit, not to weary it with scientific abstruseness.

The end of De Sanctis's account is curious. Remarking that Rossini had urged him strongly to remain in Paris rather than return to Rome, he wrote: "Embracing me, he said: 'Look, if you go back to Rome, I'll stop being your friend, and don't hope that I'll ever write to you.' And he kept his word."

Rossini's enormous correspondence during the 1860's is full of references to contemporary musical events. For example, he had not at all lost his curiosity about Verdi. Writing from Passy to Alessandro Castellani in London on June 11, 1862, he said: "You didn't tell me anything about the marches performed at the Exhibition," about the Cantata at the Queen's Theater. You know that I regard your opinion on music as an oracle." The "Cantata at the Queen's Theater" was Verdi's *Inno delle nazioni*, his first setting of a text by Boito. As Franco Faccio had gone from Paris to London to attend its *première* (at Her Majesty's Theatre, on May 24, 1862),[n] Rossini very probably had discussed this strange mélange with him and Boito.

A letter that Rossini wrote from Paris on November 11, 1862, to Nicholas Ivanoff in Bologna is wonderfully characteristic and revealing, particularly as written by a man of seventy to an internationally renowned singer then fifty-two years old:[n]

"Most Beloved Nicolino: For me to leave your last letter unanswered would be injustice and ingratitude on my part. I am late, it is true, but during the removal from the country [Passy] back to the Chaussée d'Antin and during my annual catarrh, it was impossible for me to find a snippet of time to devote to a thing so close to my heart. Bravo, Nicolino! The noble resolution that you have made to give up gambling (and all the deplorable habits that feed it) again puts you in the position of deserving my esteem and affection. I am not surprised by your action, as I know your dauntless character, but I am edified by the methods you used to shake off a *Vile Yoke* that held you prisoner too long. You have been living in a city whose sons exist by shrewdness, fraud, and lies, the Great with the little, the tiny and vile with the Great. I always regret having induced you and the good Donzelli to settle in that Sewer—may God forgive me that! ! !—and as it's too late now to change it, learn how to live with few people, and they your betters in fortune and knowledge. Offer, in speaking of your political beliefs, the smallest possible chance for the Felsinese [Bolognese] Deriders to criticize and mock. *Caffè* life is proper only for Vagabonds, for the ignorant. You, my good Nicolino (whom I do not want to reduce to an automaton), have common sense and sufficient self-esteem to take the least twisted road to your destination—as Horace says, to the Aureas Mediocritatis [*sic*], a thing to be desired only in Times of Barricades and Assassins.

"Write me about yourself and the good Liverani, to whom I shall send a letter as soon as some things that are en route shall have arrived. Olympe embraces you, and I, with the feelings of a Father and a True Friend, call myself Your affectionate G. Rossini."

Late in 1862, Baronne James (Jakob) de Rothschild asked Rossini to compose a ceremonial piece to be performed during Napoleon III's forthcoming visit to the new Rothschild residence, the Château de

Ferrières. Rossini's answer was a *Choeur de chasseurs démocrates*, for tenors, baritones, and basses accompanied by two drums and a tam-tam."
On the festive day, choristers from the Opéra duly sang this *allegro brillante* chorus, no doubt swelling to a mighty fortissimo on the closing phrase: "*Amis! Le cerf est pris!*" Beginning with the Emperor, the guests signed their names in the Rothschilds' golden book: just below Napoleon's signature appeared that of Rossini.

CHAPTER XVIII

1863-1867

D URING TWO MONTHS of the summer of 1863, life at the Rossinis' Passy villa ran less smoothly than during the past several years. Rossini had turned nervous, on occasion somewhat grumpy Olympe increased the rigidity of her guardianship: her husband was at work, for the first time since he had completed the *Stabat Mater* twenty-two years before, on a major composition. At seventy-one, he had embarked upon a Mass that he would call *Petite Messe solennelle*, an astonishing finale to his astonishing career. Its fourteen sections were composed for four (or more) vocal soloists, a chorus of eight voices, two pianos, and a harmonium. The second page of the autograph score of this first version of the Mass reads: "*Petite Messe solennelle*, in four voices with accompaniment of 2 pianos and harmonium, composed during my country stay at Passy. Twelve singers of three sexes—men, women, and *castrati*—will be enough for its performance: that is, eight for the chorus, four for the solos, a total of twelve cherubim. God, forgive me the following *rapprochment*. Twelve also are the Apostles in the celebrated *coup de mâchoire* [jaw-stroke] painted in fresco by Leonardo, called *The Last Supper*: who would believe it! Among Thy disciples there are those who strike false notes! ! Lord, rest assured, I swear to Thee that there will be no Judas at my supper and that mine will sing properly and *con amore* Thy praises and this little composition, which is, alas, the last mortal sin of my old age." The final flickerings of Rossini's mockery also include, for the *Credo*, the tempo indication "*Allegro cristiano*."

The autograph of the *Petite Messe solennelle* also contains the following "letter to God": "Good God, there we have it, complete, this poor little Mass. Is it really sacred music that I have made, or is it merely abominable music [here Rossini is punning on the word *sacrée*, meaning both sacred or holy and damned or abominable—*musique sacrée* and *sacrée musique*]. I was born for *opera buffa*, as Thou well knowest. Little skill, a little heart, and that is all. So be Thou blessed and admit me to Paradise. G. Rossini. Passy, 1863."

At two o'clock on Sunday afternoon, March 14, 1864, the *Petite Messe solennelle* was sung for the first time at the rue Moncey *hôtel* of Comte Michel-Frédéric and Comtesse Louise Pillet-Will, she being its dedicatee; the occasion was the consecration of their private chapel. Jules Cohen had rehearsed the small chorus of Conservatoire students selected by Auber. The soloists, from the Théâtre-Italien, were Barbara and Carlotta Marchisio, Italo Gardoni, and the Belgian bass Louis Agniez, known as Agnesi. The two pianos were played by Georges Mathias and Andrea Peruzzi; Albert Lavignac was at the harmonium. Rossini stood near the accompanists, indicating the tempo for each section and turning pages for Mathias. Among the small group of invited listeners were Auber, Carafa, Meyerbeer, and Ambroise Thomas.

The little group was thunderstruck by the beauty and originality of what they heard. The ailing, impressionable, intensely emotional Meyerbeer stood throughout the performance, at times excitedly raising his hands above his head, trembling, even weeping. At the end, he rushed up to Rossini and embraced him fervidly. "My poor Giacomo," Rossini protested, "don't do that! Your health will suffer; you know that you must take the greatest care of it now!" But Meyerbeer went on pouring out admiration, addressing not only Rossini, but also Auber and Carafa. The apparently impassive Rossini left the Pillet-Will *hôtel* and walked home along the boulevards. "Poor Meyerbeer!" he said to those with him. "How sensitive he is! He has always been like that. I really felt sorry for him a little while ago . . . Will his health permit these emotions? He was in bed for three days, but he absolutely insisted upon getting up to come to the Pillet-Wills'."

The enchanted Meyerbeer returned to the rue Moncey the next day, when the second singing of the *Petite Messe solennelle* was heard by a larger, very distinguished audience that included the papal nuncio, government officials, members of the Poniatowski and Rothschild families, Ernest Legouvé, Azevedo, Gilbert-Louis Duprez, François-Auguste Gevaert, Mario, and Pierre Scudo—but not, it seems, Rossini. The reports in the Paris press were breathless. Completely beside himself with ecstasy, the critic for *Le Siècle* wrote that when this Mass was orchestrated, it would provide fire enough to melt marble cathedrals. When Rossini learned that the critics were insisting upon his harmonic originality and innovations, he said: "I didn't spare the dissonances, but I put some sugar into it too."

After that second singing of the *Petite Messe solennelle*, Meyerbeer wrote Rossini this letter: "To Jupiter Rossini. Divine Master! I cannot allow the day to end without thanking you again for the enormous pleasure given me by the experience of twice hearing your latest sublime creation; may Heaven preserve you to a hundred so that you can procreate again some other, similar masterpiece, and may God grant me a like age to be able to hear and admire those new facets of your immortal genius! Your constant admirer and old friend G. Meyerbeer. Paris, 15 March 1864." But Rossini would compose no more large works and Meyerbeer had less than two months of life remaining.

News of the furor stirred up by the *Petite Messe solennelle* brought Rossini new decorations and honors. He was at once pursued with demands that he orchestrate the Mass. The labor of composing it had exhausted him, however, and at first he refused. Then, in 1866–7, saying that he himself must provide the orchestration lest others provide it later, he completed the nearly five hundred pages of full score.[n] He would not authorize a performance of this version—which many have thought inferior to the original—while he lived;[n] it was heard for the first time three months after his death, at the Théâtre-Italien on February 24, 1869, when the soloists were Marietta Alboni, Gabrielle Krauss, Nicolini (Ernest Nicolas, future husband of Adelina Patti), and Agnesi. Four of the numbers had to be repeated. Olympe Rossini, who had sold the performance rights to the impressario Maurice Strakosch (Patti's brother-in-law), wrote a letter of thanks to him and to the participating artists for having glorified anew her late husband's memory.[n]

Strakosch, who had taken in 26,000 francs (about $14,760) at that first performance, then organized a "*Petite Messe solennelle* troupe," which, after singing the Mass fourteen times in one month at the Italien, took it on a two-month tour of France, Belgium, and Holland, presenting it sixty times. The company included Alboni, Marie Battu, a tenor known as Tom Hohler, and Agnesi. Although Strakosch had paid Olympe 100,000 francs (more than $56,700) for the performance rights and Alboni the same amount for three months of singing, he said[n] that his profit after expenses amounted to 50,000 francs (almost $28,350); he carried out two similar tours in 1870. Meanwhile, the *Petite Messe solen-nelle* had spread across the world. At St. Petersburg, it was conducted by Augusto Vianesi (who would conduct Gounod's *Faust* at the perform-ance inaugurating the first Metropolitan Opera House in New York on October 22, 1883); at Moscow, the conductor was Anton Rubinstein, whose soloists included the Marchisio sisters and Roberto Stagno. In February 1870, Rossini's Mass was sung in Sydney, Australia.[n]

Referring to one of the *samedi soirs,* early in 1864 Léon Escudier wrote to Verdi:[n] "Rossini . . . who never fails to ask me for news of you and Mme Verdi, wanted Delle Sedie to sing during that soirée a com-position of yours, and himself designated the *romanza* from *Un Ballo in maschera,* which produced an immense effect. That Rossini makes these demonstrations out of courtesy or comic maladroitness does not make them any less laudatory in appearance. I know that you make fun of all this." Escudier, perhaps still smarting over long-dead events, continued to accept Rossini's hospitality while mocking him to Verdi. In another letter to Verdi (April 9, 1864), he told him that Rossini was boasting of having obtained a splendid performance of the *Rigoletto* quartet. He added that he himself had told Rossini ironically: "Verdi admires you so much that he in turn gives evenings in which he has only your music sung!"

Still pursuing the same unfriendly line, on February 10, 1865, Escudier wrote Verdi that he had gone to see Rossini and—miraculously —had found him working: "He was writing—can you guess what?—a piano ritornello for the trio from *Attila,* which Mlle Patti, MM. Gardoni and Delle Sedie were singing at his home that night. 'Don't leap to the conclusion,' he told me, 'that I permit myself to arrange Verdi's music: but as they always make noise before a new piece is begun, and as I don't want them to miss anything of this beautiful trio, I am permitting myself to add six or eight measures of ritornello.'[n] For the rest, he was negative, protesting, as always, sincere friendship for you and charging me to send his compliments to you and Mme Verdi, which I do without in the least believing in his tales of affectionate sympathy. *Voilà!*"

The composition and orchestration of the Mass by no measure indicated that Rossini had turned solemn. His humorous quirks— in-stanced, to be sure, by his having called *"Petite"* and *"solennelle"* a very long, only intermittently solemn Mass—persisted, as did his pungency of expression. Writing to the singer Caroline Unger during 1864, for ex-ample, he noted: "I have the glory of telling you that in all Paris there is only one house illuminated by oil, mine. That is the homage that I render to the century of—tenebrous—enlightenment." Azevedo reported: "One morning the humble author of this account found him [Rossini] in very bad humor. He had twelve letters of introduction to write,[n] a bunch of portrait cards to indite and sign, a multitude of albums to illustrate with some measure of his musical writing.[n] When he saw the visitor enter, he complained: 'God, fame is fatiguing! Butchers are happy men.' 'Why didn't you take up their profession?' the visitor asked him jokingly, wanting to have some fun at his expense. 'You were well prepared by an apprenticeship when, during your childhood, your parents put you out to board with one of them at Bologna.' 'I would have done so gladly,' he replied, 'but I couldn't; it wasn't my fault. *I was badly guided!*' And with those words a double burst of laughter dispersed his bad mood as if by enchantment."

On May 2, 1864, Meyerbeer—while still polishing the score of *L'Africaine*, which was already in rehearsal at the Opéra—died after a ten-day illness.[n] Rossini, who had liked the finicking German and had enjoyed his company and his extravagant flattery, was particularly saddened by the loss of a musical colleague so nearly his exact contemporary (not quite six months his senior). They had known each other for almost fifty years. Rossini responded to the loss by composing a choral *Chant funèbre* to lines beginning "*Pleure! pleure! muse sublime.*"[n] For four-part male chorus, it is accompanied only by pianissimo bass-drum rolls and taps. At the foot of the last page of the autograph score, Rossini wrote: "Some measures of funeral chant to my poor friend Meyerbeer. G. Rossini."[n]

Not all of Rossini's recorded reactions to Meyerbeer's death were in that solemn vein. Verdi told Italo Pizzi that a young nephew of Meyerbeer composed a funeral march for the dead man and then went to play it on the piano for Rossini, soliciting his approval. Verdi sat at a piano while telling this anecdote; Pizzi said that he gave a hilarious impersonation of Rossini commenting on the march: "Very good, very good! But, truthfully, wouldn't it have been better if *you* had died and your poor uncle had composed the march?" Verdi commented to Pizzi: "Thus Rossini killed."

Proving by the vigor and intelligence of his words what he denied himself in self-description, Rossini wrote to Gaetano Fabi from Passy on June 6, 1864:

"DEAR GAETANINO: I take advantage of my friend [Antonio] Peruzzi (who is making a trip to Bologna) to send you a little portrait of myself taken recently and which my Parisian friends find looks like me. However, it represents a certain vigor that is only apparent, as because of the years my feebleness increases so that now I cannot depend upon my legs; also, *Memory*, *Acumen*, *Wit*, etc., etc., are decaying. In order to avoid these miseries, we must pay the penalty of dying. Let us go on living, then, and be patient. . . ." The "little portrait" very probably was a print of one of the photographs taken by Nadar (Félix Tournachon).[n]

To one of the Rossinis' parties during 1864 were invited the American banker Charles Moulton, long a Paris resident, and his beautiful and musically talented wife, the former Lillie Greenough of Cambridge, Massachusetts, later to become known as the writer of flighty, entertaining memoirs under her second married name, Lillie de Hegermann-Lindencrone. In her book entitled *In the Courts of Memory*,[n] she wrote: "We were invited to one of Rossini's Saturday evenings. There was a queer mixture of people: some diplomats, and some well-known members of society, but I fancy that the guests were mostly artists; at least they looked so. The most celebrated ones were pointed out to me. There were Saint-Saëns, Prince Poniatowski, Gounod, and others. . . .

"Prince [Richard von] Metternich[n] told me that Rossini had once said to him that he wished people would not always feel obliged to sing his music when they sang at his house. '*J'acclamerais avec délice "Au clair de la lune*," *même avec variations*,' he said, in his comical way. Rossini's wife's name is Olga [*sic*]. Some one called her Vulgar, she is so ordinary and pretentious, and would make Rossini's home and salon very commonplace if it were not that the master glorified all by his presence. I saw Rossini's writing-table, which is a thing never to be forgotten; brushes, combs, toothpicks, nails, and all sorts of rubbish lying about pell-mell; and promiscuous among them was the tube that Rossini uses for his famous *macaroni à la Rossini*. Prince Metternich said that no power on earth would induce him to touch any food *à la Rossini*, especially the macaroni, which he said was stuffed with hash and all sorts of remnants of last week's food and piled upon a dish like a log cabin. '*J'ai des frissons chaque fois que j'y pense*.'

"Not long ago Baron James Rothschild sent Rossini some splendid grapes from his hothouse. Rossini, in thanking him, wrote, '*Bien que vos raisins soient superbes, je n'aime pas mon vin en pillules*.' . . . Rossini does not dye his hair, but wears the most wiggy of wigs. When he goes to mass" he puts one wig on top of the other, and if it is very cold he puts still a third one on, curlier than the others, for the sake of warmth." Mme Moulton was invited to sing—and chose *"Sombre forêt,"* from *Guillaume Tell.* She wrote that after she had sung it, "Auber came up flushed with delight at my success, and said to Rossini, 'Did I say too much about Madame Moulton's voice?'

" 'Not enough,' replied Rossini. 'She has more than voice; she has intelligence and *le feu sacré—un rossignol doublé en velours*; and more than all, she sings my music as I have written it. . . .'

"Auber" asked me, 'Do you know what Rossini said about me? . . . He said . . . *Auber est un grand musicien qui fait de la petite musique.*' . . . 'Well, I said,' and he hesitated before continuing, 'I said that Rossini *est un très grand musicien et fait de la belle musique, mais une exécrable cuisine.*' . . .

"Auber asked him how he had liked the representation of 'Tannhäuser'?" Rossini answered, with a satirical smile, 'It is a music one must hear several times. I am not going again.'

"Rossini said that neither Weber nor Wagner understood the voice. Wagner's interminable dissonances were insupportable. That these two composers imagine that to sing is simply to *dégoiser* the note; but the art of singing, or technic was considered by them to be secondary and insignificant. Phrasing or any sort of *finesse* was superfluous. The orchestra must be all-powerful. 'If Wagner gets the upper hand,' Rossini continued, 'as he is sure to do, for people will run after the New, then what will become of the art of singing? No more *bel canto*, no more phrasing, no more enunciation! What is the use when all that is required of you is to *beugler* (bellow)? Any *cornet à piston* is just as good as the best tenor, and better, for it can be heard over the orchestra. But the instrumentation is magnificent. There Wagner excels. The overture of Tannhäuser is a *chef-d'œuvre*; there is a swing, a sway, and a rush that carries you off your feet. . . .I wish I had composed it myself.' "

Madame Moulton records that in 1865 she was a guest at one of Princess Mathilde Bonaparte's Sunday evening receptions. "Rossini was, as a great exception, present. I fancy that he and his wife had dined with the Princess; therefore, when the Princess asked him to accompany me, saying that she desired so much to hear me sing, he could not well refuse to be amiable, and sat down to the piano with a good enough grace. I sang 'Bel Raggio,' from 'Semiramide,' as I knew it by heart (I had sung it often enough with [Manuel Patricio] Garcia"). Rossini was kind enough not to condemn the cadenzas with which Garcia had interlarded it. . . .

"I was amused at his gala dress for royalty: a much-too-big redingote, a white tie tied a good deal to one side, and only one wig.

"He says that he is seventy-three years old. I must say that this is difficult to believe, for he does not look it by ten years. He never accepts any invitations. I know I have never seen him anywhere outside his own house, and it was a great surprise to see him now. We once ventured to invite him and his wife to dinner one evening, when the Prince and Princess Metternich were dining with us; and we got this answer: 'Merci, de votre invitation pour ma femme et moi. Nous regrettons de ne pouvoir l'accepter. Ma femme ne sort que pour aller à la messe, et moi je ne sors jamais de mes habitudes.' We felt snubbed, as no doubt we deserved to be."

What took place at the Passy villa on Rossini's name-day in 1864 was reported in full by the Paris press. One paper[n] said: "After supper, the gardens of the villa were illuminated as if by magic and made merry with fireworks prepared by M. Ruggieri, the great composer's fellow townsman. Then the program of music began in the inside salon.

"Messrs. Faure, Obin, and Villaret, accompanied at the piano by Maître [François-Eugène] Vauthrot, first accompanist at the Opéra, performed to enthusiastic applause the immortal duet and trio from G. Tell. Then a great artist of the finest period of our Théâtre-Italien, the bass Tamburini, sang the duet from Il Barbiere with an English celebrity, Mme Lemmens-Sharrigton [sic],[n] who a little later performed deliciously the cavatina from Bianca e Falliero, almost forgotten in our day.

"Alongside these beautiful pages of vocal music, the pianist Louis Diémer won admiration for two instrumental pieces by Rossini, who, having seated himself at the piano, then accompanied, as only he knows how to accompany, an elegy of his, Les adieux à la vie, a moving unpublished scena [sic] written on a single note to poetry by Émilien Pacini. Mme Lemmens performed it so marvelously that a repetition was called for.

"After the music came the time for recitation. Mme Damain and Coquelin, the young and already famed actor of the Théâtre-Français, recited with great verve and uncommon ability Verconsin's Le Wagon.

"The Rossinis' salons were inundated with flowers, and alongside the pianoforte had been placed a superb marble medallion of the famous

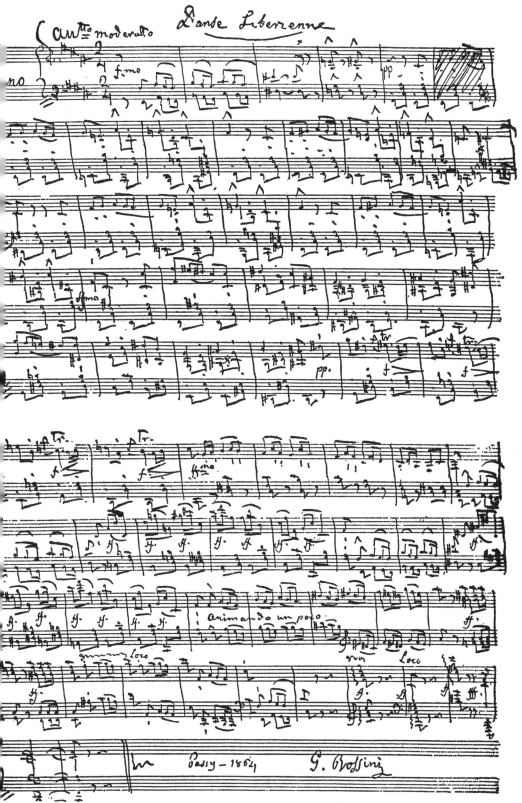

MANUSCRIPT OF THE "*Danse sibérienne,*" **DATED** 'PASSY—1864"

maître by the sculptor Chevalier. [Radiciotti's footnote: "This magnif-icent work, destined for the foyer of the Opéra, was commissioned from the renowned French sculptor by His Excellency Marshal Vaillant, Minister of the Imperial Household and of Fine Arts, at the suggestion of Senator Comte de Nieuwerkerke."] Thanks to this inspired work, to this faithful and characteristic Roman profile, which recalls that of Dante, the great figure of Rossini will live for future generations in all the splendor of his genius, which Italy and France have covered with the highest honors."

The seventy-two-year-old man thus being feted had been named a *grand officier* of the Légion d'honneur by Napoleon III on August 13; at the celebration in Passy, five of Rossini's aristocratic French friends signalized this new honor by presenting him with a lyre made of sugar. On August 20 he had been created a commander of the Order of Sts. Maurice and Lazarus by Victor Emanuel II; the decree was officially handed to the *sindaco* of Pesaro the next day by Ubaldino Peruzzi, Minister of the Interior.

Rossini's 1864 name-day had also evoked a remarkable series of celebratory events at Pesaro. The central feature of them was to be the dedication of a seated bronze statue of the most famous of all Pesarese. It had been modeled and cast by Barone Marochetti on com-mission from two directors of the Ferrovie Romane, Gustave Delehante of Paris, and the Marqués José de Salamanca of Madrid, who were giving it to the city of Pesaro. Hard by the railroad station there," a temporary pavilion and amphitheater had been erected to accom-modate the hundreds of performers and a crowd later estimated at twenty thousand. The music was conducted by Angelo Mariani; the chorus included many celebrated people, among them the musician-bibliophile-librarian Gaetano Gaspari, Cesare Badiali, and Nicholas Ivan-off. Hooded, the statue loomed up opposite the large orchestra (205 instrumentalists, 255 choristers) when it began the program with the overture to *La Gazza ladra*. Then Minister Peruzzi unveiled the statute of Rossini, evoking noisy approval from the crowd. Next came per-formances of an *Inno* that Mercadante had based on Rossinian melodies" and of the overture to *Semiramide*. The program closed on official speeches, several of which deserted Rossini to touch upon the fact that the noble city of Venice still remained in Austrian hands.

At the Teatro Rossini that evening, the newly constituted Società Rossiniana presented a second ceremonial *Inno*, this one an effort by

Giovanni Pacini, and a performance of *Guglielmo Tell*[n] which was received so enthusiastically that it was repeated on succeeding nights. Mariani again conducted, and the cast included the baritone Davide Squarcia and the German tenor Georg Stiegel (Giorgio Stigelli). That night, the streets of Pesaro—including the former Via del Duomo, now renamed Via Rossini—were illuminated; a band concert was given in the main *piazza*.[n] Later in 1864, Professore Giuliano Vanzolini of Pesaro published a full account of these celebrations.[n]

On September 2, 1864, Rossini wrote to a Bolognese friend, Vincenzo Alberti, a letter that again demonstrates the persistence of his animus against Bologna: "My dear Vincenzo, I certainly cannot delay answering your very dear and affectionate letter of the 21st of last month, in which you have painted with the brushes of a Salvator Rosa all the details of the ceremony held that same day in the Piazza del Liceo in my honor. I could not help smiling at your reflection on the lack of heart-throbs [*palpiti*] and of blood in their veins! If they were different, I was sufficiently well disposed not to have left Bologna. *Laus Deo*. . . . I have read the epigraph (written so well by you)[n] raised over the entrance to the Liceo, and now I can boast of having been *stoned*." As if underlining the point, he signed the letter "Rossini of Pesaro."[n]

Old and ailing, Rossini certainly had no desire or intention to return to Bologna. That he had as little intention to return to Florence is proved by the fact that on November 17, 1864, his Florentine attorney, Carlo Capezzuoli, signed in his name a deed selling his *palazzo* there (and the two contiguous structures) to Giacomo Servadio for 250,000 Italian lire. The three buildings later became the property of the Amministrazione Provinciale and housed public offices.

On December 14, 1864, Rossini wrote to Tito Ricordi to thank him for twenty-one piano scores of his operas. Ricordi was in the process of publishing what was meant to be a complete collection of Rossini's operas. "The edition that you have undertaken," Rossini warned him by letter, "will give rise (with reason) to many criticisms because the same piece of music will be found in various operas: the time and money granted me for composing were so *homeopathic* that I scarcely had time to read the so-called poetry to be set to music: only the upkeep of my most beloved parents and poor relatives was in my heart." He had never intended his operas for solemn perpetuation in a collected edition.

Plans for this edition had been under way at least since 1852: on February 24 of that year, writing to Giovanni Ricordi from Florence, Rossini had said: "I shall not fail to furnish Sig. Stefani everything that depends upon me for the edition of which you tell me, an edition that unfortunately will bring back to light all my lacks [*miserie*]." On June 8, 1854, he told his friend the architect Doussault:[n] "I still am furious, furious about that publication, which places all my works before the public's eyes at once; there they often will find the same pieces because I believed that I had the right to retire from my whistled-at operas those pieces which seemed to me the best, and to save them from shipwreck by placing them in new works that I was doing. A whistled-at opera seemed to me completely dead—and, behold, everything has been resuscitated!"

On March 21, 1865, Max Maria von Weber—whose famous father had called on Rossini nearly thirty-nine years before—went to see Rossini for the first time. In the article already quoted from,[n] Weber wrote: "I never have found myself embarrassed when facing the great of the Earth. Nevertheless, when, on March 21, 1865, I climbed the dark stairs of rue Chaussée d'Antin No. 2, I could feel my heartbeats. As soon as my name was announced, I was admitted. Crossing a large, rather dark antechamber, I entered the Maestro's study. He was seated at a small table covered with papers, and he came to meet me immediately, wholly different from what I had imagined him to be—the hero or the artist—and introduced his wife to me, a short, rather fat woman, but gay and spirited." Weber was struck by the notion that the man before him looked much as his own father might have looked if he had lived to be seventy-three.

"An *Oberon* will never be written again," Rossini said. "Why does one understand great men only when one is old and wise, and—the worst of it—when they usually are dead? Were he alive, I am sure that he would accept me now too. After all, we both would be old men!"[n] Rossini remarked that Weber had been right to die young: as an old man, he himself constantly had to find something amusing to do. He composed continually, he said, because he could not get out of the habit. But if he had lived in antiquity, he would have had the consolation of knowing that when he came to die, his works would be burned with him. Weber was delighted to notice German music on Rossini's desk, notably works by Mozart and Gluck. "Only the old ones!" Rossini commented, adding that perhaps Wagner was a great genius, but that he himself would never be able to understand him and would be able to comprehend his genius only if Wagner were to demonstrate it in some nonmusical way.

As Weber was leaving, Rossini invited him to dinner the following Saturday, when the other guests included Gustave Doré. He noted that Rossini and his guests were completely absorbed in appreciating the excellent dinner—and that Rossini flirted with several young women who were present. What Weber calls Rossini's new "Spanish Romances" then were performed, and he found them delightful; he noticed that Rossini became irritated when a performer departed from exactness or otherwise distorted what he had composed—an attitude that reminded him of his father's strictness in such matters.

Weber was to call upon Rossini again in the summer of 1867, this time at Passy. He had been told that the villa was at No. 20, avenue Ingres, but soon realized that not all of the properties bore numbers. Accosting a sweeper, he asked: "Friend, don't the houses in Passy have numbers?" "For whom are you looking?" "Monsieur Rossini." "Oh!" the man said, waving toward the Rossini villa, "that name is better than a house number," thus giving Weber the title for his future reminiscences. Finding Rossini in the garden, Weber soon was chatting with him about his father, Schumann, and Morlacchi. Their conversation was punctuated by the whistling of a locomotive on the nearby railroad, and Weber commented: "How these ultramodern dissonances must offend your musical ear!" "Oh, no!" Rossini replied, smiling. "That whistle always reminds me of the blessed times of my youth. My God, how much whistling I heard at the performances of my first operas, as well as at those of *La Cenerentola* and *Torvaldo e Dorliska*!" They discussed an announced plan to present Weber operas in Paris. "You should come to hear how we French [*sic*] ruin German music!" Rossini said, and added: "Perhaps I might even make up my mind to join Weber's son in listening to one of his father's operas once again!"

On Monday, April 24, 1865, the *Petite Messe solennelle* was repeated at the Pillet-Will *hôtel*. The *Revue et Gazette musicale* noted that "the composer absented himself from the ovation that the audience had prepared for him." But he was sensitive to the praise that this "learned" composition had wormed from the Paris critics. Writing to Francesco Florimo on June 10, he said: "I am happy to notify you that a month ago a Mass of mine was performed by my friend Comte Pillet-Will in his *palazzo*. Would you believe it? The Parisian doctors, because of this work, have classified me in the number of the savants and classics. Rossini a savant! Rossini a classic! Laugh, then, dear friend, and with you will also smile Mercadante and Conti (whom I embrace affectionately). If my poor Maestro Mattei were alive, he would say: Well, this time Gioachino has not dishonored my school. That's what the poor fellow wrote me at the beginning of my operatic career. When you come here, I'll show you my work, and you will decide whether Mattei judged more correctly at first or later."

Correspondence between Rossini and his "adored son"—Michele Costa—continued to cross the English Channel. A letter that Frank Walker well called "one of the most curious ever written, even by Rossini," was dated at Paris on January 3, 1865:[n]

"MY ADORED SON! I have delayed writing to you because my unsteady health does not allow me to enjoy your precious gift, The Stilton. Today, reinvigorated by that delicious cheese and pervaded by its flavor, I come to offer you feelings of lively gratitude from my Stomach and my Heart. Now more than ever I am confirmed in my Opinion, which is that eating Stilton often (as I suppose you do), one must compose Classical Oratorios and trot down to posterity with one's forehead circled with laurels. Continue on, then, my beloved son, in the Specialty that renders you unique, and thus become the Glory of the Fatherland and the consolation of your Genitor.

"I must ask a great Service of you, and here is what it deals with: A very dear friend of mine, Conte [Giuseppe] Mattei of Bologna, is the Inventor of a Medicine composed of vegetables which, if applied in time, works miraculous cures and healings in Cancerous Illnesses. Mattei is not a physician, still less a Charlatan, and is led only by a Noble Philanthropic Feeling in favor of humanity. Understand? The favor that I ask of you is limited to your being willing to ask your physician if there really exists in London a *Special Hospital* for Cancerous Diseases and what is its name and street address. I beg you to be deserving in rendering me this Service. If the thing exists, Mattei would wish to make the trip to London to perform a few experiments. Note well that your physician might profit greatly in this affair! Here in Paris, I have relieved some unfortunates who were on their way to the other world, and I can assure you of the prodigious efficacy of this Liquid. I know your heart and have no doubt that you will want to do me this favor. My wife joins me in wishing you, for the year just begun, a full measure of Contentments, Corporeal and Spiritual. I am always happy to call myself Your affectionate Father Rossini.

"Tenderly embrace Your Brother."

To Parisians, Rossini was an object of constant curiosity. Carafa told him that a Russian princess had waited two hours on the boulevard to catch a glimpse of him and, hopefully, to make his acquaintance. What ought he to do? Rossini's answer was:[n] "Tell her that I am excessively fond of asparagus. She need only go to Potel de Chabot and buy the finest bunch she can get and bring it here. I shall then rise, and after she has inspected me well in front, I shall turn around, and she can complete her inspection by taking the other view too, and then she may go."

On December 27, 1865, Rossini wrote a letter to Verdi which, otherwise commonplace, is notable for its signature and address—respectively "Rossini / Ex-Composer of Music" and "To M. Verdi / Celebrated Composer of Music. / Pianist of the Fifth Class! ! !" In the latter, Rossini probably was alluding to a well-known incident in Verdi's early life; he had been refused admission to the Milan Conservatory at least in part because his piano playing had been found insufficiently accomplished.

Some time in late May or early June 1866, a twelve-year-old girl named Teresa Carreño was brought to Rossini. As she recounted that first meeting almost sixty years later:[n] "Here [in Paris] I had opportunities of meeting many of the great musicians and celebrities of the hour, among others the great Rossini, who, curiously enough, gave me my first lesson in singing. Oh, yes, I am said to have had a good voice in my younger days, and for a fact I studied singing and actually sang a number of times in grand opera.

"At the time of my meeting with Rossini I was 12 years old, but because I was a very robust and healthy-looking girl no doubt I appeared older. Rossini looked at me critically, and then said to my father, "I believe this child can sing. Come,' he said, sitting down at the piano, 'let me hear your voice.' He gave me some advice about breathing and so on, expressed his approval, and then sent me to the famous Italian teacher, Delle Sedie, with whom I studied for a considerable length of time." Rossini was sufficiently impressed by "Teresita's" double talent as singer and pianist to write letters of introduction for her to Luigi Arditi and to the noted teacher of singing Madame Puzzi Toso, both dated June 6, 1866. In the former, he wrote of Carreño as "a pupil of Nature, who always will be the mother of the fine arts, and trained by the celebrated [Louis Moreau] Gottschalk."[n]

The orchestrated *Petite Messe solennelle* was on Rossini's mind, and he conceived the wish to hear it sung in a church. Barring fulfillment of that desire was the ban on female singers in Catholic churches. Wanting to submit a plea for cancelation of that ban in the form of a Latin memorial to Pius IX, Rossini on March 23, 1866, wrote to his old friend Luigi Crisostomo Ferrucci, a noted Latinist who was librarian of the Biblioteca Laurenziana at Florence:

"What will you think of my slowness in answering your affection-ate letters and in offering you expressions of my admiration and my thanks for the repeated proofs that you give me of a constant affection that is no longer of our times! Blame only my uncertain health. I have been afflicted for two months and more by an old-age catarrh that is preparing me for the road of the great journey. Today I am better and, as you see, can write at least this sheet to bless you and tell you that I received your Vergilian verses (so well translated), in which emerge your affection for me, your high knowledge, and the exquisite art of lying so as to honor the poor Pesarese beyond his merit. The first packet suffered some delay; the second arrived on time, and always dear. Let me, then, kiss you and thank you again, oh my beloved Ferrucci.

"You will perhaps have heard that I composed a solemn Mass performed in a large salon of my friend Comte Pillet-Will, for whom it stirred up a lot of noise. The performance was perfect. The provisional accompaniment was for two pianofortes and a harmonium (little organ). Much success despite the solicitations of the knowing and the ignorant that I should instrumentate it so that it could be performed later in some big basilica, and that despite the lack of the voices (so-called white), both soprano and contralto, without which one does not sing the Glories of the Lord! I shall explain myself . . . A pontiff whose name I don't know published a Bull that prohibited the mutilation of boys to turn them into sopranists; that measure, though it had an admirable aspect, has been fatal for the art of music, and especially for religious music (now in such decadence). Those mutilated boys, who could follow no career but that of singing, were the founders of the *'cantar che nell'anima si sente,'* and the horrid decadence of Italian *bel canto* originated with their suppression . . . Another pontiff, of whom I know neither the name nor the epoch, published a Bull that prohibited the presence of the two sexes promiscuously in choir lofts: you will recall clearly that in our churches the masculine faithful used to be on only one side and the feminine on the other; now that customs have changed completely, which is to say that men and women are all mixed together, it is ridiculous to want to observe rigorously the proscription of that later Bull; who takes the place of the sopranists and the women? They are young boys from nine to fourteen years old with voices that are sour and mostly off pitch . . . Do you think that religious music can subsist on such miserable resources? You will say to me: and the tenors and the basses no longer exist? I shall answer you by saying that they are excellent for the *De profundis* and distressing for the *Gloria in excelsis Deo* . . .

"Now I come to the point of my story: if you will counsel me, I want to write to Pius IX to get him to publish a new Bull that would allow women to sing (promiscuously with men) in the churches. I know that he loves music, I know also that I am not unknown to him because someone who heard him singing '*Siete Turchi, non vi credo*'[n] while walking in the Vatican garden approached him to compliment him upon his beautiful voice and beautiful way of using it; to which His Holiness replied: 'My dear, as a young man I always sang the music of Gioachino.' Dear Ferrucci, what do you say? Ought I to hazard a page to your old friend Pius IX? If I should obtain what I want, I would be blessed by God and men. But, I repeat, without your advice I shall remain mute. Do not be put off, I beg you, by the wording and the confusion of this prolix letter of mine. After you have read it, be charitable, throw it on the fire . . .

"If you agree that I should turn to His Holiness, send me (in Latin, of course) a model letter: I shall be still more thankful to you."

A month later (April 26, 1866), Rossini again addressed Ferrucci: "I have received your very dear letter of the 18th of this month, with a memorial for the Supreme Pontiff. If you would consider me competent, I should say that this memorial is a masterpiece, but I am sure that you would regard me as an ignoramus of the first water. I shall limit myself to blessing you and thanking you a thousand times for the care and heart that you have so generously devoted to pleasing me. However, I am proud of having turned to a born musician *cum* . . . to deal with such a question; only someone who sings so well '*Ah! quel giorno ognor rammento*'[n] could have come out so victorious from so difficult an undertaking. Let me embrace you, oh my Vergil! On the theme of making excessively gross blunders, I have followed your advice, putting at the bottom of the memorial (which you wrote in capital letters) the JOACHIM R., and yesterday I delivered it to our Nunzio Chigi (to whom your worth is well known), who promises me to see that it gets into the hands of His Holiness soon.

"May the Heavens desire that our prayers be granted. We shall see!"

Nearly six months elapsed. Then, on October 14, 1866, Rossini wrote to Ferrucci again on the matter: "Let me give you a sketch now of the correspondence of your Mastai[Pius IX's name had been Giovanni Maria Mastai-Ferretti]. In reply to your magnificent letter in Latin, *after three months* I received one, also in Latin, signed by him, in which he bestowed benedictions, eulogies, tenderness, etc., etc., upon me, but made no reference whatsoever to the assent that I had asked for, that is, to women being allowed to sing promiscuously with men in the basilicas. I understand very well that in these moments he has so many preoccupations that they do not permit him to descend to us; however, once the crisis has passed, I intend to write him in Italian, and in my poor phrasing declare to him that if it is in his power to grant my desires and he does not do it, *he will have to be accountable to God!* that if it is not in his power to grant me them, I *commiserate* with him and will not for that reason remain any less affectionate toward him, etc., etc. Do you understand, oh my Ferrucci?"

That Rossini ever wrote the jocularly threatened letter in the vulgate is unlikely. He must, however, have discussed the subject freely. A Paris paper commented upon the exchange of communications and asked: ". . . do you know what he [Pius IX] replied to the Swan of Pesaro? He sent him a long letter in which it is a question of the misfortunes of the Church, the sufferings of the Church, the final triumph of the Church. And that is the way that all affairs are treated at Rome." Resigned though Rossini may have been to not obtaining the desired permission, he did not forget the matter. In a long letter to Ferrucci written on June 21, 1867,[n] he said: "Once this damned Exposition, which makes Paris a real Babylon, is over, I shall take up the reigns of the big matter again! ! You can be very sure of that.

"Our Holy Father, in reply to our magnificent letter, answered me: he offered me benedictions and tendernesses, but the Bull so much desired by me remained (I think) in his heart. Poor religious music! ! !"[n]

Rossini's appetite for particular flavors in food had not been dulled by advancing age. On May 28, 1866, in a letter to Michele Costa in

London, he said: "The cheese sent to me would be worthy of a Bach, a Handel, a Cimarosa; imagine, then, if it is not worthy of the old man from Pesaro! ! . . . for three successive days I have enjoyed it moistened with the best wines of my cellar . . . and I swear that I never eaten any food better than your *Chedor Chiese* (damn the British orthography!)."ⁿ

During 1866, when "the Abbé" Liszt made his first appearance in clerical garb in Paris, he visited Rossini several times. One morning, Rossini having invited pianist friends for the occasion, Liszt went to the piano and improvised a long fantasy on themes from Rossini operas. The effect on the listeners was overwhelming (though some of them noticed that Liszt's fingers no longer responded to his demands upon them with the accuracy of former years). Then he read at sight some of Rossini's most recent compositions, amazing everyone by the speed with which he discerned and made clear in performance the patterns of what Rossini had writen. At times, indeed, he made pianistically effective changes in the music, emphasizing a figure that Rossini had not marked for emphasis, sometimes doubling single notes as octaves. "Is that what you would have wanted?" he asked. For reply, Rossini turned toward the other guests: "This man is a demon!" he said.

Toward the end of 1866, Rossini was more than usually unwell. For some years, winter had been extremely unwelcome to him: it aggravated his chronic catarrh and often led to long, enfeebling spasms of coughing. His heart was not so strong as his generally healthy appearance led many to suppose, and he often canceled his daily walk because of muscular weakness brought on by what was described as abundant bronchial secretions and intestinal catarrh. In December 1866, he almost certainly suffered a light stroke or thrombosis. Completely immobilized for some time thereafter, he gradually regained so much of his former strength that no external sign of the attack showed. On February 28, 1867, he celebrated his seventy-fifth birthday.

CHAPTER XIX

1867-1868

Visiting Paris in March 1867 to attend the *première* of Verdi's *Don Carlos* (March 11) at the Opéra, Tito di Giovanni Ricordi and his twenty-six-year-old son Giulio naturally called upon the Rossinis, arriving, as Rossini had suggested, at nine o'clock in the morning. Of that meeting, Giulio later wrote:[n]

"The great Maestro lived on the first floor of a house at the corner of the boulevards and the Chaussée d'Antin; I confess that my heart was thumping at the moment when I ascended the stairs: scarcely had my father and I entered an antechamber and given our names when the manservant said that we were awaited; we crossed two rooms, in one of which a grand piano stood, and reached the doorway to a small room. Directly facing the doorway, there was Rossini, seated at a table dipping a slice of bread into an *oeuf à la cocque;* his wife sat facing him. As soon as he saw my father, Rossini jumped up, quickly wiped his lips, and, extending his arms, clasped my father to his breast with great affection, exclaiming: 'Toh! toh! my good Titone! . . .'

"My presentation to the Maestro and his wife followed; naturally, I could only stammer out a few words . . .

"Rossini sat down, saying: 'After the salaams, now sit down right here near me . . . and let me finish my breakfast.'

"And Signora Rossini to my father: 'See how well Rossini is? Two *oeufs à la cocque* and a good glass of Bordeaux—there you have his hygienic collation; but at supper . . . you'll see that he always does it full honors.' "

The next day, the Ricordis dined in the Chaussée d'Antin. Giulio described the seventy-five-year-old Rossini on that occasion thus: "The

Maestro appeared to me to be a man of ordinary stature, but with powerful shoulders and a large, robust chest; the hands very beautiful, white, aristocratic; the face broad, grandiose, imposing, such as to inspire genuine respect and admiration; the physiognomy highly pleasant, smiling, with a sensuous mouth; the eyes mobile, very vivacious, with a perpetual smile reflected in them; the neck was full and fat, but did not have a bull-like aspect; the cranium very large, resembling a Michelangelesque cupola, completely bald; the light beating down upon it picked out a luminous point to which my glance turned often. Rossini noticed this and, turning toward my father, said:

" 'Your son admires my baldness . . . it's a beauty . . . what do you Milanese call it? . . . wait a moment, wait a moment . . . *crappa pelada* [peeled head].'

"Then to me:

" 'There's my headgear . . .'

"And, saying that, he reached his hand along the table and picked up an object that I had taken for a handkerchief and . . . panf! planted it on his head. It was a wig: and thus Rossini appeared to me as he commonly was seen in the official world."

Ricordi then tells of Olympe's picking up Rossini's breakfast tray and leaving the room. "Then my father . . . but here a parenthesis occurs . . . When the first Italian laws for [the protection of] literary property had been promulgated, Tito Ricordi immediately had informed Rossini, and had advised him to make the necessary payments to protect his interests in his own works in Italy; Rossini not only had accepted the advice, but also had instructed Ricordi to do whatever was needed, naming him his administrator and representative. When leaving Milan for Paris, Tito Ricordi had wanted to surprise Rossini by taking him the first payments of his auctorial rights—I close the parenthesis and start over: now my father, taking from his pocket a roll of forty-five napoleoni d'oro [about $510], handed it to Rossini, saying:

" 'Here . . . I bring you the first fruits of your rights.'

" 'What?' Rossini answered in surprise. 'My operas are still worth something in Italy.'

"But a sound of steps in the next room interrupted the conversation: Rossini quickly took the roll of napoleoni, opened a drawer, threw the roll into it, and closed it. Then, putting a finger to his mouth, he said:

" 'Sh, sh, sh . . . that's my wife coming back: I'll keep these for my pocket money . . . I'll send you the receipt tomorrow.'

"The Signora returned and the conversation started again.

"ROSSINI: 'Then, dear Tito, you have come to be present at a new triumph for our Verdi? . . . There's a man who knows where he's going! Here in Paris he has the reputation of being a bear because he doesn't lend himself complacently to all the visits, the interviews, the polite compliments! ! . . . he wants to stay fresh! When one has given so many payments on account to the art, as I did, one can do all those pretty things . . . but one must have a tranquil life in order to work seriously.'

"T. RICORDI: 'But you are always working . . .'

"ROSSINI: 'What! . . . what! . . . those are scribblings that I put down for my own amusement: they ask me so often! Maître here, Maître there . . . for you should know that music is performed in my house from time to time, and I have the honor to receive the *beau monde, le tout Paris*! . . . On those occasions, some piece by old Rossini comes forth. But . . . I don't intend to publish these sins of mine.' "

Later in the same article, Giulio Ricordi says: "I was also at two of the musical soirées at Rossini's house: at the second, especially, the crowd was so great that some thirty of the guests had to remain seated on the staircase steps! . . . My father and I wormed our way patiently through the crowd: fortunately we were escorted by Signora Rossini, who with exquisite courtesy made a path for us and led us into the music room. What a spectacle!

"Rossini truly was surrounded by *tout Paris* . . . I no longer recall the names of the *Duchesses*, the *Marquises*, the *Baronesses* who were paying court to the celebrated Maestro: there were ministers, ambassadors; in one corner of the room, standing surrounded by many people, was the Pope's cardinal legate in a great violet tunic: I don't remember the name of that ecclesiastical eminence either, but I do recall that he was a very handsome man of imposing stature and gay face.

"When Rossini saw us, he signaled for us to approach, at the same time calling to him two very attractive young fellows, the one rather skinny, the other with the fine chest of an Italian baritone.

" 'Here are two young friends of mine whom I want you to know,' Rossini said. 'Monsieur [Francis] Planté, a pianist colleague, and Monsieur [Gustave] Doré, whom the world believes to be a great draftsman, but who is in fact a great singer! . . . and therefore my colleague too . . .'

"And that was how I came to know two artists who so honor France.

"In the meantime, Gaetano Braga had approached the pianoforte; Rossini got up and induced a religious silence, and then Braga's violoncello delighted the attentive audience with a new piece by Rossini, accompanied by the composer himself.

"Then Planté played his transcription for piano of the overture to *Semiramide*, with truly extraordinary vigor and effect.

"Next, Gustave Doré sang a song; Rossini was right: Doré had a very beautiful baritone voice and sang with great taste and expression.

"I shall pass over four or five pieces that followed so as to reach the *clou* of the evening: and the *clou* was the quartet from *Rigoletto*, sung by Adelina Patti, Alboni, Gardoni, Delle Sedie, and accompanied by Gioachino Rossini.

"My very dear readers, anyone who has heard such a performance never for his whole life forgets so intense an artistic emotion! . . . And what an accompanist Rossini was . . . what an exquisite touch, neat, delicate . . . a marvel, on my honor; I know only one other individual who could compete with Rossini for the most perfect way of accompanying: the composer of *Rigoletto* himself, Giuseppe Verdi.

"Need I say that the quartet ended amid indescribable enthusiasm? . . . need I say that it was repeated? . . . No word, no superlative could succeed in giving, however pallidly, an exact idea of that ambiance saturated with musical electricity."

Shortly after the visits by the Ricordis, the German composer-writer Emil Naumann appeared at the Rossinis' with a letter of introduction from Pauline Viardot-Garcia. He later wrote:"

"I was fortunate enough to make our Master's acquaintance in Paris in April 1867 (that is, only a year and a half before his death); my talk with him characterized him too well for me to be able to resist telling you about it.

"Upon my entrance, the old gentleman, an amiable expression on his face, rose from an armchair near his desk, upon which lay the manuscript score on which he was then at work. I had just enough time to notice a flower stand to his right and an upright piano to his left. Characteristically, on each corner of the latter there were statuettes of the heroes of the two operas that have immortalized his name: Tell, with the boy, and the Barber of Seville in his Spanish costume. After we had exchanged greetings in French, and after Rossini had inquired about Mme Viardot-Garcia . . . [he] pointed to the still-wet manuscript [the orchestration of the *Petite Messe solennelle*] and said: 'You just

found me in the process of finishing a composition that I have designated for performance right after my death.' These words, spoken with
a happy, beaming expression on his face, surprised me because they
seemed to deny the renowned *joie de vivre* of the still-youthful old
man. When I made a remark to that effect, he answered: 'Oh, you
mustn't believe that I am finishing my little composition because I am
despondent or preoccupied with thoughts of death; it's only to keep it
from falling into the hands of Sax and his friends here." You should know
that I did the score for the vocal parts of this modest work some time
ago; if it were to be found among my effects, there would be Monsieur
Sax with his saxophone or Monsieur Berlioz with another monstrous
modern orchestra, and they'd want to orchestrate my Mass, killing all
my vocal lines, and thus killing me also. *Car je ne suis rien qu'un pauvre
melodiste* ["For I am nothing but a poor melodist"]! That is why I
am now in the process of adding a string quartet and a few modest
winds to my choruses and arias. That's what one always used to do, and
it will give my poor singers a chance to be heard. So, you see, you are
in the presence of a man who, like all old and increasingly weak people,
is attached to the good old times and the habits of his youth; that's why,
you young people must be patient with us [Naumann was thirty-nine]!'
The charming old man went on in that happy, ironic tone for a while;
all the mischievousness of the creator of the *Barbiere* seemed to shine
through. Suddenly he interrupted himself with the words: '*A propos,*
how is Herr Richard Wagner? Is he still the idol of Germany, or has the
fever with which he infected his compatriots subsided? But wait a
moment—I am so thoughtless—perhaps you yourself are a Wagnerian,
and if so, perhaps you don't think that you and the other Germans are
plagued by a fever, but rather that I, the old man, am?' I assured him
that he need not worry in that respect, as our great classical masters
were our ideals; nevertheless, now that Mendelssohn, Robert Schumann,
and Meyerbeer were dead, I could not refrain from declaring Richard
Wagner the most significant and independent talent among living composers. 'Oh, in that respect, I completely agree with you,' Rossini said
emphatically, 'and nothing could be farther from my mind than to
cast doubt on the originality of the creator of *Lohengrin*; but the composer occasionally makes it very difficult, in the chaos of sounds which
his operas contain, for us to find the beauties for which we are indebted
to him. *Monsieur Wagner a de beaux moments, mais de mauvais quart
d'heures* ["Monsieur Wagner has good moments, but bad quarters of an

hour"]! Nevertheless, I have followed his career up to now with the greatest interest. There is only one thing I never understood and still cannot understand: how is it possible that a people that has produced a Mozart can begin to forget him for a Wagner?' And then the old gentleman started praising Mozart, whom he called his idol, though he said that unfortunately he could not boast of always having proved himself a worthy disciple. 'The Germans,' he went on, 'always have been the great harmonists; we Italians have been the melodists; but since you Northerners produced Mozart, we Southerners have been beaten on our own ground, for this man rises above both nations: he combines the whole magic of Italy's cantilena with Germany's profound heartfelt inwardness [*Gemüthstiefe*]. This appears in the ingenious and richly developed harmony of the combined voices in his works. If Mozart is no longer regarded as the beautiful and the lofty, then we old ones, who still are left over, can be entirely happy to quit this earth. But one thing I know for certain, Mozart and his audiences will meet again in Paradise! . . .' "

Some months after Naumann's visit, Hanslick—nearly seven years after what he reasonably had feared would be his only chance to see the old Maestro—visited Rossini again in Passy. In the *Neue freie Presse*, Vienna, he published a "Musical Letter from Paris" dated July 18, 1867:

"When, seven years ago in Paris, I took leave of Rossini and Auber, I did so with the sad premonition that I probably had seen these two patriarchs of modern opera for the last time. After all, they both had reached those wintry heights of life upon which each year must be regarded as a special gift. How happy I was, therefore, to see both of my friends again, both of them healthy and happy and completely unchanged [Rossini was seventy-five, Auber eight-five]. The momentous ascending scale of seven years had scarcely affected them at all; it is barely possible to detect the difference between the octave and the root. . . ."

Hanslick had gone out to Passy with two other men—one of them the pianist Julius Schulhoff—to show Rossini a photograph of the fresco by Moritz von Schwind" with which a lunette of the new Opera at Vienna had been filled. After Rossini had studied the picture (which showed scenes from *Il Barbiere di Siviglia* and *L'Italiana in Algeri*), he asked his visitors whether or not the Mozart and Beethoven monuments at Vienna had been completed. Hanslick continued: "We three Austrians became somewhat embarrassed. 'I remember Beethoven very well,"

Rossini went on after a short pause, 'though it will soon be half a century. During my stay in Vienna, I hastened to seek him out.' 'And, as [Anton Felix] Schindler and other biographers assure us, he didn't admit you.'ⁿ 'On the contrary,' Rossini corrected me, 'I had asked the Italian poet Carpani, with whom I had visited Salieri earlier, to introduce me to Beethoven, and he received us immediately, and very politely. Of course, the visit didn't last very long, as conversation with Beethoven was really painful. That day he heard especially badly, and though I spoke as loudly as possible, he didn't understand me; furthermore, his lack of facility in Italian may have made conversation even more difficult for him.' I must admit that this information, the truth of which was corroborated by numerous details, pleased me like an unexpected gift. I had always been bothered by this incident in Beethoven's biography, as well as by those musical Jacobins who had glorified the brutal German virtue of denying admittance to a Rossini. Well, the whole story was untrue. Another example of the lack of concern with which incorrect facts are presented and repeated so that they can harden into historical truth with incredible speed. And all this while it still would be so easy to obtain authentic enlightenment from living participants! . . ."

The four men then moved to the ground floor of the villa. "It is known," Hanslick wrote, "that during recent years, Rossini has cultivated a predilection for the piano, and this belated accomplishment" furnishes him with a subject for continuous jokes (many of them stereotyped). He at once began to complain that Schulhoff refused to consider him a pianist. 'Of course, I don't practice scales every day like you young people, because if I were to play scales the length of the keyboard, I'd fall off the chair either to the left or to the right.' On Schulhoff's insistence, Rossini played one of his piano jests for us, the '*Petit Caprice* (*style Offen*bach).' An Italian once told Rossini—this is the genesis of this piece—that Offenbach had the evil eye and that one had to make the *jettatore* sign (extension of the index and fifth fingers) in his presence. 'Consequently one must play Offenbach like that,' Rossini said jokingly, and proceeded to improvize an extremely droll little thing at the piano, playing its melody masterfully with two forklike extended fingers of his right hand. I noticed a few fine original modulations, whereupon Rossini was so obliging as to play his arrangement of the old Marlborough song."￼ It is amazing that just Rossini, whose modulations never were extremely subtle, should have provided this folk melody with a wealth of clever harmonies and enharmonic surprises.

In a few other songs and piano pieces that I had heard at one of his soirées, I had been struck by Rossini's new predilection for pronounced basses and lively modulations. Although I am not inclined to lay undue stress upon this afterglow of a flame fundamentally extinguished long ago, I nevertheless find it interesting that the style of the seventy-five-year-old Pesaro minstrel is still capable of any innovation at all."

Adelina Patti's name came up in the conversation. "The Maestro speaks of the latter [Patti] with admiring esteem, and always singles her out as an exception when deploring the extinction of truly great singers," Hanslick added. " 'Look there,' he said, pointing to the scaffolding of the new Opéra, which rose outside his windows, 'now we'll soon have a new theater, but already we have no more singers. Will you be better off when your new Vienna Opera is finished? . . .'

"I regret not having got to know Rossini's new *Messe*. This work (which, like the others, has been hidden away by the composer, who refuses to publish it) is said to contain many beauties. 'That's not church music for you Germans,' Rossini scoffed. 'My most sacred music still is always just *semiseria*.' He called his *Hymne à Napoléon* (for the distribution of the awards on July 1) 'drinking music,' his operas 'antiquated stuff.' Altogether, it is not possible to talk seriously with the famous Maestro. He is comfortable only with easy humor and gentle raillery, and when he derides his compositions, one is never entirely sure whether it is at his expense or that of others. One may disapprove of the extremism of this grotesque self-denial, but it undoubtedly is caused by a motive or feeling that can only be respected when one examines the situation more closely. Rossini, you must know, lives amid uninterrupted adoration and overindulgence. Few men on earth are venerated—and nothing but venerated—in such a manner. His room never lacks visitors; the highest notables of the nobility, of the rich, and of art come and go. He is showered with costly gifts and delicate attentions; of every hundred people, ninety-nine feel obliged to flatter him. Were Rossini to accept all those admiring words with that complacent, conceited-modest smile of so many famous men, as though refusing with one hand and accepting with the other, then one could not bear to remain in his house for fifteen minutes. One would choke on the incense. Serious disapproval and anger are not in keeping with Rossini's personality; therefore he prefers to knock the censer from the admirer's hand by playful self-ridicule and then proceed to enjoy his embarrassment. 'However should I address you?' a beautiful lady breathlessly asked him recently. 'Great master? Prince of Music? Or Divine Genius?' 'I'd like it best,' Rossini replied, 'if you would call me *Mon petit lapin*! ["My little rabbit"] . . .' '*Allez vous-en*,' he recently exclaimed to one such wretch, '*ma célébrité m'embête*! ["Get on with you, my fame bores me!"].' "

At least two new compositions by Rossini were performed in public during 1867.[n] Probably his only composition to an English text, the *National Hymn* was composed for the Birmingham Festival of August 1867. The verse begins:

> *Oh! Lord most high!*
> *Who art God and Father!*
> *Hear Thou our cry*
> *While Thy children gather!*

For baritone solo with mixed chorus (unison sopranos, contraltos, tenors, and basses), it was published by Hutchings and Romer in London in 1873.

The second new composition was the *Hymne à Napoléon III et à son vaillant peuple* mentioned by Hanslick. To a bombastic text by Émilien Pacini, this occasional piece for vocal soloists, chorus, orchestra, and band was performed for the first time at the Palais de l'Industrie[n] on the occasion of the distribution (July 1, 1867) of awards and prizes for the Exposition Universelle. The score bears an inscription in French: "To Napoleon III and his valiant People.—Hymn (with accompaniment of Large Orchestra and Military Band) for Baritone (solo), a Pontiff; Chorus of High Priests, Chorus of Vivandières, of Soldiers, and of People.—Dances, Bells, Side Drums, and Cannon. Forgive the paucity!! Passy, 1867, Words by E. Pacini." When Gaetano Fabi wrote Rossini from Bologna to congratulate him on the performance of this *Hymne*, Rossini replied (July 17, 1867): "I thank you for the compliments that you offer me for the *Hymne à Napoléon III* as a kindness on your part, but not as a reward for my poor composition, which I wrote out to be sung in my garden in Passy, *en famille*, and certainly not under such solemn circumstances. What could I do? I was asked, and I couldn't refuse."[n]

At two o'clock on the afternoon of July 1, Napoleon, the Empress Eugénie, Abdul-Aziz, Sultan of Turkey, and an entourage of royalty, nobility, and other dignitaries were received at the entrance to the Palais de l'Industrie. When they had been seated, Jules Cohen stepped before 800 instrumentalists (600 civilian, 200 military) and 400 choristers and struck up the first measure of Rossini's *Hymne*. The *Revue et Gazette musicale* reported: "An introduction in two-step rhythm, a motive in quadruple time accompanied in the grand style by harp, a chorus of women, lively and gay, a peroration that brings into play all the forces, instruments, and devices invented to make noise: such is this composition, of which so much was said, and of which so much still is being said. Excusing himself 'for the paucity,' the illustrous Maestro has disarmed criticism spiritedly; but in truth he has given proof of too-great modesty, writing a piece that he supposed should not and could not be heard well amid the noise of an official festival. Nonetheless, it was sung in religious silence. The performance, under Maître Jules Cohen, was splendid." The *Hymne* was sung at least three times more before falling into disuse: at the Opéra on August 15, 1867, for the annual Festival of the Emperor; again at the Palais de l'Industrie on August 18; and at the Birmingham Festival of August 1873.

The Paris critics divided sharply on the merits of Rossini's *Hymne à Napoléon*—as they were divided less overtly by 1867 on those of the Emperor himself. Madame Olympe became terribly disturbed; in a letter in faulty French to the editor of a paper whose critic had treated the *Hymne* badly, she poured out her hurt and determination: "The *Hymne* by Rossini will be performed on August 15 at the Opéra in honor of the valiant French people, and you must publish a critique. I desire, however, that this not be done by your editor for two reasons: first because his knowledge is no greater than his veracity; then because I do not want a paper directed by you to be allowed to forget the respect owed to my name [Rossini]. I want an impartial judge, without *parti-pris* and competent, such as, for example, Berlioz, whom I do not have the honor of knowing, but whom I know able to evaluate the judgments of certain ignorant publications. I beg him to analyze this page, wholly of circumstance. The Pontiff's solo could not have been signed and paragraphed [*sic*] by anyone but the composer of the *Moïse* prayer; the chorus of *vivandières* is written with that melodic *brio* native to no one other than the composer of *Il Barbiere*. Tell me, then, who would have known how to do better? . . . For the rest, the outrage could only add one more rosette to his crown, as nothing could lower him from the pedestal on which his genius has placed him. He will remain the greatest figure of future centuries."[n] At seventy, Olympe had lost none of her unwavering devotion to Rossini and had learned nothing from his talent for public modesty.

As the winter of 1867–8 came on, Rossini's health increasingly deteriorated.

Not only did his chronic catarrh take on alarming intensity, but also he was psychologically disturbed, suffering from exacerbated nerves, anxiety, insomnia, difficulty in breathing, and a sensation of pressure in the abdomen. He was never to be passably well again; he was ordered to cut off almost all activity and to spend his waking hours in rest. Nonetheless, when the Opéra celebrated the official "five-hundredth" performance of *Guillaume Tell* on February 10, 1868,ⁿ the soloists, chorus, and orchestra went afterward to the Chaussée d'Antin to serenade Rossini. As the conductor, Georges Hainl, struck up the overture to *Tell*, the gravely ill Rossini appeared for a moment at a window of his apartment. Then Jean-Baptiste Faure and the chorus sang a number from Act I of the opera, to the enormous delight of the crowd that had gathered. Madame Olympe came down to thank the performers and then accompanied Mlle Battu, Faure, and Vilaret back upstairs, where, in the name of the Opéra personnel, they presented her husband with a wreath inscribed: "To Rossini, in memory of the 500th performance of *Guillaume Tell*, the artists of the Opéra, 1829–1868."

The February of 1868 ended with a 29th, Rossini's seventy-sixth birthday. Letters, telegrams, verses, gifts poured into the Chaussée d'Antin from all parts of the world. Ten guests sat down to dine with Rossini and Olympe: Alboni, Conte Pillet-Will, Jean-Baptiste Faure and his wife (Caroline Faure-Lefébure), Gustave Doré, Bigottini, Moïnna, Edmond Michotte, Jean-Fréderic Possoz, *maire* of Passy, and Antoine Berryer. At one side, the table was decorated with a cake sent by the Baronne de Rothschild; it had an iced inscription, *"Bonheur et santé—1868."* The other side of the table was enlivened by a confection in which a swan with spread wings upheld garlands bearing the names of Rossini's chief compositions. At the close of the dinner, Berryer made a short formal speech—which he later said had moved him more than anything similar in his whole oratorical career. After dinner, other guests arrived. Nadaud presented Rossini with one of his songs. The music-making was in the capable hands of Diémer, Battu, Delle Sedie, Faure, and Gardoni. As a souvenir of the occasion, Doré gave Olympe a fan that he had painted. On it, a bust of Rossini rose from a bed of greenery, with vines twined around five parallel lines of ribbon forming a musical staff. Numerous *amorini* were depicted as playing instruments among the foliage, their heads being placed in relation to the five ribbons so as to become the opening notes of Arnold's aria in *Guillaume Tell*, "O *Mathilde, idole de mon âme*."

In March, Rossini's health worsened still more. When he replied to a letter written to him at Florence on March 29 by Emilio Broglio, Minister of Public Education, he very probably was in no condition to realize that he was striking open a hornets' nest or that his reply would sharply irritate many Italians and set on edge the teeth of Arrigo Boito and Giuseppe Verdi. After a flowery presentation of himself, Broglio had written: "In my short existence as a minister, great good fortune has been my lot. I turned to Alessandro Manzoni, begging him to help me in a question of language; and that venerable old man, after thirty years of silence, has put himself to work, writing and publishing furiously; and what is more, he has also given me the consolation of writing me that I have rejuvenated him! See how this happy example gives me the courage to try the experiment again with you, certainly much less aged, but not less illustrious."

"Among the matters handled by my ministry, there is also music, about which I am as passionate as—woe is me!—ignorant. Of that of the past century, which might be called pre-Rossinian, as one speaks of the pre-Raphaelite painters, it is not worth talking; despite its great beauties and its songs of Paradise, as far as the theater is concerned— which is what I intend to occupy myself with here—it is all dead and buried, some rare exception aside.

"Your music, certainly, is alive and immortal; but we are now reduced to this, that it can no longer be heard because there is no longer anyone who knows how to sing it. You yourself, Maestro, would, I believe, fly ten miles from the city where there was announced, for example, a performance of *Semiramide*, because you would be certain of hearing it lacerate the paternal viscera.

"After Rossini, what can we say for forty years, what do we have? Four operas by Meyerbeer and . . ."

"How could we remedy such grave sterility. Evidently in only two ways: 1. by rebeginning from the beginning the education of singers; a long and very difficult undertaking; 2. opening the field to young *maestri*.

"These no longer can come to life; they are suffocated in their swaddling clothes for one big reason. The exterminating operas that last five hours have become a calamitous habit with the public; those colossi, those musical mastodons can only crush a nascent talent, now that the Mephistophelean presumptions . . ." But even when a young man dares to confront so Herculean an undertaking, how will be be able, except in truly extraordinary cases, to find an impresario to assume such large expenses in view of the very great probability of tossing it all away on a first night of whistlings? Then the young *maestri* can neither turn out these monstrous operas nor, once they are done, see them performed. And so, what to do? Here is where you enter the field. It is necessary, it seems to me, to establish in Italy a big musical association composed of all the dilettantes and lovers of music, who are still numerous; and which I should like to call, if you accept my proposal that you be its president, the Società Rossiniana. This society would cover all of Italy, would have committees in the principal cities, and naturally would have its good statute, in which would be clearly defined the purposes for which it would exist and the means for attaining them.

"For me to wish to indicate here, in a letter to you—to you!— what those aims and those methods of restoration and progress for the musical art should be would simply be an insane presumption, and I shall protect myself from that as the Devil from Holy Water. I shall say only, this letter already being too long, that if you accept the presidency, if you accept it with good will and the youthful drive with which Manzoni has accepted his; if, with those secretarial assistants whom the excellent Commendatore [Costantino] Nigra, the King's Minister at Paris, will have the goodness to furnish you, you would put yourself into a little correspondence with the outstanding *maestri*, writers, and musical Maecenases of Italy and, if you think it wise, also abroad; if, to sum up, you, illustrious *signore Maestro*, should be disposed to embrace ardently this, my first idea, and be willing to win this other title to the gratitude of your country, I am frankly persuaded that it would be possible to bring together the number of 2,000 or 2,500 subscribers who, at 40 or 50 lire per year, would provide a first fund of 100,000 lire, which, increased by the return from some grand concerts, in which you would permit the performance of your unpublished music, already would constitute a good foundation for covering the expenses called for by those aims and those means which would be found useful for promoting, as I said just above, the restoration and progress of the art.

"Once, then, that the Società had attained a notable and promising first development, see what could happen. I, as Minister of Public Instruction, have four or five conservatories or musical institutes, with an approved budget of about 400,000 lire. There is in Parliament, and it is natural that there should be, some opinion contrary to that curious government interference in the free evolution of the art; it would, then, be easy to get the State to wash its hands of that matter, ceding the conservatories, with their physical material and a part of the payment fixed in the budget, to the new Società, which thus could very opportunely replace the Government in this matter. Excuse the length and confusion of my letter. Your most devoted Emilio Broglio."

Rossini undoubtedly was pleased by this sign of honor from the government of Italy, but certainly he had not understood that the whole purpose of Broglio's letter lay in its final paragraph. His answer, the exact date of which cannot be determined, read: "For the love of Heaven, it was not my wish to be (involuntarily) late in answering Your Excellency's precious letter of the past March 29; the blame belongs wholly to my uncertain health and the constant wish to be able to write this poor letter of mine (in perhaps undiplomatic phraseology) with my own hand. Even though I am now in the grasp of a terrible malady of the nerves which has deprived me completely of sleep and strength for five months and more, I take courage and pick up my pen to offer Your Excellency the expressions of my warmest thanks for the generous and opportune details set forth in Your Excellency's letter, aiming not only to honor the old Pesarese, but also to raise up again an art that I have so much at heart and which for centuries was the glory of our Italy. I accept with joy and gratitude the presidency to which Your Excellency refers, and I want to be included among the annual members for the sum indicated. As for the performance of unpublished music, I must tell you that I have only a single concert piece, and that is the *Chant des Titans* for four bass voices in unison, with accompaniment of large orchestra. This piece (unpublished) was performed in Vienna in a concert given for the monument to Mozart. I was glad to lend it for so noble a circumstance (with vocal and orchestral parts, without, be it well understood, the extraction of any copy); I shall be doubly grateful, if Your Excellency thinks to make use of it, to lend it under such an important circumstance. May the present state of Italy second the noble thoughts that, with such love, come from Your Excellency's heart and breast. I shall in any case make the warmest prayers for a happy outcome. Be indulgent toward this, my writing; it is an infirm man who writes and who has the honor to call himself Your Excellency's most honest admirer.

"P.S. It is well that you should not be unaware that in Milan they want to open a so-called *experimental* theater for the young composers; Maestro [Lauro] Rossi, director of the Conservatory, is one of those promoting it."

The suggestion in Broglio's letter which Rossini had failed to understand—or at least to comment upon—was that the state should withdraw most of its financial support from the conservatories and other musical institutes. But when Broglio's letter was published in Italy, the press rose up to denounce him, not only for trying to arrange the eventual dismantling of the great music schools, but also for having insulted many operatic composers, living and dead. Verdi's correspondence shows that he became extremely agitated at once. To Broglio, who just had forwarded to him a diploma of nomination as a *commendatore* of the Order of the Crown of Italy, he wrote: "This Order was instituted to honor those who benefit Italy, whether by arms or by literature, the sciences, and the arts. A letter to Rossini from Your Excellency, though you are *ignorant* of music (as you yourself say and believe), asserts that no opera has been made in Italy for forty years. Why, then, is this decoration sent to me? The address is certainly a mistake, and I return it." Explaining to Conte Opprandino Arrivabene his return of the decoration, Verdi wrote: "Intentionally or unintentionally, the Minister's letter is an insult to Italian art. I sent back the Cross not for my own sake, but out of respect for the memory of those two [Bellini and Donizetti] who are no longer alive and who have filled the world with their melodies."

Early in the summer of 1868, from Genoa, Verdi also wrote to one of the Escudier brothers an irate letter containing references that in part are tantalizing because obscure. Referring to Rossini, he wrote: "This is the second [hurt] that he has done me, and the third will be when we shall meet in the Valley of Jehoshaphat. Do you remember, during the *Trovatore* trial," the letter written to me, and read in court by the adversary, Torribio? And now he accepts the presidency of a project that insults his country and outrages the memory of Two who were his friends [Bellini and Donizetti]! who cannot defend themselves and who deserve all respect?"

Boito, infuriated by Broglio's implied insult to, among others, Bellini, Donizetti, Verdi, and (the "Mephistophelean presumptions" and "musical mastodons") himself, attacked the Minister and his proposals by publishing in *Il Pungolo* of May 2, 1868, a "Letter in Four Para-

graphs (to His Excellency the Minister of Public Instruction).'" Brilliantly parodying the pseudo-Manzonian, stilted, bureaucratic Italian
of Broglio's letter to Rossini, Boito began his attack with a satirical
paragraph echoing the beginning of that letter: "Your Excellency naturally will not remember, but I had the honor and pleasure of meeting
you, as well as of making an arrangement with you (as our Tuscan
maestri say)," once before. And that was in the autumn of '66, on
Monte Bisbino, during a trip with the asses [*asinelli*].

"I tell you this to lessen the surprise that Your Excellency will
experience on reading this, my letter, etc., etc." Then, after a very
detailed, barbed, and funny description of that imaginary trip "with
the asses," Boito remarked that Broglio had gone only as far as Pruth
—and had proceeded to become a minister only to stop at *Semiramide*.
He continued:

"Have the grace to move ahead, don't bawl so much back there,
all of us have moved on, now you too get on from there. Get on!
Courage! There is a word that makes the world move ahead, and it is
the word '*Arri*! ["giddap"].' You will recall that you too shouted it
that day on the Bisbino, when traveling assback; the poor beast, hearing
'*arri!*' trotted ahead. At Florence, Your Excellency must often have
heard Tuscans say:

> *Il bisognino fa trottar la vecchia*
> ["The call of nature makes the old girl trot"]

and since 1300 they have said: '*Bisogno fa trottar la vecchia* ["Need
moves one"].' But the only need Your Excellency feels is to stand still.

"*Semiramide* is a great thing, but there is more: *Guglielmo Tell*—
and Your Excellency has not caught up with it yet; Rossinian though
you are, you have, without realizing it, placed it in that category
of 'musical mastodons that have become a calamitous habit with the
public.' For pity's sake, *sor ministro*, take care when you write letters
not to let phrases escape you which can displease the people who are
supposed to read them.

"You must know that Rossini is the greatest jester there ever has
been, as is proved by the reply that Your Excellency received, which
reply, beyond the fact that you had to wait for it a long time, has
irony sprinkled in its ink. Your Excellency, wishing to make yourself
more of an opera critic than a minister, has gone hunting in a thicket
of misunderstandings."

"Yesterday you were the victim of a Rossinian burlesque; today of a rebuff by Verdi, who refused the Order of the Crown of Italy."

Earlier in the "Letter in Four Paragraphs," Boito had written: "God prevent me from belittling the august figure of Rossini, but not even for his sake would it be permissible for me to belittle the history of Italian opera.

"After Rossini, what have we had?—Your Excellency asks. Eh! nothing; from '29 to now, nothing has been done but humbug! *nugæque canoræ* [roughly, "buffoons and droners"]!

"In '31, for example, there was *Norma*, a humbug that led Rossini to say:—I'll write no more—and keep his word.

"Then, in '35, *I Puritani*, more humbug! Then, in '40, *La Favorita* and in '43 *Don Sebastiano*; *nugæque canoræ*!

"In '51, *Rigoletto* and in '53, *Il Trovatore*, and the whole fascinating, glorious, fecund theater of Verdi! And, seeing that you have had the grace to name Meyerbeer, why have you not named Halévy, Gounod, Weber, Wag . . . (don't be frightened). Your Excellency can see that there is something for all tastes. But Your Excellency calls such a history sterile."

Meanwhile, Rossini had come to realize the enormity of his mistake in agreeing, out of whatever mixture of patriotism and ironic obedience, to Broglio's request. When Lauro Rossi wrote him in agitation on the subject, Rossini answered on June 21 in a letter that Rossi immediately released to a Milan newspaper. After congratulating Rossi on the condition of the Milan Conservatory, Rossini went on:

"Son of a Public Musical Establishment (the Liceo Comunale at Bologna), as I am proud of being, it pleases me to say that I always have been a friend and defender of the Conservatories, which should not be looked upon now as the cradle of geniuses, it being given only to God to make that gift (rarely) to mortals, but rather as a providential field for emulation, like a beneficent artistic proving ground, advantage of which is taken by the chapels, the theaters, the orchestras, the colleges, etc., etc.

"Furthermore, it is saddening to me to read in some respectable journals that it is the intention of Minister Broglio to abolish the Conservatories of Music! What further remains incomprehensible to me is that such an intention should be induced from the (unfortunate) ministerial letter published and addressed to me. I can swear to you, dear Maestro, on my honor that in the correspondence carried on with the above-mentioned Minister (correspondence that has not lost its importance), there was not even the smallest inkling of such a thing. Would I ever have been capable of being a secret accomplice of such disasters??? Be calm, and I promise you (if anything of the above sort were to be attempted) to be, in my small way, the warmest advocate in favor of the Conservatories, in which it is given me to hope that no roots will be put down by those new philosophical principles which would like to make of the musical art a literary art! an imitative art! a philosophical melopea, which is equivalent to recitative, now free, now measured, with various accompaniments of tremolo and so-called. . . .

"Don't let us Italians forget that the musical art is all ideal and expressive; let the cultivated public and the Glorious Crew not forget that delight must be the basis and aim of this art.

"Simple melody—clear rhythm.

"In the absence of these *accidenti* (Roman style [that is, to mean unforeseen events]), believe, then, my dearest Maestro, that these new pseudo-philosophers (whom you mention in your appreciated letter to me) are simply supporters and advocates of those poor composers of music who lack *ideas, imagination*!!!

"*Laus Deo*—I see that I have imposed upon you too long the pain of reading me. Forgive me. Count upon my sympathy, and may it please you to believe me your admirer and servant. G. ROSSINI."

Rossini also had footnoted his first unthinking reply to Broglio: on May 31, he had sent to Rome a letter that sidestepped the controversial question of the music schools but insisted upon that of the experimental theater, which he said should be "similar to the old one that existed at Venice, called the [Teatro] San Moisè. There they played exclusively little operas (set by celebrated composers) in a single act, called *farse*. That theater, further, served for the debuts of young *maestri*, as it did for Mayer [*sic*], Generali, Pavesi, Farinelli, Coccia, etc., and for myself in 1810, with the *farsa* entitled *La Cambiale di matrimonio* (with an encouragement of 100 francs!!). The impresario's expenses were minimal because, except for a good roster of singers (without choristers), the whole thing was reduced to the outlay for a single setting for each *farsa*, a very modest *mise en scène*, and to a few days' expenses for rehearsals. From all that it is easy to see that everything tended toward facilitating the debut of a beginning *maestro*, who better than in an opera of four or five acts, in a *farsa* could sufficiently display his innate imagination (if Heaven had granted it to him!!) and his technique (if he had learned it!).

"Such a farce, made up, be it well understood, of an introduction, duets, arias, a concerted piece, a finale, and a *sinfonia*, is more than is required for a debutant. However, it would be good that the so-called libretto be composed by a veteran theater poet, this with the aim of giving the timid beginning musician all those means which are of a nature to give full value to the theatrical, melodic, harmonic qualities that he possesses . . ."[n]

Rossini's part in the Broglio controversy was to be terminated by his death, Broglio's part in it by the fall of the government in which he had been serving. Nothing, unfortunately, was to come of Maestro Lauro Rossi's projected experimental theater in Milan—unless one were to regard as a remote echo of it the opening, on December 26, 1955, of the small auditorium known as the Piccola Scala.

On May 28, three days before writing his second letter to Minister Broglio, Rossini had penned, in humorous vein, the last surviving of his letters to Michele Costa:

"FRIEND, SON, AND MOST BELOVED COLLEAGUE: Your Celebrity and mine are a real Scourge! Everyone wants to know us and to have our friendship and Protection! We must needs obey destiny, and *chutt*!!! This poor Autograph of mine will be presented by a Russian Colleague of ours, *il Sig.r Cav.re* Lazarew (who perhaps will not be unknown to you); he is an Old Acquaintance of mine. He is madly devoted to music, and is almost hydrophobic. He wants to know the Great Costa, and that is why I am giving you the pain of reading me! He wants to see Say [?] and the Father of the Diva [Adelina] Patti, Quondam Marchesa—Courage.

"Don't forget Your most affectionate ROSSINI."[n]

Very probably it was during 1868, too, that Victor Emanuel II named Rossini a Grand Knight of the Order of the Crown of Italy and that, in response, Rossini composed *La Corona d'Italia*, a fanfare for military band which he forwarded to Broglio with an inscription noting that it was "offered to His Majesty Victor Emanuel II by the grateful G. Rossini."[n] In the letter of September 10, 1868, which accompanied its dispatch to Broglio, he said: "Instrumentating this little piece of music, to be performed, be it well understood, on foot, I took advantage not only of the old instruments of Italian bands, but also of the excellent new ones we owe to Sax, their celebrated inventor and maker. I cannot imagine that the leaders of Italian military bands have not adopted these instruments (as was done everywhere). If by any chance this *only advance of our days* was not embraced by them (a thing that would pain me), I beg Your Excellency to be willing to entrust my score to a good composer of military music (such as often is found among the bandleaders) so that he may adapt it to the standard instruments, preserving with judgment and patience the melodic and harmonic effects of the original fanfare. It will also be necessary to guard against copies being made, and to prohibit reproductions for whatever instrument—to respect, in short, the rights!! . . ."[n]

Broglio, evidently intending to have *La Corona d'Italia* played immediately, ordered the necessary saxophones from Paris. However, he was soon out of office. No performance of this last of Rossini's instrumentated compositions took place until ten years after the composer's death. Then, on November 25, 1878, it was played in the *piazza* outside the Palazzo Quirinale in Rome to honor the safe return of Umberto I and Queen Margherita from Naples, where they had been the objects of an assassination attempt. Three hundred musicians from two municipal bands, plus the band of the Rome Fire Department and the bands of four regiments of the line—with the addition of thirty drummers—played it to everyone's satisfaction. In all probability, it was Rossini's last completed composition.

CHAPTER XX

1868

SIXTEEN DAYS after Rossini dated the letter transmitting the score of *La Corona d'Italia* to Minister Broglio, the last of the *samedi soirs* took place at the Passy villa. The chronicle of it in *Le Ménestrel* said: "The Saturday evening [September 26] *chez* Rossini must be numbered among the most brilliant of the season . . ." Then it was time for Rossini and Olympe to move back to the Chaussée d'Antin for the autumn and winter. During October, however, the "bronchial catarrh" that had been enfeebling Rossini for many autumns and winters returned with unexampled virulence. He and Olympe were forced to stay in Passy, for he soon was too weak to make the short trip into Paris. When his personal physician, Dr. Vio Bonato—who had seen him last on September 15, then apparently in reasonably good health—returned, he found his patient extremely nervous and in low spirits.[n] What was referred to as a rectal fistula, but almost certainly was a cancer, developed rapidly. An operation became urgent. But the bedridden Rossini, who had retired into almost complete silence, lying mostly with closed eyes and speaking only when he needed something, was in no condition to undergo surgery.

The distraught Olympe received moral support and offers of assistance from many of Rossini's friends and admirers.[n] Finally, the lung inflammation having responded to treatment, Dr. Auguste Nélaton (called in at Rossini's request) decided to operate on November 3.[n] Because of the patient's heart condition, Nélaton felt that he could not be kept under chloroform very long, and therefore acted with the greatest possible speed, performing the operation in five minutes. He found what must have been a spreading cancer, removed as much as possible of the diseased tissue, stanched the hemorrhaging, and had the patient returned to his bed. For two days thereafter, Olympe dressed her husband's wound: he would not permit anyone else to touch him. On November 5, Dr. Nélaton, alarmed by the appearance of one side of the wound, decided upon a second operation. During the following three days, an appearance of normal healing led Nélaton to say: "I think that we shall save him!" Thereafter, Rossini—who at first had seemed reluctant to obey Nélaton's orders—lent himself willingly to the prescribed treatment.

Each morning, four interns came out from a Paris hospital to move the very heavy Rossini to a second bed so that the linen on the first could be changed, each of them taking one corner of the undersheet and lifting him with the greatest care. During their first visits, the dying man found them terrifying. But soon he began to respond to their arrival by saying: "Here are the young men! What fine examples of manhood you are! Let's go, my sons, courage!" Michotte told Radiciotti that these were sometimes the only words that Rossini uttered for an entire day. Soon he was in unremitting pain. Groans burst from his lips, terribly disturbing Olympe and the callers who came and went in his room.

When an assisting physican asked: "Well, dear Maestro, how do you feel this morning?" he answered: "Open the window and throw me into the garden; I'll do well there; I won't suffer any more." Michotte reported that at one point, maddened by pain, Rossini shouted: "Oh, Goodwife Death [*Comare*], Goodwife Death; but come to me, then!" He began to burn with unslakable thirst and to ask constantly for ice, which his physicians had ordered given to him very seldom. When he was not calling out: "I am burning up. Ice! Ice!" he was wheedling ice from those near him, addressing them by pet names. When someone would bend over to insert a sliver of ice into his mouth, he would caress the benefactor's head lovingly.

News of Rossini's relapse spread not only across Paris, but also to the rest of the world. Telegrams and letters piled up. A special guestbook was set out to be signed by the many callers who could not be admitted to see the patient." A messenger from the Imperial Household reached Passy each day to obtain word of Rossini's condition. An attaché of the Italian Legation sent frequent reports on it to Rome. One day, Rossini's old friend the papal nuncio Monsignor Chigi went to Passy intent upon administering the last sacraments. Olympe reluctantly allowed him to approach Rossini. But when Chigi said: "Dear Maestro, every man, however great, must sometime think of dying," Rossini summoned Olympe and said: "Olympe, take the Monsignor out."

Several times thereafter, Olympe tried vainly to induce Rossini to receive the last sacraments. Finally an assisting physician, Dr. Barthe, undertook the persuasion. "My dear Maestro, I find you more than usually agitated. My remedies, as I well know, are not enough to bring you the calm you need so badly, and for that reason I want to bring you the Abbé Gallet of St.-Roch. You know him, and he is also a friend of mine and a very mild and sympathetic man." After a show of reluctance, Rossini agreed to receive the Abbé. When the churchman entered the bedroom and spoke, Rossini said: "You have a beautiful voice, Monsieur Abbé." Gallet put the ritual questions to him, including that of his having always been a believer.

"Would I have been able to write the *Stabat* and the *Messe* if I had not had faith?" Rossini replied. "Here, I am ready. Let us begin!" Then he made his confession.

Gallet later published an account of this scene:[n]

"His confession completed, the Maestro said to me: 'Go on talking. I don't feel tired. Your voice has done me so much good. Thanks! You have freed me from a great weight. You will return soon, isn't that so?' And he kissed my hand in the Italian way.

"Madame Olympe, hearing my words of farewell, came back into the room.

" 'Come, my poor friend,' her husband said to her. 'I am thankful to you.' And they embraced, weeping.

" 'I too will confess,' she added, 'and at once.'

" 'Monsieur Abbé,' the Maestro began with a certain warmth, 'it is the Italian clergy who have lost us . . .'

" 'Oh, Maestro, your spirit is too big and you have lived in too elevated an ambiance for your convictions to depend upon the behavior of men . . .'

" 'I have seen the Italian priests from too near. If I had had to deal only with French priests, I would have been a practicing Christian.'

"Fearing to tire the patient too much—for he talked constantly—I left—or, rather, freed myself from the hand that still grasped me, and promised to return the next day and the days after that. However, I had a presentiment that they would not be many: the erysipelas [*sic: érysipèle*] had spread everywhere; his body was not more than one great sore, and he suffered horribly.

"Devoted friends watched over his deathbed; they often heard him pray: '*O crux, ave* . . . *Inflammatus* . . . *Pie Jesus* . . . *Paradisi gloria.*' In the depths of the night he invoked the Virgin in the manner of the Italians: 'What are you doing, then, Virgin Mary? I am suffering the pains of Hell and I have been calling you since early tonight! . . . You hear me . . . If you want to, you can . . . That depends upon you . . . Hurry up, then, get on with it now!' "[n]

When the Abbé Gallet returned the next evening to administer Extreme Unction, others in the room included Alboni, Tamburini, and Adelina Patti, who had just arrived from London. "After the final benediction," Gallet wrote, "and some words that I directed more toward the others than to the dying man, Tamburini, much moved, took my hand, saying: 'Monsieur Abbé, you have written a beautiful page in your history.'

" 'It is beautiful above all, and precious for the poor sick man,' I told him.

" 'The poor Maestro! Madame Alboni exclaimed. 'And unhappily his last [page]!' . . . and Patti collapsed on a sofa, sobbing.

"Sobs came from all parts of the room: one would have said that a desolated family was gathered at the deathbed of the best of parents."

It was now Friday, November 13. Lapsing into a semicoma, the delirious and fevered Rossini was heard to murmur distantly: "*Santa Maria!* . . . *Sant'Anna!* . . ." The latter was his mother's name. At about ten o'clock that night, lying with his spent eyes wide open, Rossini said: "Olympe." At quarter after eleven, Dr. D'Ancona said to Olympe: "Madame, Rossini has stopped suffering." Olympe threw herself upon her husband's body, exclaiming: "Rossini, I shall always be worthy of you!" She could be pulled away only with difficulty.[n]

As Rossini had lain dying, a truly Rossinian event had taken place in Bologna. On the preceding August 2, a twenty-six-year-old Parmesan conductor composer named Costantino Dall'Argine had written to Rossini to say that he had composed a new setting of Sterbini's libretto for *Il Barbiere di Siviglia*—and would like Rossini's permission to dedicate the opera to him. Answering from Passy on August 8, Rossini had written: "I duly hasten to advise you that your highly valued letter of the 2nd of the current month has reached me. Although your name was not unknown to me, given that some time back there reached me the widespread report of the brilliant success that you had obtained with your opera *I Due Orsi*,[n] it is nonetheless dear to me to see that you (a daring young man, by your own words!) hold me in some esteem, intending as you are to dedicate to me the opera that you are now completing. I find only the word 'daring' superfluous in your very courteous letter: I certainly did not consider myself daring when I set to music (in twelve days) after Padre Paisiello the very charming comedy of Beaumarchais. Why should you be so, coming after half a century and more, and with new styles, in setting a *Barbiere* to music?

"Not long ago, Paisiello's was performed in a Paris theater; being, as it is, a gem of spontaneous melodies, of theatrical spirit, it won a very happy and well-merited success. Many polemics, many disputes have risen and always exist between old and new music lovers; you should take to heart (I advise you) the old proverb that says *between two contending parties, the third party benefits*. You may be certain that I do not wish that third to be the winner.

"May, then, your new *Barbiere* join your opera *I Due Orsi* ["The Two Bears"] as a big bear to form a musical triumvirate and assure you, as its creator, and our common century imperishable glory. These are the warm good wishes offered you by the old Pesarese who has the name Rossini.

"P.S. Confirming the above, I shall be happy to accept the dedication of your new work. Please accept in anticipation the most heartfelt thanks."

When Rossini's Beaumarchais opera had received its first performance at Rome on February 20, 1816, Paisiello had had less than four months to live. Fifty-two years later, Rossini had but two days of life remaining when, on November 11, 1868, Dall'Argine's *Il Barbiere di Siviglia* was sung for the first time at the Teatro Comunale, Bologna. Like Rossini's opera, this one stirred up a tempest of controversy; like Rossini, Dall'Argine was accused of offense to his predecessor; unlike Rossini's opera, Dall'Argine's quickly sank into oblivion." Paisiello's *Barbiere* is played sometimes, Rossini's always, Dall'Argine's never.

Epilogue

O
N SATURDAY MORNING, November 14, 1868, Gustave Doré made two sketches of Rossini on his deathbed. The etching that he later based on one of them shows a bewigged Rossini, his head deep in a soft bolster, a crucifix on his chest, his extremely peaceful face strongly suggesting well-known portraits of Dante, but showing a hint of a smile. Two days later, the corpse was embalmed, with Dr. D'Ancona's assistance, by Falcony, inventor of a liquid for which he made the claim that, introduced into the blood vessels, it would hold back corruption forever. The corpse then was placed in a double coffin of precious wood bearing a gold plaque:

GIOACCHINO ANTONIO ROSSINI
NÉ À PESARO LE 29 FÉVRIER 1792
MORT À PASSY LE 13 NOVEMBRE 1868

That evening, November 16, the coffin was placed in a temporary tomb in the Madeleine, where the funeral ceremonies had been planned for five days later. But the capacity of the Madeleine was only about 3,000, and some 5,000 people had asked for invitations to the ceremony. The funeral therefore was set for the Église de la Trinité for Saturday noon, November 21, by which time an announced delegation from Pesaro would have arrived. The musical aspect of the rite was put in the hands of a committee presided over by the eighty-six-year-old Auber. The huge chorus was to be conducted by Jules Cohen; it was to be swelled by the most renowned singers in Paris. On Friday evening, November 20, the coffin was borne from the Madeleine to a catafalque in La Trinité, where two nuns prayed over it throughout the night.

In his will,* Rossini had specified that his burial should be modest, to cost no more than 2,000 francs. But at noon on November 21, more than 4,000 people had jammed themselves into La Trinité. No orchestra supported the music, but the hundreds of singers—many of them stars of the Opéra, the Opéra-Comique, and the Théâtre-Italien[n]—were joined by the entire body of Conservatoire students. Achille de Lauzières, the poet-librettist, wrote: "There was heard, first, on the organ, the instrumental phrases of the shades from *Moïse*. . . . The *Introibo* had been taken from Jommelli's *Messa dei morti*, a work and composer much admired by Rossini, and performed by all the massed voices. The *Dies irae* followed the *Introibo*. The words of this tremendous and austere canticle had been adapted to the *Mater dolorosa* from the *Stabat*, and were sung, in four parts, by [Christine] Nilsson, [Rosine] Bloch, Tamburini, and Nicolini, and backed by the choruses.

"The duet from the *Stabat*: *Quis est homo qui non fleret*, was sung (as it never was another time) by Alboni and Patti . . . To the *Quid sum miser* of the Mass for the Dead had been adapted the music from another strophe of the *Stabat* (*Pro peccatis suae gentis*), sung by the baritone Faure; after which came the *Lacrymosa* from Mozart's Requiem. Then Nilsson sang for the offertory the *Vidit suum dulcem natum*, from Pergolesi's *Stabat*. . . . Next, the Elevation. A full and majestic chant was required. It was offered by the final strophe of the *Stabat*: *Quando corpus morietur*, sung in four parts by [Gabrielle] Krauss, [Eleanora] Grossi,[n] Nicolini, and Agnesi. For the *Agnus*, the inimitable prayer from *Moïse* had been chosen. . . . And the Mass was ended.

"The prayer for final absolution remained. While the priest spoke it near the catafalque, Sax's wind instruments performed Beethoven's Funeral March as especially arranged by Gevaert. You would have thought that you were hearing the sevenfold blasts of the Angels of the Last Judgment. . . .

"The sky seemed draped in mourning. Never had Paris appeared so dull, so sad, so gelid. The cortège, emerging from the church at about two o'clock, was preceded by two line battalions and by the bands of the two legions of the Garde Nationale, which played the Funeral March from *La Gazza* [*ladra*], the Prayer from *Moïse*, and fragments of the *Stabat*.

"The ribbons of the funeral car were held in turn by Conte Nigra, the Italian ambassador, by Camille Doucet, by Baron Taylor, Prince Poniatowski, Auber, Ambroise Thomas, Perrin, Saint-Georges, by the Deputy D'Ancona, by the Italian consul Cerutti, etc.

"Along the entire stretch of the rue de la Trinité to the Cemetery of Père-Lachaise, the populace was thick; the windows, despite the north wind, were full, and a huge throng followed the remains of the lamented composer. The Institut de France, the Conservatoire, the diplomatic corps, the press, the arts, the stage—all were well represented. At the cemetery, many speeches were pronounced; by Doucet for the Académie; by Thomas for the Institut; by D'Ancona for Italy, by Perrin for the theater; by Saint-Georges for the composers; by Baron Taylor for the artists; by Pougin for the professors; by Elwart for the Conservatoire. Then the throng, gradually thinning out, slowly, sadly dispersed. Rossini alone remained in the funeral precinct; he reposes there, not far from Cherubini, from Hérold, from Boieldieu, from Chopin, and, above all, from his beloved Bellini, who was to Rossini what Raphael was to Michelangelo."[n]

Rossinian performances were to have been given that night at the Théâtre-Italien, the Théâtre-Lyrique, and the Opéra. At the Italien, Krauss, Grossi, Nicolini, and Agnesi sang the *Stabat Mater* with a chorus in which many other noted singers took their places near a wreathed bust of Rossini. In the interval between the parts, mourning wreaths were deposited around the bust and Krauss sang the *Requiem æternam* as adapted to the gondolier's song from *Otello*. At the Lyrique, a performance of *Le Barbier de Séville* was filled out with other music by Rossini and with poetic recitations. The Opéra had announced *Guillaume Tell*, but postponed it to the following Saturday because of illness among the singers.

On November 28, however, *Tell* was sung at the Opéra. Étex's statute of Rossini in the entrance vestibule and Chevalier's large medallion of him suspended above the foyer were topped with memorial wreaths; a bust of Rossini by Dantan stood in a stage box. At the second intermission, the singers placed wreaths on the bust and sang the finale of the opera ("Your voice is stilled forever . . . The universe will repeat your songs, and immortality b͜e͜ ͜'ns!"). From Mme Rossini's loge, the deputation from Pesaro looked and listened.

Related ceremonies were staged elsewhere in France, in London,[n] in Leipzig, and throughout Italy. On December 14, a solemn ritual was held in the Italian national pantheon, the Church of Santa Croce in Florence. This was attended by ministers, senators, deputies, members of the diplomatic corps, councilors of state, the *sindaco* of Florence, and all the local civil and military dignitaries. The performance of

Mozart's Requiem was participated in by the best-known musicians then in Florence, including Teodulo Mabellini, Prince Carlo Poniatowski, the tenor Napoleone Moriani, and the violinists Antonio Bazzini and Camillo Sivori, the latter of whom, during the Elevation of the Host, performed the Prayer from *Mosè in Egitto* "on his fourth string."[n]

On November 17, 1868, four days after Rossini's death, Giuseppe Verdi had written from his estate at Sant'Agata to Tito Ricordi:[n]

"My DEAREST RICORDI: To honor Rossini's memory, I should like the outstanding Italian composers (Mercadante at the head, even if only for a few measures[n]) to compose a Requiem Mass to be performed on the anniversary of his death.

"I should like not only the composers, but the performing artists as well, not only to donate their work, but also to offer their obol to pay the necessary expenses.

"I should like no foreign hand, nor any extraneous to the art, be it as powerful as you wish, to lend aid. In that case, I should retire from the association at once.

"The Mass should be performed in S. Petronio of the city of Bologna, which was Rossini's real musical homeland.

"This Mass should not be an object of curiosity or of speculation; but, once performed, it should be sealed up and placed in the archives of the Liceo Musicale of that city, whence it should never be removed. Perhaps exception could be made for his anniversaries, when posterity might think of celebrating him.

"If I were in the good graces of the Holy Father, I would beg him to permit, at least this time, that women should take part in the performance of this music, but as I am not, it will be advisable to find someone better suited to the purpose than I am.

"It will be good to establish a commission of intelligent men to regulate the arrangement of this performance, and above all to select the composers, distribute the pieces, and supervise the general form of the work.

"This composition (however good the single pieces can be) will necessarily lack musical unity; but if it will be defective in that sense, it will nonetheless serve to demonstrate how great the veneration in all of us was for that man, over whose loss the whole world weeps.

"*Addio*, and believe me Most affectionately, G. VERDI."

By May 1869, the commission suggested by Verdi had selected the composers for the thirteen sections of the proposed Requiem.[n] It had decided upon the length, form, tonality, and tempo for each section; many of the sections had been completed. The intention had been to make use of the orchestra and chorus of the Teatro Comunale at Bologna, but when L. Scalaberni, then its impresario, was approached in what the commission had assumed was good time, he refused to cooperate." Verdi and the commission then regarded the entire plan as doomed. In November 1869, when performance of the Requiem had been foreseen, the commission announced the impossibility of performance. As Verdi wrote on June 17, 1878, that failure had not been "the fault of the *maestri* destined to compose, but of others' indifference or ill will."

Rossini's death had thrown Verdi into agitated correspondence besides that concerning the projected Requiem. On November 18, 1868, he had written to Senator Giuseppe Piroli: "Here they want to stage solemn funeral rites for Rossini, and that is good. Yesterday evening, the Pesarese delegation left for Paris, charged with attending the funeral and with asking the widow for the body of the deceased. I feel that this lady is very little disposed to concede it, also because they say that she is much averse to Italians. Rossini also thought of his own cadaver, leaving in his will that the widow can dispose of it as she wishes . . ."

Two days later, again to Piroli, Verdi wrote: "I greatly praise the Minister's project concerning the funeral ceremonies and the monument to Rossini [both were to be in Santa Croce, Florence]. They'll not have the body if that depends upon Mad.me Rossini. No Frenchman loves the Italians, but Mad.me Rossini by herself detests them as much as all the French put together. I have written to Ricordi, sending him a project for the composition of a Requiem, to be done and performed by only Italian musicians. You will see it and tell me whether I have done well or badly . . ."

Still pursuing Olympe with his scorn, on December 12, Verdi wrote Piroli: "I was mistaken in saying to you, in my last letter, that Mad.me Rossini would not give the cadaver of her husband. That is to say, I was half mistaken, as she hopes thus to be placed in that temple [Santa Croce] in which lie those great men whom I don't even dare to name after having named Mad.me Rossini. Our ministers would be capable of permitting this also? . . . Tell me what has become of the march that Rossini recently sent to Broglio, entitled the '*Corona d'Italia.*' It is said to be something miserable; it is also said that it is the '*Largo al factotum*' transcribed for band. He was capable of this joke, but I don't believe that he did it . . ."

At Pesaro, the next year, the city authorities carried to a bright conclusion a four-day Rossini memorial (August 21–5). They had dispatched a commission to Passy to invite Olympe to attend it as their guest. She had replied on June 30 that to leave Passy was beyond her strength and that they must represent her. By the hands of the returning commissioners, she sent to the *sindaco* of Pesaro a thousand francs to be distributed among the poorest of her late husband's surviving relatives. On August 21, Cherubini's D-minor Requiem was sung in the Church of San Francesco, about one hundred voices taking part; on August 22 and 23, the *Stabat Mater* was sung in the Teatro Rossini; on August 25, that theater housed a vocal-instrumental concert of Rossini's music. Bologna sent to Pesaro its renowned Banda Nazionale under the direction of Alessandro Antonelli; among the artists who lent their services were Verdi's friend Teresa Stolz, the contralto Rosa Vaccolini, the tenors Giuseppe Capponi and Lodovico Graziani, the baritones Francesco Graziani, Antonio Cotogni, Davide Squarcia, and Francesco Angeli, and the bass Luigi Vecchi. Angelo Mariani conducted the orchestra, in which many of Italy's outsanding instrumentalists played.

Olympe Rossini, who suffered greatly during the ordeal of the Paris Commune in 1870, lived until March 22, 1878, dying at nearly eighty-one after a six-month illness. Thereafter, the articles of Rossini's will were put into effect. The Liceo Musicale at Pesaro was established in what had been the Convento dei Filippini, its first director being Carlo Pedrotti. It was officially opened on November 5, 1882." Its later directors have included Arturo Vambianchi, Pietro Mascagni, and Amilcare Zanella. Among the pupils to emerge from it into professional musical life have been the singers Celestina Boninsegna, Alessandro Bonci, and Umberto Macnez; the violinist Gioconda De Vito; and the composers Francesco Balilla Pratella and Riccardo Zandonai.

The Rossini Prizes provided for in the will were announced in late June 1878 (the prize for a text to be awarded on December 31). The musical contest was to open on January 1, 1879, each entrant to be handed for setting a copy of the prize-winning text. The prize for each was 3,000 francs [about $1,700]. The first winners were Paul Collin for his *La Fille de Jaïre*, and the Vicomtesse de Grandval, who set it to music. The jury had included Ambroise Thomas, Napoléon-Henri Réber, Ernest Reyer, and Jules Massenet.

Carrying out a desire expressed to her by Rossini, Olympe in her will left the Welfare Agency of the City of Paris about 200,000 francs

—an amount which, as increased by interest over the next five years, proved sufficient to build the Maison de Retraite Rossini, a home for disabled or superannuated operatic performers. The chosen site was in Auteuil, near the Bois de Boulogne. Work was initiated in 1883; the rest home was ready for occupancy in January 1889,[n] by which time twenty-six performers were admitted to the new building on the rue Mirabeau, at the edge of the Parc des Saints-Perrins.[n]

Olympe had looked forward eagerly—and, be it said, understandably—to being buried beside Rossini in Père-Lachaise. She had rejected the first demands—from both Florence and Pesaro—for her husband's body. Then, enraging Verdi, she had agreed to the removal of Rossini's remains to Florence—if she could be buried beside him there in Santa Croce.[n] The Italian authorities naturally could not accept this naïve proviso, and the negotations were therefore suspended for some years. After a hard search of her mind and heart, however, Olympe finally agreed to the demand from Florence, putting the following into her will: "I desire that my body be deposited finally and forever in the Cimetière de l'Est [Père-Lachaise], in the tomb in which at present are to be found the mortal remains of my venerated husband. After their removal to Florence, I shall remain there alone: I make this sacrifice in all humility; I have been glorified enough by the name that I bear. My faith, my religious feelings, give me the hope of a reunion that escapes the earth."

Three months after Olympe's death in 1878, a committee was formed in Florence to arrange for elaborate solemn rites on the arrival of Rossini's remains.[n] The national government promised to pay the cost of transporting Rossini's coffin from Paris to Florence. But then the ministry fell, and it was not until December 4, 1886, that a new Minister of Public Instruction, Filippo Mariotti, put a motion to Parliament to reinstate the earlier government's promise; adopted unanimously, the motion became law on December 26. The Academy of the Royal Institute of Music at Florence (now the Conservatorio Luigi Cherubini) constituted itself a committee, presided over by the Marchese Filippo Torrigiani, to arrange the ceremonial. It agreed with Rome that May 3, 1887, should be the date for Rossini's entombment in Santa Croce.

Accompanied by Torrigiani, Boito, and other members of an official escort, Rossini's remains reached the Santa Maria Novella railroad station at Florence on May 2, 1887. At one o'clock the next afternoon, the coffin was installed upon a huge triumphal hearse and drawn through the streets amid representatives of the King, the government, the province, the City of Pesaro, and the City of Florence, and the massed military bands of Tuscany. As it was borne into Santa Croce, a chorus of about 500 voices[n] led by Jefté Sbolci twice sang *"Dal tuo stellato soglio,"* from *Mosè in Egitto.*

At two o'clock on the afternoon of May 4, Rossini's *Stabat Mater* was sung in the Salone del Cinquecento of the Palazzo Vecchio. Its performance had been prepared by Rossini's old friend Teodulo Mabellini; it was conducted by Sbolci; the soloists were Marie Louise Durand, Barbara Marchisio, Giovanni Sani, and Romano Nannetti.[n] After the *Stabat,* the orchestra played the overture to *Guillaume Tell.* The musical memorial continued through a *"gran concerto"* in the Teatro Pagliano on the evening of May 9.[n]

Although the centenary of Rossini's birth was duly marked in Florence on February 29, 1892, the musical citizens of that city remained uncomfortably aware that no appropriate monument marked Rossini's burial place in Santa Croce. A first open contest, held in 1897, produced no design for the tomb which the commission found acceptable. A second contest was held in 1898, and the new commission— which included Arrigo Boito's brother Camillo—decided that a design submitted by the sculptor Giuseppe Cassioli could be altered and made to serve. Cassioli's second submission was approved. The resulting monument[n] was dedicated on June 23, 1902. Standing against the north wall of Santa Croce, it bears this inscription: GIOACHINO ROSSINI. At its base, three dated cartouches read: "Pesaro," "Firenze," "Parigi," thus disposing, negatively but officially, with the just claim of Bologna to a large share in Rossini's enduring renown.

APPENDIXES

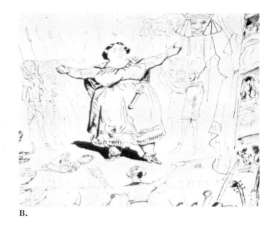

B.

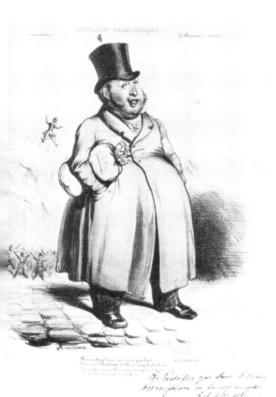

CARICATURES

A. ROSSINI, BY BENJAMIN

B. MARIETTA ALBONI AS
   SEMIRAMIDE, BY GIRAUD

C. ROSSINI, BY DANTAN (?)

D. ROSSINI, BY ANDRÉ GILL

A.

C.   D.

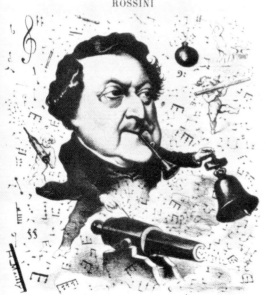

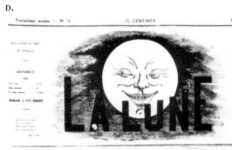

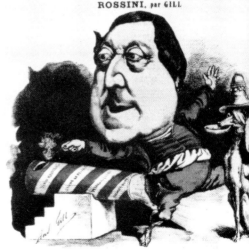

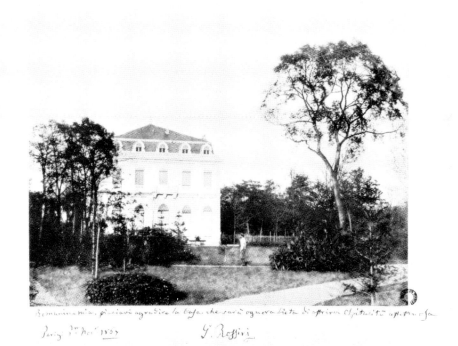

Rossini mio, piaciavi agradire la bafa, che farà ognora lieta di offrirvi spiritosi apetitosi

Paris 1.º Nov.ª 1867   G. Rossini

The Villa Rossini, Passy

Building at the boulevard des Italiens and the rue de la
Chaussée d'Antin, Paris (Rossini's apartment indicated by star)

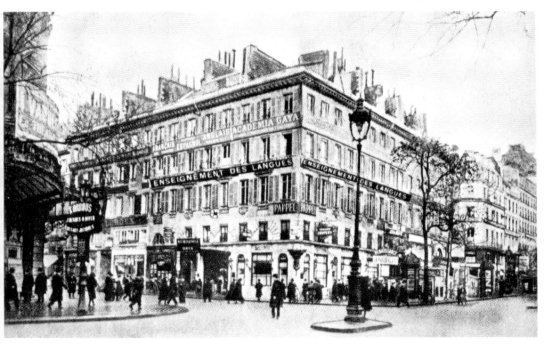

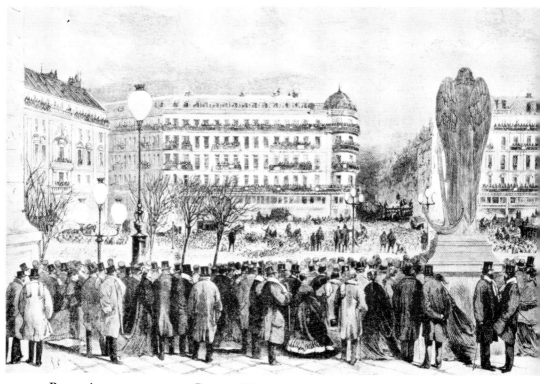

ROSSINI'S FUNERAL CORTEGE, PARIS, 1868

ROSSINI'S REBURIAL CORTEGE OUTSIDE SANTA CROCE, FLORENCE, 1887

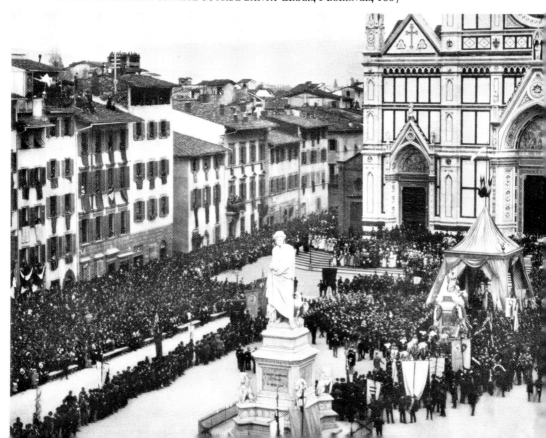

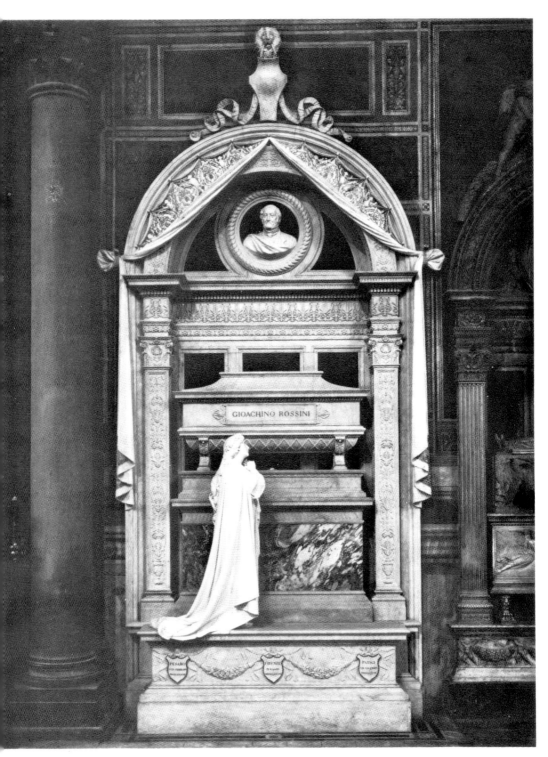

ROSSINI'S TOMB, SANTA CROCE, FLORENCE

Appendix A

Text of contract signed by Rossini and Duca Francesco Sforza-Cesarini for an opera (*Il Barbiere di Siviglia*)

NOBILE TEATRO DI TORRE ARGENTINA ROME, DECEMBER 15, 1815

By the present act, done as a private agreement, but which shall have the force and validity of a public contract, there is stipulated between the contracting parties everything hereinbelow:

The *signor duca* Sforza-Cesarini, impresario of the aforementioned theater, engages the *maestro* Gioachino Rossini for the forthcoming Carnival season of the year 1816; said Rossini promises and binds himself to compose and stage the second opera (*buffa*) to be presented during the aforementioned season at the theater indicated, and to whichever libretto, be it new or old, shall be given him by the aforementioned Duca, impresario.

Maestro Rossini binds himself to deliver the score by the middle of the month of January and to adapt it to the voices of the singers; and further binds himself to make all those changes which may be considered necessary both to the good success of the music and to the advantage and demands of the singers.

Maestro Rossini also promises and binds himself to be present in Rome to carry out the present contract not later than the end of the current December, and to turn over to the copyist the first act of his opera, entirely completed, by January 20, 1816. (January 20 is specified to the end of being able to carry out the rehearsals perfectly and to be able to go on stage the day that shall please the impresario, the performance being fixed for about February 5.) And also Maestro Rossini, equally, must deliver his second act to the copyist at the desired time, so that there may be time to prepare it and carry out the rehearsals early enough to be able to go on stage on the evening indicated above; otherwise, Maestro Rossini will expose himself to all damages, as it should be thus and not otherwise.

Further, Maestro Rossini will be obliged to conduct his opera as is customary and to be present in persons at all the vocal and orchestral rehearsals as often as may be necessary, whether in the theater or elsewhere, at the demand of the director, and also binds himself to attend the first performances to be given consecutively and to conduct the performance at the cembalo, etc., because it should be thus and not otherwise.

In payment for his labors, the director binds himself to pay the total sum and quantity of 400 Roman scudi once the first three performances that [Rossini] should conduct at the cembalo have been concluded.

It is agreed that during months when the theater is interdicted or closed, whether by act of the authorities or for another unforeseen reason, the practices of the Roman theaters and those of all other countries in similar cases will be observed, etc. As a guarantee of the exact carrying-out of the present contract, it will be signed by the above mentioned impresario and by Maestro Gioachino Rossini; further, the impresario grants living quarters to Maestro Rossini for the entire duration of the contract, in the same house assigned to Signor Luigi Zamboni."

Appendix B

The Bologna physician's report on Rossini which Olympe Rossini sent to Hector Couvert in 1842

MONSIEUR ROSSINI, endowed with a temperament lymphatic rather than sanguine, with a very sensitive nervous system, abused Venus from his earliest youth. That is why he frequently contracted gonorrheas that he almost always treated with astringents and more often with mild laxatives [*raffraichissants*] and purges. At the age of 44, he tempered his passions for women, stopped the abuse of liquors and heating foods. But well before that period there manifested themselves in him hemorrhoids, during the emanation of which his health improved greatly. It was about four years ago that M. R. was seized by a flow of mucous matters through the urethra, often white, often yellowish or greenish yellow. During the emission of urine, he did not suffer any dysuria; the urine was and always has been limpid, but nearly always bifurcated, which suddenly became a simple and natural jet. M. R. often enough used cooling medicines and purgatives, but without obtaining any improvement. In the month of February and March 1840, he was advised to use emollients introduced through the urethra—such as injections of sweet almond oil, of milk, of mallow, of gum, etc. A month later the sick man complained of a sensation of weight which, starting at the bulb of the urethra, reached to the anus, the matter emerging was always of mucous nature, thick, greenish, and sometimes streaks of blood made their appearance. The flow was more abundant, and the urine no longer could come out except drop by drop. In that situation, the physicians decided to apply leeches to the hemorrhoids and to the perineum, having noticed that the hemorrhoids had not fluctuated for three years as they previously had with him. This application was made for two days, but two hours after the second application, a complete ischuria of urine set in; a half bath not having brought any alleviation, the sick man, beside himself with alarm, sought a surgeon, who at once introduced an elastic catheter into the bladder; the bladder contained only a very small quantity of urine. The catheter was left in for 48 hours, and although no symptom of fever or inflammation manifested itself in the sick man, bleeding was practiced. After the catheter was removed, the urines came out in abundance, but with dysuria.

Despite complete tepid baths of fresh water and refreshing drinks, of which a long dosage was made, it was not possible [illegible word—*vamere?*] and the urethral flow reappeared. Two months later, a psoriasis manifested itself on the scrotum, an eruption that caused him strong itching without the flow becoming any less abundant. The spring season then being well advanced, his physician had him take a strong decoction of sarsaparilla and complete baths of fresh water for four days, but he reaped no advantage from this treatment except in the matter of the psoriasis. One should remark here that the ischuria no longer manifested itself and that the sick man's fears were almost wholly dissipated. Eight days before leaving for Venice, where M. R. had to spend the Carnival of 1841, he was for a whole night under the influence of a diarrhea so abundant that he took two drams of magnesia and a purgative broth. Then, finding himself cured, he left for Venice, where he spent twenty days, going to the toilet three or four times each day. He returned to Bologna during the first days of Lent with symptoms of gastricism which were very pronounced and which were followed immediately by diarrhea that continued for three or four months despite all the remedies used in such a case, but not always using powerful astringents. This new malady was attributed not so much to abuse of food as to the water that he drank in Venice, because every time that M. R. has stayed in Venice he always had ended up by having a relaxation of the bowels, which, however, never has been of such long duration. One should observe here that no alteration of fever was manifested in the sick man and that his pulses have almost always been in a normal state. The celebrated Professor Carus of Dresden passed through Bologna in the month of April 1841; he was consulted by M. R. He was of the opinion that the slow and chronic phlogosis of the urethra was intimately connected in rapport with the hemorrhoidal system, and that consequently flowers of sulphur mixed with cream of tartar and taken over a long lapse of time could be of great usefulness, that some applications of leeches to the hemorrhoids from time to time will be one of the most appropriate means of combatting this chronicity, that castor oil will be preferable as a special purgative to the saline substances that M. R. has been using; and further he was sure that by using the baths at Marienbad he had seen many similar sick men cured.

In the month of July 1841, the Bologna physicians sent M. R. to the baths of Poretta, located between Bologna and Tuscany in the Apennines. These sulphurous, hydrogenous, thermal waters are used for drinking [and] for external and internal baths. M. R. was completely cured of the psoriasis by these waters, but on the contrary the flow became even more abundant, the matters that came out being only less thick. And additionally the sick man grew noticeably thinner and began to complain of a great weakening of his physical powers; the least exercise tired him. In such a condition, the physicians again had recourse to flowers of sulphur, no longer mixed with cream of tartar, but with magnesia, because the former, even though administered in a small dose, caused him copious evacuations, his intestinal tube being very sensitive to the action of purgatives and, above all, to saline substances. One should observe that the bowels eject twice a day regularly, but that the stools are always liquid and smooth. After two months of continuous use of flowers of sulphur mixed with magnesia, his nutrition is noticeably improved, but the flow from the urethra is always the same and increases at the least heating-up of the body and after exciting foods.

M. R. having always feared a contracting of the urethra, himself introduced, for seven or eight years, each day for a month and for fifteen or twenty minutes, the catheter into the bladder—this without any dysuria resulting, despite the fact that at the first introduction he suffered difficulty in introducing the catheter. One should remark that the dysuria that M. R. fears has been combatted by all the means possible, but without any positive result other than that given after the stay of 48 hours of a foreign body in the bladder.

Has there been any laceration of the flesh? Has it made any ulcerations in the bladder? Or does the external psoriasis extend to the interior? These are the sick man's apprehensions. Is it the hemorrhoids, as was M. Carus's opinion, which cause the general disorder? These are the apprehensions of the Bologna physicians, who find themselves completely in accord with those of Professor Carus. The observations are these:

1st) that for three years the hemorrhoids have not protruded more

2nd) that the emission of urine is made more freely and with less dysuria, though the mucous flow from the urethra is in abundance and that the contrary happens if the flow diminishes

3rd) it should be observed to the consultants that this dysuria causes no painful sensation except at the commencement of the emission of urine.

Appendix C

Rossini's will and its codicils

Rossini's estate was estimated at 2,500,00 francs (about $1,420,000). When his will was opened, on November 18, 1868, it was found, with its codicils, to read as follows:

Paris, July 5, 1858.

This is my testament, in the name of the Father, the Son, and the Holy Ghost, Amen.

In the certainty of having to abandon this mortal life, I have determined to make my final dispositions.

Upon my death, the sum of two thousand lire at most will be spent for my funeral; my body will be interred where my wife esteems it fitting.

Under the classification of legatee, and for one time only, I leave to my maternal uncle Francesco Maria Guidarini, living in Pesaro, six thousand francs; to Maria Mazzotti, my maternal aunt living in Bologna, five thousand francs; and to my two cousins living in Pesaro, Antonio and Giuseppe Gorini, two thousand francs to each. These legatees are my only and unique wish and will be paid immediately after my death, if the money is available; in the contrary case, my testamentary executors will take the necessary time, in harmony with the interest of 5 per cent. If the aforesaid legatees should predecease me, the sums willed will pass to their male and female children in equal parts.

To my much-loved wife Olympe Descuillier, who was an affectionate and faithful companion, and to whose merit every praise would be inferior, I leave in absolute ownership all the household furniture, linens, carpets, draperies, porcelains, vases; all my autographs of music, carriages, horses, all the objects of the stable, of the harness room, of the cellar; copper, bronze, pictures, and finally other things that may be found in my home, whether that in the city or that in the country; excepting only the objects that I shall mention hereinbelow. I further declare to be the exclusive property of my wife all the silverware, as I wish to be recognized as her property whatever object she declares to belong to her, even though it be found in my room or among my effects.

The boxes, the rings, the chains, the pins, the canes, the pipes, the medals, the clocks—except, however, a small clock from the factory of Brêguet, which is my wife's; a small battle scene in silver by Benvenuto Cellini, framed in gold and ivory; another object in silver bas-relief, my violins, piccolo, oboe, ivory syrinx, toilet articles, sketches in albums, will be sold privately or by means of public auction, as my testamentary executors judge best, and the money to be earned by this sale will be put to profit in increasing the inheritance.

I leave to my wife the full and entire power to choose and opt among my real-estate properties or my movable assets that one or those which will suit her best as repayment of the dowry that was assigned to me at the moment of the marriage. I name my very dear and much-loved wife, for the duration of her natural life, the usufructory heir of all other goods, effects, and substances.

As heir to the property, I name the Comune of Pesaro, my homeland, to found and endow a Liceo Musicale in that city after the death of my wife. I prohib˙ the magistrature or the communal representatives of that city from having any species of control or of intervention in my estate, wishing my wife to enjoy it in complete and absolute liberty and not wishing her to have to give any security or be obliged to make a special use of the goods that I shall leave behind me, and of which I leave her the usufruct.

I nominate as my testimentary executors in Italy the Marchese Carlo Bevilacqua and the Cavaliere Marco Minghetti of Bologna, where they live, giving them the fullest power and begging them to accept the burdens that my choice imposes upon them, thus giving me this last proof of benevolence and friendship. Further, I nominate as my testamentary executors in France, Monsieur Vincenzo Buttarini, living at rue Basse du Rempart, 30, and Monsieur Aubry, boulevard des Italiens, 27, begging them to accept as a token of remembrance 100 ounces of silver each, to be delivered to them within the space of one year after the date of my death.

I wish that after my death and that of my wife there be founded in perpetuity in Paris, and exclusively for the French, two prizes of three thousand francs each to be distributed annually, one to the composer of a piece of religious or operatic music which shall have been distinguished principally for its melody, now so much neglected; the other to the author of the words (prose or verse) to which music could be applied and be perfectly appropriate, and observing the laws of morality, of which writers do not always take sufficient count. These productions will be submitted to examination by a special commission set up by the Académie des Beaux-Arts of the Institut, which will judge who shall have merited the prize called ROSSINI, which shall be awarded in public session after the performance of the composition, whether at the Institut or at the Conservatoire.

My testimentary executors shall obtain from the ministry the authorization to invest at 3 per cent a capital necessary to produce an annual return of six thousand francs. I have desired to leave to France, from which I had so benevolent a welcome, this testimony of my gratitude and of my desire to see perfected an art to which I have devoted my life.

I leave as a contribution to the Establishment for shelter and for the derelicts of Bologna, twenty scudi for one single time, and the same to the Monte di Pietà.

I leave to my manservant Antonio Scanavini, who served me with precision and fidelity, the monthly sum of fifty lire for the duration of his life, and all my old wearing apparel. I reserve the right to make additions and modifications in the present testament, and I intend that they be executed literally and observed as if they were written in the present document. I annul any other testament.

Done, written, and signed by my hand today.
Paris, July 5, 1858.

Signed: Gioachino Antonio Rossini

Codicil to the Above

This is my codicil.

I add what follows to the dispositions that I already have made in favor of my dear wife in my testament.

I transmit to her and leave her all my rights and portions in the property in Passy resulting from our contract with the city of Paris: in consequence, all that which can or may in the future come either to me or to those who succeed to my rights to whatever title as a sequel of the acquisitions in usufruct, constructions, works, and whatever cause and whatever title there may be, shall pass to my wife in complete ownership; and if even during our lifetime we shall have returned our usufruct to the city of Paris in virtue of the terms of the contract, my wife shall withdraw from my succession the price that I shall have received.

I annul the disposition that I made in favor of Antonio Scanavini, my manservant, which shall be without effect.
Paris, February 4, 1860.

Signed: Gioachino Antonio Rossini

Other Codicils to the Above

In my Montmorency writing table in Paris there is a large black leather portfolio containing all the obligations and the weekly statements of the Paris Works Fund; there also are to be found all my credit titles and those of the Italian real estate, and, finally, my testament.

In the mirrored armoire in my bedroom in Paris there is a large book in which are entered all my credits formed in Paris and the accounting of the related earnings; also in the same armoire there are important letters and receipts.

In the above-mentioned black leather portfolio is to be found, on blue paper, a record in the hand of my agent Gaetano Fabi (Bologna), in which will be seen what are the repaid loans and what the existing: from the letter of my agent Angelo Mignani (Bologna) can be determined which are delinquent and why! The accounts of the sums withdrawn and of the trimonthly expenses of Gaetano Fabi complete the work.

Monsieur Possoz is *au courant* with everything concerning the Paris Works fund.

Monsieur Bigotti, further, is *au courant* with my obligations of the Orléans and Lyon railroads (amalgamation).

Monsieur Pillet-Will, further, is *au courant* with everything that concerns the public debt of the 3 and 4½ [?], as he possesses the titles that belong to me.

I should like to recall that in the aforementioned book, and which is in the mirrored armoire in my bedroom in Paris, is listed the creation of the dowry of my wife Olympe, received at Bologna, and that, furthermore, I wrote in my own hand what follows.

I declare by these lines (as if they were by notarial act) that I give all my unpublished musical compositions, both vocal and instrumental, together with all my autographs, to my much-loved wife Olympe in sign of affection and gratitude. After my death, she may make whatever use of them seems best to her.

And let this be in codicil.

Paris, June 15, 1865

(*Signed*): GIOACHINO ROSSINI

Let what follows be held as a codicil to my testament.

I wish that after my death the commune of Pesaro (in arrangement with my wife Olympe) take possession of my real estate and investments in Italy, alienating them, if that is thought useful, and reinvesting them in its province, paying, be it well understood, to my aforementioned wife Olympe during her natural life the income at the rate of five per cent: my wife thus will have no administrative bother and the commune of Pesaro thus will enter into possession of the patrimony that I have conferred upon it in my testament. I hope to find full agreement to all this.

Paris, June 1, 1866

(*Signed*): GIOACHINO ROSSINI

If the abovementioned things be affected, I desire that my good Olympe make a present to my agents (who will be freed of the handling of my affairs), G. Fabi and A. Mignani.

(*Signed*): G. ROSSINI

Most important recommendation that I make to my wife Olympe.

Gathering together the few autographs remaining to me of my operas, it has been impossible to find that of the opera *Otello*, composed by me in Naples. Has this autograph been simply mislaid? Or was it stolen from my house? If the purloiner should be discovered, I mean that a suit be brought against him, and I swear and declare never to have given it to anyone, nor to have had it sold. May the thief be found and punished!"

Paris, December 31, 1867

G. ROSSINI

Appendix D

A note on present-day equivalent values of some currencies of Rossini's time

WHEN COMPLETING my biography of Donizetti in 1963, I was enabled, through the kindness of Signora Luisa Ambrosini, Rome, who put me in touch with Dottoressa Maria Vismara of the Società per l'Organizzazione Internazionale, Rome, to present an approximation of the then buying power of currencies mentioned in that book (p. 311). The mathematics represented a consensus of several Italian and other economic historians and economists.

The problem is more complex with Rossini, who was born earlier than Donizetti and who lived seventy-six years. Allowing for economic fluctuations during his lifetime and for the decrease in buying power of the United States dollar over the past several years, I have attempted below to give another approximation: to that of present-day (1967) buying powers of currencies mentioned by and in connection with Rossini. I believe that these are reasonably accurate, and therefore useful, but I know that other interpretations of the values are not merely possible, but also likely. The following figures supply, then, only a general guide.

currency	value in 1967 United States dollars
bajocco, or baiocco (Rome, pontifical)	$ .102985
carantino (Austria)	?
ducato (Two Sicilies)	2.40
franc (France)	.567776
franc (in northern Italy, synonym for lira)	.515677
lira (Austria)	.475512
lira (Tuscany)	.475512
luigi, or luigi vecchio (Lombardo-Veneto)	12.376248

napoleone d'oro (Sardinia and Piedmont)	11.355
paolo, silver (Rome, pontifical)	.13
piastra, silver (five-lira piece)	2.578385
scudo (Austria)	3.022952
scudo (Rome, pontifical)	3.157124
zecchino, gold (Rome, pontifical)	6.64297

NOTES

Notes

FULL TITLES and publication data of books cited in the notes are given in the bibliography. Books, other publications, and collections of music mentioned frequently are referred to by initials in the notes, the lists of Rossini's compositions, and the bibliography:

AZ—Azevedo, Alexis-Jacob: *G. Rossini: Sa Vie et ses oeuvres*, Paris
BdPCR—*Bollettino del Primo Centenario Rossiniano*, Pesaro
BdCRdS—*Bollettino del Centro Rossiniano di Studi*, Pesaro
BdS—*Il Barbiere di Siviglia* (periodical), Milan
FdD—*Fanfulla della domenica*, Rome
FR—Branca, Emilia: *Felice Romani*, Turin, Florence, Rome
GdI—*Giornale d'Italia*, Rome
GR—*Grove's Dictionary of Music and Musicians*, 5th edn., London, New York
LCM—*La Cronaca musicale*, Pesaro
LdR—Mazzatinti, Giuseppe, and Manis, F. and G.: *Lettere di G. Rossini*, Florence
LfS—Les Frères Escudier: *Rossini: Sa Vie et ses oeuvres*, Paris
LGMF—*La Gazzetta musicale*, Florence
LGMM—*La Gazzetta musicale di Milano*, Milan
LRM—*La Rassegna musicale*, Rome, etc.
LSM—Florimo, Francesco: *La Scuola musicale di Napoli*, Naples
LTI—Soubies, Albert: *Le Théâtre-Italien*, Paris
LVdW—Michotte, Edmond: *La Visite de R. Wagner à Rossini*, Brussels
MdO—*Musica d'oggi*, Milan
NA—*Nuova Antologia*, Rome
Of—*Onoranze fiorentine a Gioachino Rossini*, Florence
Pdv—*Péchés de vieillesse* (published only in part), Pesaro
PmR—Hiller, Ferdinand: *Plaudereien mit Rossini*, Leipzig
QR—*Quaderni Rossiniani*, Pesaro
RAD—Radiciotti, Giuseppe: *Gioacchino Rossini*, Tivoli

RG—Righetti-Giorgi, Geltrude: *Cenni di una donna già cantante sopra il maestro Rossini*, Bologna

RMI—*Rivista musicale italiana*

RNI—Pougin, Arthur: *Rossini*, Paris

ROG—Rognoni, Luigi: *Rossini*, Parma

ROS—*Rossiniana*, Bologna

SIL—Silvestri, Lodovico Settimo: *Della Vita e delle opere di Gioachino Rossini*, Milan

Sm—*Soirées musicales*, Paris

UScR—Michotte, Edmond: *Souvenirs: Une Soirée chez Rossini à Beau-Sejour (Passy)*, Paris

XVM—*XV Maggio Musicale Fiorentino* (program), 1952, Florence

ZAN—Zanolini, Antonio: *Biografia di Gioachino Rossini*, Bologna

NOTES TO INTRODUCTION

p. xv, l. 25 "this century" Lord Derwent's *Rossini and Some Forgotten Nightingales*, published almost simultaneously with Toye's biography (both London, 1934), is an entertaining commentary on Rossini and his times rather than a formal biography.

p. xvi, ll. 21-2 "doublebass accompaniment" *"Undici Lettere inedite di G. Rossini,"* Of, 10.

p. xvi, l. 27 "in 1960" "Rossiniana in the Piancastelli Collection," *Monthly Musical Record*, London, 7-8/1960, 140.

p. xvi, l. 36 "through 1829" From before 1815, I have seen only the application that the fourteen-year-old Rossini sent to the Accademia Filarmonica, Bologna, in 1806. Giuseppe Radiciotti, in *RAD*, quoted from (I, 145 and cited (I, 159, footnote 2) a letter of May 15, 1815, to Luigi Prividali which I have been unable to locate.

p. xvii, l. 10 "since 1957" *Life of Rossini by Stendhal*, translated and annotated by Richard N. Coe, London and New York, 1957.

NOTES TO CHAPTER I

p. 4, l. 17 "Ferdinand Hiller" *PmR*.

p. 4, ll. 24-5 "her appearance" *RAD* I, 7.

p. 4, l. 38 "twenty scudi" See Appendix D, p. 386, for table of currencies mentioned in this book.

p. 5, ll. 23-4 "and background" *"L'Infanzia di Gioacchino Rossini (Da documenti inediti dell'Archivio storico del Comune di Pesaro),"* in *BdCRdS* 1958, 6, 103; 1, 6; 2, 28 (because the first two issues of the first series of this valuable *Bollettino* were issued late in the year 1955, the first issue of 1956 and of each succeeding year was numbered 3, the order of issues within a single year therefore being 3, 4, 5, 6, 1, 2). Padre Albarelli also pointed out that he found no mention of Giuseppe Rossini as either an inspector of abattoirs or a forester—pursuits attributed to him by some writers—and added that Giuseppe himself had not mentioned these public positions.

p. 5, l. 38 "Jesuit refugee" The Rossinis later occupied all four of the rooms now shown.

p. 6, l. 9 "Rossini's baptism" *"Rassini in patria."*

p. 8, l. 6 *"Capricciosa corretta"* Like Mozart's *Don Giovanni* and Martín y Soler's *Una Cosa rara* (which is quoted in the final act of *Don Giovanni*), this intermezzo had a libretto by Lorenzo da Ponte. It had first been sung at His Majesty's Theatre, London, in 1795 as *La Scola de' maritati*.

p. 8, l. 39 "and Latin" *RAD* I, 15, lists the three priests as "Don

Innocenzo, who taught him to read and write, Don Fini [in] arithmetic, and Don Agostino Monti [in] Latin."

p. 9, ll. 16–17   "index finger"   This perhaps factually accurate but very Rossinian description is unfair to Prinetti, who in 1788 was recitative cembalist at the Teatro Comunale, Bologna, and who composed sacred music, some of which has survived in the library of the Conservatorio at Bologna.

p. 9, l. 34   "Vecchio Teatrofilo"   *Memorie del Teatro Comunale di Trieste dal MDCCCI al MDCCCLXXVI* (Trieste, n.d., but 1876?).

p. 10, l. 9   "broke out"   When expressing disapproval during a performance, Italians commonly whistle rather than boo.

p. 11, l. 4   "of Lugo"   The chief documents of this amusing, pointless argument are: Giuliano Vanzolini's *Della Vera Patria di Gioacchino Rossini*, written in 1871, published at Pesaro in 1873, and Luigi Crisostomo Ferrucci's *Giudizio perentorio sulla verità della patria di Gioachino Rossini impugnata dal Prof. Giuliano Vanzolini*, published at Florence in 1874. Ferrucci, a native of Lugo, gave interesting information on the background of the Rossini family: "He [Vanzolini] is not obliged to know that by a street called *of the Russinis*, along the terraces of Lugo a little more than half a mile, one comes to the *ripe* [banks]—that is, to the confines of Cotignola; and that through it nearly all the people were Russinis, who, with various nicknames, owned the adjacent lands up to the Senio River, where there was a Russini called *della Chiusa* [of the dam or barrier]. No more is he obliged to know that at an earlier time a Franciscan *padre* named Baffi (in an oration *on the nobility of Lugo* read to the General Chapter of his Order) named some families of noble and distinguished origin as *Baldratiam* (Baldrati), *Gregoriam* (Gregori), *Russiniam* (Russini)." Ferrucci then described the Russini coat of arms, which he had found on the largest bell in Cotignola, and which Rossini had carved as his seal by the "very celebrated Castellani at Rome . . . The Russini arms consist of an arm holding up a rose on which a nightingale sits, with three stars in the upper part of the field." The coat of arms is given here as reproduced on page 3 of Ferrucci's pamphlet:

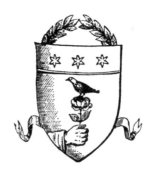

p. 11, l. 9 "the horn"   The mature Rossini was to have a special feeling for and mastery of the horn. See, for example, the introduction to the cavatina *"Languir per una bella,"* in *L'Italiana in Algeri* (1813); the fanfare for six horns in *La Donna del lago* (1819); the passage for four horns in the andantino section of the overture to *Semiramide* (1823); and the Gessler fanfare in *Guillaume Tell* (1829).

p. 11, l. 13 "prominent families"   Giuseppe Malerbi later became a member of both the Accademia Filarmonica, Bologna, and the Accademia di Santa Cecilia, Rome. A sister or cousin of the Malerbi brothers became the mother of Luigi Crisostomo Ferrucci, who wrote of Anna Rossini: "I saw her a few times in the home of my mother (Malerbi) seated at the table and after dinner dispensing the favors of her snuffbox."

p. 11, l. 21 "the cembalo"   On October 18, 1868, four weeks before his death, Rossini wrote Ferrucci: "Nothing could be more welcome to me than your mention of the *gravicembalo* or *spinetta* still surviving in the hands of your cousin Malerbi. You will know that during my adolescence, while living in Lugo, I practiced daily on that barbarous instrument . . ." This cembalo, dated 1707 and bearing the name of its maker, Augustinius Henrichini Silesiensis, was exhibited in Florence in 1876; it was sent to the St. Louis (Missouri) Exposition of 1904, where it was sold.

p. 11, l. 27 *"tournedos Rossini"*   For anyone wanting to try this most familiar of several dishes named for Rossini, this recipe is given by Joseph Donon (*The Classic French Cuisine*, New York, 1959): "Brown in hot butter as many tournedos [one-and-a-half-inch-thick slices of beef filet or tenderloin] as are required, and season them. Put each steak on a freshly made piece of toast trimmed to fit it. Top with a slice of *foie gras* or a bit of truffle. Serve with Madeira sauce."

p. 12, ll. 6–7 "musical life"   In addition to the internationally known Liceo Musicale (now the Conservatorio G. B. Martini) and the Accademia Filarmonica, Bologna had two other musical societies: the Accademia Polimniaca and the Accademia dei Concordi.

p. 12, l. 31 "the theater"   This was a Marchese Cavalli, later impresario of the Teatro San Moisè, Venice. Carpano was almost certainly his mistress: Henri Blaze de Bury remarked that "this was a right acquired by every self-respecting theatrical director."

p. 13, l. 6 "in Bologna"   According to *ZAN* (p. 7, footnote 1), Rossini had first sung this minor role at the Teatro Zagnoni (Bologna) when only eight or nine years old.

p. 13, l. 17 "Washington, D.C."   Casella published, through Carisch of Milan in 1951, the third of these sonatas for two violins, cello, and double-bass. The whole set was published at Pesaro in 1954 as the first of the *Quaderni Rossiniani* (QR), under the editorship of Alfredo Bonaccorsi; several of them (the third in Casella's arrangement) have been recorded more than once.

p. 13, l. 20 "Monsieur Mazzoni"   Possibly Giuseppe Mazzoni, who sang in Rossini's *Bianca e Falliero* at Siena during the summer of 1868.

p. 13, l. 32 "Matteo Babbini"   Babbini (or Babini, 1754–1816) had abandoned the stage in 1803 after a wide-ranging career. Alexis-Jacob Azevedo (*AZ*) wrote that when Rossini first reached Paris (1823), he astonished Cherubini by singing from memory a *Giulio Sabino* aria that Babbini had taught him.

p. 14, l. 13 "Lorenzo Gibelli"   Gibelli (1719?–1812?), whom Dr. Charles Burney described as a good harmonist devoid of melodic gift, was one of the last pupils of Padre Martini: he was referred to as "*Gibellone dalle belle fughe.*" Carlo Pancaldi, in his *Vita di Lorenzo Gibelli . . .* (p. 27), said: "The celebrated *cavaliere* Rossini had the first principles of music from the priest Don Angelo Tesei, another of the disciples of Martini; but then, when the Liceo Filarmonico was opened to him, Rossini, being put among the students in the schools of violin, violoncello, pianoforte, and counterpoint, also had to attend those [Gibelli's] of solfeggio and singing, as it was always the excellent basic rule of the establishment that these schools must precede any others and must be attended with them simultaneously later."

p. 14, l. 20 "Dorinda Caranti"   Caranti later sang secondary roles in opera in several theaters. She may have been in the cast of the *première* of Rossini's *L'Inganno felice* (1811), as she was on the roster of the Teatro del Corso troupe when that opera was given there.

p. 15, l. 10 "Clément wrote"   *Les Musiciens célèbres depuis le XVI*e *siècle jusqu'à nos jours.*

p. 15, l. 13 "Padre Mattei"   Rossini later told Ferdinand Hiller: "His [Haydn's] quartets are ravishing works. What marvelous motion of the parts and what finesse in modulation! All good composers offer beautiful cadences, but Haydn's have a special attraction for me."

p. 15, l. 21 "at Bologna"   After childhood studies in Madrid, Colbran had been awarded a scholarship by Queen María Luisa for study abroad. In 1801, she had sung in Bordeaux and Paris. She and her father, Giovanni Colbran, appear thereafter to have lived in Sicily for some time. Emigrating to northern Italy, they lived for a time in Bologna—in the records connected with their having lived there at No. 399 (later No. 18) Via Barberia, they are described as "musical virtuosos of the King of Spain and of the Indies." Isabella sang at Bologna in 1807 and at Milan in 1808; she also sang in opera at the Teatro Comunale, Bologna, in 1809, at Venice during that year, and at Rome in 1810. She made her Naples debut (San Carlo, August 15, 1811) in Pietro Raimondi's cantata *L'Oracolo di Delfo*; her first operatic role there (September 8, 1811) was that of Giulia in the Italian *première* of Spontini's *La Vestale*.

p. 15, l. 33 "Spanish woman"   Even before her first performance in Italy, Colbran had been elected to membership in the Bolognese Accademia Filarmonica (November 1806).

p. 16, l. 10 "wife, Vincenza"   Vincenza (or Vincenzina) Viganò Mombelli was a niece of Luigi Boccherini and a sister of the choreographer Salvatore Viganò, for whom Beethoven composed *Die Geschöpfe des*

Prometheus. Mombelli's first wife, Luigia (or Luisa) Laschi, who had died in 1791, had created the role of the Contessa Almaviva in Mozart's *Le Nozze di Figaro* (Vienna, 1786).

p. 16, l. 19 "by Portogallo. . . ." Marcos Antonio da Assumpção (or Ascenção), who called himself "Portugal" ("Portogallo" in Italy), was born in Lisbon in 1762 and died at Rio de Janeiro in 1830. Rossini told Hiller (*PmR*): "My first wife, Mme Colbran, had about forty pieces by him in her repertoire."

p. 17, l. 9 *"opera seria"* Some horn duets that Rossini composed to play with his father also belong to his pre-Liceo days. So probably does the *arietta buffa* beginning "*Se il vuol la molinara*," which contains a passage that seems to echo Mozart—a passage that Rossini would recall when composing the introduction to Roggiero's "*Torni alfin ridente e bella*" in *Tancredi* (1813).

p. 17, l. 12 "and Syrians" Vincenza Mombelli had derived the situations in this libretto from the *Demetrio* of Metastasio—who, according to Bruno Mombelli (*Tutte le opere di Pietro Metastasio*, 5 vols., Milan, 1954, Vol. I, p. 1476), may have been influenced in turn by Pierre Corneille's *Don Sanche d'Aragon.*

p. 17, l. 24 "Azevedo wrote" *AZ.*

p. 17, l. 28 "Edmond Michotte." Michotte (1830–1914), a wealthy Belgian amateur composer-pianist, became a close friend of Rossini's during the composer's later years in Paris. He gave his important collection of Rossiniana to the Conservatoire Royal de Musique, Brussels. Michotte communicated details about Rossini to Radiciotti and others; in addition to *UScR*, he wrote *La Visite de R. Wagner à Rossini (LVdW).*

p. 17, l. 38 "Battista Giusti" Giusti wrote the poem that Rossini set as *Inno dell'Indipendenza*, which was sung at the Teatro Contavalli, Bologna, in April 1815. He also made an Italian translation of Sophocles' *Œdipus Rex* and paid Rossini to compose incidental music for a private performance of it (see p. 232 and note for that page).

p. 18, l. 2 "the Bologna')" Alfredo Bonaccorsi, annotating a recording of this *Sinfonia* (as "revised by Lino Livabella"), wrote: "The historic form is as follows: Introduction, Exposition (first theme, modulating bridge, second idea), central part, Re-exposition. One notes the resemblance of the first theme (a little march) to the duet '*Cinque . . . dieci . . . venti*' in Mozart's *Le Nozze di Figaro*, Act I. In this brief *Sinfonia*, Rossini was displaying with finesse an eighteenth-century art form."

p. 18, l. 7 "Mattei's corrections" Radiciotti pointed out (*RAD* I, 48) that a C-minor passage at the end of the instrumental introduction includes a harmonic progression that Rossini was to repeat several times later: in the introduction to *La Cambiale di matrimonio*, in the storm music of *Il Barbiere di Siviglia*, and in the "plague of shadows" in *Mosè in Egitto.*

p. 18, l. 25 "Lord Burghersh" John Fane, Lord Burghersh, later Earl of Westmorland (1784–1859), soldier and diplomat, composed a large body of music, including seven operas. He became president of the Royal

Academy of Music, London, upon its foundation in 1822; from 1832 on, he was also a director of the Concert of Antient Music.

p. 18, ll. 35–6 "not transcribed"   Two sets of transcriptions of the quartet arrangements also were published—by Schott for flute, violin, viola, and cello; by Breitkopf & Härtel for piano solo. The quartet arrangements are in major keys: G, A, B, B-flat, and D.

p. 19, l. 4 "December 23, 1808"   The "Bologna" *Sinfonia* is scored for flute, two oboes, two C clarinets, bassoon, two D horns, two D trumpets timpani, and strings. The Library of the Conservatorio at Bologna has a score of this *Sinfonia* prepared from the original autograph parts by Rossini's fellow-student Giuseppe Busi and most of the parts as copied out by another fellow-student, Benedetto Donelli. The horn and second oboe parts are missing. The *Sinfonia* has been published and recorded.

p. 19, l. 28 "been published"   *QR* IX, 1959, 1.

p. 20, l. 8 "operatic cavatinas"   This set of *Variazioni* was published by Breitkopf & Härtel (1904) as transposed from C major to B-flat; and in the original tonality in *QR* VI, 1957, 57. It has been recorded.

p. 21, l. 38 "Gaetano Rossi"   Gaetano Rossi, a Veronese (1780–1855), typified the mediocre scribblers who labored for Italian opera impresarios during the first half of the nineteenth century (only Jacopo Ferretti and Felice Romani rose much above that level of mediocrity or worse). Of the numerous operas made from his librettos, the most enduring are Rossini's *Semiramide* (1823) and Donizetti's *Linda di Chamounix* (1842). In addition to *La Cambiale di matrimonio* and *Semiramide*, Rossi would write for Rossini's use the libretto of *Tancredi* (1813) and poems for cantatas. The five-act play that served him as the basis for *La Cambiale* had been adapted earlier by Giuseppe Checcherini for an opera by Carlo Coccia, *Il Matrimonio per cambiale* (1807), which has been a failure.

p. 22, l. 13 "November 3, 1810"   At the south end of the Calle del Teatro a San Moisè, Venice, an incised stone in the wall of a building reads: "On this site, where the Teatro San Moisè formerly stood, the genius of Gioachino Rossini, then eighteen years old, joyfully took flight toward immortal glory on November 3, 1810, with the presentation of his first opera, *La Cambiale di matrimonio*. The Municipality." In the cast of that 1810 *première* had been Rosa Morandi (Fanny—spelled "Fanni" in the printed libretto), Clementina Lanari (Clarina), Tommaso Ricci (Edoardo Milfort), Luigi Raffanelli (Sir Tobia Mill), Nicola De Grecis (Slook), and Domenico Remolini (Norton). Clementina Lanari and Tommaso Ricci seldom appear in operatic chronicles. Luigi Raffanelli, born at Lecce about 1752, had been a successful singer in Paris when, in 1813, toward the end of his career, he also created for Rossini the title role of *Il Signor Bruschino*. Nicola De Grecis, a *primo buffo*, was to sing in the *premières* of Rossini's *La Scala di seta* (1812) and *Il Signor Bruschino*. Domenico Remolini appears to have remained a *comprimario*.

p. 22, l. 35 "and December 1"   Reports in the *Quotidiano Veneto* establish that *La Cambiale di matrimonio* was sung with *Non precipitare i giudizi* on November 3 and 6, and with *Adelina* on November 14, 15, 17, 19, 22, 23, 26, 27, and 29 and December 1. The *Quotidiano* was not published on Sunday; other performances that it did not report may have taken place. As noted earlier, Rossini used as a preluding *sinfonia* for *La Cambiale di matrimonio* the *Sinfonia a più strumenti obbligati concertata* that he had composed as a student piece in 1809; he would use it again in 1817 for *Adelaide di Borgogna*. Elements of Fanny's aria *"Vorrei spiegarvi il giubilo"* would be metamorphosed into the Rosina-Figaro duet in *Il Barbiere di Siviglia* beginning *"Dunque io son."*

  p. 23, l. 4 "Della Corte noted"   *"Fra gorgheggi e melodie di Rossini."*

Notes to Chapter II

  p. 24, l. 14 "until 1818"   See p. 86. References to a nonexistent Rossini cantata called *Didone abbandonata* resulted from Ricordi's publication of two arias from *La Morte di Didone* (*"Se dal ciel pietà non trovo"* and *"Per tutto l'orror"*) as being from an 1811 Rossini opera by that title. Aware that no opera called *Didone abbandonata* existed, commentators assumed that Rossini must have composed an 1811 cantata by that name.

  p. 24, l. 17 "in Bologna"   During the agitated Napoleonic period, three new theaters were opened in Bologna within nine years: the Teatro del Corso (1805), the Arena del Sole (1810), and the Teatro Contavalli (1814).

  p. 24, l. 19 *"Ser Marcantonio"*   Pavesi (1779–1850) flourished between the decline of Paisiello's productivity and the emergence of Rossini and Donizetti. *Ser Marcantonio*, his most popular opera, ran up fifty-four consecutive performances at La Scala, Milan, after its *première* there on September 26, 1810. Giovanni Ruffini and Donizetti later reworked Angelo Anelli's libretto for *Ser Marcantonio* into that of *Don Pasquale* (1843).

  p. 24 l. 22 "spelled Gasbarri)"   *RAD* called the librettist of *L'Equivoco stravagante* "a very mediocre bungler of librettos living in Florence." He should not be mistaken for the Bolognese composer-librarian Gaetano Gasparri (1807–81).

  p. 24, l. 27 "October 26, 1811"   Almost every printed source gives the date of this *première* as October 29, 1811, but reports of it in the Bolognese press establish that it occurred on October 26. The correct date, with related substantiation of it, is given in Adelmo Damerini's *"La Prima Ripresa moderna di un'opera giovanile di Rossini: 'L'Equivoco stravagante'* (*1811*)." The cast of the first performance of *L'Equivoco* was: Marietta (Maria) Marcolini (Ernestina), Angiola (Angela) Chies (Rosalia), Domenico Vaccani (Gamberotto—spelled "Gambarotto" in the printed libretto), Paolo (Pablo) Rosich (Buralicchio—spelled "Buralecchio" in the libretto), Tommaso Berti (Ermanno), and Giuseppe Spirito (Frontino). Marcolini, a leading mezzo-soprano (really soprano-contralto), would create roles in Rossini's *Ciro in Babilonia* (1812), *La Pietra del paragone* (1812), *L'Italiana in Algeri* (1813), and *Sigismondo* (1814). Chies, a soprano, occupies small space in operatic annals. Vaccani, a *basso cantante*, had a long career: he was singing Melchthal in *Guglielmo Tell* at Siena in 1835. Rosich, a *basso buffo*, would be the first Taddeo in *L'Italiana*; for him, during November 1816 Florence performances of *Il Barbiere di Siviglia*, Pietro Romani would compose the aria "*Manca un foglio*," long substituted for Rossini's "*A un dottor dell mia sorte.*" Berti, a tenor, also would create roles for Rossini in *L'Occasione fa il ladro* (1812) and *Il Signor Bruschino*. Spirito, another tenor, would be the first Haly in *L'Italiana*.

p. 25, l. 17   "*L'Equivoco stravagante*"   See preceding note.

p. 25, l. 26   "its allegro"   In reply to a letter in which I wrote that the Florentine overture seemed to me to be a *pastiche* put together later, Dr. Guglielmo Barblan replied: "My opinion . . . agrees with yours: that for the manuscript copy to be found at the Florence Conservatory, recourse was had to a '*pastiche*' *sinfonia*; while for the Ricordi edition, recourse was had to Rossini's most popular *sinfonia* [that to *Aureliano in Palmira, Elisabetta*, and *Il Barbiere*]. The scrupulous Radiciotti, then, was correct."

p. 25, l. 30   "merely wrote"   *Cenni di una donna già cantante sopra il maestro Rossini in risposta a ciò che ne scrisse nella state dell'anno 1822 il giornalista inglese in Parigi e fu riportato in una gazzetta di Milano dello stesso anno*, Bologna, 1823. The "English journalist in Paris" to whom Righetti-Giorgi was replying was actually the more than usually pseudonymous Henri Beyle.

p. 26, l. 5   "the libretto"   The music of *L'Equivoco stravagante* was adapted to another libretto and presented at Trieste in 1825 under the original title. Thereafter, the opera had few, if any, other stagings until it was revived at Siena on September 17, 1965, in a version "prepared" by Vito Frazzi. Adelmo Damerini, in the article cited above, remarked that the libretto had a marked modernity and no longer shocked.

p. 26, l. 9   "Domenico Puccini"   Domenico Vincenzo Puccini (1771–1815), grandson of the founder of the Luccan musical dynasty, was the grandfather of Giacomo Puccini. His *Il Trionfo di Quinto Fabio* (Leghorn, 1810) had elicited a letter of commendation from Paisiello (see Alfredo Bonaccorsi's *Giacomo Puccini e i suoi antenati musicali*, p. 21).

p. 26, l. 24   "his teens"   Bruno Riboli, while president of the Fondazione Rossini at Pesaro, published an article in *LRM* entitled "*Profilo medico-psicologico di G. Rossini.*" The detailed medical data in it were from letters written between May 1839 and June 1843 by Olympe Pélissier, later Rossini's second wife, and from a four-page report in French (probably dating from 1842) by a physician. Riboli originally had published that report in a psychiatric journal, in an article entitled "*Malattia di Gioacchino Rossini secondo una relazione medica del 184.*" For a complete translation of the report, see Appendix B, p. 379.

p. 27, l. 7   "Maria Foppa"   Foppa (1760–1845), a Venetian, also provided the librettos of *La Scala di seta* (which Radiciotti incorrectly assigns to Gaetano Rossi), *Il Signor Bruschino*, and *Sigismondo*.

p. 27, l. 9   "by Paisiello"   In the strictest interpretation it might be called the second time: in 1765, at the Teatro Rangoni in Modena, Paisiello had presented a *Demetrio* using the Metastasio libretto from which Vincenza Mombelli later borrowed the materials for her *Demetrio e Polibio* libretto.

p. 27, l. 15 "the loges"   In the first cast of *L'Inganno felice* were Giorgi-Belloc (Isabella), Raffaele Monelli (Bertrando), Filippo Galli (Tarabotto), Luigi Raffanelli (Batone), Vincenzo Venturi, and Rossini's former classmate Dorinda Caranti. The printed libretto merely says: "*Prima Donna Buffa*—Teresa Giorgi Belloc; *Primo Mezzo Carattere*—Raffaele Monelli; *Primi Buffi a Vicende* [i.e., in turn]—Luigi Raffanelli and Filippo Galli; *Altro Primo Buffo*—Vincenzo Venturi; *Seconda Donna Assoluta*—Dorinda Caranti," without specifying the roles that they sang in this opera. Maria Teresa (Trombetti) Giorgi-Belloc, often written Belloc-Giorgi (1784–1855), a contralto and mezzo-soprano who often sang soprano roles, had made her operatic debut at Turin in 1801; she retired in 1828. For her talents, Rossini was to shape the role of Ninetta in *La Gazza ladra* (1817). Raffaele Monelli of Fermo would create the role of Dorvil in *La Scala di seta* (1812); he is often confused with his brother Savino, another leading tenor. Filippo Galli (1783–1853) was a great *basso cantante* and one of the busiest singers of his era. Having made his operatic debut as a mediocre tenor in 1804, Galli took the advice of the *castrato* Luigi Marchesi to develop his deepest range; his success in *L'Inganno felice* when he was still less than thirty instituted a spectacular career during which he created leading bass roles in, among many other operas, Rossini's *La Pietra del paragone* (1812), *L'Italiana in Algeri* (1813), *Il Turco in Italia* (1814), *Torvaldo e Dorliska* (1815), *La Gazza ladra*, *Maometto II* (1820), and *Semiramide* (1823), as well as the Enrico VIII of Donizetti's *Anna Bolena* (1830). Almost nothing is known of Venturi.

p. 27, l. 29 "March 14), 1812"   The cast included Marietta Marcolini (the travesty role of Ciro), Elisabetta Manfredini (Amira), Anna Savinelli (Argene), Eliodoro Bianchi (Baldassare), Giovanni Layner (Zambri), Francesco Savinelli (Arbace), and Giovanni Fraschi (Daniello). Elisabetta (Elisa) Manfredini-Guarmani, a soprano, had made her debut in 1809; her beautiful voice was said to be used with little expressiveness. She was to create roles in *Tancredi*, *Sigismondo*, and *Adelaide di Borgogna* (1817). The Savinellis left almost no traces in operatic annals. Eliodoro Bianchi, a tenor, had made his debut in 1799; he was to sing also in the *première* of Rossini's *Eduardo e Cristina* (1819). He was a teacher of Rossini's close friend the Russian tenor Nicholas Ivanoff. Layner and Fraschi appear to have remained secondary singers.

p. 28, l. 8 "her triumph"   For a similarly underprivileged singer (or perhaps just as a lark), Rossini later composed *Les Adieux à la vie* (*Élégie sur une seule note*) and an *Ave Maria* for contralto and piano in E-flat in which the vocal line consists entirely of contiguous G's and A-flats. As with "*Chi disprezza gl'infelici*," these make their musical points by constant modulation and other changes in the accompaniment. *Les Adieux à la vie,* one of the *Péchés de vieillesse*—Rossini's name for numerous small pieces that he composed in his old age—is No. 9 of the *Album français*. The two-note *Ave Maria* is No. 7 of the *Album per canto italiano*; it has been published (*QR* V, 1955, p. 51).

p. 28, l. 17 "*di Seta*"   Foppa had derived it either from *L'Échelle de soie*, a play by François-Antoine-Eugène de Planard, or, more likely, from a libretto after that play which Pierre Gaveaux had set in 1808.

p. 28, l. 22 "(about $130)"   The original cast of *La Scala di seta* probably included Maria Cantarelli (Giulia), Carolina Nagher (Lucilla), Raffaele Monelli (Dorvil), Gaetano Del Monte (Dormont), Nicola De Grecis (Blansac), and Nicola Tacci (Germano). These ascriptions cannot be documented, but seem very likely. The printed libretto reads: "*Prima donna*— Maria Cantarelli; *Primo mezzo carattere*—Raffaele Monelli; *Primi Buffi*— Nicola de Grecis & Nicola Tacci; *Seconda Donna*—Carolina Nagher; *Secondo Tenore*—Gaetano Del Monte; *Terza Donna*—Teresa Cantarelli." The Cantarellis appear to have made little impression upon their contemporaries. Carolina Nagher would create roles for Rossini in *L'Occasione fa il ladro* and *Il Signor Bruschino*. Gaetano Del Monte (del Monte, Delmonte, even Dalmonte) would be in the first casts of *L'Occasione fa il ladro* and *Il Signor Bruschino*. Nicola Tacci would create a role in *Il Signor Bruschino* and the leading part in Donizetti's *L'Ajo nell'imbarazzo*.

p. 29, l. 1 "to Cera"   The text of the "letter to Cera" did not appear in Giuseppe Mazzatinti's *Lettere inedite e rare di G. Rossini*; it was published by G. Paloschi in *LGMM* on February 29, 1892, the centenary of Rossini's birth. Then Mazzatinti and L. and G. Manis reprinted it as the first document in *LdR*, giving no location for the autograph. Two of Radiciotti's denunciations of the letter occur in *RAD* (I, 90, footnote 1; I, 303).

p. 29, l. 23 "Frank Walker"   In Walker's much-annotated copy of *LdR*, now in the present writer's possession, he wrote "fake" alongside the text of the supposed letter to Cera.

p. 29, l. 28 "World War II"   *La Scala di seta* was revived for the Maggio Musicale Fiorentino of 1952 and at the Piccola Scala, Milan, on February 6, 1961, when the cast included Graziella Sciutti (Giulia), Cecilia Fusco (Lucilla), Luigi Alva (Dorvil), Angelo Mercuriali (Dormont), Franco Calabrese (Blansac), and Sesto Bruscantini (Germano).

p. 30, l. 3 "Lodovico Olivieri"   For the genesis of this opera and for the Mombellis, see. p. 17. Marianna (Anna) Mombelli left the stage in 1817 after her marriage to the musical journalist Angelo Lambertini. Ester Mombelli (later the wife of the impresario Conte Gritti) sang until 1827. She was the Madama Cortese of the *première* performance of Rossini's *Il Viaggio a Reims* (1825); for her, too, Rossini composed *La Morte di Didone*. She sang several Rossinian roles and from 1817 on was a noted Cenerentola. The bass Olivieri holds almost no place in operatic annals.

p. 30, l. 5 "first performance"   Only one other of Rossini's operas reached its *première* without his personal intervention: *Adina* (see pp. 89 and 150).

p. 30, l. 24 "in Milan" Talking forty-three years after the *première* of *Demetrio e Polibio*, Rossini had forgotten the Roman performance in May 1812 (which he would have been unlikely to forget if he had attended it). The Milanese staging did not occur until July 1813 (Teatro Carcano). Mombelli may have composed one or two numbers for this opera, perhaps the tenor cavatina "*Presenta in questi doni*" and the contralto aria "*Perdon ti chiedo, o padre.*" The circumstances of the opera's composition and first stagings suggest that Mombelli also probably supplied linking recitative. *RAD* I, 34, footnote 1, said that the Milan Conservatory had an autograph *Sinfonia all'opera Demetrio e Polibio* wholly different from the overture in the published piano score; in December 1965, however, Dr. Guglielmo Barblan wrote me that no such autograph could be located in the Conservatory library.

p. 30, l. 32 "in 1814" Stendhal was in Paris at the time of the Como performance that he describes so vividly. He said of the Mombelli sisters: "Without being pretty, the two Mombellis are generally attractive in appearance; but they are of a savage virtue." *Demetrio e Polibio* did not remain the exclusive property of the Mombellis for more than a few years: the libretto printed for a staging of it at the Teatro San Benedetto, Venice, in the spring of 1817 lists this cast: Luigi Campitelli (Eumene), Luciano Bianchi (Polibio), Catterina Liparini (Lisinga), Benedetta Rosmunda Pisaroni (Demetrio), Annetta Liparini (Almira), Agostino Trentanove (Onao); the music is attributed to Rossini, but no librettist's name is listed.

p. 31, l. 29 "outlying towns" The first-season popularity of *La Pietra del paragone*, which came within one performance of the 1810 run of Pavesi's *Ser Marcantonio*, was not exceeded at La Scala until 1842, when Verdi's *Nabucco* ran up fifty-eight performances during its first season. In 1822, *La Pietra* returned to La Scala for a seasonal run of thirty-seven performances.

p. 31, l. 32 "of Italy" The first cast of *La Pietra del paragone* consisted of Marietta Marcolini (La Marchesa Clarice), Carolina Zerbini (La Baronessa Aspasia), Orsola Fei (Donna Fulvia), Filippo Galli (Asdrubale), Claudio Bonoldi (Giocondo), Antonio Parlamagni (Il Conte Macrobio), Pietro Vasoli (Pacuvio), and Paolo Rossignoli (Fabrizio). Carolina Zerbini and Orsola Fei seem to have remained secondary singers. Claudio Bonoldi, a tenor, was to create roles in Rossini's *Sigismondo*, *Armida*, and *Bianca e Falliero*. Parlamagni, a renowned Neapolitan *buffo*, sang with success in Rome in 1818, when past sixty; he would create the role of Isidoro in Rossini's *Matilde Shabran*. Of the Pacuvio of Vasoli, another *buffo* (he would create roles in *Aureliano in Palmira* and *Il Turco in Italia*), Stendhal wrote: "The public's good will extended even to poor Vasoli, an aged grenadier of the Army of Egypt who made a reputation in the 'Mississippi' [actually 'Missipipì'] aria." During the little more than seventeen years of Rossini's active career as a composer of operas, La Scala gave 1,316 performances of twenty-five of his operas, an average of seventy-eight per year.

p. 33, l. 2 "November 24, 1812" The first cast of *L'Occasione fa il ladro* included Giacinta Canonici (Berenice), Carolina Nagher (Ernestina),

Gaetano Del Monte (Don Eusebio), Tommaso Berti (Conte Alberto), Luigi Pacini (Don Parmenione), and Luigi Spada (Martino). Canonici, passionately admired by Stendhal, would create a role in Donizetti's *La Zingara*. Luigi Pacini (Paccini in the libretto) a *buffo*, was the father of the composer Giovanni Pacini; he would create the role of Geronio in *Il Turco in Italia*; like Filippo Galli, he was a tenor turned bass. Luigi Spada left few traces in operatic chronicles. *ZAN* includes Teresa Batarelli in the first cast of *L'Occasione*, but her name does not appear in the printed libretto.

L'Occasione gave rise to extraordinarily numerous confusions and misstatements. Azevedo (*AZ*) mistook its subtitle for the title of a separate opera: he put *Il Cambio della valigia* in the Carnival season of 1811-12, *L'Occasione fa il ladro* in the autumn season of 1812. Zanolini (*ZAN*), stating that he listed the singers as given in the first printed libretto, omitted Pacini. In a published piano-vocal score, the libretto is attributed to Foppa. Early books on Rossini by Enrico Montazio (*Giovacchino Rossini*) and the Escudiers (*LfS*) express doubt that the opera ever was staged at all.

p. 33, l. 6 "in 1834" Radiciotti erred in saying (*RAD* I, 87, footnote 1) that *L'Occasione fa il ladro* "never left Italy" (he himself listed a staging at Lisbon—*RAD* III, 195). But he died (1931) too early to have had the benefit of the late Alfred Loewenberg's *Annals of Opera* (1943; rev. edn. in 2 vols., 1955), a prime source book on operatic *premières* and performances which lists five non-Italian productions of this opera. Stendhal made a more peculiar error, as Radiciotti noted: "By mistake, Stendhal wrote Graciata Canonici instead of Giacinta Canonici, and that error has been repeated by many in the usual way; even in aggravated form, as someone has made of a single person two different artists: *la Graciata* (!) and *la Canonici!*"

p. 33, l. 27 "January 1813" The first cast of *Il Signor Bruschino* included Teodolinda Pontiggia (Sofia), Carolina Nagher (Marianna), Luigi Raffanelli (Bruschino *padre*), Gaetano Del Monte (Bruschino *figlio* and Un Delegato di Polizia), Nicola De Grecis (Gaudenzio), Tommaso Berti (Florville), and Nicola Tacci (Filiberto). Between 1811 and 1815, Pontiggia sang secondary roles at La Scala, Milan, and the San Carlo, Naples—at the latter several times in casts with Colbran. Azevedo (*AZ*) insisted that the name of this opera was *I Due Bruschini* and wrote that at its *première* the role of Sofia was sung by Maria Cantarelli; he had confused this first performance with that of *La Scala di seta* eight months earlier.

p. 34, ll. 17-18 "their disapproval" For a complete discussion of this story, see Radiciotti's " '*Il Signor Bruschino*' ed il '*Tancredi.*' "

p. 34, l. 24 "the Pesarese . . ." *ROG*, pp. 41-2.

p. 35, l. 3 "was begun" Other unfounded legends clustered about the composition and *première* of *Il Signor Bruschino*. The diverting, unreliable memoirs of Giovanni Pacini state that Raffanelli, the Signor Bruschino of the first cast, not only had presented the idea for the libretto to Foppa (*sic*)—who merely had versified it—but also had given the musical ideas to Rossini, who thereupon had dubbed him "the new Orpheus" and had merely written them down, thus arranging "that monstrous jumble which is called *Bruschino*." He added that at the first performance, Rossini had put two small

"Pulcinello" dolls on the cembalo and had made them appear to bow ac-knowledgments to each howl of disapproval from the audience.

NOTES TO CHAPTER III

p. 36, l. 5   "Gaetano Rossi"   For Rossi, see footnote to page 21.

p. 36, l. 20   "February 6, 1813"   The first cast of *Tancredi* included Adelaide Malanotte-Montresor (Tancredi), Elisabetta Manfredini-Guarmani (Adelaide), Teresa Marchesi (Isaura), Carolina Sivelli (Roggiero), Pietro Todràn (Argirio), and Luciano Bianchi (Orbazzano). Malanotte-Montresor, a contralto of aristocratic family, had made her debut in her native Verona in 1806. Hérold, the composer of *Zampa* and *Le Pré aux clercs*, who lived in Italy from 1812 to 1815, described her as superb in appearance and said that she sang stupendously, with perfect intonation and very refined taste, but added that the timbre of her voice too closely resembled that of an English horn, "an unpleasant singularity without which Malanotte would figure honorably among first-rank artists. However, habits unseemly in a *signorina* were attributed to her, such as that of overuse of tobacco and brandies." Her first wide fame resulted from her portrayal of the travesty role of Tancredi. Teresa Marchesi was not a singer of importance. Pietro Todràn left relatively few traces in operatic annals. Luciano Bianchi of Pesaro was to create Rossinian roles in *Sigismondo* and *Eduardo e Cristina*.

p. 37, l. 7   "and Argirio"   Manfredini and Todràn repeated their roles at Ferrara, but the Tancredi was Francesca Riccardi Paër, temporarily the wife of Ferdinando Paër.

p. 37, l. 16   "throughout Italy"   The third staging of *Tancredi* appears to have been that with which the Teatro Re, Milan, was inaugurated in December 1813.

p. 37, ll. 18–19   "across Europe"   The first of Rossini's operas to be translated—and in many instances the first heard in foreign ciites—by 1843, *Tancredi* had been sung in German, Polish, Czech, Spanish, French, Hun-garian, Swedish, Russian, and English. A few months after the Vienna *première* (December 17, 1816), Artaria published a four-hand piano arrange-ment of its overture (the one that Rossini had brought over from *La Pietra del paragone*).

p. 37, l. 29   "and Vienna"   *AZ* reports that "*Di tanti palpiti*" came to be called "the rice aria" because Rossini once remarked that he had composed it in the time needed for boiling rice. In the anonymously published booklet *Rossini e la sua musica: Una Passeggiata con Rossini*, Zanolini wrote: "Mal-anotte, at the final rehearsal of *Tancredi* having taken it into her head not to sing the first-act aria as Rossini had composed it, he had to write her another during the very night that preceded the first performance, and he added that song full of suavity with which Malanotte and [Giuditta] Pasta excited their listeners' transports." The story could well be true.

p. 38, l. 7   "more pains"   I am indebted to Leslie A. Marchand, biog-rapher of Byron, for calling this passage and footnote to my attention.

p. 38, l. 13   "Giuseppe Carpani"   Carpani (1752–1825), journalist,

librettist, translator, biographer, and critic, provided Paër with the libretto
of his long-popular opera *Camilla* (1799). He also made the standard Italian
translation—*La Creazione*—of the text of Haydn's *Die Schöpfung*. At Padua
in 1824, he published a monograph entitled *Le Rossiniane, ossia Lettere
musico-teatrali*. Stendhal, under the pseudonym of Louis-Alexandre Bombet,
plagiarized large sections of Carpani's earlier *Le Haydine* (1812) in his
*Lettres écrites de Vienne en Autriche, sur le célèbre compositeur Joseph
Haydn, suivies d'une vie de Mozart et de considérations sur Métastase et l'état
présent de la musique en France et en Italie*. Carpani denounced the plagiarism in a brochure entitled *Lettere dell'autore delle Haydine* (Vienna, 1815),
but that exposure did not dissuade Stendhal from reissuing his book in 1817
as *Vies de Haydn, Mozart et Métastase*—which is no more reliable than his
Vie de Rossini, a condition for which no blame should be attached to Giuseppe Carpani.

p. 38, l. 29 "Angelo Anelli" Anelli (1761–1820), a native of Desen-
zano, was the prolific librettist whose text for Pavesi's *Ser Marcantonio*
(1810) later became—as revised by Giovanni Ruffini and Donizetti—that of
Donizetti's *Don Pasquale* (1843).

p. 38, l. 30 "the Magnificent" Or perhaps on the story of an aristocratic Milanese girl named Antonietta Frapolli Suini, whom Algerian pirates
abducted from a ship in 1805. She appears thereafter to have been confined
in several harems, but was returned to Italy a few years later on board a
Venetian ship without any ransom money having been paid. In a footnote
to stanza 80 of Canto IV of *Don Juan*, Byron wrote: "A few years ago a
man engaged a company for some foreign theatre, embarked them at an
Italian port, and carrying them to Algiers, sold them all. One of the women,
returned from her captivity, I heard sing, by a strange coincidence, in Rossini's opera of *L'Italiana in Algieri* [*sic*], at Venice, in the beginning of 1817."
L'Italiana seems (despite *RAD* III, 200) not to have been sung in Venice in
1817, but Byron was still there in 1818, when the opera was staged in the
spring at the Teatro San Luca (with a Signora Losetti as Isabella) and in the
autumn at both that theater and the San Benedetto (with Fanny Eckerlin
as Isabella in both cases). Byron's anecdote, then, is incorrect in detail.

p. 39, l. 9 "May 22, 1813" The original cast of *L'Italiana in Algeri*
consisted of Marietta (Maria) Marcolini (Isabella), Luttgard Annibaldi
(Elvira), Annunziata Berni Chelli (Zulma), Filippo Galli (Mustafà), Serafino Gentili (Lindoro), Paolo (Pablo) Rosich (Taddeo). Luttgard Annibaldi had created the role of Dorina in Pavesi's *Ser Marcantonio* at La Scala,
Milan, in 1810. Berni Chelli (or Chelli Berni) also had sung at La Scala in
1810. Serafino Gentili (1786–1835), a tenor, had made his debut in 1807; for
twenty years thereafter, he was a valued performer.

p. 39, l. 15 "was reported" *LfS*, p. 15.

p. 39, ll. 30–1 "to Zanolini" Zanolini (1791–1877) knew Rossini well.
His Rossini biography was first published by Nicolò Bettoni in the periodical
L'Ape italana rediviva (Paris); it was reissued in *Annali universali delle
scienze ed industrie* (1837), and also in *Moda* during that year. In 1841 at

Florence, a booklet entitled *Rossini e la sua musica: Una Passeggiata con Rossini*, described on its title page as "articles extracted from the *Ricoglitore fiorentino*," was published anonymously, though it had been written by Zanolini. Later editions of his original biography were issued at Bologna in 1875 and 1879, the latter with an appendix by Gioachino Paglia. In a bibliographical note on the 1875 edition, Radiciotti wrote (*RAD* III, 311): "Here is added another writing by the same Zanolini: *Una passeggiata in compagnia di Rossini* [*sic*], which appeared for the first time in the periodical *Il Raccoglitore*. This is the truest and most exact (though incomplete) of the biographies to appear up to now [1929], especially with regard to the first years of the Maestro's life. In 1853, Rossini himself replied to the compiler of a biographical dictionary who had asked him from what source to obtain dependable information about his life: 'Abide, if you will say something about my early years, by what my friend Zanolini wrote . . . That text was read by me before it was printed.' On the critical side, however, it is valueless." Curiously, Radiciotti (who listed the anonymous 1841 booklet without comment) gives no indication of having recognized that *Una Passeggiata con Rossini*, as extracted from the *Ricoglitore fiorentino*, and "*Una passeggiata in compagnia di Rossini*," as extracted from "*Il Raccoglitore*," were identical—and that the anonymous script was written by Zanolini.

p. 40, l. 8 "*La Cenerentola*" During 1813, *L'Italiana in Algeri* was staged at the Teatro Carignano, Turin, with Rosa Morandi as Isabella, and began its long tour of other Italian opera houses. Geltrude Righetti-Giorgi wrote (*RG*): "On thirty-nine occasions in Rome I repeated the rondo '*Pensa alla patria*.' I shall not be considered vain because I record a fact."

p. 40, l. 16 "Carnival season" As the Carnival season extended from December 26 (Santo Stefano) to Ash Wednesday, it varied in length from year to year.

p. 40, ll. 19–20 "or Romanelli)." For the intricate, convincing reasons behind this almost-certainty, see Mario Rinaldi's *Felice Romani*, p. 34.

p. 40, ll. 22–3 "Alessandro Rolla" Rolla (1757–1841), violinist and composer, had been Paganini's teacher at Parma. While serving as court violinist to Eugène de Beauharnais, Viceroy of Italy, he became one of the first instructors at the Milan Conservatory (1807).

p. 40, l. 27 "coldly received" The first cast of *Aureliano in Palmira* consisted of Lorenza Correa (Zenobia), Luigia Sorrentini (Publio), Giambattista Velluti (Arsace), Luigi Mari (Aureliano), Gaetano Pozzi (Oraspe), Pietro Vasoli (Licinio), and Vincenzo Botticelli (Gran Sacerdote d'Iside). Rossini had begun the role of Aureliano in the belief that it would be sung by the great tenor Giovanni David, who, however, had contracted measles. Act II therefore was completed with Mari in mind for the role. Although changes very probably were made in Act I to accommodate it to the inferior capabilities of Mari, a noticeable difference remains between the difficulty of Aureliano's vocal line in Act I and the comparative simplicty in that for Act II. Lorenza Correa, a Portuguese soprano, had made her debut at Madrid in 1790; she was forty-two at the time of the first *Aureliano*. Azevedo (*AZ*) spoke of her "beautiful voice and good method" as redeeming "the negative beauty of her physique." Sorrentini appears to have remained a *comprimaria*. Velluti (1780–1861) was the last notable operatic *castrato*. He had made his debut at Forlì in 1800; Rossini had heard him in Bologna in 1809. Arsace is the only *castrato* role in a Rossini opera. Luigi Mari would be singing tenor roles at La Scala as late as 1831. Pozzi would create the role of Albazar in *Il Turco in Italia*. Vincenzo Botticelli, a bass, would create the role of Fabrizio Vingradito in *La Gazza ladra*.

p. 40, l. 36　"long period . . ."　Only eleven months had passed since the *première* of *Tancredi*, seven since that of *L'Italiana in Algeri*.

p. 40, l. 39　"that season"　Sections of *Aureliano in Palmira*, in part as refashioned later, remain familiar as transferred by Rossini to *Il Barbiere di Siviglia*. They begin with the famous overture (which he also would use for *Elisabetta, regina d'Inghilterra*), and include the opening chorus ("*Sposa del grande Osiride*"), the first eight measures of which lead off Almaviva's "*Ecco ridente in cielo*"; Arsace's rondo ("*Non lasciarmi in tal momento*"), the first eight measures of which recur in Rosina's "*Una voce poco fa*"; and elements of the introduction to the Zenobia-Arsace duet which became the opening of "*La calunnia*." Careful study of the score of *Aureliano* led Bonaccorsi (*LRM*, p. 219) to write that "the acts were composed after the overture —came, that is, from the overture and with notable internal affinities, and therefore not the other way round, as usually occurred if the overture had to summarize the salient points of the opera, in which case it evidently was composed after the drafting of the acts." This of course suggests that the overture may have existed some time earlier—and may even have been composed, as has been suggested, for *L'Equivoco stravagante* in 1811.

p. 41, l. 5　"Felice Romani"　Romani (1788–1865) was perhaps the most accomplished Italian librettist during the long period between Metastasio and Boito. He was a distinguished journalist and an appreciable force in the intellectual life of northern Italy. In addition to providing Rossini with the librettos of *Il Turco in Italia* and *Bianca e Falliero*, he wrote about 120 others, several of which served more than one composer. They included eleven texts used by Donizetti (among them, those for *Anna Bolena, L'Elisir d'amore*, and *Lucrezia Borgia*) and seven used by Bellini (*Il Pirata, La Straniera, Zaira, I Capuleti ed i Montecchi, La Sonnambula, Norma*, and *Beatrice di Tenda*). Mercadante set sixteen Romani librettos, Meyerbeer two of them, and Verdi one (*Un Giorno di regno*—later called *Il Finto Stanislao*).

p. 41, ll. 14–15　"August 14, 1814"　The cast at the first performance of *Il Turco in Italia* was made up of Francesca Maffei-Festa (Fiorilla), Adelaide Carpano (Zaida), Giovanni David (Narciso), Filippo Galli (Selim), Luigi Pacini (Geronio), Pietro Vasoli (Prosdocimo), and Gaetano Pozzi (Albazar). The soprano Maffei-Festa (1778–1836) was a sister of Giuseppe Festa, the violinist-conductor at the Teatro San Carlo, Naples; she had a voice of intense sensuous appeal. Rossini had encountered Adelaide Carpano at Sinigaglia some years before (see p. 12); she seems to have remained a secondary singer. The great tenor Giovanni David (or Davide, 1790–1864) was the son of a very famous Bergamasque tenor, Giacomo David (1750–1831). His range extended from the C below the staff to high G and even A. He had made his debut at Brescia in 1810; he sang until about 1841.

p. 41, l. 36 "Teatro Carcano"   Long-standing custom allowed both Italian and foreign impresarios to insert into *Il Turco* irrelevant numbers from other Rossini operas, and even from operas by other composers. Radiciotti pointed out that piano-vocal scores published in France and England were full of such interpolations. Vladimir Nabokov (*Eugene Onegin*, New York, 1964, III, 306) wrote that on July 8, 1824, Alexander Pushkin was discharged from the civil service for "bad behavior" and ordered to his mother's manor. "On the night of July 30," Nabokov wrote, "he was for the last time at the Italian opera in Odessa, where he saw Rossini's *Il Turco in Italia* (1814)." The opera had been sung in Russian in St. Petersburg in 1823; its production in Odessa little more than a year later emphasizes the speed with which a well-liked Italian opera then sped across the world.

p. 42, l. 3 "*ed Irene*"   *Egle ed Irene* remains of some interest because a piece of its score recurs in *Il Barbiere di Siviglia*, in the second-act Rosina-Almaviva duet, at the words "*Dolce nodo avventurato/ Che fai paghi i miei desiri*," music originally used with echo effect in the cantata at the text words "*Voi che amate, compiangete*."

p. 42, l. 9 "into composing"   Rossini avowedly disliked supernatural interventions in libretto stories. Only *Mosè* and *Armida* among his operas notably include them. He probably therefore did not relish the ghostly apparitions that play some part in the texts of *Sigismondo* and *Semiramide*.

p. 42, l. 15 "December 26, 1814"   The first cast of *Sigismondo* was made up of Marietta (Maria) Marcolini (Sigismondo, re di Polonia), Elisabetta Manfredini-Guarmani (Aldimira), Marianna Rossi (Anagilda), Claudio Bonoldi (Ladislao), Luciano Bianchi (Ulderico, re de Boemia, and Zenovito), and Domenico Bartoli (Radoski). Marianna Rossi seems to have remained a *comprimaria*. Domenico Bartoli, a tenor, never attracted much attention.

p. 42, l. 17 "best opera"   The Fenice musicians, of course, would have had no way of hearing several other Rossini operas. The low opinion that some composers held of reactions by orchestral players is epitomized in a story told by Radiciotti about the Maltese Niccolò Isouard (1775–1818). After a rehearsal at the Opéra-Comique, Paris, he is said to have gone home in consternation: the orchestra had applauded three numbers in his new opera, and he therefore felt it necessary to recompose them.

p. 42, l. 29 "fine *fiasco*"   A *fiasco* is a bottle or flask. The use of the word to mean a failure resulted from the fact that bottles coming out so defective that they would not stand upright were wrapped in woven straw to provide a flat surface at the bottom.

p. 43, l. 12 "its due)"   Radiciotti (*RAD* I, 145) quotes two passages from this unpublished letter. In the first, Rossini says: "What are Perucchini, Ancillo, Buratti, Maruzzi, Arnoldi, Suardi, Straolino, Capello, Topetti, Stroti, Papadopoli doing? . . . Do they speak of me? Do these great buffoons remember me? if these rascals have forgotten me so soon, I send them all to Hades! . . ." I have been unable to locate the autograph or full text of this letter (May 15, 1815), the earliest from Rossini about which dependable information exists.

p. 44, ll. 9–10 "several years"   See p. 107.

p. 44, l. 35 *"are worth!"*   Given here in the translation by William Weaver published with a recording of *L'Italiana in Algeri* by Angel Records, the lines are all from Act II of that opera: the first three are sung by Isabella, the last two by the chorus of Italians.

p. 45, l. 5 "another poem)"   The text to which Rossini was reported to have fitted the music of the *Inno dell'indipendenza* was by Vincenzo Monti, a poet of distinction who "deserted" to the Austrians in 1815. The hymn (really a cantata) incorrectly attributed to Rossini existed: it was composed to Monti's text by the Hungarian Joseph Weigl and sung for the first time, in the presence of the Emperor Francis II and the Empress Maria Theresa, at La Scala, Milan, on January 6, 1816. A long-current legend had it that when Rossini's original hymn aroused the suspicions of the Austrian authorities, Padre Mattei warned his ex-pupil to hide and offered him funds with which to flee Bologna.

Notes to Chapter IV

p. 46, l. 4 "Ferdinand IV"   Confusingly, Ferdinand was Ferdinand IV of Naples, Ferdinand III of Sicily. Only with the disappearance of Napoleon's power and after the Congress of Vienna did he become Ferdinand I of the Two Sicilies—that is, of Sicily and of Naples, the latter referring not merely to the city, but also to the large area of southern Italy which it controlled.

p. 47, l. 13 "of Music)"   The Royal School of Music was transferred from the ex-Nunnery of San Sebastiano to the ex-Monastery of San Pietro a Maiella in 1826.

p. 47, l. 25 "(1778–1841)"   That Barbaja died in his villa at Posillipo on October 19, 1841 (and not on October 16, 1842, the date often given) is proved by 1841 newspaper accounts of his death and elaborate obsequies.

p. 47, l. 34 "the city"   On June 2, 1836, after an interruption in his management, Barbaja signed a contract as impresario of the Royal Theaters of Naples for four years.

p. 47, l. 36 "and gourmet"   What Italians now call *granita di caffè* long was known as *barbajata* because Barbaja was credited with its invention.

p. 49, l. 4 "would lapse"   Arthur Pougin wrote (*RNI*): "Rossini received from Barbaja, not at all 12,000 francs per year [about $7,100], but 200 ducats [about $480] per month, representing a little less than 900 francs; on the other hand, his interest in the gambling rose much higher than the 30 or 40 louis of which Stendhal speaks, and he earned annually about 1,000 ducats, or 4,400 francs [from that]. It should be added that whenever the composer took leave to go to mount a new opera in another city, the generous

Barbaja, who owed him the success of his enterprise, conscientiously suppressed his remuneration for the whole term of his absence." But why should
Barbaja have paid Rossini to mount operas for other impresarios?

p. 49, l. 17   "and *Cora*"   Mayr's *Medea in Corinto* (1813) had been
sung at the San Carlo late in 1813 with a cast including Colbran, Manuel
Garcia, and Andrea Nozzari. His *Alonso e Cora* (1803), as revised to a new
libretto entitled *Cora* (by the Marchese Francesco Berio di Salsa, future
librettist of Rossini's *Otello* and *Ricciardo e Zoraide*), had received its
première at the San Carlo, with much the same cast, on March 27, 1815.

p. 49, l. 20   "Federico Schmidt"   Many writers (including Ada Melica,
BdCRdS 1958, 2, 28) have attributed this libretto to Andrea Leone Tottola.
But the libretto as published for the *première* of *Elisabetta* includes an *Av-
vertimento* signed by Schmidt which makes certain his having been the
librettist. Schmidt, a Tuscan (1775?–1840?), wrote about one hundred librettos for the San Carlo and the Fondo; for La Scala, Milan; and for La Fenice,
Venice. For Rossini, he supplied, besides the libretto of *Elisabetta*, that of
Armida; also, the text of Rossini's *Eduardo e Cristina* was a reshaping by two
other writers of a libretto that Schmidt had written for Pavesi in 1810.
Azevedo wrote: "This Schmidt essentially lacked gaiety and never talked
about anything but unhappiness and catastrophes. Rossini, whose verve was
quenched by his conversation, found it necessary, so as to be able to work,
to beg Barbaja to spare him any interviews with this distressing person."

p. 50, l. 6   "October 4, 1815"   The first cast of *Elisabetta* was made
up of Isabella Colbran (Elisabetta), Girolama Dardanelli (Matilde), Maria(?)
Manzi (Enrico), Andrea Nozzari (Leicester), Manuel Garcia (Norfolc), and
Gaetano Chizzola (Guglielmo). Girolama Dardanelli Corradi also sang in
Rossini's cantata *Le Nozze di Teti e di Peleo*. One or more of the numerous
Manzis singing in Naples at about the time of this *première*—and that it
was Maria is in each case no more than a careful guess—also created for
Rossini the roles of Madama La Rosa (*La Gazzetta*), Emilia (*Otello*), Amenofi
(*Mosè in Egitto*), Fatima (*Ricciardo e Zoraide*), Cleone (*Ermione*), and
Albina (*La Donna del lago*). Nozzari (1775–1832) was a leading tenor of the
period (Carpani called him "more baritone than tenor, but gifted with un-
common strength and with a wide extension of voice"). For Rossini, he also
created the title role in *Otello*, Rinaldo (*Armida*), Osiride (*Mosè in Egitto*),
Agorante (*Ricciardo e Zoraide*), Pirro (*Ermione*), Rodrigo di Dhu (*La
Donna del lago*), Erisso (*Maometto II*), and Antenore (*Zelmira*). Manuel
del Popolo Vicente Garcia (1775–1832), Spanish composer and outstanding
tenor, became the father of the famous singing teacher Manuel Patricio
Garcia (1805–1906) and of Maria Malibran and Pauline Viardot-Garcia. In
1816, he was to create the role of Conte Almaviva in Rossini's *Il Barbiere di
Siviglia*. Gaetano Chizzola, one of the busiest secondary tenors of his time,
would create numerous roles for both Rossini and Donizetti. In addition to
Guglielmo, his Rossinian firsts were The Doge (*Otello*), Eustazio, Carlo,
and Astarotte (*Armida*), Mambre (*Mosè in Egitto*), Attalo (*Ermione*),
Serano (*La Donna del lago*), Selimo (*Maometto II*), and Eacide (*Zelmira*).

p. 52, l. 9 "Cesare Sterbini" Sterbini (1784?–1831), who achieved his measure of immortality by writing the libretto of *Il Barbiere di Siviglia*, was a notable linguist. Jacopo Ferretti described him as "very expert in the Greek tongue, Latin, French, and German"; his familiarity with French was useful to him when deriving the *Barbiere* libretto in part directly from Beaumarchais's play.

p. 52, l. 14 "December 26, 1815" The cast at the *première* of *Torvaldo e Dorliska* consisted of Adelaide Sala (Dorliska), Agnese Loyselet (Carlotta), Domenico Donzelli (Torvaldo), Raniero Remorini (Giorgio), Filippo Galli (Il Duca d'Ordow), and Cristoforo Bastianelli (Ormondo). Sala, a mezzo-soprano, was very young at this time; she earned considerable success in later years. Agnese Loyselet later would create a role for Donizetti in *L'Ajo nell'imbarazzo*. Donzelli (1790?–1873) was, with Rubini, the most renowned of all the "Bergamo" tenors; he was to become a very close friend of Rossini as well as his landlord. He also sang in the *première* of Rossini's *Il Viaggio a Reims* (1825), created roles in three Donizetti operas, and was the first Pollione in Bellini's *Norma*. Remorini, a bass, would create the role of Faraone in Rossini's *Mosè in Egitto*. Bastianelli remained a *comprimario*.

p. 52, l. 29 "was recognizable" Rossini's later borrowings from *Torvaldo e Dorliska* were not large or numerous. The *agitato* section of the Duca d'Ordow's aria *"Ah! qual voce d'intorni ribombi!"* became the chief melody of the Otello-Rodrigo duet *"L'ira d'avverso fato"* in *Otello*; the final measures of the orchestral introduction to Torvaldo's cavatina in Act I, Scene 7 likewise reappeared in *Otello* (final scene).

p. 53, ll. 3–4 "the Valle" Looked upon as a relative failure, *Torvaldo e Dorliska* nonetheless had by 1842 been staged not only in about twenty Italian theaters, but also in Paris, Budapest, Prague, Madrid, Moscow, Berlin, Frankfurt-am-Main, St. Petersburg, Mexico City, Malta, and Oran. Radiciotti's statement (*RAD* I, 178, footnote 3) that Maria Malibran made her (unofficial) debut in this opera at the Théâtre-Italien, Paris, in May 1825 cannot be documented.

p. 53, l. 9 "in 1815" See Appendix A, p. 377, for the complete text of this contract.

p. 54, l. 1 "Cesare Sterbini" For Sterbini, see p. 52 and note for that page.

p. 54, l. 4 "*de Séville*" Stendhal asserted that the pontifical censor had rejected several subjects submitted by Sforza-Cesarini and had finally suggested the Beaumarchais comedy—an incredible tale in view of Beaumarchais's widespread reputation as a revolutionary propagandist.

p. 54, l. 11 "in America" Paisiello's was not the only earlier opera with a libretto derived from *Le Barbier de Séville*. In 1776, a German translation of the play had been staged at Dresden with an overture, ten arias, two duets, and a chorus by Friedrich Ludwig Benda (1752–92); in that same year, an opera on the subject by Johann André (1741–99) had been produced at Berlin. Many others have followed, one of the most recent, by Alberto Torazza, having been staged at Sestri Ponente in 1924.

p. 54, l. 14   "to repeat"   Beaumarchais had called Bartolo's two farcical servants *"La Jeunesse, vieux domestique de Bartholo"* and *"L'Eveillé, autre vallet de Bartholo, garçon niais et endormi."* Petrosellini had turned them into "Il Giovinetto" and "Lo Svegliato"; Sterbini assigned their minor functions to a character of his own devising, Berta.

p. 54, l. 29   "his libretto . . ."   If (as Stendhal stated) Paisiello replied —he was seventy-five, ailing, and very unhappy at the time, and would die on the following June 5—his letter appears not to have survived.

p. 55, ll. 13–14   "Settimo Silvestri)"   Ortigue, *Dictionnaire de la conversation et de la lecture*; Montazio, *Giovacchino Rossini*; Félix Clément, *Musiciens célèbres depuis le XVIe siècle*; Silvestri, *SIL*.

p. 55, ll. 15–16   "Radiciotti wrote"   *RAD* I, 86.

p. 55, l. 21   "and *concertazione*"   No English equivalent exists for this word, which implies finally putting all components into performable state. The man in charge of these multifarious details is the *maestro concertatore*.

p. 56, l. 4   "in existence' "   German musicians generally have agreed with Verdi and other Italian musicians in considering *Il Barbiere di Siviglia* to be the finest of Rossini's operas. Hans von Bülow wrote (*Briefe und ausgewählte Schriften*, Leipzig, 1906, III, 356): "This model comic opera can only please not only the public and the dilettantes, but also the musicians, as much, furthermore, as *Die Zauberflöte* or *Die Meistersinger*. Eternal youth lives in this opera; it is all a bouquet of flowers that never wither and always preserve their perfume; it is all a champagne intoxication without a tomorrow; and, above all, it is a truly classic opera and will remain such because whatever pleases everywhere and always merits that name."

p. 56, l. 13   "in 1815"   The version of the overture used with *Aureliano in Palmira* lacked the trombones and timpani called for in that used with *Elisabetta* (the version now traditionally part of *Il Barbiere*). Also, the two versions differ by an interesting eighth note in the third measure of the *allegro vivo* section:

Aureliano in Palmira   *Elisabetta, regina d'Inghilterra*

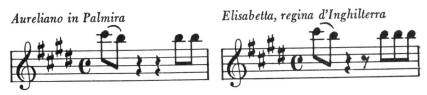

p. 56, l. 24   "wrote him"   I am grateful to Mr. Cecil Hopkinson, London, for sending me a photostatic copy of this letter, then in his possession.

p. 56, l. 31   "that way"   Francis Toye wrote (*Rossini*, p. 57, footnote): "The score would seem, however, to have been in existence in 1865, when [Luigi] Arditi announced in the prospectus of his promenade concerts at Her Majesty's Theatre [London] an 'overture in B flat, originally written for *Il Barbiere di Siviglia* (first performance in England).' Unless, of course, Arditi was the victim, conscious or unconscious, of a hoax."

What may well be the overture announced by Arditi (but is very unlikely to be the missing original Rossini overture) is included in a piano transcription of *"Der Barbier von Sevilla"* owned by the present writer. It contains no Lesson Scene, but begins with an overture in B-flat that is not at all Spanish or notably Rossinian. The edition is described as *"Komische Opera in 2 Aufzügen von G. Rossini für das Piano-Forte ohne Singstimme eingerichtet"* and as being published *"in Wien bey Tranquillo Mollo"* (who had been Beethoven's publisher early in the century); the principal melody of its overture, *allegro vivace*, reads:

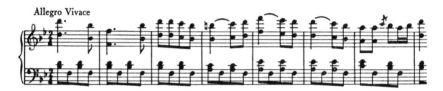

    p. 59, l. 2   "February 20, 1816"   Stendhal put the date of the *Almaviva première* at December 26, 1816, perhaps because that date (Santo Stefano) was the traditional one for the opening of the Carnival season, perhaps because it was the correct date for the first performance (1817) of *La Cenerentola*. Other writers have put it at February 1, 1816; still others, aware that an approximate date (February 5, 1816) for the *première* was stipulated in the contract, gave that as the date of the actual first performance. But Principe Agostino Chigi-Albani, under date of February 21, 1816, wrote in his diary: "Yesterday evening a new *burletta* entitled *Il Barbiere di Siviglia* [the dodge of calling the opera *Almaviva*, then, proved a futile precaution indeed, and from the beginning] by Maestro Rossini went onto the stage of the Argentina; an unhappy event." Conte Cesare Gallo, "a fervent patriot from Osimo in the Province of Ancona," also made an entry in his diary: "20 February 1816, a new opera by Rossini entitled *Il Barbiere di Siviglia* whistled at at the Argentina."

    p. 59, l. 6   "Biagelli (Fiorello)"   Geltrude Righetti (1793?–1862) of Bologna, who married a Dr. Luigi Giorgi, had become a much-admired contralto after her Rome debut in 1814. She retired to Bologna in 1822 because of ill health, thereafter presiding over a salon frequented by fashionable people and artists. In 1823 she published her *Cenni di una donna già cantante sopra il maestro Rossini*, a reply to a biographical article that had been published in *The Paris Monthly Review* (London) as by "Alceste," a pseudonym of Henri Beyle (Stendhal). She was contracted to create the role of Rosina at the last moment because the singer originally wanted, Elisabetta Gafforini, had made demands that Sforza-Cesarini found excessive. Righetti-Giorgi's voice, which Louis Spohr described as "full, powerful, and of rare extension, rising from the F below the staff to the B-flat above it," had been urged upon Sforza-Cesarini as early as September 1815, in vain. She would also create the title role of *La Cenerentola* (1817). Elisabetta Loyselet remained a secondary singer. Zamboni, a childhood acquaintance of Rossini's from Bologna, where he had been born about 1767 (died at Florence, 1837), had made his debut in 1791. He went on to become a greatly admired *buffo cantante*. Bartolommeo (or Bartolomeo) Botticelli was described by Radiciotti as "not rising much above mediocrity." Vitarelli—who, though a singer in the Sistine Chapel, had an "evil eye" reputation—would also create the role of Alidoro in *La Cenerentola*. Paolo Biagelli made no recorded impression upon his contemporaries.

p. 59, l. 21 "was finished" Rossini, of course, was writing forty-four years after the event; it is possible, but very unlikely, that he spent about thirteen *working* days on the task.

p. 59, l. 35 "to Azevedo" *AZ.*

p. 60, l. 12 " 'Calumny' aria" Giulio Fara (*Genio ed ingegno musicale: Gioacchino Rossini*, p. 137) pointed out that *"La calunnia è un venticello"* resembles the related aria in Paisiello's opera in that they both have the same time signature, 4/4; the same tempo indication, allegro; and the same mode, major. "They have also the, so to speak, same principal phrase, and which in Rossini's *calunnia* begins the piece, to which it gives all the crafty flavor of Jesuitical hypocrisy, and [in] which they are as alike as two drops of water, not only in melodic and rhythmic design, but also in instrumental color, for both of them are assigned to the unctuous sonority of the fourth string of the violin."

p. 60, l. 14 "his hand" Don Basilio's flourishing of his handkerchief has remained traditional.

p. 61, l. 7 "sleeping tranquilly" Doubt was cast on Rossini's peaceful repose after the catastrophic *première*—first by Giulio Fara and then by Radiciotti. But Rossini himself related the story of that night to Salvatore Marchesi di Castrone (husband of Mathilde Marchesi and father of Blanche Marchesi), who quoted him, assertedly verbatim, in his *"Souvenirs de Rossini"* (*Le Ménestrel*, Paris, February 10, 1889). That account of the occasion is very close to Righetti-Giorgi's. She said that she had found Rossini sleeping (she would have changed into street clothes, allowing for the lapse of some time), and she very probably was writing the truth.

p. 61, l. 10 "the cembalo" To prevent a repetition of what had ensued when Garcia had tuned his guitar onstage and then sung music of his own devising, Rossini insisted that Garcia sing the aria he himself had composed for Almaviva. Garcia complied during the rest of the Argentina performances; in appearances elsewhere, he interpolated his own music in its place.

p. 62, ll. 30-1 "Adolphe de Mareste" *Stendhal: Correspondance,* ed. Henri Martineau, Paris, 1934, p. 382.

Notes to Chapter V

p. 64, l. 9 "who reported" In "Rossini in Naples: Some Major Works Recovered," *The Musical Quarterly,* New York, July 1968, pp. 316–

340. The singers in what appears to have been the only performance of this cantata were Colbran (Cerere), Margherita Chabrand (Teti), Girolama Dardanelli (Giunone), Giovanni David (Peleo), and Andrea Nozzari (Giove). Chabrand, a *prima donna*, sang at Naples from about 1802 to at least 1820; she was also at La Scala, Milan, in 1802; she created the role of Lisetta in Rossini's *La Gazzetta* at the Teatro dei Fiorentini, Naples, in 1817. A well-known anecdote about Matteo Porto and his role in *Le Nozze di Teti e di Peleo*, first told by Azevedo (*AZ*, pp. 122–4) and retold in the first printing of the present book, was shown by Mr. Gossett to be apocryphal.

p. 65, l. 6 "Leone Tottola" Goldoni's comedy, dating from 1763, had been made into an opera, to a libretto by Gaetano Martinelli, by Niccolò Jommelli (1766). Discussing eighteenth-century Italian opera with Ferdinand Hiller at Trouville in 1855, Rossini said of Jommelli: "He was our most inspired composer of that time. No one could treat melody as he did. His slow movements especially are often of marvelous melodic beauty." Palomba (birth and death dates unknown) was a nephew of Antonio Palomba (1705–69), who had supplied Pergolesi with the text of *La Serva Padrona*; he himself had written the librettos of Cimarosa's *Le Astuzie femminili* (1794) and Fioravanti's *Le Cantatrici villane* (1798). In 1816 he was near the end of a career during which, according to Ulderico Rolandi (*Il Libretto per musica attraverso i tempi*, Rome, 1951), he became the most prolific of librettists, supplying 313 texts in about sixty years.

p. 65, l. 10 "old rigmaroles" Naples, it should be remembered, thus far had had only one Rossini *première*: that of *Elisabetta, regina d'Inghilterra* (1815). The "old rigmaroles" heard earlier that year at the Fiorentini had been Giuseppe Mosca's *Il Disperato per eccesso di buon core*, Valentino Fioravanti's *I Virtuosi ambulanti* and *Adelson e Salvini*, and Stefano Pavesi's *La Festa della rosa*. After the singing of Rossini's cantata on April 24, 1816, the operas heard at the Fondo had been Paisiello's *Nina, ossia La Pazza per amore*, Sebastiano Nasolini's *Il Ritorno di Serse*, Boieldieu's *Jean de Paris* (in Italian), Carafa's *Gabriella di Vergy*, and Paër's *Eleonora*.

p. 65, ll. 16–17 "September 26, 1816" The cast of the first performance of *La Gazzetta* consisted of Margherita Chabrand (Lisetta), Francesca Cardini (Doralice), Maria(?) Manzi (Madama La Rosa), Alberico Curioni (Alberto), Carlo Casaccia (Storione), Felice Pellegrini (Filippo), Giovanni Pace (Anselmo), and Francesco Sparano (Monsù Traversen). Chabrand (spelled "Chambrand" in the first printed libretto of this opera) was a long-time favorite of the Neapolitan theaters. Cardini was a *comprimaria* at the San Carlo from about 1813 to 1832. Curioni (1790?–1860?—listed in this libretto as Alberigo Cozioni) was called the handsomest tenor in Italy; he became a favorite with composers, audiences, and critics. His career, taking him to most Italian opera houses and to many abroad, was of extraordinary duration: having made his debut early in the century, he was still singing at the San Carlo in 1855. Carlo Casaccia, member of a Neapolitan dynasty of comic singers and actors, was described vividly by Stendhal as he appeared in Pietro Carlo Guglielmi's *Paolo e Virginia* at the Teatro dei Fiorentini in

1817: "The good Domingo appears; it is the famous Casaccia, the Brunet of Naples, who speaks the people's jargon. He is enormous, a fact that gives him opportunity for considerable pleasant buffoonery. When seated, he undertakes to give himself an appearance of ease by crossing his legs; impossible; the effort that he goes through topples him onto his neighbor; a general collapse. This actor, commonly called Casacciello, is adored by the public; he has the nasal voice of a Capuchin. At this theater, everyone sings through his nose." Casaccia and his son Raffaele were to create roles in many of Donizetti's Neapolitan operas. Felice Pellegrini (1774–1832) had made his debut at Leghorn in 1795; at the Fiorentini from 1803 to 1818, he was listed as *primo buffo toscano assoluto*. He would be one of the leading interpreters of Rossinian roles at the Théâtre-Italien, Paris, in the 1820's. Giovanni Pace would create many roles in Donizetti's Naples operas. Francesco Sparano left no traces in operatic chronicles.

　　p. 65, l. 18 "*opera buffa*" Journalists referred to Rossini's new opera as *La Gazzetta, ossia Il Matrimonio per concorso*, or even just by its subtitle. The printed libretto carries neither the subtitle nor Tottola's name as reviser.

　　p. 65, l. 20 "Rossini's lifetime" *La Gazzetta* has received a few performances since World War II, and a noncommercial recording of it has had some circulation.

　　p. 65, l. 38 "of 1820, said:" *Italy* III, 278. Lady Morgan's text, with its erratic spelling, is quoted verbatim.

　　p. 66, l. 31 "of Naples" Antonio Canova (1757–1822) was the internationally renowned sculptor. Gabriele Rossetti (1783–1854), poet, critic, and patriot was the father of Dante Gabriel, William Michael, and Christina Rossetti. For Cesare delle Valle, Duca di Ventignano, librettist of Rossini's *Maometto II*, see p. 102 and note for that page. Melchiorre Delfico (1744–1835) wrote a once famous book on Roman jurisprudence; he was almost certainly a relative (grandfather?) of another Melchiorre Delfico, a caricaturist, librettist, and operatic composer whose caricatures of his friend Giuseppe Verdi are well known. Urbano Lampredi (1761–1838) carried on a long polemic battle with the poet Vincenzo Monti. I have been unable to identify Salvaggi. Luigi Blanc (Blanch—1784–1872) wrote on Neapolitan and military subjects. Cavaliere Antonio Micheroux was a diplomat and civil servant.

　　p. 67, l. 20 "*Moro di Venezia*" Some early editions of *Otello* give the subtitle as *L'Africano di Venezia*.

　　p. 67, l. 24 "December 4, 1816" The first cast of *Otello* was made up of Isabella Colbran (Desdemona), Maria(?) Manzi (Emilia), Andrea Nozzari (Otello), Michele Benedetti (Elmiro Barberigo), Giovanni David (Rodrigo), and Giuseppe Ciccimarra (Jago). The first printed libretto assigns the role of Jago to Ciccimarra, but its creation often is credited to Manuel Garcia. An undated Ricordi edition of *Otello* in my possession (perhaps reflecting the 1817 San Carlo cast) assigns Jago to Garcia, "*Un Gondoliere*" to Ciccimarra, and lists as unknown the singers of Emilia, Lucio, and the Doge. Michele Benedetti, a very popular bass, was also to create roles in *Armida, Mosè in Egitto, Ricciardo e Zoraide, Ermione, La Donna del lago,* and *Zelmira,* as well as in several of Donizetti's operas. Giuseppe Ciccimarra (or Cicimarra) would also be in the first casts of *Armida, Mosè in Egitto, Ricciardo e Zoraide, Ermione,* and *Maometto II.* Donizetti mentioned him as singing in Mayr's cantata *Atalia* under Rossini's direction at the San Carlo in March 1822.

p. 67, l. 29 "in 1817" The rebuilt San Carlo opened (January 13, 1817) with Mayr's *Il Sogno di Partenope;* five days later, *Otello* was sung there by the 1816 Fondo cast, except that Manuel Garcia now certainly was the Jago. *Otello* also was heard during the first season of the Teatro Carlo Felice, Genoa (spring 1828); the Rodrigo was the mezzo-soprano Brigida Lorenzani, who interpolated a cavatina composed for her by Bellini. Four years later, *Otello* provided Maria Malibran with her Neapolitan debut role (Teatro del Fondo, August 6, 1832), initiating a season during which she also was heard at the San Carlo in *Otello, Il Barbiere di Siviglia, La Gazza ladra,* and Vaccaj's *Giulietta e Romeo.*

p. 67, l. 38 "him well . . ." Translated from the French edition of 1956, p. 54.

p. 68, l. 2 "we read:" The passage from the 1826 edition is given as published in the English edition of 1959, translated by Richard N. Coe, p. 376.

p. 68, l. 24 "Pergolesi, *Orfeo*" Pergolesi's chamber cantata *Nel chiuso centro* was also known as *L'Orfeo.*

p. 68, ll. 31–2 "*tuo pensiero* . . .]" What Verdi thought of Rossini's *Otello* seventy years later is implied in a letter about his own *Otello* which he wrote to Boito on January 21, 1886: "They talk and they always write to me of *Jago*!!! . . . He is (it is true) the Demon who moves everything; but Otello is the one who acts: he loves, is jealous, kills, and commits suicide . . . For my part, it would seem to me hypocrisy not to call it *Otello.* I should prefer that they say *He has dared to struggle with the giant* [Rossini] *and has come out crushed* rather than *He wanted to hide under the title of Jago.* If you agree with me, let's begin, then, to baptize it *Otello.*"

p. 68, l. 35 "in Berlin" Translated by Sam Morgenstern from *Giacomo Meyerbeer: Briefwechsel und Tagebücher* I, ed. Heinz Becker, Berlin 1960, p. 359.

p. 69, l. 24 "of Italy" Rossini, writing from Naples on August 13, 1819, to Pietro Cartoni at the Argentina in Rome, said: "It remains understood that when I come to Rome, I'll bring you all the music of *Otello,* not to mention the adjustments, which are well along, and for which I shall be owed the sum of 150 zecchini d'oro [about $1,000], which you will turn over to me when I pass through, and precisely at the moment when I shall deliver all of the music to you." The "adjustments" included a new ending for the opera. In it, Desdemona calls out, as Otello raises his dagger to kill her: "Unhappy man, what are you doing? I am innocent!" Otello's reply is: "Innocent? But is that true?" And Desdemona asserts forcefully: "Yes. I swear it!" Convinced, Otello takes her by the hand to lead her downstage, where they sing the duet "*Cara, per te quest'anima,*" from *Armida,* after which the curtains close.

p. 70, l. 4 "mid-December" One of the liveliest and most attractive of the fabrications or multiple confusions that have infested biographies of Rossini concerns Stendhal's first meeting with him, Stendhal's account of which I translate here from the 1956 French edition of *Rome, Naples et Florence*, p. 35:

"At Terracina [we read under date of January 9, 1817], in the superb inn erected by Pius VI, it was suggested that we sup with the travelers arriving from Naples. I noticed among the seven or eight people a very handsome blond man, a little bald, of thirty or thirty-two years. I asked him for news of Naples, and above all about music. He answered me with clear-cut, brilliant ideas. I asked him if I could still have any hope of seeing Rossini's *Otello* at Naples; he smiled as he answered. I told him that in my eyes Rossini is the hope of the Italian school: he is the only man born with genius, and he bases his success, not on richness of accompaniments, but on the beauty of song. I noticed that my man seemed slightly embarrassed; his traveling companions smiled; in short, it was Rossini himself. Happily, and by the merest chance, I had not spoken of this fine genius's laziness.

"He tells me that Naples wants a different music from Rome, Rome a different music from Milan. They are so poorly paid! He must run ceaselessly from one end of Italy to the other, and the most beautiful opera does not earn him a thousand francs. He tells me that his *Otello* is only half successful, that he is on the way to Rome to do a *Cinderella*, and from there to Milan to recompose *The Thieving Magpie* at La Scala.

"This poor man of genius interests me, not that he is not very gay and rather happy—but what a pity that he does not find in this unhappy country a sovereign to give him a pension of two thousand écus and place him in a position to wait for the hour of inspiration for writing! [That Stendhal could imagine the twenty-four-year-old Rossini awaiting inspiration demonstrates his misunderstanding of his idol's musical nature.] How have the courage to reproach him for making an opera in fifteen days? He writes on a poor inn table in the noise from the kitchen and with clogged ink brought him in an old pomade jar. He is the Italian in whom I find the most intelligence, and certainly he cannot doubt it: for in this country the reign of the pedants still endures. I told him of my enthusiasm for *L'Italiana in Algeri*; I asked him whether he loved *L'Italiana* or *Tancredi* the more; he answered *Il Matrimonio segreto*. This was charming: for *The Secret Marriage* is as completely forgotten as, in Paris, Marmontel's tragedies. Why does he not receive royalties from the troupes that perform his thirty operas? He shows me that such a thing cannot even be proposed in the era's disorder.

"We stayed drinking tea until past midnight: it was the most delightful of my Italian evenings, as his is the gaiety of a happy man. Finally I parted from the great composer with a feeling of melancholy. Canova and he— there you have, thanks to those who govern, everything that the land of genius now possesses. I repeat to myself, with a sad joy, Falstaff's exclamation: 'There live not three great men in England; and one of them is poor and grows old'—*King Henry IV, Part I*, Act 2, Scene 4."

But Rossini was not in Terracina en route from Naples to Rome on

January 9, 1817; he had reached Rome in mid-December, certainly some days before December 23, to busy himself with preparations for the new *opera buffa*, the subject of which he did not know until after reaching Rome, and which was staged there on January 25, 1817. Nor was Stendhal in Terracina on January 9, 1817; actually, the two men met for the first time in Milan late in 1819. Nor had Rossini composed thirty operas: *La Cenerentola* would be his twentieth. Nor did Stendhal quote Shakespeare correctly (this probably was deliberate): what Falstaff says is: "There live not three good men unhanged in England; and one of them is fat, and grows old." In the second (1826) version of *Rome, Naples et Florence*, moreover, the details of the Terracina anecdote are very different. The entry is now dated February 7, 1817—by which date Rossini could not possibly have been en route from Naples to Rome to produce *La Cenerentola*, which was staged there on January 25. Rossini now is described as looking twenty-five or twenty-six rather than thirty or thirty-two; he is accused of extensive plagiarism as well as of laziness; the amount that his "noblest opera" could not earn him is now two thousand francs; the writer whose tragedies had been forgotten in Paris is Jean-François Ducis; and the number of operas upon which Rossini is not collecting royalties is "about twenty." The anecdote is as fictional as *Le Rouge et le noir*.

p. 70, ll. 12–13 "late delivery"   A clause in this contract refers for the first time to the possibility of Rossini's composing an opera for London. He did not reach London until 1823—and he never completed an opera there.

p. 70, l. 15 "Jacopo Ferretti"   *Un Poeta melodrammatico romano: Appunti e notizie in gran parte inedite sopra Jacopo Ferretti e i musicisti del suo tempo, con ritratti e fac-simili*, Milan, n. d. (but 1898).

p. 70, l. 31 "upon me"   See p. 53 for the rejection of a subject suggested, and in part treated, by Ferretti, only to be discarded in favor of Sterbini's *Il Barbiere di Siviglia*.

p. 71, l. 3 "Alighieri's Farinata"   Farinata Degli Uberti, a leader of the Ghibelline party in Florence, rises suddenly and unexpectedly (*Inferno*, Canto X, verse 31) when Dante asks Vergil if he may talk with one of the heretics: "*Ed ei mi disse: Volgiti: che fai?/Vedi là Farinata che s'è dritto:/ Dalla cintola in su tutto il vedrai . . .*"

p. 71, l. 14 "La Cenerentola"   In a note printed in the first libretto of *La Cenerentola*, Ferretti stated that the supernatural element had been eliminated from the story because of a "necessity of the Teatro Valle's stage." However, Rossini's dislike of magic in a libretto was well known.

p. 71, l. 28 "by Rossini"   Agolini's contributions to the score actually were limited to two *arie del sorbetto*—one beginning "*Vasto teatro è il mondo*" and sung by Alidoro disguised as a pilgrim in Act I, Scene 7, and one sung by Clorinda in Act II, Scene 9, "*Sventurata! mi credea*"—and an introductory chorus to the second act, "*Ah! della bella incognita.*" When *La Cenerentola* was staged in Rome for the fourth time (Carnival season, 1820–21), Rossini replaced Agolini's "*Vasto teatro è il mondo*" with an aria of his own to new lines by Ferretti; this aria for Alidoro was lost until Cametti found a copy of it among manuscripts at the Accademia di Santa Cecilia, Rome. Ricordi published it in piano-vocal score in 1917; the autograph is in the Conservatorio G. Rossini, Pesaro. Most modern performances of *La Cenerentola* avoid the problem by omitting to have Alidoro sing any aria whatever.

p. 72, *l. 1* "*più felice*" In present-day performances of *Il Barbiere di Siviglia*, "*Ah! il più lieto*" commonly is dispensed with; the second *finaletto*, "*Da sì felice innesto*," is made to serve in its place.

p. 72, *l. 13* "his journal" Louis Spohr's *Selbstbiographie*, 2 vols., Kassel, 1860–1.

p. 72, *l. 32* "Mario Rinaldi" *Felice Romani: Dal melodramma classico al melodramma romantico*, Rome, 1965.

p. 73, *l. 5* "Vitarelli [Alidoro]" The basso buffo Andrea Verni, who sang at La Scala from about 1800 to 1816, was described by Giuseppe Carpani as more distinguished for his natural, vivacious acting than for his singing, Giuseppe De Begnis (1793–1849), a *buffo comico*, had made his debut at Modena in 1813 in Pavesi's *Ser Marcantonio*. He and his French wife, the famous Giuseppina (Claudine) Ronzi, were to be more important to Donizetti than to Rossini. After having directed opera in Bath and Dublin, De Begnis was to die in New York. Giacomo Guglielmi, eighth son of the composer Pietro Alessandro Guglielmi, had made his debut at Rome in about 1803 and had sung in Paris in 1809; he was described as having a weak, seductive voice. Caterina Rossi and Teresa Mariani were *comprimarie*; Rossi later sang in Paris.

p. 73, *l. 24* "*Qui pro quo*" Spohr, who heard Romani's opera at the Teatro Valle with Meyerbeer in 1816, reported that it contained so many borrowed ideas that the audience several times called out: "*Bravo, Rossini!*"

p. 73, *l. 39* "*prime donne*" Before 1817 ran out, *La Cenerentola* was staged in Genoa (with Righetti-Giorgi again much applauded); at La Scala, Milan (with Francesca Maffei-Festa in the title role, Filippo Galli as Don Magnifico) for forty-four performances; and in five other Italian cities. Numerous productions of it followed, both in Italy and abroad. Before Rossini's death in 1868, this opera would have been sung in Italian, English, German, Russian, Polish, French, and Czech. On February 12, 1844, in English, it became the first opera to be staged in Australia. Its popularity diminished after 1895, but rose again after the title role was sung at Turin in 1921–2 by Conchita Supervia. Since World War II, it has been staged often; it has been recorded more than once. Giulietta Simionato sang its title role at Pesaro on the 164th anniversary of Rossini's birth there (February 29, 1956).

p. 74, *l. 17* "was over" Rossini composed two more comic operas. But *Adina* was written for Lisbon and *Le Comte Ory* was composed to a French libretto for performance at the Paris Opéra. In one sense, *Il Viaggio a Reims*, also composed for Paris, almost might be called comic.

p. 75, *l. 15* "Giovanni Gherardini" Gherardini (1778–1861) was a

Milanese lawyer, philologist, and lexicographer; his most noted publication was a *Supplemento al vocabolario italiano.*

p. 75, l. 30   "May 31, 1817"   In the cast of the *première* of *La Gazza ladra* were Teresa Giorgi-Belloc (Ninetta), Teresa Gallianis (Pippo), Marietta Castiglioni (Lucia), Savino Monelli (Giannetto), Vincenzo Botticelli (Fabrizio Vingradito), Filippo Galli (Fernando Villabella), Antonio Ambrosi (Gottardo, the *podestà*), Francesco Biscottini (Isacco), Paolo Rossignoli (Giorgio), and Alessandro De Angeli (Ernesto). Teresa Gallianis sang numerous contralto roles at La Scala in 1817–18. Marietta Castiglioni left no traces in operatic annals. Savino Monelli, tenor brother of the more famous Raffaele, was noted for his good looks; he would create a role in Rossini's *Adelaide di Borgogna.* Antonio Ambrosi (often written Ambrogi), who acquired the sobriquet "*Podestà*" from his role in *La Gazza ladra*, later created roles for Rossini in *Adelaide di Borgogna*, *Zelmira*, and *Matilde Shabran.* Biscottini would have a minor role in the first performance of Rossini's *Bianca e Falliero.* Alessandro De Angeli would be the first Doge Priulì in *Bianca e Falliero.*

p. 76, ll. 2–3   "La Scala"   The libretto for the La Scala revival of *La Gazza ladra* on April 22, 1820, carried this note: "Various changes have been made in the present *melodramma.* The author had no part in them." When it was staged there again on March 3, 1823, the libretto said: "Fernando's aria in Scene 5 of Act II has been expressly composed by Maestro Rossini himself in Naples." By the end of 1829, *La Gazza ladra* had been heard 139 times at La Scala.

p. 77, l. 14   "someone else"   Giulio Confalonieri wrote (*Enciclopedia dello Spettacolo* VIII, column 1240): "The story of the girl unjustly accused together with her father, but then completely exculpated, will find an echo in Bellini's *La Sonnambula* and, in certain pathetic connections between father and daughter, also in some episodes of Verdi's *Rigoletto.*"

NOTES TO CHAPTER VI

p. 80, l. 10   "faulty text"   Librettos based upon the Rinaldo-Armida encounter and other episodes from *Gerusalemme liberata* were spaced out from that for Benedetto Ferrari's *Armida* of 1639 to that of Dvořák's *Armida* (1904). Wagner was remembering Armida when he wrote the section of his *Parsifal* poem which deals with Kundry and her Magic Garden.

p. 80, l. 15   "November 11, 1817"   The cast of the *première* of *Armida* consisted of Isabella Colbran (Armida), Andrea Nozzari (Rinaldo), Giuseppe Ciccimarra (Goffredo), Michele Benedetti (Idraste), Claudio Bonoldi (Gerando and Ubaldo), and Gaetano Chizzola (Eustazio, Carlo, and Astarotte).

p. 81, l. 29   "the San Carlo"   One of the early compositions of Franz Liszt, done when he was twelve or thirteen, was an *Impromptu brillant pour le Piano-Forte, sur des Thèmes de Rossini & Spontini . . . Opéra 3.* The Rossini themes are from the *Armida* first-act duet "*Amor! Possente nome*" and from the finale of Act I of *La Donna del lago*. Lizst later derived the openings both of No. 7 of his *Grandes Études* and of the "*Eroica*" (No. 7) of his *Études d'exécution transcendante* from the first measures of this early *Impromptu brillant*.

p. 81, l. 40   "(December 27)"   In the first cast of *Adelaide di Borgogna* were Elizabetta Manfredini-Guarmani (Adelaide), Elizabetta Pinotti (Ottone), Anna Maria Muratori (Eurice), Luisa Bottesi (Iroldo), Savino Monelli (Adalberto), Antonio Ambrosi (Berengario), and Giovanni Puglieschi (Ernesto). Alberto Cametti wrote of Elisabetta Pinotti: "The role of Ottone, by one of those strange customs of the time, was sustained by a woman; it was the contralto part, also called that of the *primo musico*, a denomination that explains itself when we think that the contralto *donna* had taken the place of the elephant songbirds [*castrati*] of the seventeen-hundreds . . . The part was interpreted by one of the two Pinotti sisters, Elisabetta, of the robust, wide-ranged voice, who was a little unsteady. The part that Rossini wrote for her rises from a deep B to the high F, and a few times pushes from the deep G to the high B-flat." Anna Maria Muratori was a *comprimaria*. Luisa Bottesi cannot be otherwise identified. Many writers—and the libretto issued for the first performances of *Adelaide di Borgogna*—list the role of Berengario as being sung by Gioacchino Sciarpelletti, a bass who sang chiefly at Rome. On December 27, 1817, however, Principe Chigi-Albani noted in his diary: "The theaters opened this evening. Argentina: the *dramma* is *Adelaide di Borgogna*, music by Rossini. . . . Everything turned out rather badly except a third, added [singer, a] *buffo* named Ambrogi [Ambrosi], who found favor instead." Ambrosi, then, apparently replaced Sciarpelletti at a late hour. Giovanni Puglieschi, a tenor, would create the role of Pippetto in Donizetti's *L'Ajo nell'imbarazzo* (1824).

p. 82, l. 11   "Michele Carafa"   Michele Enrico Carafa, Principe di Colobrano (1787–1872), a Neapolitan noble, had served Napoleon's government in Italy and had been an aide to Murat in 1806. After the Bonapartist collapse, he devoted his energy to music, eventually composing—among church pieces, Masses, cantatas, and ballets—some thirty operas, the most popular of which were *Gabriella di Vergy* (1816) and *Masaniello* (1817). The latter ran up 136 permormances at the Paris Opéra despite the production there, during its run, of Auber's very successful opera on the same subject, *La Muette de Portici*. Carafa's willing assistance to Rossini on this and other occasions would be handsomely repaid at the time of the 1860 production of *Semiramide* in Paris (see p. 281).

p. 82, l. 22   "in recitative)"   The printed libretto indicates an aria ("*Si, mi svena, o figlio ingrato*," Act II, Scene 6) for one of them, but this was omitted from the piano score published by Ricordi.

p. 82, l. 23   "December 27, 1817"   It shared a double bill with *La Morte di Ciro* (also called *Ciro e Tomiri*) to music by Rossini and others. Curious errors were to be committed with regard to *Adelaide di Borgogna*. Zanolini (*ZAN*) spoke of "*Ottone, re d'Italia*" and *Adelaide* as if they were separate operas. Stendhal cited "*O crude stelle*" as the finest piece in the opera, though the phrase occurs neither in the printed libretto nor in the score. The opera seems to have been obliterated from sight and sound after a staging at Leghorn in 1825 except as nine of its numbers were borrowed by Rossini for *Eduardo e Cristina* (see pp. 91–2).

p. 82, l. 34   "advanced disrepair"   The Teatro del Sole dated from 1637. In 1655, it had been the scene of an elaborate spectacle to honor a visit to Pesaro by Queen Christina of Sweden. The first Rossini opera sung there had been *Tancredi* (Carnival 1815). During the 1816 Carnival, the Sole housed two Rossini operas: *L'Inganno felice* and *L'Italiana in Algeri*. It was replaced in 1818 by the Teatro Nuovo (later Rossini).

p. 83, l. 28   "Signor Panziere"   This was almost certainly the dancer-choreographer Lorenzo Panzieri, long active at La Scala.

p. 83, ll. 34–5   "Leone Tottola"   Tottola, often called "the Abbé Tottola," was a full match for the inept Foppa and Schmidt. Raffaele D'Ambra described him as "an illustrious upholder of the most corrupt taste"; in 1881, P. Raffaeli, pouncing joyfully upon a rhyme, wrote:

> "*Fu di libretti autor, chiamossi Tottola;*
> *Un'aquila non era, anzi fu nottola.*"
> ("He was the author of librettos; he was called Tottola;
> An eagle he wasn't; he was, in fact, a screech-owl.")

Tottola had revised a Palomba libretto for Rossini's *La Gazzetta* (1816); he also wrote for Rossini's use, besides *Mosè in Egitto*, the librettos of *Ermione*, *La Donna del lago*, and *Zelmira*—and was one of the collaborating authors of that for *Eduardo e Cristina*. He had begun his writing career in 1796; he was to end it in 1831 after having turned out dozens of librettos, for each of which he was said to have been paid sixty lire (less than $30).

p. 83, l. 36   "Francesco Ringhieri"   Ringhieri (1721–87), an Olivetan monk, from 1746 on wrote poetic tragedies and *azioni sacre* that won acceptance from the public but were deprecated by critics because of the lurid liberties that he took with Biblical and other sanctified sources.

p. 84, l. 8   "March 5, 1818"   The first cast of *Mosè in Egitto* was made up of Isabella Colbran (Elcia), Frederike Funk (Amaltea), Maria(?) Manzi (Amenofi), Michele Benedetti (Mosè), Andrea Nozzari (Osiride), Giuseppe Ciccimarra (Aronne), Raniero Remorini (Faraone), and Gaetano Chizzola (Mambre). Frederike Funk was on leave from the Dresden Hofoper, where she sang leading soprano roles—including Rossini's Desdemona, Elisabetta, and Zoraide—up to 1826.

p. 85, l. 2   "Morlacchi's example?"   Morlacchi later became, at Dresden, director of Italian opera for the King of Saxony, as which he was to be the *bête noire* of the King's director of German opera, Carl Maria von Weber, like Rossini a "radical" subjected to bombast from the right.

p. 85, l. 16   "the anti-Rossinians"   The *Notizie del giorno* (Rome) had reported the opening of the Teatro Valle's spring season with Generali's "twin farces," *Adelina* and *Cecchina*: "Both of them offer many musical beauties, in which have been recognized some feathers from the celebrated bird of ill omen"—that is, Rossini.

p. 85, l. 17 "Lady Morgan" *Italy* III, 287. The quotation is verbatim.

p. 87, l. 26 "100; *Musico*" The *musico* (a castrato; also, later, a female singer of male roles) in this case was Anna Ferri. But, misinterpreting the word to mean "musician," Tommaso Casini and some writers who have consulted him have said that Rossini himself was the one to receive only 150 scudi.

p. 88, l. 4 "Vanzolini related" *Della vera patria di Gioacchino Rossini*, p. 29.

p. 88, l. 24 "his father" After the death of George III in 1820, Caroline returned to London, hoping to re-establish her relationship with her cousin-husband George IV—and thus achieve recognition as queen. Instead, she was tried for adultery with Bergami, with whom she was said to have been seen "sleeping on deck under an awning." The trial was broken off, however. Caroline tried to force her way into Westminster Abbey to participate in her husband's coronation in 1821, but was prevented from entering. She died a few weeks later.

p. 89, l. 23 "quoted intact" On September 16, 1800, Boieldieu's opera *Le Calife de Bagdad*, with a libretto by Claude Godard d'Aucour de Saint-Just, was heard at the Opéra-Comique, Paris, thus initiating a long stay on French and other stages. Using Andrea Leone Tottola's Italian version of its French text, Manuel Garcia composed *Il Califfo di Bagdad*, which had its *première* at the Teatro del Fondo, Naples, on September 30, 1813, and proved to be the most popular of the famous tenor's operas.

p. 89, l. 27 "June 22, 1826" See p. 150 for the first staging of *Adina*.

p. 89, l. 28 "A letter" Translated by Sam Morgenstern from *Giacomo Meyerbeer: Briefwechsel und Tagebücher* I, ed. Heinz Becker, Berlin, 1960, p. 360.

p. 89, l. 33 "the Catalanis" Angelica Catalani and her husband, Paul Valabrègue, had been directors of the Théâtre-Italien, Paris, for a brief period during 1814-15.

p. 90, l. 16 "Niccolò Forteguerri" Forteguerri (1674-1735) was an Arcadian priest-poet. His *Ricciardetto*, in thirty cantos, is a satirical attack on the profligacy of the clergy.

p. 90, ll. 17-18 "December 3, 1818" The first cast of *Ricciardo e Zoraide* was made up of Isabella Colbran (Zoraide), Benedetta Rosmunda Pisaroni-Carrara (Zomira), Maria(?) Manzi (Fatima), Raffaela De Bernardis (Elmira), Giovanni David (Ricciardo), Andrea Nozzari (Agorante), Michele Benedetti (Ircano), and Giuseppe Ciccimarra (Ernesto). Pisaroni (1793-1872), whose name is spelled Pesaroni in the 1818 San Carlo libretto (as often elsewhere), had made her debut at Bergamo in 1811 in Mayr's *La Rosa bianca e la rosa rossa*. Two years later, despite her notorious ugliness—which resulted in part from a disfiguring smallpox—she was considered one of the finest contraltos in serious roles. Raffaela De Bernardis sang many secondary roles in the Neapolitan theaters.

p. 90, l. 32 "an illness" Confusion impossible to dissipate has been caused by references to this and another cantata that Rossini prepared some months later. One or both of them is referred to as *Partenope*, as *Igea*, and as *Partenope ed Igea*. A manuscript of the cantata sung on February 20, 1819, is in the library of San Pietro a Maiella at Naples; it consists of fifty-two pages without a title, being headed only *"Cantata con cori—1818."* That date indicates that Rossini probably had composed it right after the première of *Ricciardo e Zoraide*. In 1960, a manuscript of twenty-six folios was found in the library of the Conservatoire de Musique, Paris; it is marked *"Cantata in occasione della ricuperata salute di S. Maestà Ferdinando 1° Re delle Due Sicilie . . . nel 1818."*

The gala performance of the cantata on February 20, 1819, was staged under the guidance of the court architect, Antonio Niccolini, who also had supplied the scenario. The evening consisted of a ballet called *Gerusalemme liberata*, the first act of *Ricciardo e Zoraide*, and the cantata. Interpolated dances were choreographed by Philippe Taglioni, father of the famous Marie, to a set of Rossini variations; these were performed by all of the San Carlo's leading dancers. The orchestra had been supplemented by a band of 120 instrumentalists directed on the stage by Luigi Calegari. The solo part in the cantata was sung by Isabella Colbran. Rossini had expended no real creative effort on his part in all this: he merely had responded to Barbaja's wishes and had been respectful toward the King.

p. 91, l. 2 "different story" *Vie de Rossini* (Martineau edition, 1929) II, 106.

p. 91, l. 9 "Louis Engel" *From Mozart to Mario*, 2 vols., London, 1886, II, 72.

p. 92, l. 3 "March 27, 1819" The first cast of *Ermione* was made up of Isabella Colbran (Ermione), Rosmunda Pisaroni (Andromaca), Maria(?) Manzi (Cleone), De Bernardis *minore* (Cefiso), Andrea Nozzari (Pirro), Giovanni David (Oreste), Michele Benedetti (Fenicio), Giuseppe Ciccimarra (Pilade), and Gaetano Chizzola (Attalo). "A Pupil of the Royal School of Dance" had the role of Astianatte. De Bernardis *minore* seems to have been a daughter of Raffaela De Bernardis.

p. 92, l. 18 "of Byron:" In an unpublished article of which Professor Marchand kindly lent me a copy; an altered version of the article ("Byron and Rossini") later was published in *Opera News*, New York (March 31, 1965).

p. 92, l. 28 "years later" In *La Vie de Lord Byron en Italie*, a manuscript surviving among the Gamba Papers in the Biblioteca Classense, Ravenna; quoted in Marchand: *Byron: A Biography*, New York, 1957, II, 781.

p. 93, l. 1 "Naples, 1810)" The 1819 Venice libretto for *Eduardo e Cristina*, so spelled, reads: *"Dramma per musica in due atti di T. S. B.,"* the initials standing for Tottola, Schmidt, Bevilacqua-Aldobrandini.

p. 93, l. 9 "its cast" The cast of the *première* of *Eduardo e Cristina* was made up of Rosa Morandi (Cristina), Carolina Cortesi (Eduardo), Eliodoro Bianchi (Carlo, re di Svezia), Luciano Bianchi (Giacomo, principe di Scozia), and Vincenzo Fracalini (Atlei). Nothing further is known of Cortesi. Fracalini (or Fraccalini, or even Fracabini) was singing at Bergamo in 1819 and 1820; he seems to have remained a *comprimario*.

p. 93, l. 15 "on June 25" *Edoardo e Cristina*—now so spelled—was transferred to La Fenice in 1820, during which year it also was staged in many cities in Italy and abroad. For obvious reasons, it was not produced in Naples, but it reached La Scala, Milan (with Caroline Unger as Edoardo), on January 26, 1828. Few if any stagings of it were undertaken after 1840.

p. 94, ll. 17–18 "in Rome" Conte Cassi's letter is quoted in full in *BdPCR* 3, 3/17/1892, 17.

p. 95, l. 20 "this theater" *BdPCR*, 3/17/1892, 19.

p. 95, l. 30 "the Academy" Some months later, the academicians authorized Conte Perticari to order the bust of Rossini. He selected the sculptor Adamo Tadolini (1792–1868), a pupil of Canova, who was to be paid 100 scudi (about $315) for his work. Because Tadolini lived in Rome, he waited to complete the bust until Rossini could sit for him there in March 1820 (see p. 99).

p. 96, l. 6 "under Cherubini" Batton became a teacher of singing after achieving some success with operas of his own and as co-composer with nine other men (including Auber, Boieldieu, Carafa, Cherubini, Hérold, and Paër) of *La Marquise de Brinvilliers* (1831), to a libretto by Scribe and Castil-Blaze dealing with the seventeenth-century specialist in poisoning.

p. 96, l. 20 "right away" Translated from *RAD* I, 376.

p. 96, l. 21 "the Channel" From Rossini's *La Donna del lago* (1819) to Alick McLean's *Quentin Durward* (published in 1894, produced in 1920), some twenty operas were composed to Scott-derived librettos. They included Boieldieu's *La Dame blanche*, Donizetti's *Elisabetta al castello di Kenilworth* and *Lucia di Lammermoor*, Bizet's *La Jolie Fille de Perth*, and Sir Arthur Sullivan's *Ivanhoe*. The fact that the full title of Bellini's last opera was *I Puritani di Scozia* unquestionably reflected Scott's ability to convince Continental Europeans that his native land was a wildly romantic place.

p. 96, l. 33 "September 24, 1819" The first cast of *La Donna del lago* consisted of Isabella Colbran (Elena), Rosmunda Pisaroni (Malcolm Groeme—so spelled in the first printed libretto, though "Graeme" elsewhere), Maria(?) Manzi (Albina), Giovanni David (Giacomo V, re di Scozia, alias Cavaliere Uberto), Andrea Nozzari (Rodrigo di Dhu), Michele Benedetti (Douglas d'Angus), Gaetano Chizzola (Serano), and Massimo Orlandini (Bertram). Orlandini, a bass who would also create a role in Rossini's *Zelmira*, sang at the San Carlo intermittently between 1819 and 1826; his brother Antonio was a tenor.

p. 96, l. 38 "untrue. Azevedo" *AZ*, 155.

p. 98, l. 12 "used before" The overture consists of a new *allegro vivace*; an andante borrowed from *Edoardo e Cristina* (for which it had been refashioned from *Ricciardo e Zoraide*); a melody from the first duet in *La Donna del lago*; and a crescendo from the overture to *Edoardo e Cristina*. In reverse, the new *allegro vivace* would turn up again, transposed from D

major to C, as the first twenty-eight measures of the superior overture to
Le Siège de Corinthe; the introductory chorus of Act I *("Viva Fallier'!")*
would reappear in the introductory scene of *Moïse et Pharaon.*

p. 98, ll. 14–15 "December 26, 1819;" The cast of the *première* of
Bianca e Falliero was made up of Violante Camporesi (Bianca), Carolina
Bassi (Falliero), Adelaide Chinzani, or Ghinzani (Costanza), Claudio Bonoldi
(Contareno), Alessandro De Angeli (Friulì, doge di Venezia), Giuseppe
Fioravanti, a son of the composer Valentino Fioravanti (Capellio), and
Francesco Biscottini (Un Concellerie—so listed in the first printed libretto).
Camporesi (1785–1839) was a prominent Roman soprano; she had sung
privately for Napoleon and was very popular at the King's Theatre, London.
Carolina Bassi-Manna, a Neapolitan contralto, had made her debut at Naples
in 1798; she retired about 1830. Adelaide Chinzani or Ghinzani appears to
have made little impression upon her contemporaries.

NOTES TO CHAPTER VII

p. 100, l. 13 "to Raimondi" Raimondi's skill as a contrapuntalist
led him to fantastic displays of ingenuity, culminating in his *Giuseppe,* sung
at the Teatro Argentina, Rome, on August 7, 1852, one year before his death.
Giuseppe consisted of three "lyric dramas"—*Putifar, Giacobbe,* and *Giuseppe*
—sung seriatim and then simultaneously by soloists and a chorus of 250
singers, with instrumental support from 150 players. In a letter from Paris
dated October 7, 1861, Rossini urged Michele Costa to get *Giuseppe* performed and published in London for the benefit of Raimondi's destitute
children; he reported that its success at Rome had been "colossal."

p. 100, ll. 23–4 "1820, wrote" Quoted in Johann Amadeus Wendt's
Rossini's Leben und Treiben. Miltitz (1781–1845), a composer of operas
and religious music, contributed articles on musical subjects to several German publications. They were assembled in his *Oranienblätter,* 3 volumes,
1822–5.

p. 102, l. 6 "is possible" Tadolini did not carry out this commission.
A monument elaborating Rossini's rough sketches was placed in the Certosa
at Bologna, but it was the work of a Carraran sculptor named Del Rosso.

p. 102, l. 12 "Duca di Ventignano" The Duca di Ventignano was
reputed to be a powerful *jettatore,* or wielder of the evil eye. Because of that
reputation, the superstitious Rossini was reported, while composing the duke's
libretto for *Maometto II,* to have formed horns with the index and little
fingers of his left hand, a gesture effective in warding off such black magic.
Of Rossini's superstitions, Radiciotti wrote: "Nor was this the only super-
stition that Rossini had. A calamity if at table he saw a salt cellar or oil
cruet overturned! A calamity if a mirror was shattered into fragments! If
possible, he began nothing on Friday or the 13th of a month. And to think
that he died precisely on Friday, November 13!"

p. 103, l. 23 "December 3, 1820" The cast of the *première* of *Maometto II* was made up of Isabella Colbran (Anna), Adelaide Comelli (Calbo),

Andrea Nozzari (Paolo Erisso), Filippo Galli (Maometto II), Giuseppe Ciccimarra (Condulmiero), and Gaetano Chizzola (Selimo). Adelaide—or Adele—Chaumel, called "Comelli" in Italy, recently had married Giovanni Battista Rubini (she later was billed as Comelli-Rubini). She is sometimes said to have been a page in the *première* of Rossini's *Elisabetta, regina d'Inghilterra.*

p. 104, l. 2 "in 1826"   Much of the very great popularity of *Le Siège de Corinthe* was to result from the very numbers that had been insufficient to make the fortune of *Maometto II* in Italy in 1820–1—and which Italian operagoers were to appreciate only when hearing them, from 1828 on, in *L'Assedio di Corinto*, the Italian version of *Le Siège*. And yet, *Maometto II* did not require Rossini to send his mother another drawing of a *fiasco*.

p. 104, l. 17 "that season"   Mercadante's *Scipione in Cartagine* at the Teatro Argentina and Filippo Grazioli's *Il Pellegrino bianco* at the Apollo.

p. 104, ll. 23–4 "*Matilde Shabran*"   *Matilde Shabran* was the original title of Rossini's opera, as is proved by both the 1821 Rome libretto and that printed in Milan in 1822. Only later did it acquire the particule *di*, becoming *Matilde di Shabran* or *Shabrand* or even *Chabran* in later librettos.

p. 104, l. 34 "[Luigi] Vestri"   Vestri (1781–1841), considered the foremost Italian actor of his era, had been engaged by Giovanni Torlonia, duca di Bracciano, owner of the Teatro Valle, to bring his company to the theater for three weeks. In view of the resulting success, Vestri himself formed two acting troupes at Rome and became impresario of the Valle, with Torlonia remaining in control. The results were disastrous: Vestri lost all his money and had to pledge future earnings to pay off the large debts he had incurred.

p. 105, l. 2 "earlier operas"   For the overture to *Matilde Shabran*, Rossini used the one that he had prepared the preceding year for *Edoardo e Cristina*, which in turn had included a mélange of motives from the overtures to *Ricciardo e Zoraide* (1818) and *Ermione* (1819). From *Ricciardo*, he also borrowed (for Ferretti's lines beginning "*Anima mia, Matilde*") the opening of a soprano-contralto duet; from it, too, he took a soldier's chorus, using it for a chorus beginning "*Che ne dite? Pare un sogno.*" He also had Ferretti supply a text—to music that he already had composed—for the beginning of a duet for the two chief protagonists of *Matilde Shabran*.

p. 105, l. 2 "Giovanni Pacini"   Pacini (1796–1867), like Vincenzo Bellini a Sicilian from Catania, had studied, like Rossini and Donizetti, at the Bolognia Liceo under Padre Stanislao Mattei. He brought out his first opera, *Annetta e Lucinda*, at Vienna in 1813, and thereafter composed more than forty operas in twenty-two years. When the last of them was poorly received, he opened a music school; treatises that he wrote while teaching long remained in use. He returned to opera in 1838, composing forty more stage pieces. He also wrote large amounts of nonoperatic music. When his lively, unreliable autobiography, *Le Mie Memorie artistiche*, was published in Florence (1865), it had been revised and extended by others. A son of the noted *basso buffo* (and onetime tenor and baritone) Luigi Pacini, Giovanni Pacini in turn was the father of Émilien Pacini, poet and librettist. The Paris music-publisher Antonio Pacini was not a member of this family.

p. 105, ll. 5–6 "Francesco Regli"   In his *Dizionario biografico*.

p. 105, l. 11 "the Tordinona"   The Teatro Apollo had formerly been the Teatro Torre di Nona or Tordinona.

p. 105, l. 12 "Duke Torlonia"   Giovanni Torlonia, duca di Bracciano, owned the Teatro Apollo.

p. 105, l. 16 "to work"   Ferretti wrote: "Nor did Pacini's notes find less good fortune than those of the Pesarese Orpheus. The proof is that no one who did not know this story ever suspected anything." According to *LGMM* 2/29/1892, "Rossini later remade all the pieces of which he was not the author, and the score reproduced and given to the printer bore no traces of this practical collaboration."

p. 105, ll. 21–2 "February 24, 1821"   The cast of the *première of Matilde Shabran* was made up of Caterina Lipparini (Matilde), Annetta Parlamagni (Edoardo), Luigia Cruciati (Contessa d'Arco), Giuseppe Fusconi (Corradino), Giuseppe Fioravanti (Aliprando), Antonio Parlamagni (Isidoro), Antonio Ambrosi (Ginardo), Gaetano Rambaldi (Egoldo and Rodrigo), and Carlo Moncada (Raimondo). Lipparini (or Liparini) was a very high soprano; she would create a role in Donizetti's *Otto Mese in due ore* (Naples, 1827). Annetta (Anna) Parlamagni would be singing in *Il Barbiere di Siviglia* at Siena as late as 1835. She was a daughter of Antonio Parlamagni, the Neapolitan *buffo* who had been the first Macrobio in *La Pietra del paragone* (1812). Luigia Cruciati is not otherwise identifiable. Giuseppe Fusconi, a lyric tenor, sang in many Italian theaters; his known repertoire includes only Rossinian roles except for Don Ottavio in *Don Giovanni*. Carlo Moncada is listed in the 1821 Rome libretto of *Matilde Shabran*; Luigi Rognoni, however, assigns this role to the tenor Gioacchino Moncada, apparently repeating an error in *RAD* (I, 271).

p. 107, l. 30 "Pacini wrote"   *Le Mie Memorie artistiche*, p. 21.

p. 107, l. 36 "Pellegrino bianco"   By Filippo Grazioli, who also composed *I Taglialegna di Dombar* (Rome, 1828). *Il Pellegrino bianco* had not been a success.

p. 108, l. 6 "also reported"   *Le Mie Memorie artistiche*, p. 24.

p. 108, l. 12 "d'Azeglio wrote:"   *I Miei Ricordi* II, p. 146.

p. 108 l. 22 "to music"   The text of this "blind men's song" was published in facsimile by Gino Monaldi in *Noi e il mondo* (August 1925). The verse runs to fourteen lines; the music opens with a theme that Rossini had used in *Ricciardo e Zoraide*.

p. 109, l. 37 "del Lago"   The writer was misinformed: the plan was to present in Vienna not *La Donna del lago*, but the still-unperformed *Zelmira*.

p. 110, l. 10–11 "the nobility"   The soloists in the first performance of *La Riconoscenza* were Adelaide Comelli-Rubini (Argene), Girolama Dardanelli (Melania), Giovanni Battista Rubini (Fileno), and Michele Benedetti (Elpino).

p. 111, l. 14 "February 16, 1822" The singers in the *première* of *Zelmira* were Isabella Colbran (Zelmira), Anna Maria Cecconi (Emma), Antonio Ambrosi (Polidoro), Giovanni David (Ilo), Andrea Nozzari (Antenore), Michele Benedetti (Leucippo), Gaetano Chizzola (Eacide), and Massimo Orlandini (Gran Sacerdote). Cecconi, a contralto, was the mother of Barbaja's son Pietro.

p. 112, l. 12 "really is" Guido Zavadini: *Donizetti,* p. 231.

p. 112, l. 29 "at Castenaso" Giovanni Colbran had bought the Castenaso villa in 1812; by the time of his death in 1820, it had become Isabella's property. When I visited Castenaso in May 1966, the villa was a ruin.

p. 113, l. 16 "the Maestro" Stendhal: *Correspondance* II, p. 164.

Notes to Chapter VIII

p. 115, l. 3 "of *Zelmira*" The Vienna cast was that of the Naples *première* except that Fanny Eckerlin sang Emma and Vincenzo Botticelli was the Leucippo. Eckerlin had created a role in Donizetti's first publicly performed opera, *Enrico di Borgogna* (Venice, 1818).

p. 115, l. 6 "Vienna theater" Of the Kärnthnertortheater, Rossini, like Colbran accustomed to the acoustics of the San Carlo at Naples, said: "The chorus was excellent. The orchestra was very good too, but lacked power. Possibly that may have been the fault of the hall."

p. 116, l. 1 "fantastic exaggerations" Carpani may not have been an altogether disinterested party with regard to the quality of *Zelmira.* Azevedo asserted that he had provided the text for an aria that Rossini interpolated into the Vienna production of it for Fanny Eckerlin.

p. 118, l. 3 "his wife" *Briefe von und an Hegel,* Leipzig, 1887, p. 154.

p. 119, l. 19 "in 1860" *LVdW.*

p. 119, l. 21 "and Rossini" Ernest Newman, in *The Life of Richard Wagner,* 4 vols., London and New York, 1933-46, II, 12, at first refers slightingly to Michotte: "In 1906 one E. Michotte published a brochure in which he claimed that he had been a member of the small circle of literary men who gathered round Wagner in Paris in 1860, that it was he who took Wagner to Rossini's house and introduced him, and that his brochure is based on notes made at the time of the conversation between the two." Then, having granted that Wagner's "own accounts of his meeting with Rossini—in the autobiography [*Mein Leben*] and in the *Recollections of Rossini* which he wrote for the Augsburg *Allgemeine Zeitung* of the 17th December, 1868, a month after the Italian master's death—agree in essence with that of Michotte," Newman admits that "biographers and historians will hardly expect from any man a minutely accurate recollection of a conversation of nearly half a century earlier." (Michotte nowhere claimed to have "recollected" the conversation; as Newman himself just had written, he stated that he had kept notes of it.) But then Newman swings around completely: "All in all, however, when full allowance has been made for Michotte's mistakes [not specified] and embroideries, there seems little reason to doubt that he was present at the interview, and that the talk was substantially as he represents it to have been"—an opinion that the present writer shares.

p. 119, l. 28 "his theories" *LVdW*, p. 19, footnote 1.

p. 119, l. 31 "of Beethoven" *LVdW*, p. 22.

p. 119, l. 33 "up again" *LVdW*, p. 25.

p. 120, l. 4 "slightly fogged" Rossini was describing the fifty-one-year-old Beethoven of 1822, the year during which he labored on the *Missa solemnis* (completed in 1823) and composed the C-minor Piano Sonata, opus 111.

p. 120, l. 18 Rossini later told his architect-friend Doussault: "He [Beethoven] didn't understand the theater; he knew only the orchestra and treated the singing lines in the same way as those for flutes and clarinets. *Fidelio* is composed like a symphony. There's a great distance between him and Mozart in the field of opera."

p. 121, l. 11 "of instinct" This became one of Rossini's most-quoted remarks. Michotte's footnote on it (*LVdW*, p. 29, footnote 1) is revealing: "*I had facility* . . . Most chroniclers, struck by this reply, which Wagner himself has reported, have thought to see some malicious intention in it, a spurt of malice imagined by the Monkey [*Singe*] of Pesaro (as Rossini sometimes called himself) in order to have sport with the German master by persuading him to take this avowal at face value . . . [points of omission in original]

"Nothing could be less exact; the same is true of the attitude attributed to Wagner by other publicists, that of having prostrated himself humbly before Rossini—confessing an outright *mea culpa* with regard to his doctrines.

"The reply in question, I assert, led up to quite naturally in the course of the conversation—as we just have seen—could not leave behind any doubt as to its sincerity.

"Furthermore, it is *true*. It is identical to the declaration that the Maestro was in the habit of making to his close friends when he talked to them about himself and his works."

p. 121, l. 34 "had ended" *LVdW*, p. 31.

p. 123, l. 11 "thus ends" *LVdW*, p. 33.

p. 123, l. 17 "*opere semiserie*" Of Rossini's thirty-nine operas as usually classified, twenty-five are *opere serie* of one variety or another; only fourteen are *opere buffe*.

p. 124, l. 2 "written himself" During his stay in Vienna, Rossini also composed for military band a *Passo doppio* that he would remember in 1829, when he adapted it for orchestra to form the concluding *allegro vivace* of the overture to *Guillaume Tell*.

p. 124, l. 17 "Carnival season" In March 1821, Rossini had signed with the "Teatro Italiano" (King's Theatre) of London an agreement that could have required his presence in England at this time had he not insisted that it include an escape clause, which he now invoked.

p. 124, l. 23 "in 1827" Schlesinger (Berlin) later published an expanded version of these lessons, the added materials being ten new vocalizations for mezzo-soprano or baritone. A *Traité de composition* in the Bibliothèque Nationale, Paris, sometimes attributed to Rossini, certainly is not his work, as Jean-Baptiste-Théodore Weckerlin noted when he wrote on its first page: "*Ce n'est pas de lui.*"

p. 124, l. 27 "Via Mazzini)" Rossini had been living with his parents and Isabella at No. 248, Strada Maggiore (now included in the buildings numbered 16 and 18, Via Mazzini). Some time after his mother's death in 1827, he, Isabella, and his father began to live in the *palazzo* at No. 243, Strada Maggiore (now Via Mazzini, 26). After Giuseppe Rossini's death in 1839, however, Rossini—by then legally separated from Isabella—moved out of the *palazzo*. He lived briefly at No. 268, Strada Maggiore (now No. 29, Via Mazzini); during the summer, no longer able to go to Castenaso, he rented the Villa Cornetti, just outside the Porta Castiglione. He next lived at No. 79, Strada Santo Stefano (now No. 42); and then in the *palazzo* at No. 101, Strada Santo Stefano (now No. 57) belonging to Severino Degli Antonj. He was still living there when his *Stabat Mater* was sung in Bologna for the first time in 1842—when his landlord's wife, Clementina Degli Antonj, sang the contralto solo. Only in August 1846, probably just before his marriage to Olympe Pélissier, did he move into his last Bologna residence, No. 239 Strada Maggiore (now No. 34, Via Mazzini), a *palazzo* belonging to his friend the tenor Domenico Donzelli.

p. 124, l. 30 "of 1829" Then, as now, the building showed this motto incised into the top of its front façade: NON DOMO DOMINUS—SED DOMINO DOMUS (a slightly altered abridgement of a sentence in Cicero's *De Oficiis* 1, 39, 139: "*Nec domo dominus—sed domino domus honestanda est*" —"The house does not bring honor to its master, but the master to his house"). Another inscription, on the flank of the building, quotes a verse and a hemistich from Book VI of the *Aeneid* (lines 646 and 658): "*Obloquitur numeris septem discrimina vocum/Inter odoratum lauri nemus*" (given in C. Day Lewis's translation published by the Oxford University Press in 1952 as "To accompany their measures upon the seven-stringed lyre/Amidst a fragrant grove of bay trees").

p. 124, ll. 34-5 "told Hiller" *PmR*, 68-70.

p. 125, l. 6 "compose five" On the cover of the special supplement to *LGMM* published on the centenary of Rossini's birth (February 29, 1892), Ricordi presented a "*Prospetto cronologico delle opere di Rossini*"; it listed four cantatas as having been composed for the Congress of Verona: *L'Augurio felice*, *Il Bardo*, *La Sacra* [*Santa*] *Alleanza*, and *Il Vero Omaggio*.

p. 125, l. 19 "Gaetano Rossi" For other uses by Rossini of texts by Rossi, see p. 21 and note for that page.

p. 125, ll. 29-30 "*Tebaldo e Isolina*" Rossini told Ferdinand Hiller that Metternich was fanatically interested in music and that at Venice in 1823 he had come every evening to La Fenice for the rehearsals of *Semiramide* there.

p. 125, l. 37   "*Santa Alleanza*"   The *podestà* asked the colonel of the local hussars for sixteen cavalrymen; the infantry major was requisitioned for sixteen soldiers for the procession and eighteen more "who must act as genii, and therefore must be of the youngest, without mustaches." In a letter of November 28 to Meyerbeer in Venice, Gaetano Rossi mentioned as singing in *La Santa Alleanza* both Eliodoro Bianchi and Trentanove (either Agostino Trentanove or Niccola Trentanove-Cenni).

p. 126, l. 14   "Teatro Filarmonico"   Unlike the free public performance of *La Santa Alleanza*, that of *Il Vero Omaggio* was a profit-making venture. The invited dignitaries were not numerous enough to prevent the sale of many tickets, receipts from which were divided equally between the Royal Chamber of Commerce and Conte Leandro Giusti, impresario of the Teatro Filarmonico.

p. 126, l. 18   "Mazzanti remarked"   *Rossini a Verona durante il Congresso del 1822.*

p. 126, l. 26   "olive branches"   The soloists in the singing of *Il Vero Omaggio* on December 3, 1822, were Adelaide Tosi, replacing Isabella Colbran, who was indisposed (Argene), the *castrato* Giambattista Velluti (Aleco), Gaetano Crivelli (Genio dell'Austria), Luigi Campitelli (Fileno), and Filippo Galli (Elpino). Describing Rossini's score for this cantata, the *Allgemeine musikalische Zeitung* detected borrowings from *Sigismondo*, *Ricciardo e Zoraide, Bianca e Falliero*, and *Elisabetta, regina d'Inghilterra*; the writer naturally had failed to recognize music brought over from Rossini's 1821 cantata *La Riconoscenza*. Twelve hundred ten copies of the libretto were printed, fifty of them being bound in silk to sell for 900 lire (about $465) each. A copy of it survives in the library of the Conservatoire Royal de Musique, Brussels.

p. 127, l. 32   "*L'Inganno felice*"   In a letter of November 28, 1822, to Meyerbeer in Venice, Gaetano Rossi listed the singers in *L'Inganno felice* as "la Passerina" (Carolina Passerini), Eliodoro Bianchi, Luigi Campitelli, Filippo Galli, and Trentanove (either Agostino Trentanove or Niccola Trentanove-Cenni).

p. 127, l. 34   "in Venice"   A letter from Rossini to a Veronese musician named (Alessio? Antonio?) Mortellari, dated at Venice on December 9, 1822, is in the Library of Congress, Washington, D.C.

p. 128, l. 24   "[*sic*] *tragico*"   Very popular during Rossini's youth had been the posthumous *La Vendetta di Nino* of Alessio Prati, with a text derived from Voltaire's *Sémiramis*. The availability of the Semiramis legend in Italy had begun in 1593, when Muzio Manfredi had published his *Semiramide* at Bergamo. The number of operas using librettos based upon that legend is beyond computing. Perhaps the earliest Italian opera on the subject was Francesco Paolo Sacrati's *Semiramide in India* (1648). The century-long popularity of Metastasio's *Semiramide* almost passes belief: beginning with a setting of it by Leonardo Vinci (1729), it was used by dozens of composers before Meyerbeer set it in 1819. Even Paisiello's *La Semiramide in villa* (1772), a parody of Metastasio, preserved many of its original verses.

p. 128, l. 34   "an article"   "*G. Rossini,*" *Omnibus,* Naples, 10/5/1839.

p. 129, l. 5   "*L'usato ardir*"   Introduced by a recitative beginning "*Dei! qual sospiro!*" the trio opening with these words is sung by Semiramide, Arsace, and Assur in the finale of Act I.

p. 129, ll. 8–9   "February 3, 1823"   The cast of the first performance of *Semiramide* was made up of Isabella Colbran (Semiramide), Rosa Mariani (Arsace), Matilde Spagna (Azema), Filippo Galli (Assur), John Sinclair (Idreno), and Luciano Mariani (Oroe). Rosa Mariani, a contralto, was to make a specialty of the travesty role of Arsace. Matilde Spagna had sung Lucia in *La Gazza ladra* at Siena in the spring of 1822; little more is known of her. Sinclair (sometimes Saint-Clair, 1791–1857) was a Scottish tenor; having made his operatic debut in London in 1810, he sang for Rossini in Naples in May 1821. Mariani, a fine bass, later created the role of Conte Rodolfo in Bellini's *La Sonnambula* (1831).

p. 129, l. 10   "later performances)"   Colonel J. H. Mapleson, describing a visit of his opera troupe to Washington, D.C., in February 1883, speaks of a performance of *Semiramide* in which Adelina Patti and Sofia Scalchi were, respectively, Semiramide and Arsace, and adds: "In a letter to the papers the following morning a mathematician stated that by carefully counting the notes in the part of *Semiramide*, and dividing the result by the sum paid nightly to Patti for singing that part, he discovered that she received exactly 42⅝ cents for each of the notes that issued from her throat. This was found to be just 7¹⁄₁₀ cents per note more than Rossini got for writing the whole opera" (*The Mapleson Memoirs* I, 313).

p. 129, l. 32   "Theatre, London"   In May 1823, Benelli had taken over the King's Theatre from John Ebers for £10,000. This acquisition, effected in mid-season, included the lease (which ran until 1825) and all the existing scenery, costumes, and other stage properties. Benelli also took on Ebers's contractual responsibilities for the rest of that season and agreed that Ebers should remain manager until it ended.

p. 129, l. 34   "*Figlia dell'aria*"   *La Figlia dell'aria* may never have been worked on at all, and certainly never was finished. Instead, Rossini worked on a lost opera entitled *Ugo, re d'Italia.* For this information I am particularly indebted to Mr. Andrew Porter, who sent me an offprint of his article "A Lost Opera by Rossini."

NOTES TO CHAPTER IX

p. 131, l. 5   "Ferdinando Paër"   Paër was born at Parma on June 1, 1771, and died in Paris on May 3, 1839. His operatic career began at Parma with a French *mélodrame, Orphée et Eurydice* (1791). He married the singer Francesca Riccardi, who later left him. While living in Vienna, he composed perhaps his best opera, *Camilla, ossia Il Sotterraneo* (1799). Paër became *maître de chapelle* to Napoleon in Paris in 1807, and for a time served as director of the Opéra-Comique. In 1812 he was appointed to succeed Spontini as director of the Théâtre-Italien, a position that he held intermittently—for a short time in uncomfortable tandem with Rossini—until 1826, when he had to resign because he was blamed for the troupe's financial difficulties. In his own defense he published (1827) a pamphlet, *M. Paer, ex-directeur du Théâtre Italien à MM. les dilettantes.* Besides *Camilla*, his successful operas included *Griselda, ossia La Virtù al cimento* (Parma, 1798), *Agnese di Fitz-Henry* (Ponte d'Attaro, 1809), and the one-act *opéra-comique* entitled *Le Maître de chapelle, ou Le Souper imprévu* (Paris, 1821), which was sung in France and England down to recent decades.

p. 132, l. 2   "the Italien"   In 1822, for example, of the sixteen operas sung at the Italien, eight were by Rossini; they accounted for 119 out of that year's 154 performances. By 1911, the total number of performances of seventeen Rossini operas at the Italien reached 2,209. The Rossini operas heard there before his first visit to France had been *L'Italiana in Algeri* (February 1, 1817); *L'Inganno felice* (May 13, 1819); *Il Barbiere di Siviglia* (October 26, 1819); *Il Turco in Italia* (May 23, 1820); *Torvaldo e Dorliska* (November 21, 1820); *La Pietra del paragone* (April 5, 1821); *Otello* (June 5, 1821); *La Gazza ladra* (September 18, 1821); *Elisabetta, regina d'Inghilterra* (March 10, 1822); *Tancredi* (April 23, 1822); *La Cenerentola* (June 8, 1822); and *Mosè in Egitto* (October 20, 1822).

p. 132, l. 12   "Comtesse Merlin"   Née Mercedes Jaruco and born in Havana, the Comtesse Merlin had become a renowned Parisian *salonnière.* She studied singing with Manuel Garcia: Arthur Pougin said of her (*Marie Malibran*, p. 17) that "she could sing, not amateurishly, but really like a great artist. She also wrote with grace and facility, and in 1836, Sainte-Beuve published an encomium of her *Souvenirs d'une créole*, which just had appeared." She was also part-author of *Memoirs of Madame Malibran, by the Countess de Merlin and Other Intimate Friends, with a Selection from Her Correspondence and Notices of the Progress of the Musical Drama in England* (2 vol., London, 1840).

p. 138, l. 34   "Henri-Montan Berton"   Berton (1767–1844), orginally a violinist, had begun his career in opera with *Les Promesses de mariage* (1787). Reacting with violent distaste to the Parisian acclaim for Rossini's operas, he published two polemic tracts attacking the Italian and defending his own abstract ideas and theories: *De la Musique mécanique et de la musique philosophique* (1826) and *Épître à un célèbre compositeur français, précédée de quelques observations sur la musique mécanique et la musique philosophique* (1829). Boieldieu expressed displeasure at being the addressee of the latter pamphlet. Ferdinand Hiller reported that at Trouville in 1855, Rossini told him: "Old Berton even made poems about me in which he called me 'M. Crescendo.' That all passed without endangering my life."

p. 134, l. 9   "Il Barbiere"   *Lettre à un compositeur français,* Paris, 1827, p. 24.

p. 134, l. 11   "Charles Maurice"   Boieldieu's letter is quoted from Georges Favre: *Boieldieu* I, 227.

p. 135, l. 29   "Rossini operas"   *Elisabetta, regina d'Inghilterra* (April 30, 1818); *L'Italiana in Algeri* (January 26, 1819); *L'Inganno felice* (May 13,

1819); *La Cenerentola* (January 8, 1820); *Tancredi* (May 4, 1820); *La Gazza ladra* (March 10, 1821); *Il Turco in Italia* (May 19, 1821); *Mosè in Egitto* (as *Pietro l'eremita*, April 23, 1822); *Otello* (May 16, 1822); *La Donna del lago* (February 18, 1823); *Ricciardo e Zoraide* (June 5, 1823); and *Matilde di Shabran* (July 3, 1823). During the 1823 season, the King's Theatre presented nine operas, six of them by Rossini; the 1824 repertoire would consist of twelve operas, eight of them by Rossini and conducted by him.

p. 135, l. 34 "Carlo Coccia" Coccia (1782–1873), a Neapolitan, began his operatic career at Rome in 1807 with *Il Matrimonio per lettera di cambio* (with a libretto based on the same Federici comedy that had supplied Rossi with the basis for the text of Rossini's *La Cambiale di matrimonio*). His success dated from 1809 and the first of ten successive operas heard at Venice. In 1828, he returned to Italy, mostly abandoning *opera buffa* for *opera seria*. After Rossini's death, Verdi invited Coccia to compose the *Lacrymosa* and *Amen* for the projected Requiem Mass. Coccia died at Novara in 1873.

p. 135, l. 40 "to £10,950." Somewhat different figures were cited by *RAD* II, 26, as from the *Quarterly Musical Magazine*. The list given here is cited as "from a periodical work" in Ebers: *Seven Years of the King's Theatre*, p. 229, where the total amount paid to members of the ballet, headed by Le Gros at £1,200, is given as £9,400.

p. 136, l. 5 "ushered out" Rossini congratulated the leader of the band, Franz Cramer (brother of the pianist-pedagogue Johann Baptist Cramer), on the success with which he had transcribed the overture and led the band in performing it.

p. 136, ll. 27–8 "January 24, 1824" The cast of *Zelmira* included Colbran (Zelmira), Lucia Elizabeth Vestris (Emma), Manuel Patricio Garcia (Ilo), and Matteo Porto (Polidoro). Mme Vestris was the daughter of Gaetano Bartolozzi, son of the noted engraver Francesco Bartolozzi and of Theresa Jansen, a friend of Haydn, who had attended Lucia Elizabeth's first wedding, in May 1795, when she had been only sixteen, to Auguste-Armand Vestris, dancer-son of the more famous Auguste Vestris. Her second husband (1838) was Charles James Mathews, the actor-playwright who managed Covent Garden from 1839 to 1842 with her assistance. Manuel Patricio Garcia, son of the original Almaviva in *Il Barbiere* and brother to Maria Malibran and Pauline Viardot-Garcia, had been born in 1805; he died in 1906. Abandoning the stage in 1829, he became a teacher of singing and invented the laryngoscope. He taught very briefly at the Paris Conservatoire, but in 1848 returned to London, where he was at the Royal Academy of Music until 1895.

p. 137, ll. 9–10 "Benelli's troubles" Benelli's season was made up of twelve operas. Those by Rossini were *Zelmira*; *Otello*, with Jago's role transposed for bass; *Il Barbiere di Siviglia*; *Ricciardo e Zoraide* (which seems to have provided Colbran with her last operatic appearance); *Il Turco in Italia*; *La Donna del lago*; *Tancredi*; and *Semiramide*. The other operas were Mayr's *Il Nuovo Fanatico per la musica*, with Angelica Catalani; Mozart's

Don Giovanni and *Le Nozze di Figaro*; and Zingarelli's *Giulietta e Romeo*.

p. 138, l. 5 "fair voice"   The London press reported that Rossini conducted three concerts at Prince Leopold's palace, receiving a fee of £525 and a diamond cravat pin.

p. 138, l. 15 "the grave"   A contemporary caricature showed George IV in the act of genuflecting before Rossini as though begging him for a musical favor, probably that of being permitted to sing a duet with him. The caption reads: "His Majesty would do better to conserve his voice to raise it in favor of his subjects."

p. 138, l. 24 "creak horribly"   One name appearing in the notations is that of Sir Thomas Charles Morgan, a noted physician, husband of the Sydney Morgan who had met Rossini in Naples and had written about him in her *Italy*.

p. 139, l. 6 "orchestral accompaniment"   The Byron cantata was divided into a recitative, an adagio, an invocation, and a peroration. No full score of it was published, but T. Boosey & Co. issued a piano reduction of it with Rossini's dedication to the Honorable Henry F. De Roos, whose family name appears several times in Rossini's *Almanack and Cash Account*.

p. 140, l. 7 "Andrew Porter"   "A Lost Opera by Rossini."

p. 140, l. 12 "*Figlia dell'aria*"   Edmond Michotte quoted Rossini as having told him: "I had begun to write an opera on a subject entitled *La Figlia dell'aria*, but after I had completed the first act, I did not go ahead with it for various reasons. Later, I adapted for other operas various of the pieces already written; thus I had reason to say that I was de-composing." The possibility exists, then, that Rossini dropped *La Figlia dell'aria* to begin *Ugo, re d'Italia* and perhaps transferred sections of the completed act of the former to the latter. Some possibility exists, too, that we hear (however transmuted) ideas from either *La Figlia dell'aria* or *Ugo, re d'Italia* (or both) in Rossini's Paris operas.

p. 141, l. 8 "December 18, 1830"   This letter, in English, is not in Rossini's script, but its signature is, as is also "*le 18*" in its date ("*Paris, le 18* December 1830").

p. 141, l. 9 "Mr. Obicini"   Signor A Obicini took over Rossini's interests in London when the composer went to Paris in July 1824.

p. 141, l. 14 "should still"   Rossini appears, then, to have tried earlier to recover the score.

p. 141, l. 18 "considerable loss"   This letter belongs to Lord Kinnaird, whom Mr. Porter thanked for permission to publish it.

p. 141, l. 22 "Kinnaird & Co."   Mr. Porter pointed out that no bank of this name existed, "but the Hon. Douglas Kinnaird was the principal partner of Ransom & Co., and there is little doubt that the bank was often called Kinnaird and Co." Messrs. Ransom later was absorbed by Barclays Bank Ltd.

p. 142, ll. 28-9 "vanished completely"   A considerable collection of Rossini's scores was incinerated in the fire that destroyed the Salle Favart (Théâtre-Italien) on January 14-15, 1838; the score of the unfinished London opera well may have been among them.

p. 142, l. 34 "December 1, 1823" This document—*Bases de l'engagement que Rossini pense pouvoir proposer au Gouvernement français*—is in the Bibliothèque Nationale, Paris; written in French by someone else, it is signed by Rossini. It is quoted in full in Albert Soubies: *Le Théâtre-Italien de 1801 à 1913*, p. 28.

p. 143, l. 9 "ten articles" The contract of February 27, 1824, provided that: (1) Rossini would reside in Paris for one year and compose an evening-long French *grand opéra* in three, four, or five acts and a two-act Italian *opera semiseria* or *opera buffa*; (2) that the French libretto would be selected jointly by Rossini and the administration of the Opéra; (3) that the Italian libretto would be selected by the administration of the Italien; (4) that Rossini would adapt for the troupe of the Italien and stage at the Salle Louvois one of his existing operas not yet heard in Paris, the opera to be agreed upon jointly by him and the administration; (5) that the Rossini benefit mentioned in Article 6 would be held during the final four months of the agreement; and that the French and Italian operas would not be staged simultaneously—for which reason they would be made ready during the first nine months of his engagement so that he could supervise the staging and rehearsal of both; (6) that Rossini was to be paid 40,000 francs at the rate of 3,500 francs monthly; that the administration would pay for the new librettos; that Rossini would own the score of the French opera, with the Opéra retaining rights to its performance; and that Rossini would be accorded a benefit night at the Opéra; (7) that the benefit would be made up of (a) an Italian opera not yet presented in Paris, together with divertissements and other accessories; and that it would be presented so that it could enter the repertoire of the Italien, for which reason its total cost would be kept within the proportions established by other operas being performed at the Louvois; and (b) a ballet from the current repertoire; (8) that the agreement would run one year from the date in July 1824 at which Rossini would be in Paris; (9) that during the year covered by the agreement, Rossini would live in Paris and work exclusively for the Opéra and the Théâtre-Italien; and that he would not allow any other old or new work of his to be performed in France during the life of the contract; and (10) that in case of disagreements or difficulties regarding matters specified in the agreement, Rossini would abide by the decisions of the Ministry of the Royal Household, as was required of all artists in its employ.

p. 143, l. 24 "Bolognese friends" During this brief stay in Bologna, Rossini went ahead with the reconstruction and decorating of the *palazzo* that he had bought in 1822, entrusting the construction work to one Conti, the decoration to the architect Francesco Santini. It seems likely, too, that while in Italy, Rossini gave thought to singers who might serve in Paris.

p. 143, l. 29 "Charles X" The contract of November 26, 1824, provided that (1) Rossini would conduct the musical and stage affairs of the Italien, his authority to extend over all stage and orchestral personnel and, during performances, over all functionaries and employees of the establishment (this article established his precedence over Paër without eliminating Paër's position); (2) Rossini's title was to be Directeur de la musique et de la scène du Théâtre Royal Italien, carrying with it a payment of 25,000 francs per year; he was to be granted lodgings in a building appertaining to the Beaux-Arts; (3) the administration of the Italien was, as before, to be united with that of the Opéra, with all matters concerning properties, the police, and bookkeeping to continue under the administrative authority of the Opéra; (4) Rossini was to "compose the works that may be asked from him, whether for the Théâtre Italien or the Opéra," his remuneration to be 5,000 francs for operas in one act, 10,000 francs for those in more than one act, to be paid after the production of each opera; the administration was to pay all the rights and honoraria for the French librettos; and Rossini was to own any scores composed by him for the Italien, but was not to have the right to have them performed in other French theaters; and (5) the agreement was to become effective on December 1, 1824; Rossini was to give at least six months' notice of any intention to terminate the agreement; and the agreement was to be revocable by the King without any indemnity to Rossini.

p. 144, l. 16   "anti-Rossinians"   This version of *Der Freischütz*, its text and its music both sadly mangled, was in fact received badly by its first audience. Castil-Blaze thereupon withdrew it, reworked it, and presented it again, this time papering the Odéon liberally until it caught on. Then, running up 327 consecutive performances, it helped to convert to German romanticism many French romantics, Victor Hugo included. Its success induced Castil-Blaze to prepare *La Forêt de Sénart, ou La Partie de chasse* (to a text based on a long-popular play, *La Partie de chasse de Henri IV*), with a score patched together out of Beethoven, Rossini, and Weber (*Euryanthe*). Produced at the Odéon on January 14, 1826, *La Forêt de Sénart* almost duplicated the popularity of *Robin des bois*. But when Castil-Blaze's own substantially complete translation of *Euryanthe* was sung at the Opéra five years later (April 6, 1831), it survived for only four performances.

p. 144, l. 32   "Luigi Balocchi"   Balocchi (1766–18?), himself a composer, had written the libretto for Valentino Fioravanti's *I Virtuosi ambulanti* (1807). For Rossini, besides writing the libretto of *Il Viaggio a Reims*, he helped remake the libretto of *Mosè in Egitto* into that of *Moïse et Pharaon*.

p. 144, l. 39   "June 19, 1825"   The singers in the first performance of *Il Viaggio a Reims* were Giuditta Pasta (Corinna), Laure Cinti-Damoreau (La Contessa di Folleville), Ester Mombelli (Madama Cortese), Adelaide Schias(s)etti (La Marchesa Melibea), Domenico Donzelli (Il Cavalier Belfiore), Marco Bordogni (Il Conte di Libenskof), Carlo Zucchelli (Lord Sidney), Felice Pellegrini (Don Profondo), Vincenzo Graziani (Il Barone di Trombonok), Nicholas-Prosper Levasseur (Don Alvaro), Pierre Scudo (Don Luigini), Maria Amigo (Delia), Rossi (Maddalena), Dotty (Modestina), Giovanola (Zefirino), Auletta (Antonio), and Amigo (a sister of the Delia?), Dotty, Giovanola, and Scudo (Quattro Virtuosi ambulanti). Pasta (1798–1865) was one of the greatest sopranos of her era. Cinti-Damoreau (1801–63), a soprano, had made her debut at the Italien in 1816; she would also create for Rossini the roles of Pamira (*Le Siège de Corinthe*), Anaï (*Moïse et Pharaon*), the Comtesse Adèle de Formoutiers (*Le Comte Ory*), and Mathilde (*Guillaume Tell*). Schiassetti (1800?-?), a contralto, had sung in Munich (1818-24) and at the Italien; she was a close friend of Stendhal. Giulio Marco Bordogni (1788-1856), a tenor who had studied at Bergamo with Mayr, had made his debut in Rossini's *Tancredi* at the Teatro Re, Milan, in 1813; a close friend of Donizetti, he later taught at the Paris Conservatoire, where his pupils included Henriette Sontag, Laure Cinti-Damoreau, and Mario Zucchelli (1793-1879), who had been born in London of Italian-English parents, had made his debut at Novara in 1814; he became a leading *basso cantante* and *basso buffo*. It seems impossible to identify Graziani. Levasseur (1791-1871), an outstanding bass, would also create for Rossini the roles of Moïse (*Moïse et Pharaon*), Le Gouverneur (*Le Comte Ory*), and Walter Fürst (*Guillaume Tell*). Pierre Scudo, a dilettante singer, became a noted music critic (see bibliography). Two sisters named Amigo sang at the Italien; the older, a mezzo, generally sang secondary roles, whereas the younger, a soprano, was a minor *comprimaria*. The Rossi who sang the role of Maddalena very probably was Caterina Rossi, who had created the role of Clorinda in *La Cenerentola* (Rome, 1817). It has proved impossible to find further information about Dotty, Giovanola, and Auletta.

p. 145, l. 1 "the score" For Rossini's later use of large sections of the score of *Il Viaggio a Reims* in *Le Comte Ory*, see page 158. For the adaptation of *Il Viaggio a Reims* as *Andremo a Parigi?* see page 247 and note to that page. Although the statement made immediately after the *première* of *Il Viaggio a Reims* (by the *Journal des débats*) that the opera lacked a *sinfonia* long was credited, a nonautograph copy of such a *sinfonia* survives at Pesaro; it has been performed a few times, but has not been published (see Alfredo Bonaccorsi's preface to *QR* IX, v). According to the *Enciclopedia dello Spettacolo* VIII, column 1248, a version of *Il Viaggio* was presented in Vienna on April 26, 1854, under the title of *Il Viaggio a Vienna ossia l'Albergo di . . . ai Bagni di . . .*, *Melodramma d'Occasione con Quadro allusivo*; but it is unlikely to have had reference to the original *cantata scenica* except in its text.

p. 145, ll. 9-10 "really is" *L'Opéra-Italien*, p. 423. Castil-Blaze must be approached with unsleeping skepticism; with reason, Arthur Pougin wrote (*Marie Malibran*, p. 27): "*Historiens de l'avenir, méfiez-vous de Castil Blaze!*"

p. 146, l. 7 "del lago" *La Donna del lago*, its libretto translated into French by Jean-Baptiste Villet d'Épagny, Auguste Rousseau, and H. Raison, also was sung (as *La Dame au lac*) at the Odéon on October 31, 1825; it had been "arranged" by Jean-Frédéric-Auguste Lemière de Corvey.

p. 146, l. 18 "noisy enthusiasm" Born in 1789, daughter of a Hungarian violinist, Joséphine Fodor had married an actor named Mainvielle. Her brilliant successes in England, Paris, Naples, and Vienna had been climaxed during the season of 1824-5 in Vienna, where she had sung the title role of *Semiramide* sixty times. At the age of sixty-eight (1857), she would publish her still-interesting *Réflexions et conseils sur l'art du chant.* She died in 1870.

p. 148, l. 10   "of Rossini"   "*Ein Name besser als eine Hausnummer: Erinnerungen an K. M. von Weber und Rossini.*"

p. 148, ll. 30–1   "later said"   *Life of Moscheles,* adapted from the original German by A. D. Coleridge, p. 275.

p. 148, l. 33   "bass voice"   Rossini had composed it for a contralto in travesty.

p. 149, l. 1   "as saying"   *LVdW*, p. 21.

p. 150, ll. 23–4   "first performance"   The 1826 Lisbon libretto lists the cast for *Adina* as João Oracio (Giovanni Orazio) Cartagenova (O Califa), Luiza (Luigia) Valesi (Adina), Luiz (Luigi) Ravaglia (Selimo), Gaspar(e) Martinelli (Alì), and Filippe (Filippo) Spada (Mustafà). "*A Musica he de JOAQUIM ROSSINE.*" The statement that *Adina* had been staged at La Scala, Milan, earlier (1825) is incorrect. As Mario Rinaldi remarked, the error probably represented confusion with Giuseppe Rastrelli's *Amina* (La Scala, March 16, 1824). Cartagenova (1800–41), a bass, was especially noted for the intelligence of his interpretations; his most popular role was that of Cardenio in Donizetti's *Il Furioso all'isola di San Domingo.* Valesi, a *prima donna buffa,* sang in the Italian and Spanish provincial theaters for some years; she was the wife of the *basso* Stefano Valesi. Ravaglia sang at La Scala, Milan, in 1827–8, joining Henriette Méric-Lalande, Caroline Unger, and Giovanni David in thirty-one performances of Rossini's *Elisabetta, regina d'Inghilterra.* Martinelli, a tenor, sang at La Scala in the early years of the century. Spada had sung Orbezzano in *Tancredi* at Siena in 1814; he seems to have been singing at La Scala, Milan, as late as 1832.

p. 150, l. 39   "that house"   Before resigning, Rossini heard an echo of his London visit. John Ebers wrote (*Seven Years of the King's Theatre,* p. 310): ". . . in the autumn of 1826, I went to Paris for the usual purpose of forming engagements. Here I was in frequent intercourse with Rossini and Meyerbeer; the former of whom continued to fill the situation of director, and took every opportunity of assisting and obliging me. Rossini was in great repute at Paris, and mixed a great deal in society, to which his social and happy temperament inclines him. He was living in a handsome style, had a villa about three miles from Paris [Aguado's at Petit-Bourg?], and spent his time in an agreeable union of the occupations of the director and the *bon vivant.* Our intimacy led to a proposition, which, however, was never carried into effect,—that he, Barbaja, and myself, should become partners in the management of the King's Theatre. Had this been effected, the direction of the music and the performances would have devolved upon Rossini, and the engagements would have been transacted by Barbaja, who, from his numerous theatrical concerns, was better calculated than any other man in Europe, to engage performers with advantage. The arrangements for the ballet, letting the boxes, and attending to the subscribers, would have been my department. Rossini appeared very anxious that this proposal should have been acted on, in which case, he, as Director of the Italian Opera at Paris, would have afforded additional assistance to that of London. A proposal was about the same time made to me, by Mr. Glossop, Barbaja's partner." Glossop, husband of the soprano Elisabetta Ferron, was the father of Augustus Harris, long stage manager at Covent Garden, who in turn was the father of Sir Augustus Harris.

p. 152, l. 8 "called *Ivanhoé*" The first cast of the Rossini-Antonio Pacini *Ivanhoé* included Mlle Lemoule, Gilbert-Louis Duprez, and M. Lecomte. This mélange also was staged at Strasbourg in 1826 and at Coburg in 1833.

p. 152, l. 14 "and *Zelmira*" Confusion between this *Ivanhoé* and the opera *Ivanhoé* by Giovanni Pacini infests Italian and other chronicles of the late 1820's and 1830's. The two Pacinis were not related. Giovanni Pacini, however, was the father of Émilien (Emiliano) Pacini, who made the French translation of *Der Freischütz* for the 1841 Berlioz version, collaborated on the French translation of Verdi's *Luisa Miller*, and himself translated *Il Trovatore* into French (1856).

p. 152, l. 19 "mild success" Besides *Ivanhoé*, Paris heard at least four other pastiches using Rossini music during 1826 and 1827. *La Fausse Agnès* (Odéon, June 13, 1826), an "*opéra-bouffon*" in three acts, arranged by Castil-Blaze after a one-act play by Destouches (Philippe Néricault), was a revival, it having been staged earlier at the Théâtre de Madame, Paris; it made use of music by Cimarosa, Meyerbeer, and Rossini. *Le Neveu de Monseigneur* (Odéon, August 7, 1826), with a libretto by Jean-François-Alfred Bayard, Romieu, and Thomas-Marie-François Sauvage, was more successful, perhaps because Duprez sang in it; it boasted music by Fioravanti, Morlacchi, Pacini, and Rossini arranged by Luc Guénée. *Ivanhoé* followed on September 15. Then came *Le Testament*, an "*opéra*" in two acts with a libretto by Joseph-Henri de Saur and Léonce de Saint-Géniès, its music adapted by Jean-Frédéric-Auguste Lemierre (Lemière) de Corvey from Rossini operas—cast undetermined, except that it included Duprez. It was a failure. And at the Odéon on February 24, 1827, *M. de Pourceaugnac*, another "*opéra-bouffon*" arranged by Castil-Blaze, succeeded, in part because of its basis in Molière, in part because it deftly mixed Rossini and Weber. Several other similar pastiches were to come and go.

Notes to Chapter X

p. 153, l. 2 "October 9, 1826" The cast of the *première* of *Le Siège de Corinthe* was made up of Laure Cinti-Damoreau (Pamyre), Mlle Frémont (Ismène), Louis Nourrit (Cléomène), Adolphe Nourrit (Néoclès), Henri-Étienne Dérivis (Mahomet II), Ferdinand Prévost (Omar), M. Prévost (Hiéros), and M. Bonel—sometimes Bonnel (Adraste). Mlle Frémont appears to have remained a secondary singer. Louis Nourrit (Nourrit *père*, 1780–1831) was a dealer in diamonds and the Opéra's leading tenor—in which position his son Adolphe (1802–39) succeeded him just after the *première* of *Le Siège*. Among the roles that Adolphe Nourrit would create were Comte Ory, Arnold (*Guillaume Tell*), Robert (*Robert le Diable*), Masaniello (*La Muette de Portici*), Raoul (*Les Huguenots*), and Eléazar (*La Juive*). He left the Opéra after the rapid rise of Gilbert-Louis Duprez and committed suicide at Naples when he could not sing the leading role that Donizetti had designed for him in *Poliuto* because the Bourbon censorship prohibited performances of that opera. Henri-Étienne Dérivis (1780–1856) was the father of the more renowned bass Prosper Dérivis (1808–80). Alex Prévost, known as Ferdinand-Prevôt, was the son of Ferdinand Prévost; both were basses. Alex was to create the role of Orphide in *Moïse et Pharaon* and that of Leuthold in *Guillaume Tell*, Ferdinand that of Gessler in *Tell*. Bonel would be the first Osiride in *Moïse*, the first Melcthal in *Tell*.

p. 153, l. 18 "Maestro's windows . . ." The Rossinis were living at No. 10, boulevard Montmartre. That Colbran was in Paris and had not stayed behind in Bologna after the 1824 visit there, as some writers have maintained, is proved by remarks in several of Rossini's letters. On January 13, 1826, for example, he wrote to Domenico Donzelli: "Isabella sends you lots of good wishes"; on July 24, 1827, writing to Gaetano Conti, he said: "Isabella embraces you and so does my Father [then visiting in Paris]."

p. 154, l. 2 "in 1850" After the *première* of Auber's *La Muette de Portici* (Opéra, February 29, 1828—Rossini's thirty-sixth birthday), Rossini urged Troupenas to acquire publication rights in it. Troupenas did so; the success of Auber's opera contributed largely to his prosperity. After the delighted response to *Moïse* in 1827, Troupenas decided to publish it too. Rossini asked how he had done up to then with *Le Siège de Corinthe*. When Troupenas answered that it still represented a loss of several thousand francs, Rossini agreed to accept 2,500 francs (about $1,485) for the later opera, thus guaranteeing Troupenas a profit from it while he waited for *Le Siège* to become profitable.

p. 154, l. 34 "late 1820's" Laget's articles, appearing first in *La Revue de Toulouse* and elsewhere, were collected in a book, *Le Chant et les chanteurs*, Paris and Toulouse, 1874.

p. 155, l. 8 "de Corinthe" Laget is referring to "*La flamme rapide, le glaive homicide*," a march with chorus in Act I of *Le Siège de Corinthe*. What no critic of the time seems to have mentioned was Rossini's self-borrowing in one of the "new numbers" of *Le Siège*: the first twenty-eight measures of its impressive overture had served first in the *sinfonia* for *Bianca e Falliero*.

p. 155, l. 11 "Guillaume Tell" See p. 166.

p. 155, l. 14 "a friend" Nourrit's letter is translated from a quotation in *Music Autographs* ("Music Catalogue 98") issued by Richard Macnutt Limited of Tunbridge Wells, England.

p. 155, l. 34 "Légion d'honneur" The success of *Le Siège de Corinthe* blotted out memory of the disastrous staging of another of the pastiches put together with Rossini's permission from snippets of older operas. Called *Le Testament*, it had a two-act libretto by J. H. de Saur and Léonce de

Saint-Géniès; its score had been assembled by Jean-Frédéric-Auguste Lemière de Corvey. As its *première* at the Odéon dragged on (January 22, 1827), the audience became restive. At a juncture requiring the chief protagonist to designate his heir after almost everyone in the cast had refused the inheritance in advance, someone in the theater called out: "Leave it to the Jesuits!" Thereafter, the rumblings of audience disapproval swelled. Before this unhappy pastiche could reach its foredoomed conclusion, the hissing became so loud that the singers could not be heard. Nothing further is recorded of *Le Testament*.

p. 155, l. 37 "to Ebers" This letter, in the present writer's possession, was written in French by someone else and signed by Rossini.

p. 156, l. 8 "*Mer Rouge*" In 1821, at the urging of Hérold, Rossini had written to Giovanni Battista Viotti, then director of the Opéra, to suggest revising *Mosè in Egitto* to a French libretto; he would, he said, write "new numbers in a style more religious than that of those which my oratorio contains."

p. 156, l. 10 "March 26, 1827" The first cast of *Moïse et Pharaon* was made up of Laure Cinti-Damoreau (Anaï), Mlle Mori (Marie), Louise-Zulme (Leroux) Dabadie (Sinaïde), Adolphe Nourrit (Amenophis), Alexis (Pierre-Auguste) Dupont (Eliezer), Alex Ferdinand-Prevòt (Orphide), Nicholas-Prosper Levasseur (Moïse), Henry-Bernard Dabadie (Pharaon), and M. Bonel—sometimes Bonnel (Osiride). Mori, a member of an Italo-English family of musicians, had been born in London; she later sang with success in Italy. Mme Dabadie, wife of Henry-Bernard Dabadie, would also create the minor role of Jemmy in *Guillaume Tell*. Sometimes known simply as Alexis, Dupont would also sing in the second (partial) performance of Rossini's *Stabat Mater* in 1841. Alex Ferdinand-Prevòt (1814–45) was the son of Ferdinand Prévost; he would also be the first Leuthold in *Guillaume Tell*. Dabadie, a notable baritone, would create the roles of Raimbaut (*Le Comte Ory*), Guillaume Tell, and Bertram in Meyerbeer's *Robert le Diable*.

p. 157, l. 5 "French shouting" The *Enciclopedia dello Spettacolo* IX, column 1305, thus defines what Italians called the *urlo* (or *grido*) *alla francese*: "In eighteenth-century opera, this was a realistic effect which, dramatically interrupting the line of the singing, tended to express a culmination of pathetic intensity. On the technical level, it was obtained by forcing the voice to the point at which the sound became indeterminate. That expedient, of French origin (Rousseau says in the *Dictionnaire*: 'French music must be *cried*; its greatest expressiveness resides in that'), came into use in Italian opera with [David] Pérez, [Domingo] Terradellas, Rinaldo da Capua, and, above all, with Jommelli and Traetta, in the periods during which French rationalistic culture and the new operatic style exercised a powerful influence upon all of Europe. For example, in *La Sofonisba* (1762), Traetta adopted the *urlo* and indicated it in the score (cf. DTB [*Denkmäler der Tonkunst in Bayern*] XVII, 87, 90, and 146, where it is called 'expression in the French style'). However, satirical appellations for the *urlo* were not lacking on the part of those opposed to the style of French singing."

Despite the seeming exactness of these data, the term was used loosely; at times it meant nothing more than the French way of emphasizing sound values of sung words somewhat at the expense of sensuous vocal tone.

p. 157, l. 24 "her death"   On February 26, 1827, Giuseppe Rossini wrote to Francesco Maria Guidarini: "Regarding Gioacchino, then, he would have been here some time ago, but he was advised not to do it because if he came, it was sure that she would die in his arms, two years ago when he came to Italy, finding herself just merely seeing him, from the happiness she remained sick in bed more than two weeks . . ."

p. 157, l. 30 "his father"   None of Rossini's letters to his father, to Isabella Colbran, or to Olympe Pélissier can now be located. Their contents can be known now only from earlier quotations from or facsimiles of them.

p. 158, l. 2 "my manservant"   This was Isabella's Spanish manservant, Francisco Fernández. How long Giuseppe Rossini remained in Paris is not clear. Rossini, writing to Dr. Gaetano Conti in London on May 3, 1827, mentioned that his father was with him in Paris. At least one letter that Giuseppe himself wrote from Paris is dated July 1827. He was back in Bologna in July 1828, when he wrote from there to Francesco Maria Guidarini that he still was prey to melancholy and was considering doing what he had done the year before: journeying to Paris in the company of Francisco.

p. 158, ll. 5–6 "Signor Aguado"   Alejandro María Aguado, Marqués de Las Marismas (1784–1842), a naturalized Frenchman who became Rossini's very close friend, financial adviser, and generous patron—and who indirectly begot the *Stabat Mater*.

p. 158, l. 25 "later dates"   The Rossini letters to Barbaja are dated November 16, 1834, and January 15, 1836 (both in the Raccolta Piancastelli, Forlì), and May 17, 1835 (quoted in full in Franco Schlitzer: *Rossiniana*, p. 20.)

p. 159, l. 13 "a penny"   Four years before the date of Stendhal's letter of December 1819, of course, Rossini already was comfortably established in Naples.

p. 159, l. 38 "August 20, 1828"   The cast of the *première* of *Le Comte Ory* was made up of Laure Cinti-Damoreau (Comtesse de Fourmoutiers), Constance Jawureck (Isolier), Mlle Mori (Ragonde), Adolphe Nourrit (Comte Ory), Henri-Bernard Dabadie (Raimbaut, also called Robert), and Nicholas-Prosper Levasseur (Le Gouverneur). Jawureck (1803–58), daughter of a German musician at Paris, had made her debut at the Opéra in 1822; continuing to sing there until 1837, she then became a leading singer at Brussels.

p. 160, l. 35 "Étienne de Jouy"   Operas dealing with the legendary Swiss hero Wilhelm Tell had antedated Schiller's drama (1804). They had included Grétry's *Guillaume Tell* (1791) and Bernhard Anselm Weber's *Wilhelm Tell* (1795). On April 18, 1796, Benjamin Carr's *The Archers, or Mountaineers of Switzerland*—the earliest American opera of which the music has survived—was performed. It had a libretto by William Dunlap from his *Wilhelm Tell*, which in turn had been adapted from *Helvetic*

Liberty or The Lass of the Lakes, an anonymous text published in London in 1792 and Philadelphia in 1794.

   p. 161, l. 7   "completed opera"   Marrast (1801–52), a writer of some distinction, later became a member of the 1848 provisional government, Mayor of Paris, and President of the National Assembly.

   p. 161, l. 38   "Rossini's position"   The original of this letter is in the Bibliothèque Nationale, Paris.

   p. 163, l. 21   "and Italy"   As far as research can determine, this was not a statement of fact. No one in England, Germany, Russia, or Italy seems to have offered Rossini anything approaching the terms he was now demanding; no one in any country had offered him a lifetime annuity.

   p. 164, l. 32   "wrote them"   Zanolini (*ZAN*) wrote: "It is entirely believable that Rossini's sharp intelligence and long practical experience gave him a presentiment or feeling about what was being plotted against Charles X." The documents concerning the drawing-up of the contract are quoted in detail in Vauthier: *"Le Jury de lecture de l'Opéra . . . d'après les papiers de la Maison du roi," La Revue musicale*, Paris 1910, 1–3; and in Henri de Curzon: *Rossini*. Rossini later reported many of the attendant circumstances to Ferdinand Hiller.

   p. 164, ll. 36–7   "and women"   An *affiche* for the *première* of *Guillaume Tell* listed the singers as: "M^rs Ad.-Nourrit, Dabadie, Levasseur, Bonel, Prévost, Alexis, Ferdinand-Prevôt, Massol, Pouilley, Trevaux; Mmes Cinti-Damoreau, Dabadie, Mori, Didier." The libretto printed for sale in connection with the first performances listed the cast this way: Guillaume Tell (M. Dabadie), Arnold Melcthal (M. A. Nourrit); Walter Furst (M. Levasseur), Melcthal (M. Bonel), Jemmy (Mme Dabadie), Gesler (M. Prévost), Rodolphe (M. Massol), Ruodi (M. Alex. Dupont), Leuthold (M. Ferd. Prevôt), Mathilde (Mme Cinti-Damoreau), Hedwige (Mlle Mori). Eugène-Etienne-Auguste Massol later would create roles in Donizetti's *Les Martyrs* and *Dom Sébastien*. The *affiche* (reproduced in *ROG*, op. p. 97) also lists the dancers: "Messieurs Albert, Paul, Lefebvre, Montessu, Simon, Daumont, Frémol; Mmes Noblet, Legallois, Montessu, [Marie] Taglioni, Elie, Buron, Alexis, Dupuis, Perceval."

   p. 165, l. 12   "the score"   In *Petits Mémoires de l'Opéra*, p. 302, Charles de Boigne wrote: "The first twelve performances [of *Tell*] brought in 71,247 francs 40 centimes, that is to say, 5,937 francs per performance— which, added to the 800 francs from annual subscriptions, make a total of 6,737 francs, about the same figures as today. If we place against these receipts for *Guillaume Tell* the receipts from the first twelve performances of *Robert le Diable, La Juive, Les Huguenots, Le Prophète, Jérusalem* [the French version of Verdi's *I Lombardi alla prima crociata*], *Les Vêpres siciliennes*, those for *Guillaume Tell* are very inferior. Ought we to conclude on the basis of these figures that Rossini is inferior to Meyerbeer, Halévy, Verdi? I should have great difficulty in resigning myself to that notion, above all if, returning to the charge, I leaf through the Opéra's accounts; and if I go back to the year 1837, to that year which witnessed the debut of Duprez and the restaging of *Guillaume Tell*, then the first ten performances rise to 121,000 [francs]."

p. 165, l. 22   "in the score"   The famous scene with the apple, then, had been excised.

p. 165, l. 28   "a work"   On September 17, 1834, nonetheless, *Guillaume Tell* had had its official hundredth performance at the Opéra, with its original cast except that Cornélie Falcon was now the Mathilde, Gosselin the Hedwige, Prosper Dérivis the Melcthal. How the continuing popularity of *Tell* touched Richard Wagner was told by him in *Mein Leben*. Speaking of 1846, he wrote ("Authorized Translation," New York, 1911): "While I was first planning the music to *Lohengrin*, I was disturbed incessantly by the echoes of some of the airs in Rossini's *William Tell*, which was the last opera I had had to conduct. At last I happened to hit on an effective means of stopping this annoying obtrusion: during my lonely walks I sang with great emphasis the first theme from the Ninth Symphony [Beethoven], which had also quite lately been revived in my memory. This succeeded!" Wagner remembered the scene of the apple ("*Sois immobile*") from *Tell* well enough to cite it to Rossini during their only conversation, in 1860.

p. 165, l. 35   "*whole thing?*"   *Guillaume Tell* was not treated worse than several other operas. Auber's very popular *Gustave III*, first sung at the Opéra on February 27, 1833, received forty-one performances up to April 27, 1834. Thereafter, its first four acts were temporarily dropped and its spectacular Act V—the masked ball—was appended to singings of other repertoire operas. Charles Bouvet reported that this ball scene had been presented by itself seventeen times. On March 30, 1847, Delacroix noted in his journal: "To the Théâtre des Italiens with Mme de Forget: the first act of *Il Matrimonio segreto*, the second of *Nabucco*, the second and third of *Otello*."

p. 166, l. 1   "Boigne wrote"   *Petits Mémoires de l'Opéra*, p. 302.

p. 166, l. 7   "us dear"   Boigne implied that Meyerbeer's great popularity alone had driven Rossini into retirement. That long-held belief will not withstand the test of contemporary evidence.

p. 166, l. 12   "their Sabbath"   This undocumented anecdote is undated. If it derived from Rossini's talks with Édouard Robert and Carlo Severini, codirectors of the Théâtre-Italien, at Bologna in the early 1830's, it can refer only to Meyerbeer; but if it dated from later, the Jewish composers may also have included Halévy and Offenbach.

p. 166, l. 27   "immediate predecessors"   "*Fra Gorgheggi e melodie di Rossini.*"

p. 167, l. 30   "longer existed"   Forty years after the *première* of *Guillaume Tell*, Giuseppe Verdi wrote to Camille Du Locle: "Certainly no one would deny genius to Rossini! Well, then: despite all his genius, in *Guglielmo Tell* one detects that fatal atmosphere of the Opéra, and at times, though less often than with other composers, one feels that there is something bigger and something smaller and that the musical working-out is not so sincere and secure as in *Il Barbiere*." Verdi almost certainly was apologizing unconsciously for one area of his own composing life; the lack of security that he detected in *Guillaume Tell* was to be found—and for closely related reasons—in his own Paris operas and revisions: *Jérusalem* (*I Lombardi*), *Les Vêpres siciliennes*, the revised *Macbeth*, and *Don Carlos*, not one of which is a successful artistic whole.

p. 168, l. 2 "Joseph Méry" François-Joseph Méry (1797–1865), a *marseillais*, became one of the most prolific writers of his time, producing huge quantities of journalism, poetry, fiction, and librettos. A passionate admirer and close friend of Rossini, he made the French translation of Rossi's libretto for *Semiramide* (1854) and wrote an introduction to the Brothers Escudiers' life of Rossini. Having written librettos for setting by Félicien David and Ernest Reyer, he had begun to prepare a text for Verdi's *Don Carlos* when he died (it was completed by Camille Du Locle). In *Voyageurs et romanciers*, Barbey d'Aurevilly said of Méry that "he always had the facility of genius, even on days on which he did not have its power."

p. 168, l. 27 "with Rossini" The complete text of this letter is given in Francesco Pastura: *Bellini secondo la storia*, p. 220.

p. 169, l. 17 "the Cantùs" The family of Giuditta Cantù Turina, Bellini's mistress.

NOTES TO CHAPTER XI

p. 170, l. 6 "see page 110)" The singers for *Il Serto votivo* were Annetta Fink-Lohr (Argene), Ippolita Ferlotti (Melania), Francesco Regoli (Fileno), and Gennaro Simoni (Elpino).

p. 170, ll. 19–20 "Francesco Sampieri" Sampieri, a close friend of Rossini's, was an accomplished semiprofessional musician and composer.

p. 170, i. 22 "of Geronio" Writing (September 29, 1829) to Paris about difficulties over engaging Malibran for the Théâtre-Italien (she was demanding what she eventually obtained: 1,075 francs per performance and exclusive rights to the roles in her repertoire), Robert said: "At Milan, I again encountered the *urlo francese*, which Rossini had rid us of at the Opéra, and which seems to have established its empire in Italy. I am scandalized, and Rossini no longer goes, as it was not like this in his time. Such delicious talents as Rubini and Tamburini are not listened to when they sing in a ravishing manner. Now the Italians listen to music like the English and neither applaud nor call out the actors except when they shout like demons; also, these unhappy singers are worn out; they lose their talent and shorten their careers. What would become of our dear Mme Malibran in these theaters, and with so barbarous and vandalous a public?"

p. 171, l. 14 "La Rochefoucauld" The autograph of this letter is in the Bibliothèque Nationale, Paris.

p. 171, l. 21 "to Severini" Andrea Cipriano Ghedini, Severini's brother-in-law, seems to have introduced the young former Bolognese tax collector to Rossini in Paris, wanting to assist his young relative in establishing himself there. Severini soon became attached to the Théâtre-Italien, and by 1830, though officially sharing the directorship with Édouard Robert, was in effect its managing director.

p. 172, l. 9 "Lord Burghersh"   For Burghersh, see p. 18 and note for that page.

p. 172, l. 11 "Lorenzo Bartolini"   Bartolini (1777–1850) attempted to lead Italian sculpture back to "realistic" models, calling himself an anti-classicist. At his funeral in 1850, Rossini held one of the ribbons attached to the funeral coach.

p. 175, l. 25 "when Crescentini"   One of Colbran's early teachers had been the great sopranist, composer, and singing teacher Girolamo Crescentini (1762–1846).

p. 175, l. 28 "to death"   Isabella had been whistled at during a performance of *Maometto II* at Venice in December 1822 (see p. 128), though hardly "to death."

p. 175, l. 39 "and grumbling"   *"Rossini," La Revue musicale*, Paris, 9/1902, 374.

p. 176, l. 29–30 "abandoned wife"   This letter is in the Raccolta Piancastelli, Forlì, which also contains several letters that Isabella wrote to such close friends of Rossini as Carlo Severini and Principessa Maria Hercolani. Mostly these are inquiries about the condition of Rossini's health.

p. 178, l. 24 "the Queen"   María Cristina, Ferdinand VII's fourth wife, was a sister of Francis I of the Two Sicilies, who had died the previous year.

p. 178, l. 38 "his wife"   Francisco de Paula, Duque de Cádiz, had married Luisa Carlota, like his brother's queen a sister of Francis I of the Two Sicilies.

p. 179, l. 23 "Giovanni Tadolini"   Tadolini (1793–1872) was a Bolognese choral conductor and composer who had been a fellow student of Rossini's under Mattei at the Liceo. By 1831, he was a conductor and *maître de chant* at the Italien. Besides chamber music and religious pieces, Tadolini wrote operas that were staged between 1815 and 1827. His wife was the famous operatic soprano Eugenia (Savorini) Tadolini.

p. 181, l. 18 "desperately bored"   The tone of a letter from Rossini to a Mme de la Tour de St.-Ygest at Bordeaux, dated June 9, 1832, at Bayonne (original in the Bibliothèque Nationale, Paris), strongly suggests an apology for unceremonious departure after intimate relations. The fact that in another letter to the same lady, dated from Pau on June 17, 1832 (Piancastelli Collection, Forlì), Rossini asks that she thank her husband for a proof of friendship does not rule out that possibility.

p. 181, l. 22 "come back"   Robert's letter is quoted in *LTI*, p. 58.

p. 181, l. 27 "in October"   Writing to Rossini on about October 20, 1832, his father said: "I am infinitely pleased to learn from your dear letter of the 7th of the present month that you have arrived at Petitbergo [Petit-Bourg] in company with the amiable Aguado . . ." A letter from Rossini to Giuseppe Ancillo, introducing Eugenia Tadolini, is dated at Paris on November 10, 1832.

p. 181, l. 31   "at Aix-les-Bains"   Emanuele Muzio, writing to Antonio Barezzi, Verdi's father-in-law (*Giuseppe Verdi nelle lettere di Emanuele Muzio ad Antonio Barezzi*, ed. A. Garibaldi, Milan, 1931, p. 146), said that Rossini had met Olympe at Horace Vernet's home while she was living with the painter, which is possible, though he seems more likely to have met her first outside Paris. In a wildly inaccurate article (*"Le Salon de Rossini"*), Victor du Bled decribed Olympe as "a very ordinary actress, accomplished woman of affairs, who, it would seem, had a partly artistic, partly political, partly gallant, salon, rue Neuve-du-Luxembourg, and refused to marry Balzac, who drew her portrait in *La Peau de chagrin* . . ." In *Prométhée, ou La Vie de Balzac* (Paris, 1965), André Maurois stated that Olympe had been the mistress of Eugène Sue; that her salon was frequented by "such distinguished figures as the Duc de Fitz-James, Horace Vernet, and Rossini"; that, though she was not the original of Foedora in *La Peau de chagrin*, the famous bedroom scene in that story "is said to have been enacted in real life between Balzac and Olympe Pélissier"; and that Balzac had often visited Olympe "in the charming village of Ville-d'Avray." None of this is documented. Olympe had been born on the 20th Floréal of the Fifth Year of the Republic—that is, on May 20, 1796.

p. 182, l. 15   "*et Holopherne*"   Jarro (Giulio Piccini) said that the recalled model for this Judith was Colbran (*Giovacchino Rossini e la sua famiglia*, p. 7); he had confused the two Mmes Rossini.

p. 183, l. 2   "(see page 304)"   *Giovanna d'Arco* in its original piano version has been published (*QR* XI, Pesaro, 1965, which also includes a fragment of the 1852 version with accompaniment of violins, violas, and doublebasses).

p. 183, l. 19   "Gioacchino Rossini' "   "*Profilo medico-psicologico di Gioacchino Rossini*," *LRM*, 7–9 1954, p. 292.

p. 183, l. 23   "the pyknic"   "Stout; fat; characterized by a large abdomen, squatness, and general roundness of form."—*Webster's New International Dictionary*, 2d edn.

p. 184, ll. 8–9   "a cyclothymic"   Cyclothymia describes "a temperament characterized by alternation of lively and depressed moods, believed to predispose the individual toward manic-depressive insanity . . ."—*Webster's New International Dictionary*, 2d edn.

p. 184, l. 31   "Donizetti replied."   Donizetti's letter is in the Raccolta Piancastelli, Forlì; it is quoted in full in *Studi Donizettiani* I, Bergamo, 1962, p. 21. The letter from Rossini to which Donizetti was replying seems not to have survived.

p. 185, l. 29   "*di Siviglia*"   Signed "B," the item in *BdS* 8/16/1834, p. 263, contains this paragraph: "Signora Tadolini sang many things with uncommon mastery and almost always displayed happily her beautiful soprano voice. But those changes of *fioriture* in the cavatina, those arbitrary ornamentations of the character passages in the other pieces, if they seemed gems to many, certainly did not seem such to those who, like me, consider it sacrilegious to ruin the texture and nature of any role, above all of a role like that of *Rosina*, already clothed by its sublime author in so much and such pure and characteristic elegance."

p. 187, l. 5 "lifetime annuity"   The Bibliothèque Nationale, Paris, has a long letter written in French by someone else and signed by Rossini, dated June 27, 1833, in which Rossini pursues the question of the annuity with Baron de Schonen, "*Commissaire liquidateur de l'ancienne Liste Civile.*"

p. 188, ll. 22–3 "Rossini's affairs"   These "affairs" evidently were related to Isabella Rossini's landholdings and other assets in Sicily.

p. 188, ll. 36–7 "January 24, 1835"   The genuinely all-star cast of this *première* was headed by Giulia Grisi (Elvira), Giovanni Battista Rubini (Arturo), Antonio Tamburini (Riccardo), and Luigi Lablache (Giorgio).

p. 189, l. 10 "to now"   Rossini wrote at the top of a page on which Bellini then also wrote to Santocanale.

p. 189, l. 24 "that opera"   Radiciotti also pointed out (*RAD* I, 351) that the adagio section of "*I Marinai*" was borrowed from the chorus in Act II of *Ricciardo e Zoraide*, where it is heard during Zoraide's imprisonment.

p. 189, ll. 29–30 "accomplished dilettantes"   In 1838, Liszt also wrote his piano transcription of the overture to *Guillaume Tell*, which was published in 1846.

p. 189, l. 33 "himself included"   Mme Benazet and her husband are mentioned in a letter of August 18, 1863, from Rossini to either Andrea or Antonio Peruzzi, now in the Bibliothèque Nationale, Paris. The album, which was rediscovered by the Milanese collector Natale Gallini, contains eighteen separate numbers. The composers represented include Cherubini, Sir Michael Costa, Mercadante, Meyerbeer, Morlacchi, George Onslow, Paër, Spontini, Giovanni Tadolini, and Rossini. Rossini's "*Mi lagnerò tacendo*" is a setting of the text from Act II, Scene 1 of Metastasio's *Siroe* which he set hundreds of times. The entire Louise Carlier album has been recorded.

p. 190, l. 13 "Opéra directorship"   In a letter of August 8, 1835, to Carlo Severini (then in Italy), Rossini wrote from Paris: "You will have learned that at a review for the anniversary of [the] July [Revolution], they tried with an infernal machine to kill the King and the Princes around him. Fortunately, the blow failed." On July 28, the Corsican Giuseppe Maria Fieschi had made an unsuccessful attempt upon the life of Louis-Philippe, killing eighteen bystanders. Fieschi and his accomplices were executed on February 16, 1836.

p. 192, l. 3 "dear friend"   At Frankfurt-am-Main in mid-June 1836, Lionel de Rothschild (1808–79) married his cousin Charlotte Rothschild in a splendid ceremony attended by members of their family from London, Naples, Vienna, and Paris, and by the eighty-five-year-old widow of Meyer Amschel Rothschild, founder of the banking dynasty and grandfather of the groom.

p. 192, l. 10 "several days"   One part of the *Péchés de vieillesse*, the *Album des enfants dégourdis*, contains a "*comique-imitatif*" entitled "*Un*

Petit Train de plaisir," not all of which is comic. The indications above its sections reflect Rossini's reactions to the ride by train from Antwerp to Brussels in 1836: "*Cloche d'Appel—Montée en Wagon—En avant la machine —Sifflet satanique—Douce mélodie du Frein—Arrivée à la Gare—Les Lions Parisiens offrant la main aux Biches pour descendre du Wagon—Suite du Voyage—Terrible déraillement du convoi—Premier Blessé—Second Blessé —Premier mort en Paradis—Second mort en Enfer—Chante funèbre—Amen —On ne m'y attrapera pas. G. R.—Douleur aiguë des héritiers—Tout ceci est plus que naïf c'est vrai.*" "*Un Petit Train de plaisir*" was published (*QR* II, Pesaro, 1954); Alfredo Bonaccorsi, in his preface to it, pointed out that at the time when Rossini probably composed it (1860–5), drawings of trains plunging over precipices were common and may have influenced him.

p. 192, l. 36 "Hiller wrote" *PmR.*

p. 194, l. 6 "wrote operas" Actually, Mendelssohn had composed one opera and one "*Liederspiel*" that was almost an opera. The former, *Die Hochzeit des Camacho,* had been performed once (Berlin, April 29, 1827); the latter, *Die Heimkehr aus der Fremde* (known in England as *Son and Stranger*), had been performed privately in 1829; it was staged publicly in Leipzig on April 10, 1851.

p. 194, l. 17 "brief cure" A two-line musical autograph to a "M.r Revenaz"(?), dated at Kissingen on August 16, 1836, survives in the Bibliothèque Nationale, Paris.

p. 194, l. 34 "Lauzières wrote" "*Memorie di un giornalista,*" in *Capitan Fracassa,* Rome, September 1885.

p. 195, l. 36 "La Fenice . . ." The opera chosen to reopen La Fenice was no gayer or more festive or less full of "miseries" than *Guglielmo Tell:* it was Donizetti's *Lucia di Lammermoor.*

NOTES TO CHAPTER XII

p. 197, l. 1 "were rooms" The added buildings cost Rossini a total of 3,100 scudi (about $9,787). When he came to sell them, along with the *palazzo* itself, he obtained 10,500 scudi (about $33,150), 2,250 scudi more than the three purchases together had cost him; the sale, however, represented a net loss to him because of the elaborate work he had done to and in the *palazzo.*

p. 197, l. 36 "successive addresses" When Olympe arrived in Bologna in 1837, her quarters were at No. 1046, Via dei Libri (later Nos. 3–5, Via Farini); in 1839, she moved to No. 1094, Borgo Salamo (later No. 10, Via Farini); and from 1840 until her marriage to Rossini, she was at No. 83, Strada Santo Stefano (now No. 36). Isabella's winter residence, to which Olympe probably went to meet her, was at No. 2593, Via San Donato (later No. 34, Via Zamboni); from May 1839 on, she lived in the Palazzo Fantuzzi, No. 118 Via San Vitale (now No. 23); and in 1842 she lived at No. 879, Via San Vitale (later Via Guido Reni, 3) when not at Castenaso.

p. 200, l. 4 "winter season" During November 1837, Mercadante's opera *I Briganti* was so little liked by audiences at La Scala that it was sung only four times. On December 26, 1837, those present at the *première* of Mercadante's *Il Giuramento* at La Scala loudly disapproved of it. And on January 9, 1838, Carlo Conti's opera *Gli Aragonesi di Napoli* (1827) aroused a Scala audience to noisy complaint; it was not repeated.

p. 200, l. 9 "Madame Pasta"   At the end of her career, Pasta was living in her villa on Lake Como, where Rossini and Olympe spent five days with her in November 1837 (letter from Olympe to Antonio Zoboli, November 29, 1837, quoted in *BdCRdS* 1960, 3, 46).

p. 201, l. 7 "at length"   An undated letter from Rossini to Robert in the Raccolta Piancastelli at Forlì almost certainly is the one of January 23, 1838, mentioned by Robert in a letter to Rossini quoted in *LTI*, p. 100.

p. 201, l. 31 "by Rossini"   The singers included Santina Ferlotti-Sangiorgi, Giovanni Conforti, Paolo Ambrosini, and Giuseppe Bruscoli.

p. 202, l. 8 "Branca girls"   Paolo Branca had four daughters: Cirilla, who married the musical biographer Isidoro Cambiasi; Emilia, who married the librettist-editor Felice Romani; Luigia, who married a man named Wereb; and Matilde, who became Signora Juva.

p. 202, l. 9 "cousin Tonino"   Both of the counts Belgiojoso were good amateur musicians. Pompeo was a close friend of Rossini, who designed the *Quoniam* of the *Petite Messe solennelle* with his voice in mind; he would sing the bass solo in the *Stabat Mater* at its first performance in Italy (Bologna, 1842).

p. 202, l. 11 "a biography"   *Felice Romani ed i più riputati maestri di musica del suo tempo, cenni biografici ed aneddotici raccolti e pubblicati da sua moglie.*

p. 203, l. 20 "January 1839"   A letter from Rossini to Ippolito Rosselini (1800–43), dated January 1, 1839 (Raccolta Piancastelli, Forlì), indicates an intimate friendship with the great Egyptologist, but no further details of the relationship seem available to research.

p. 203, ll. 29–30 "February 1842"   See Appendix B. The postmarks on this document read "Bologna" and "8 Fevr." but show no year. However, on December 15, 1841. Olympe had written Couvert to ask him to arrange a consultation for Rossini with the leading Paris specialists in urinary diseases; in it, she mentioned that a man whom she described as "more friend than physician to Rossini" was preparing a report summarizing the stages of her husband's illness. And on February 6, 1842, she wrote a letter that almost certainly accompanied the report itself: "Here is the consultation or, more exactly, the observations made by his ordinary physician on the condition of my dear invalid."

p. 204, l. 7 "unidentifiable friend"   Letter in the Raccolta Piancastelli, Forlì.

p. 204, l. 18 "a letter"   Letter in the library of the Conservatorio G. B. Martini, Bologna. It was photographically reproduced in *Rossiniana* between pp. 16 and 17. Ugo Pesci rightly described it as "very different from his [Rossini's] others, which generally are very slipshod in style, and also often in orthography." Pesci's opinion was that Rossini "had had it written by Paolo Giordani" ("*Nel Primo Centenario del Liceo Musicale in Bologna*").

p. 207, l. 9 "of 1840" Pietro Romani conducted from the harpsichord; the cast was listed as including Luigi Maggiorotti, Nicholas Ivanoff, Luigi Biondini, and Antonio Giacomelli.

p. 208, ll. 11–12 "many autographs!!!!" *Rodolfo di Sterlinga* was not put on at La Fenice. *Guglielmo Tell* as such finally was staged there during the 1856 summer season. Rossini and Ancillo kept up a running joke about Ancillo's collecting Rossini autographs.

p. 208, l. 31 "Liceo Comunale" The Accademia, wanting to notify Rossini of this honor on his name-day, withheld notification for five months. On September 6, Rossini wrote to the Marchese Antonio Bolognini Amorini of the Accademia, referring to Bologna as "my sweet home," an opinion he was to change in 1848.

p. 209, l. 33 "*la musique*" The first edition of Fétis's *Biographie universelle* appeared in 1833–34, the second in 1860–5. After Fétis's death in 1871, two supplementary volumes (1878–80) were edited by Arthur Pougin. Rossini long had been a favorite with compilers of biographical data. The so-called "Sainsbury," a two-volume work entitled *A Dictionary of Musicians* (London, 1824, a compilation by its publisher, John H. Sainsbury), had devoted twelve and a half two-column pages to him.

p. 211, l. 30 "your career" Did Rossini remember this conversation with Fétis in 1863–4, when composing the *Petite Messe solennelle*?

p. 211, l. 34 "his *Stabat. . . .*" If Fétis's statement is correct, he visited Rossini in September 1841: on September 22 of that year, Rossini signed with Troupenas an agreement concerning the *Stabat Mater*. Neither Fétis nor Rossini, of course, could foresee the *Petite Messe solennelle*.

p. 214, l. 29 "final chorus" Rossini thus had reduced the number of sections in the *Stabat Mater* to ten: 1. "*Stabat Mater dolorosa*," chorus with tenor solo; 2. "*Cujus animam gementem*," tenor aria; 3. "*Quis est homo qui non fleret*," soprano duet; 4. "*Pro peccatis suae gentis*," bass solo; 5. "*Eja Mater, fons amoris*," unaccompanied chorus with bass solo; 6. "*Sancta Mater, istud agas*," quartet for two sopranos, tenor, and bass; 7. "*Fac ut portem Christi mortem*," cavatina for second soprano; 8. "*Inflammatus et accensus*," aria for first soprano with chorus; 9. "*Quando corpus morietur*," unaccompanied quartet; 10. "*In sempiterna saecula—Amen*," four-voice fugue for vocal quartet.

p. 215, l. 10 "*Gazette musicale*" Maurice-Adolphe (Mortiz Adolf) Schlésinger (1797–1871) was a son of Martin Adolf Schlesinger, who at Berlin (1810) had founded the Schlesingersche Buch- und Musikalienhandlung and the influential *Berliner Allgemeine Musikalische Zeitung* (1824–1830)—and who had published Bach's *Matthäuspassion* shortly after its 1829 revival by Mendelssohn. In 1834, Maurice Schlésinger launched a Paris music-publishing house and began to issue *La Gazette musicale*, which the following year was combined with Fétis's *Revue Musicale* (1827–35) as *La Revue et Gazette musicale* (1835–80). Financial difficulties forced Schlésinger to sell his business in 1846; thereafter, he returned to Germany. The woman known as Mme Maurice Schlésinger (1810–88, born Élisa Foucault) was the wife of one Jacques-Émile Judée, whom she had married in 1829, and who died in 1839; in 1840, Schlésinger, a Jew, became a Catholic so that they could be legally married. At Trouville in 1836—Schlésinger long owned the Hôtel Bellevue there—the fifteen-year-old Gustave Flaubert had fallen deeply in love with the twenty-six-year-old "Mme Schlésinger"; his intense, probably Platonic attachment to her endured for the rest of their lives. Flaubert portrayed Mme Schlésinger several times—in *Novembre*; in *Mémoires d'un fou*; as Émilie Renaud in the first version of *L'Éducation sentimentale*; and as Marie Arnoux in the published final version (in which Schlésinger appears as Jacques Arnoux, Flaubert himself as Frédéric).

    p. 215, l. 22   "and Aulagnier"   The *Revue et Gazette musicale* lent all possible support to the Aulagnier-Schlésinger cause; the Escudiers' *France musicale* favored Rossini and Troupenas.

    p. 215, l. 39   "the Escudiers"   *LfS*, p. 261.

    p. 218, l. 19   "first performance"   Heine: *Sämtliche Werke* VII, 217.

    p. 220, ll. 20–1   "still reverberating"   In May 1837, Heine, writing to August Lewald, had contrasted the music of Rossini and that of Meyerbeer. He saw Rossini as a composer of and in melody, for which reason his music appealed to subjective, spontaneous, isolated emotions such as joy, sorrow, love, hate, jealousy, longing, and tenderness. Meyerbeer, on the other hand, was a composer of harmony, for which reason reactions to his music submerged personal emotions in such public reactions as patriotism and love of liberty. Heine added that this explained why each composer appealed to one historic period: Rossini could not have been appreciated during the Napoleonic era, when emotions surged up *en masse*. Significantly, he said, the time of Rossini's greatest triumphs in France had been the Restoration (*Französische Maler* I, 220).

    Richard Wagner attacked Rossini and the *Stabat Mater* "maliciously and with heavy Teutonic humour" (Ernest Newman: *The Life of Richard Wagner* I, 383) in a pseudonymous article signed H. Valentino, in the *Neue Zeitschrift für Musik* of December 28, 1841. Three decades later, he included the article in his *Gesammelte Schrifte* I.

NOTES TO CHAPTER XIII

    p. 221, l. 16   "Carlo Bevilacqua"   The Marchese Carlo Bevilacqua, active in the affairs of the Liceo Musicale, was to be an executor of Rossini's will and to inherit the autograph manuscript of the *Stabat Mater*, which, after his death, members of his family presented to the Liceo (1875).

    p. 222, l. 7   "superannuated musicians"   Decades later, the Fondation Rossini, a similar institution, was built in Passy with funds willed by Olympe Rossini. It, in turn, well may have been one inspiration for the Casa di Riposo that Verdi's will was to establish in Milan.

    p. 223, l. 14   "brother-in-law) wrote"   *Gaetano Donizetti: Biografia*, Rome and Turin, 1904, p. 89.

p. 224, l. 28 "his companions" Bolognese interest in the *Stabat Mater* continued so great that in March 1853, Principessa Maria Hercolani (who in 1829 had married as her second husband the great actor Francesco Lombardi) had it performed in her palace to the accompaniment of piano and strings under the direction of Domenico Liverani. Her daughter, Principessa Teresa Angelelli-Simonetti, accompanied at the piano; the chief singers were the twenty-five-year-old soprano Virginia Boccabadati; the contralto Marietta Aldini, a "dilettante"; the tenor Pietro Neri; and the bass Filippo Coliva. Clementina Degli Antonj took part in the concluding quartet; the chorus included such notable singers as Domenico Donzelli, Nicholas Ivanoff, Antonio Poggi, and Carlo Zucchelli. Meanwhile, the *Stabat Mater* had begun its unfailingly victorious journeys across the world. Radiciotti (*RAD* II, 260) listed twenty-seven cities in addition to Paris and Bologna in which the *Stabat Mater* was heard before the end of 1842—and even so omitted Vienna, where it was sung in May. At many of its early singings, it was preceded by a potpourri overture that Mercadante had arranged on its chief melodies. Rossini, who much disliked that innovation, said to the critic Alessandro Biaggi: "If my *Stabat* had needed an overture, I should have been aware of that, and would have composed it myself." But see p. 246.

On March 22, 1842, at a meeting of the Bologna magistracy, a motion was passed to place in the Liceo Comunale a marble bust of Rossini to be carved by Cincinnato Baruzzi. At a later date, the authorities decided that the planned installation would overbalance the room originally selected for it, and decided to install the bust in the Archiginnasio. For many reasons, the entire project was dropped in the autumn of 1843. Zanolini believed that much of Rossini's later rancor against the Bolognese was caused by that failure, but that belief is impossible to share in view of the more obvious causes of Rossini's feeling. On the first anniversary of Rossini's death, the memorial stone still to be seen in the Archiginnasio auditorium was dedicated. Its incised inscription reads:

IN THIS HALL ON THE DAY MARCH 18, 1842
FOR THE FIRST TIME IN ITALY
RESOUNDED IN FULL CONCERT
THE DIVINE MELODIES OF THE STABAT MATER
OF
Gioachino Rossini
THE ORCHESTRA AND THE SINGING WERE DIRECTED BY
GAETANO DONIZETTI
INTERPRETER WORTHY OF THE COMPOSER

———————————

THE MUNICIPALITY, BY UNANIMOUS VOTE OF THE COUNCIL,
INSTALLED THIS MEMORIAL ON THE DAY NOVEMBER 13, 1869
FIRST ANNIVERSARY
OF THE DEATH OF ROSSINI

p. 226, ll. 2-3   "[Camillo] Pizzardi"   The Marchese Camillo Pizzardi, mentioned elsewhere in Rossini's letters, was one of his Bologna intimates.

p. 226, l. 7   "Gioachino Rossini"   Valuable for the light that it plays on the musical customs of 1842 and on Donizetti's character, a transcript of the page with the emendations mentioned by Rossini is given in *LdR*, p. 127, footnote 1. The points established by Donizetti's original proposals and the emendations were chiefly: (1) Donizetti was to teach both counterpoint and composition; (2) he was to have between ten and fifteen students in each class; (3) he was to be in Bologna for the school opening between October 5 and 9; (4) he was to be present for the *festa* of San Petronio, could be absent from his duties on special leave for no more than two months each year, and was to make up for classes missed by holding them at other times; (5) he must provide a substitute teacher during his absences; (6) he was to supply one new composition each year, the costs of copying to be paid by the *cappella* of San Petronio; (7) he was to be supplied with decent lodgings or the equivalent in money; (8) the *cappella* would agree to any leaves granted by the Liceo; (9) he would have the use of Liceo pupils for playing or singing gratis any music that he gave in San Petronio; (10) the *cappella* was to furnish the proper number of singers and players for all performances; (11) at the theater, Donizetti was to be responsible for every performance that he conducted. The twelfth clause deserves translation in full: "(12) My annual honorarium, the *cappella* and the Liceo combined, will be 720 Roman scudi. The director of the Naples Liceo receives 100 ducats, lodgings, and food each month, and has no other duty." The comment on that reads: "The honorarium would always be inadequate for the most distinguished merit of the *signor cavaliere* Donizetti. If Bologna could have the resources of Naples, it too would make it proportionate; because, further, at the Conservatory-boarding school [San Pietro a Maiella] of that capital the cares and responsibility of the director are extensive and permanent. But Bologna is a provincial city that has for itself and its establishment nothing but its good fortune and Rossini. These do not suffice to overcome every difficulty; but it is to be hoped with all confidence that it is more than sufficient to deal with the most gentlemanly *signor cavaliere* Donizetti."

p. 226, ll. 8-9   "have survived"   Donizetti made his Vienna debut on May 4, 1842, conducting Rossini's *Stabat Mater* in the presence of the Emperor, Empress, and Dowager Empress. Two days later, he wrote to Antonio Vasselli: "Two days ago at court to perform the *Stabat* with two pianofortes, sixteen choristers, la [Eugenia] Tadolini, la [Marietta] Brambilla, [Napoleone] Moriani, [Domenico] Donzelli, [Cesare] Badiali, and [Prosper] Dérivis. It went very well, and His Imperial Highness the Emperor and the two Empresses (the widow and the reigning), all the brothers, and their wives, besides the Prince of Salerno, came to me over and over again to testify to their pleasure in so perfected a performance and to the sensations that they had experienced." On May 30 and June 8, Donizetti conducted the first two public performances of the *Stabat Mater* in Vienna, at the Redoutensaal, these with orchestra.

p. 227, l. 5 "hours later" A naturalized Frenchman, ennobled by the King of Spain as Marqués de las Marismas, this very rich patron of painting and music had been a Maecenas to Rossini and others, had supported the Théâtre-Italien in Paris, and had formed a notable collection of paintings. He left an estate valued at about 60,000,000 francs (about $31,000,000), made largely in speculative banking after his retirement in 1815 from services as aide-de-camp to Marshal Soult.

p. 227, l. 19 "Giovanni André" This transcription was published and sold by the Bolognese music dealer Valentino Zinotti.

p. 228, l. 17 "G. Rossini" Rossini's letter to Costa of September 12, 1842, is in the Raccolta Piancastelli at Forlì. As Frank Walker well wrote ("Rossiniana in the Piancastelli Collection"), "Outstanding among all the Rossini autographs at Forlì is a group of forty-four letters to Michele Costa, the Neapolitan conductor and composer who, after Rossini's death, became Sir Michael Costa and a naturalized Englishman. No fewer than twenty-four of them are letters of introduction, presented by musicians visiting London from Italy or Paris, but the variety of styles, the humour and oddity displayed, prevent any monotony. When Rossini wished to please he was irresistible, however badly he wrote or spelt. In this case he very much wished to please. It was a profound need of his nature to feel himself surrounded always by affection and friendship. His quasi-paternal relationship with Nikolay Ivanov in the '40s and early '50s was succeeded by a similar relationship with Costa in the '60s. In the collection at Forlì there are seven letters spread over the twenty-three years from 1836 to 1859; then there are thirty-five letters dating from 1860 to 1868, in which Costa is addressed as though he really were Rossini's son. . . . In the correspondence with Costa, Rossini produced some of his masterpieces in epistolary *buffo* style; nowhere else does he appear so engaging, so truly lovable."

p. 228, l. 23 "the report" See Appendix B, p. 379, for the text of this physician's report.

p. 229, l. 2 "Poniatowski family" The Poniatowskis were close friends of Rossini. Prince Stanislao Poniatowski, a grandson of Stanislas II Augustus, King of Poland, had settled in Rome in the late eighteenth century. Marrying a Roman girl, he had had four children: Giuseppe (Józef Michał, 1816–73), who became a naturalized Tuscan in 1847, later removed to Paris (where he was made a senator by Napoleon III), and composed Masses and operas; Prince Carlo, whom Rossini called "first in merit among musical amateurs"; a daughter who became a Marchesa Piccolelli; and a daughter Costanza who married the Marchese Daniele Zappi. Writing from Florence on October 3, 1851, to Prince Carlo, Rossini was to say: " P.S. Last night I dreamed that Donna Elisa [Prince Carlo's wife, born Montecatini], whom I adore and revere, weary of country life, arrived unexpectedly at the [Teatro della] Pergola, drove the present *prima donna* from the stage, and performed the role of Desdemona with that voice of hers which one feels in one's spirit, and thus rejuvenated *Otello*, which, like its composer, is in the plenitude of its decrepitude."

p. 229, l. 15   "Jean Civiale"   Civiale was thus described by Arturo Castiglioni (*A History of Medicine*, 2nd edn., New York, 1947, p. 872): "Lithotripsy [the breakup of bladder stones], studied by Fournier (1783–1845) and Gruithuisen, was perfected by Jean Civiale (1792–1867) with the use of better instruments, which were still further improved upon by Mercier, Charrière, and Collin. Civiale, a master of his subject and a skilful technician, created the urological service at the Necker Hospital, where the school was founded from which emerged many of the world's greatest urologists, such as J. D. d'Étiolles (1798–1860) and C. L. Herteloup (1793–1864)."

p. 229, l. 18   "Alessandro Mombelli"   Mombelli, who taught singing at the Liceo after being brought there by Rossini, was a son of Rossini's old friends Domenico and Vincenza (Viganò) Mombelli.

p. 230, ll. 12–13   "and Donizetti"   The triumphant *première* of *Don Pasquale* had taken place at the Théâtre-Italien on January 3, 1843.

p. 231, l. 6   "Emmanuel Dupaty"   Emmanuel Mercier-Dupaty had written numerous French librettos from 1792 on for such composers as Boieldieu, Dalayrac, and Isouard.

p. 231, l. 12   "*Robert Bruce*"   See p. 238.

p. 231, l. 17   "September 20, 1843"   A curious honor was bestowed upon Rossini on this same day *in absentia*. In Lugo, where he once had lived briefly, a movement had been initiated in October 1841 to nominate him a "*consigliere comunale*" in the place of the recently deceased Grand Chamberlain to His Imperial and Royal Majesty, Commendatore Bolis. When the first vote was taken at the sitting of the *consiglieri*, however, Rossini's nomination was rejected. When the proposition was resubmitted and another vote was taken (September 20, 1843), the tally was twenty-two votes in favor of it, eleven opposed. And so Rossini became a Communal Councilor of Lugo. He later was to say that if he was "the swan [*cigno*] of Pesaro," he was also "the wild boar [*cignale*] of Lugo."

Ten days before Rossini's departure from Paris, he dated and signed a six-page autograph piano solo without title. Written in a reasonably clear, firm hand on special staff-paper with elaborate decorations printed down the left side of each page, it bears this inscription: "*Petit Souvenir offert à Madm. la Baronne Charlotte Nathaniel de Rothschild par son très devoué G. Rossini/ Paris 10 Sett 1843.*" The autograph is in the Bibliothèque Nationale, Paris.

p. 232, l. 3   "at Colonos"   This music was described by Natale Gallini in "*La Musica di scena dell''Edipo a colono' di Sofocle ritrovata nella sua integrità.*" Gallini showed that Radiciotti's account of the music, based on insufficient information, was badly garbled. The original Rossini incidental music consists of: (1) a *sinfonia*; (2) a *preludietto*; (3) a recitative beginning "*A questa terra illustre*"; (4) a chorus beginning "*Dall'alma celeste*"; (5) a recitative beginning "*Ed altra esimia lode*"; (6) a *concerto per basso e coro* beginning "*Per te novella gloria*"; (7) an arioso for bass beginning "*Fussi pur io là dove*"; (8) a chorus beginning "*O Giove egioco*";

(9) a recitative beginning *"Nudo è colui di senno"*; (10) a bass aria beginning *"Meglio fora non mai"*; (11) a bass aria beginning *"Ecco il misero stato"*; (12) a bass arioso beginning *"Se a me non è vietato"*; (13) a bass aria beginning *"A te innocente e misero"*; and (14) a final chorus *"O tu dell'Orco custode indomabile."* The score calls for flutes, oboes, clarinets, trumpets, trombones, bassoons, strings, timpani, and bass drum.

p. 232, l. 22 "successor, Brandus" Natale Gallini published the text of a document showing that Masset later inscribed the manuscript of *Œdipus at Colonos* to Brandus as a souvenir of friendship.

p. 232, l. 39 "Villa Cornetti" This copy of the new chorus, now in the Bibliothèque Nationale, Paris, is inscribed: *"Gioachino Rossini à son ami Troupenas. —Bologne, ce 22 Juin 1844."*

p. 233, l. 3 "by Troupenas" Troupenas also published (as part of a publication also containing two Rossini *"ariettes"*) a bass aria from the *Œdipus at Colonos* music; this aria was also published in 1850 at Leipzig by Breitkopf & Härtel as *Oedipus, Arie für Bassstimme mit Begleit[ung] des P[ianoforte]*.

p. 233, l. 18 "ruin him" As *La Fede, La Speranza, La Carità*—now in Italian and very remote from both Sophocles and Giusti—the choruses were heard at a concert of the Società Filarmonica, Florence, in January 1845. Rossini conducted their first Bologna singing (March 14, 1845) in the palace of Principessa Maria Hercolani. Thereafter, following singings at Rome and Turin, the choruses made a brief tour of other Italian towns. In 1852, they were sung at Florence again, at a concert of the Società Filarmonica which Rossini attended. Ricordi published (n.d.) the three choruses in an Italian translation by Geremia Vitali. In that edition, they are subtitled "three religious choruses" and are specified as being "for three-part female chorus" with solo-piano accompaniment. An autograph of the third chorus in the Conservatorio Luigi Cherubini, Florence, almost certainly is the original composition of 1844: it has the doggerel text to which Rossini composed it. This autograph was presented by Rossini to the violinist Giuseppe Manetti; the inscription is dated April 19, 1852, probably the occasion of the second Florentine performance. Notable in *"La Charité"* is the dissonance between the vocal line and its accompaniment when the choral section returns after the solo. From Rome on February 19, 1864, Liszt wrote to Ricordi: "A very exceptional circumstance is turning up in which I shall have good use to make of my transcription of Rossini's *'Charité.'* You would oblige me greatly if you would send me this piece as soon as possible . . ." The transcription, for voice and organ, was one of the *Deux Transcriptions* published in 1848 by both Schott and Brandus (the other transcription, for organ and trombone, was of the *Cujus animam* from Rossini's *Stabat Mater*).

p. 234, l. 21 "Le Désert" The *première* of *Le Désert*, by the thirty-four-year-old David (1810–76), at the Paris Conservatoire on December 8, 1844, aroused such extraordinary enthusiasm that it was performed at the Salle Ventadour to cheering audiences for an entire month. The Rossini letter to Elena Viganò is in the Raccolta Piancastelli at Forlì.

p. 235, l. 14   "Felice Romani"   An account of the ceremony was published in pamphlet form in Milan. The musical program was repeated at La Scala on June 8, 1846, as a benefit for the local Pio Istituto Filarmonico.

p. 238, l. 5   "and *Moïse*"   *Robert Bruce* begins with a potpourri overture based upon themes from several Rossini operas. The Introduction to Act I, for bass, originally had been a tenor cavatina in *Zelmira*. The soprano cavatina "*Calme et pensive plage*" is a free version of "*O mattutini albori*," from *La Donna del lago*, which also was the source of the succeeding soprano-tenor duet. Verses sung by the contralto were borrowed from *Armida*. The second tenor's aria, "*La gloire est belle*," came from *La Donna del lago*; the finale of Act I had served in *Zelmira*. In Act II, the tenor's cavatina originally had been "*Dunque invano i perigli e la morte*," in *Torvaldo e Dorliska*. The soprano's chief aria, "*O saint amour!*" was a new version of "*O quante lagrime*," again from *La Donna del lago*. The soprano-bass duet was an arrangement of "*Soave conforto*," from *Zelmira*. The trio had been a quintet in *Zelmira*, from which was also borrowed what became the romance "*Anges sur moi penchés*." The dance airs were brought over from *Moïse*. The well-known quartet in *Bianca e Falliero* here became a sextet; the new finale was merely one section of the original finale of *La Donna del lago*.

p. 238, l. 7   "for Pillet"   The original of Rossini's letter is in the Bibliothèque Nationale, Paris.

p. 238, l. 21   "Rosine Stoltz"   The cast of the *première* of *Robert Bruce* included Rosine Stoltz (Marie), Marie Nau (Nelly), Moisson (Un Page), Paul Barroilhet (Robert Bruce), Louis Paulin (Édouard II), Raffaele Anconi (Douglas-le-Noir), Geremia Bettini (Arthur), Rommy (Morton), and Bessin (Dickson). Stoltz (whose real name was Victoire Noël) was a Parisian (1815–1903); reputed to be Léon Pillet's mistress, she later led a highly publicized, gaudy, and title-filled life. María Dolores Benedicta Josefina Nau, of Spanish parentage, had been born in New York in 1818. After studies in Paris with Cinti-Damoreau, she made her debut at the Opéra in 1838 as Urbain in *Les Huguenots*. She became a renowned Lucie de Lammermoor at the Opéra and later visited England and America before retiring in Paris in 1856. Certain identification seems impossible for Moisson, Rommy, and Bessin. Geremia Bettini (1820–65) later won considerable renown. Paul Barroilhet (1810–71), who became equally prominent in Italy and France, created roles in several of Donizetti's operas. Louis Paulin sang widely throughout Europe.

p. 241, l. 9   "[feel] blessed"   Muti-Papazzurri seems not to have conducted. On January 21, 1847, in another letter to Spada, Rossini remarked: "I should have been flattered if the Marchese Muti had not, on this occasion, remained so Mute. Poor Devil!!!"

p. 241, l. 15   "January 1, 1847"   Domenico Alari conducted; the soloists were Luigia Finetti (La Speranza), Pietro Caldani (L'Amore pubblico), Benedetto Laura (Il Genio cristiano), and Fortunato Silvestro (Corifeo); the chorus contained 200 singers. A pamphlet by E. Fabri-Scarpellini, entitled

Della Cantata eseguita nel Campidoglio la sera del l. ° gennaio 1847 in onore del clementissimo pontefice PIO NONO, was issued at Rome. Luigi Spada, who inherited a copy of the Rossini score, also published an account of it: "*Rossini e la cantata per Pio IX*," in the *Giornale d'Italia*, Rome, March 21, 1916. The autograph of the huge orchestra-band score was left to the Library of the Brussels Royal Conservatory by Edmond Michotte.

NOTES TO CHAPTER XIV

p. 244, l. 29 "*fatto onore*" "The beautiful style that has done me honor" (Dante: *Inferno*, Canto I, verses 84–5).

p. 246, l. 35 "than 400" Among the singers were Cesare Badiali, Domenico Donzelli, Nicholas Ivanoff, Francesco Pedrazzi, Antonio Poggi, and Carlo Zucchelli. The instrumentalists included the oboist Baldassare Centroni and the trombonist Gaetano Brizzi.

p. 247, l. 2 "of Tuscany" At Florence on June 29, 1848, the *Coro* was sung under the direction of Prince Carlo Poniatowski during a benefit performance for families of Florentine soldiers dead in recent fighting. The program (reproduced in full in *Of*) carried a note that Rossini had attended the rehearsals and would be present at the performance. The autograph score of the *Coro* long was believed lost, but was recovered some time after 1910 by Ottino Ranalli, then director of civic concerts at Bologna; it is now in the Library of the Conservatorio G. B. Martini at Bologna. Ranalli had it sung—again for the benefit of survivors killed in battle—in Bologna's Giardini Margherita.

p. 247, l. 37 "October 26, 1848" The cast included Fanny Tacchinardi-Persiani, Jeanne-Anaïs Castellan, Angiolina Bosio, Sara Clara-Bellini, Giorgio Ronconi (then codirector of the Italien), Filippo Morelli (baritone), Paul (Pablo) Bordas, and Arnoux (bass). Persiani and Castellan interpolated into Act II of *Andremo a Parigi?* a duet from Donizetti's 1841 opera *Maria Padilla*. The bilingual Franco-Italian title page of the printed libretto for *Andremo a Parigi?* lists the characters as: La Contessa di Folleville; Corina, a famous singer; La Marchesa Melibea; Il Cavalier Belfiore; Vittorio Derigny, a young student; Lord Sidney; Pandolfo, a Paris *bourgeois*; Prudenzio, a physician of the spa; Madama Cortese, owner of the spa; Maddalena, a servant; domestics; and travelers. The scene is the Inn of the White Horse at Plombières.

p. 248, l. 28 "in Paris" Of Marliani's opera *Il Bravo*, with a libretto derived from James Fenimore Cooper, first heard at the Italien on February 1, 1834, Vincenzo Bellini had written his friend Alessandro Lamperi (February 12, 1834): "If every composer were to reclaim what is his, nothing but a few measures that are his [Marliani's] would remain in the score."

p. 248, l. 33 "of music" Collection of the late Conte Guido Chigi-Saracini, Siena.

p. 249, ll. 4–5 "a Poniatowski" In an account of the *Inno alla Pace* published in *BdCRdS* 1960, 4 and 5, Alfredo Bonaccorsi announced his intention to publish the hymn in *QR*, which he edited (ten issues) from 1954 to 1960 and then reinstituted with No. XI in 1966. As of 1967, the *Inno* was announced for publication in its original form—for vocal soloists and chorus, with piano accompaniment—in one of the four new issues of *QR* to be issued at Pesaro in 1968 for the centenary of Rossini's death.

p. 249, l. 14 "in Tuscany"   In Florence, the Rossinis had been living at No. 3, Borgo Ognissanti.

p. 250, l. 1 "of Rossini"   In a letter, now in the Library of the Bologna Conservatory, to Angelo Catelani, a learned Modenese musician friendly with Rossini.

p. 250, ll. 11–12 "ill-fated story"   The sale of the property and goods that Rossini had inherited from Isabella—including the land and villa at Castenaso—had been an added reason for his 1850–1 visit to Bologna. It was consummated in March 1851.

p. 250, l. 31 "behind them"   Giovanni Rosadi ("*Rossini a Firenze nella casa che fu sua*," *Il Marzocco*, Florence, February 13, 1916) wrote that the principal *palazzo*, then designated as No. 6040, Via Larga, later became Nos. 7 and 9, Via Cavour. The adjacent buildings were designated as No. 6039 *bis*, Via Larga (later No. 5, Via Cavour) and No. 6004, Via dei Ginori. Rosadi appears to have thought that Rossini had actually lived in them. Remarking that "one of those posthumous vivisectors of geniuses" had believed that Rossini's illness had been aggravated by the large loss sustained when he sold the properties to Giacomo Servadio in 1864, Rosadi cited the facts that they had cost Rossini 300,000 Tuscan lire (about $142,600) and that he had sold them for 250,000 Italian lire. The Tuscan lira of 1853 had had approximately 86 per cent of the value of an Italian lira of 1864—so that Rossini's loss on the sale (admittedly not counting what he had spent on improving the properties) was exactly 8,600 lire (approximately $4,730). That loss certainly had no appreciable effect upon Rossini's health in 1864.

p. 250, l. 35 "some time)"   Honors still came to the retired Rossini. By a decree dated August 19, 1851, Leopold II, Grand Duke of Tuscany, named him a Knight of the Order of San Giuseppe. Later that year, he was elected Honorary President of the Cercle Lyrique of Marseille. Writing on January 10, 1852, to thank the Cercle, he seemed to express some desire to return to France, which he did not do until May 1855.

p. 251, ll. 11–12 "about him"   Unlike the *Choeur* or *Chant funèbre* that Rossini, in 1864, improvised in memory of Meyerbeer—and which Alfredo Bonaccorsi published in *QR* VII, 84—this one appears not to have been written down.

p. 252, l. 27 "your success"   Verdi certainly composed two arias especially for Ivanoff: one that the tenor sang in *Ernani*, first at Parma in 1845, and another that he used first in *Attila* at Trieste in 1846. It is possible that he composed a third aria for Ivanoff in 1848, but no indication survives that he supplied a special interpolation for *Rigoletto* in 1852.

p. 253, l. 2 "for voices"   This letter, obviously incomplete, was quoted in an article entitled "*Di giorno in giorno*," in *La Nazione* (Florence), April

12, 1893, in which the columnist ("Miss Prunella") stated that Ferrucci had given it to the Empress of Brazil (Teresa of Naples), who had lent a copy of it for publication. It is also reprinted in *LdR*, p. 207. Certainly written between 1848 and 1855, it very probably dates from 1852.

p. 253, l. 38 "of Nicham-Iftihar" Donizetti, whose brother Giuseppe was chief musician to the Sultan, had received this order in 1841; he too had composed a military march for Abdul Medjid. Giuseppe Donizetti well may have had a hand in the awarding of both decorations. Rossini's *Marcia militare* was published by Brandus in arrangements for piano, two hands, and piano, four hands (*Marche du Sultan Abdul Medjid*); copies of both versions survive in the Bibliothèque Nationale, Paris.

p. 255, l. 17 "sent me . . ." Bellentani of Modena has frequently run, in recent years, an advertisement headed "*Anche Gioacchino Rossini era un cliente di Bellentani*," with a fanciful portrait of Rossini writing a letter. The advertisement also reproduces a letter that Rossini wrote from Paris on December 14, 1858, to Bellentani (*LdR*, p. 223, footnote 1), ordering "*6 Capelli di prete . . . 4 Zamponi . . . 4 cotechini*"—and drawing sketches of each item so that no mistake could be made.

p. 256, l. 6 "Filippo Mordani" *Della vita privata di Giovacchino Rossini.*

p. 256, l. 23 "in 1847 . . ." Mordani commented: "I think it certain that here he meant to allude to what happened to him in Bologna." But Rossini's troubles began long before 1847, and in any case the demonstration against him had occurred in 1848.

p. 257, l. 11 "of Montecatini" In the *Giornale dei Bagni Montecatini*, Anno X, No. 15, September 23, 1908, under the heading "*La Locanda Maggiore*," several famous earlier visitors are described. "In 1853, Gioacchino Rossini was here, and he went down into the kitchen to prepare—*de visu*—the menu of his supper, which invariably began with a plate of *maccheroni al Pomodoro* (Rossini, as in everything, took the cure in his way) . . ."

p. 257, l. 35 "do it" After this quotation, Branca inserted "(*storico*)" to indicate that she was retailing fact, not gossip.

Notes to Chapter XV

p. 260, l. 4 "rue Basse-du-Rempart" Now vanished, the rue Basse-du-Rempart was in the *quartier Montmartre*, not far from the present Opéra.

p. 260, l. 18 "June 13, 1855" *La Gazzetta musicale* (Naples) printed the suggestion that Rossini had gone to Paris in order to attend the *première* of *Les Vêpres siciliennes*. Cesarino De Sanctis sent word of this "news" to Verdi, who replied: "Where the Devil did the *Gazetta* [*sic*] *musicale* in Naples get such news? How many fanfaronades! When one sees so many *blagues*, it seems that this journal must be compiled in Paris. If Rossini comes to Paris, it will be to attend *I Vespri*? Bah! ! I am certain that he'll not put a foot inside the theater . . ." Verdi was almost certainly correct: Rossini seems not to have attended the *première*.

p. 261 ll. 6-7 "be invincible" One of Tonino's phrases became a byword among Rossini's friends. Not understanding French well, but having heard the concierge tell people to pull a cord that would open the door ("*Cordon, s'il vous plaît*"), he would refuse entrance to an unwanted caller by saying "*Pas cordon*," believing it to mean that no one was at home. Telling one another that Rossini was out, his friends therefore would say: "*Il n'est pas cordon.*"

p. 261, ll. 23–4 "the Théâtre-Italien" *L'Opéra-Italien de 1548 à 1856*, Paris, 1856.

p. 261, l. 29 "*Crudele sospetto*" Actually a quartet (Elena, Albina, Rodrigo, Douglas), "*Crudele sospetto*" occurs near the opening of the finale to Act I of *La Donna del lago*.

p. 262, l. 3 "the Choron" Alexandre-Étienne Choron (1771?–1834) was an important musical theorist and editor of classic works. He was also briefly director of the Paris Opéra.

p. 263, l. 26 "second volume" *PmR*.

p. 264, l. 28 "[Giuseppe] Baini" The Abbate Giuseppe Baini (1775–1844) had become *maestro di cappella* at St. Peter's Rome, in 1818. The best-known of his own compositions was a ten-voice *Miserere*. He began publication of a complete edition of Palestrina, but completed only two volumes of it. Of first importance to Palestrina studies was his *Memorie storico-critiche della vita e delle opere di Giovanni Pieruluigi da Palestrina* (Rome, 1818).

p. 265, l. 31 "is insufferable" Cimarosa's *Le Trame deluse*, with a libretto by Giuseppe Maria Diodati, was first heard at the Teatro Nuovo, Naples, in September 1786; it held various stages until about 1822.

p. 265, ll. 31–2 "oratorio *Isacco*" Cimarosa seems not to have composed an oratorio entitled *Isacco*, which may have been an alternative title for (or Rossini's way of recalling) *Il Sacrificio d'Abramo*.

p. 266, l. 34 "with *Mosè*" Differing from the version of *Mosè* which had been sung at the Italien in 1822, this was in effect a translation into Italian of the French *Moïse*, but without ballet. It was not very successful, despite which the Cuban manager of the Italien, Torribio Calzado, would open his following season with a revival of *La Cenerentola*.

p. 267, ll. 29–30 "Jacques-Léopold Heugel" This villa was the Rossinis' summer residence for four years. It was located at No. 24, rue de la Pompe, in the quarter known as Beauséjour, a group of villas which had been started by Père François de La Chaise ("Père Lachaise") in the seventeenth century, and which by 1856 had become the favored summer retreat of many noted Parisians.

p. 268, l. 13 "life ahead" After the death of Olympe in 1878, Paris recovered the Passy property as foreseen and then resold it. Thereafter, a new owner tore down the Villa Rossini.

p. 268, l. 27 "it too" Rossini's letter of October 13, 1856, to André is in the Raccolta Piancastelli at Forlì. In a postscript he asks André to let him know if the autograph of *Die Zauberflöte* is in his possession and, if it is, the conditions under which he would be disposed to part with it.

p. 269, l. 8 "April 15, 1857" *Musique anodine* was published in *QR* V, 60, where it is divided as follows (translation verbatim): "N. I (contralto), N. II (baritono), N. III (soprano), N. IIII (soprano), N. IIIII (mezzo soprano), N. IIIIII (baritono)." It also has been recorded complete. Azevedo (*AZ*, p. 199) wrote: "One does not exaggerate matters by estimating at three hundred the number of cantilenas composed by him [Rossini] on these verses ["*Mi lagnerò tacendo . . .*"]." That estimate well may have been too low.

p. 269, l. 31 "in wood" Rossini believed this instrument to be sixteenth-century, but Alessandro Biaggi, who heard it in 1859, said that the harmonies it produced were modern. After Rossini's death, this mechanical organ was sold at auction at the Drouet Rooms. Rossini sometimes remarked that the monkeys formed a model orchestra because they did not "assassinate" music.

p. 270, l. 19 "of Rossini" Bartolini's last completed work, this bust was one of the few likenesses of Rossini to show him with a mustache— which he said made him look like a smuggler.

p. 270, l. 31 "arrived mail" The amount of mail at times became so huge that the Paris postal authorities arranged especially for its delivery; friends then were called in to help Olympe to open and dispose of it.

p. 271, l. 38 "he leaves" This anecdote appears in a different version in *UScR*. Speaking of Tamberlik, Rossini there is quoted as saying: "Last week, he asked to come to see me. I received him. But, fearing a second, and aggravated, edition of the Duprez adventure, I cautioned Tamberlik please, when he came to see me, to agree to deposit his C-sharp on the halltree and pick it up again, guaranteed intact, when he left."

p. 272, l. 27 "Saturday nights" A very incomplete list of people who attended one or more of the Rossini *samedi soirs* includes: Luigi Agnesi; Marietta Alboni; Jean-Sylvanie Arnould-Plessy; Auber; Charles Aubry; Azevedo; Paul Barroilhet; François-Emanuel Bazin; Antonio Bazzini; Sir Julius Benedict; Antoine Berryer; Charles-Ernest Beulé; Arrigo Boito; Adelaide Borghi-Mamo; Angiolina Bosio; Gaetano Braga; Carafa; Cesare Casella; Paul-Joseph Chenavard; Sir Michael Costa; Félicien David; Eugène Delacroix; Enrico Delle Sedie; Émile and Antony Deschamps; Louis Diémer; Ernest and Gustave Doré; Alexandre Dumas *père*; Giovanni Dupré; Alexandrine and Gilbert-Louis Duprez; Franco Faccio; Jean-Baptiste Faure; Mme Fodor-Mainvielle; Achille Fould; Erminia Frezzolini; Italo Gardoni; Charles Gounod; Giulia Grisi; Eduard Hanslick; Ferdinand Hiller; Joseph Joachim; Wilhelm Krüger; Albert Lavignac; Ernest Legouvé; Nicholas-Prosper Levasseur; Franz Liszt; Barbara and Carlotta Marchisio; Mario; Georges Mathias; Prince and Princess Richard von Metternich; Meyerbeer; Edmond Michotte; Marie Miolan-Carvalho; Gustave Nadaud; Panseron; Adelina Patti; Comte and Comtesse Frédéric Pillet-Will; Francis Planté; Prince Carlo Poniatowski; Tito di Giovanni and Giulio Ricordi; Gustave-Hippolyte Roger; Jacob Rosenhain; Anton Rubinstein; Camille Saint-Saëns; Pablo de Sarasate; Raffaele Scalese; Pierre Scudo; François Servais; Camillo Sivori; Giuseppe Stanzieri; Marie Taglioni; Enrico Tamberlik; Antonio Tamburini; Sigismond Thalberg; Ambroise Thomas; Giuseppe Verdi; Eugène Vivier; and Giovanni Zucchini.

Saint-Saëns wrote (in *École buissonière*, p. 265): "With [Giuseppe] Stanzieri, a charming young man whom Rossini loved well and who did not live [long]; with M. [Louis] Diémer, still very young, but already a great virtuoso, I was pianist-in-ordinary to the house. Often, one or the other of us had to play, at the big soirées, the little piano pieces that the Maître amused himself by scribbling down to occupy his idleness. I gladly accompanied the singers when Rossini himself did not accompany them, which he did admirably, for he played the piano to perfection."

p. 272, l. 31 "Francesco Florimo" In a letter written in 1859 to Florimo at Naples, Rossini said: "Unhappily, the *macheroni* [*sic*] have never arrived . . ." The letter is signed "disconsolately, G. Rossini without *macheroni*" (quoted in Rocco Pagliara: "*Rossini e i maccheroni*").

p. 272, l. 32 "Ascoli Piceno" Several Rossini letters to the Ascoli Piceno cellist Giovanni Vitali on the subject of olives survive.

p. 275, l. 19 "to weep? . . ." Radiciotti (*RAD* II, 365, footnote 1) rightly remarked: "And to think that some people (see, for example, an article by C[orrado] Ricci published in *L'Illustrazione italiana* of 1892, wholly intended to create the belief that the Pesarese 'had no heart' and that 'after 1829, he thought of nothing but eating') have been able to take seriously these comic laments of Rossini's and to deduce from them conclusions about his avidity for money!"

p. 275, l. 35 "*wife*, etc. . . ." The Offenbach parody is either the "*Petit Caprice (style Offenbach)*," No. 6 of the *Miscellanée pour piano* (published in QR II, 1) or the *Andantino sostenuto* that is No. 21 of *Quelques Riens pour album*, which has a note reading: "*In tempo à l'Offen* . . . ." The tarantella mentioned by Diémer is "*Tarentelle pur sang (avec traversée de la Procession)*," No. 9 of the *Album de château*; it was published in QR II, 83. "*Un Profond Sommeil—Un Reveil en sursaut*" is No. 7 of the *Album de chaumière*. The culinary pieces are not now included in *Quelques Riens pour album* (pieces inscribed in autograph albums); they now are in an album headed *Quatre hors d'oeuvres et quatre mendiants*. "*Les Anchois (Thème et variation)*" *is the second of the* "*hors d'œuvres*"; "*Les Radis*" is the first of them. "*Une Caresse à ma femme*" is No. 7 of the *Album des enfants dégourdis*; it was published in QR II, 37.

p. 276, l. 2 "*du Tyrol*" "*L'Orpheline du Tyrol*" is No. 11 of the *Album français*; it was published in QR V, 31.

p. 276, ll. 5–6 "La Sonnambula . . ." Patti actually was nineteen when she made her Italien debut in *La Sonnambula* in 1862.

p. 276, l. 19 "to play" The Rossini trifles mentioned by Diémer are also from the *Péchés de vieillesse*, 158 pieces sorted out into fourteen albums, miscellanies, or collections: I. *Album per canto italiano*; II. *Album français*; III. *Morceaux réservés*; IV. *Quatre hors d'œuvres et quatre mendiants pour piano*; V. *Album de chaumière*; VI. *Album pour les enfants adoles-*

cents; VII. *Album des enfants dégourdis;* VIII. *Album de château;* IX. *Album pour piano, violon, violoncelle, harmonium et cor;* X. *Miscellanée pour piano;* XI. *Miscellanée de musique vocale;* XII. *Quelques Riens pour Album;* XIII. *Musique anodine;* XIV. *Compositions diverses et esquisses.* Volumes IV to VIII of the *Péchés de vieillesse* are headed *Un Peu de tout* and are described by Rossini as "Collection of 56 semicomic pieces for the piano—that is, *Four Relishes, Four Hors d'œuvres* [and] four albums of twelve numbers each. I dedicate these sins of old age to the pianists of the fourth class, to which I have the honor to belong. G. Rossini, Passy—my autographs."

Many of the *Péchés* bear humorous—at times biting—marginal glosses and superscriptions. Thus, No. 9 of the *Album pour les enfants adolescents,* entitled "*La Lagune de Venise à l'expiration de l'année 1861!!!*" is marked *pppppppp* and has this note: "The shadow of Radetzki! ! ! Arrival of H[is] M[ajesty]! ! ! The Lagoon being lowered by a third." No. 1 of the *Compositions diverses et esquisses,* a "*Canone antisavant à 3 voix,*" is "Dedicated to the Turks by the Monkey [*Singe*] of Pesaro. Words and Music by the Monkey, Passy"; the words are "*Vive l'Empereur, de France la splendeur! Vive! Vive! Vive! Vive!*" The gloss on No. 8 of this Volume XIV, "*Tourniquet sur la gamme chromatique ascendante et descendante,*" reads: "Whirligig on the chromatic ascending and descending scale. The run-through (homeopathically and *à la pésarèse*) of all the tones of the chromatic scale"; midway in the piece, noticing that he had not provided a passage in E major, Rossini added: "Great-sharp [*gran-dièze*] E, pardon me for having forgotten you! Take heart, I still am in time to cover you during my little promenade. Follow on, and you'll see . . ."

The song sung by Alboni very probably was "*Les Adieux à la vie—Élégie (sur une seule note),*" No. 9 of the *Album français;* this was published in *QR* V, 75. The four-hand march for piano may have been one of three such marches which Rossani had composed in 1823; or it may have been the four-hand arrangement of the *Marche du Sultan Abdul Medjid* (see p. 253). "*Un Mot à Paganini (élégie pour violon)*" is No. 4 of the *Album pour piano, violon, violoncelle, harmonium et cor.*

p. 276, l. 27 "Saint-Saëns wrote:" *École buissonière,* p. 265.

p. 277, l. 3 "Strakoschonized it" According to Louis Engel (*From Mozart to Mario* II, 79), what Rossini actually said was "*extra-cochonnée*" (ek-Strakoschonnée), a pun on *cochonnée,* piggishly botched.

p. 277, l. 11 "Since then" Rossini, who both regarded Patti as a great singer and became very much attached to her personally, did not regard her as on an artistic level with the greatest singers he had heard earlier. In *UScR,* the music publisher Heugel asks Rossini: "Regarding Patti whose name you just mentioned . . . what, dear Maître, is your final opinion of her talent?" Rossini's reply is: "My opinion is that she is charming and that I love her very much." Heugel persists: "And then? . . ." And Rossini answers: "And then . . . that fate, very gallant toward her, has saved her from the danger of being contemporary with, for example, Sontag . . . not to mention others."

p. 278, l. 7 "Weckerlin reported" In *Nouveau Musicana,* Paris, 1879.

p. 279, l. 9.   "*Tell* overture"   In measure 37 of the first andante, the cellos were marked to play the entire trill in major, whereas the autograph score required them to go into the minor (with G-natural) at that point and return to the major in measure 38, a much less bland, more interesting effect than a steady major.

p. 280, l. 6   "Scudo wrote"   In *L'Année musicale*, 1859.

p. 281, ll. 25-6   "G. Rossini"   Carafa's original music for this production of *Semiramide* survives in the Library of the Conservatorio di San Pietro a Maiella, Naples.

p. 282, l. 25   "[Louis-Henry] Obin"   Obin (1820–95), who had studied with Levasseur, had made his Opéra debut in Rossini's *Otello* in 1844 and later had sung the title role of *Moïse* there (1851). He was to create roles in Verdi's *Les Vêpres siciliennes* (Giovanni di Procida) and *Don Carlos* (Phillippe II). He sang at the Opéra regularly until 1868 and made later guest appearances there; he taught at the Conservatoire for nearly twenty years.

p. 282, l. 35   "at eighty-five"   When being installed as a teacher of singing at San Pietro a Maiella, Naples, in February 1892 (almost exactly on the centenary of Rossini's birth), Barbara Marchisio sang the rondo finale of *La Cenerentola* and the *Agnus Dei* from the *Petite Messe Solennelle*. She taught until 1912, the most successful of her numerous pupils being Toti Dal Monte and Rosa Raïsa.

NOTES TO CHAPTER XVI

p. 283, l. 10   "Edmond Michotte"   Wagner's meeting with Rossini is described in almost stenographic detail in *LVdW*. Wagner himself wrote of it in "*Erinnerungen an Rossini*," published in the *Allegemeine Zeitung*, Augsburg, on December 17, 1868, five weeks after Rossini's death.

p. 285, l. 14   "to me?"   In another passage, Michotte wrote: "He [Rossini] suffered from that bitter publicity, which often passed the boundaries of malice and became frankly perfidious at his expense. He often complained, and then someone would answer: 'You know, Maestro, one lends only to the rich.' 'To tell the truth,' he would sigh, 'I'd like better a little more *poverty* and a little less *generosity*. In the process of wanting to give to me, they overload me, obstruct me! And what gifts, good Lord!— garbage that splashes on me even more than it hits the other! That exasperates me: *ma così va il mondo.*' "

p. 285, l. 15   "Chaussée d'Antin"   In a footnote, Michotte said: "It has been established that about a century earlier than the composer of *Il Barbiere*—O, coincidence!—the composer of *Le Nozze di Figaro*, Mozart, then staying in Paris, had lodged in a building that then occupied the same location as the one on which today the large house mentioned above rises. That was the home of Grimm (1778), with whom Mozart took refuge after having left the rue du Gros-Chenet, where he had lost his mother."

p. 287, l. 18   "court theater . . ."   See p. 148 *et seq.* for quotation from Michotte's report of that part of the Wagner-Rossini conversation which dealt with Weber, p. 119 *et seq.* for that dealing with Beethoven.

p. 295, l. 31 "in peace" In January 1866—six years after the conversation with Wagner—Rossini at nearly seventy-four, looking back thirty-seven years to his abandonment of operatic composition, wrote to Giovanni Pacini: "Dear Giovanni, be at peace; keep in mind my philosophic intention to abandon my Italian career in 1822, the French in 1829; this foresight is not given to all; God accorded it to me, and I always bless Him." It had not, of course, been so simple as that, and elsewhere in the same letter to Pacini, as though still feeling the need to justify his retirement from the stage, Rossini spoke of music as "this art which has as its only basis the Ideal and Emotion," adding that it could not be separated "from the influence of the times in which we live. Today the ideal and feeling are directed exclusively toward *steam, rapine*, and the barricades . . ."

NOTES TO CHAPTER XVII

p. 300 l. 5 "it reads:" Translated from the article as reprinted in Hanslick's *Aus dem Concertsaal.*

p. 303, l. 32 "of them" "*À Grenade*" (text by Émilien Pacini) and "*La Veuve andalouse*," which later were published by Escudier as *Deux Chansons espagnoles*. Rossini had sent "*À Grenade*," with an inscription, to Queen Isabella II of Spain, "*La Veuve andalouse*" to the director of her court concerts. The recipients had handed them on to a charitable organization, which had had them published for its profit.

p. 305, l. 22 "*l'ancien régime*" Rossini later changed these titles to "*Spécimen de l'avenir*," "*Spécimen de mon temps*" (which, still earlier had been called "*Prélude prétentieux*"), and "*Spécimen de l'ancien régime*." The first in No. 12 of the *Album de château; it was published in QR X,* 104. The second is No. 6 of that same album; it was published in QR X, 38. The third is No. 1 of the same album; it was published in QR II, 59.

p. 306, l. 5 "and Gounod" The Rossini pieces and excerpts on this occasion were: "*Toast pour le nouvel an*," for chorus; "*Tirana [alla spagnola 'Rossinizzata']*," sung by Marie Battu; the chorus "*La Charité*," with Marie Sass-Castelmary as soloist; the *Inflammatus* from the *Stabat Mater*, again with Sass-Castelmary; "*Tarentelle pur sang (avec traversée de la Procession)*," performed by Diémer and chorus; "*Les Adieux à la vie (sur une seule note)*," sung by Battu; an aria from *Le Siège de Corinthe*, sung by Jean-Baptiste Faure and chorus; "*Départ des Promis (Tyrolienne sentimentale)*," for chorus; and a duet from *Guillaume Tell*, sung by Villaret and Faure. Marie Miolan-Carvalho sang "*Voi che sapete*," from *Le Nozze di Figaro*, and the "*Valse de l'hirondelle*," from Gounod's *Mireille*; she also joined Faure in an unspecified duet.

"*Toast pour le nouvel an*," an "*ottetino*" for pairs of sopranos, contraltos, tenors, and basses, is No. 1 of the *Album français*; it was published in QR VIII, 50, and has been recorded. "*Tirana alla spagnola 'Rossinizzata'*" is No. 3 of the *Album per canto italiano*; it was published in QR IV, 30. "*Tarentelle pur sang (avec traversée de la Procession)*" is No. 9 of the *Album de château* (where it appears as a piano solo, without chorus); it was published in *QR* II, 83. *Les Adieux à la vie (sur une seule note)*," subtitled "*Élégie*," is No. 9 of the *Album français*; it was published in *QR* V, 75. "*Départ des Promis (Tyrolienne sentimentale)*" is the second of the *Deux Nocturnes* (the first is "*Adieu à l'Italie*") published by Schott (Mainz) in 1836 with the texts in French, German, and Italian.

p. 306, l. 8 "and Sass-Castelmary" Marie Sasse (1838–1907), a Belgian soprano, adopted the name Sax, which she later changed to Saxe. When the instrument inventor Adolphe Sax, her compatriot, obtained a court order prohibiting her from using his name, she styled herself Sass or—with reference to her having been married to a singer named Castan but called Castelmary—Sass-Castelmary. She was the Elisabeth of the notorious performances of Wagner's *Tannhäuser* at the Paris Opéra in 1861; she created the roles of Selika in Meyerbeer's *L'Africaine* (1865) and Elisabetta in Verdi's *Don Carlos* (1867).

p. 306, l. 17 "Chinese scale" This was "*L'Amour à Pekin*," text by Émilien Pacini, No. 5 of the *Morceaux réservés*; it was published in *QR* V, 81, and has been recorded. It carries this description: "Rising and descending scales; two Chinese scales followed by an analogous song. The whole dedicated to my friend M.r Jobart, millionaire (always some humbug). 1st rising and descending Chinese scale. 2nd rising and descending Chinese scale. *L'Amour à Pekin*—little song on the Chinese scale."

p. 306, l. 19 "A-sharp, C" Rossini notated the scale as C, D, E, F-sharp, A-flat, B-flat, C. In either notation, it is a whole-tone scale.

p. 307, l. 8 "excellent Peruzzi" "*Il Fanciullo smarrito*" is a setting of a sonnet by Antonio Castellani. When presenting a copy of the song to Castellani on March 10, 1861, Rossini included in the inscription a warning that it was "for his exclusively personal use." The "*Rien*" played by Lavignac cannot be singled out from among the twenty-four "*Riens*" in Volume XII of the *Péchés de vieillesse*. The "*Barcarolle vénitienne*" may have been either the "*Barcarolle*" that is No. 7 of the *Album des enfants dégourdis* or "*La Vénitienne*," a "*chansonette pour pianoforte*" which is No. 3 of Volume XIV of the *Péchés*. "*Valse de boudoir*" cannot be identified.

p. 308, l. 2 "later wrote" *Life of Moscheles*, adapted from the original German by A. D. Coleridge, II, 270.

p. 308, ll. 6–7 "his works" This photograph was undoubtedly the ceramic-framed portrait now in the Fondation Rossini, Passy, reproduced here as the frontispiece.

p. 309, l. 13 "singers Ponchard" This could have been either Louis-Antoine Ponchard (1787–1866) or his son Charles-Marie (1824– ?).

p. 311, l. 14 "Giovanni Caselli" Caselli (1815–91) invented the *pantelegrafo*, an early variety of telestereograph for transmitting documents by wire; the *cinemografo*, which measured the speed of railway locomotives; and an automatic rudder for ships.

p. 311, l. 37 "real subject" The letters to Costa mentioned are in the Raccolta Piancastelli at Forlì.

p. 312, l. 5 "noble hospitality" Failing to obtain the desired composition from Rossini, the English authorities turned to Verdi, who provided the *Inno delle nazioni.* See page 321 and note to that page.

p. 312, l. 25 "October 5, 1861" This letter is misdated October 15 in *LdR.* The date on the autograph, in the Bibliothèque Nationale, Paris, unquestionably is October 5.

p. 313, ll. 21–2 "occur soon" The autograph of this letter canont be located. The present translation was made from its text as published by Arthur Pougin in *Le Temps* (Paris) on September 5, 1894.

p. 313, l. 30 "Italian style)" This was published, as *La Notte del Santo Natale: Pastorale,* with text in Italian and French, for bass solo, mixed chorus of eight voices, piano, and harmonium, in *QR* V, 102; it has also been recorded. In its original form, it is No. 6 of the *Album français.*

p. 314, l. 22 "the composer" *Le Chant des titans* also was sung in England, at the Birmingham Festival of August 1873, at which time a transcription for voice and piano was published in London. There have been later performances. The composition was published in full score, with the original French text, in *QR* VIII, 66.

p. 314, l. 37 "the end" The score calls for piccolo, two flutes, two oboes, two B-flat clarinets, four bassoons (two of them *ad libitum*), two F horns, two C horns, two C trumpets, three trombones, an ophicleide, twenty-four first violins, twenty-four second violins, six violas, six cellos, six doublebasses, timpani, and tam-tam.

p. 315, l. 15 "Arrigo Boito" Faccio (1840–91), later prominent as a conductor (he was on the podium at La Scala, Milan, for more than a thousand performances, including the *première* of Verdi's *Otello* in 1887), had collaborated with Boito on a cantata, *Le Sorelle d'Italia,* which had been sung by students at the Milan Conservatory while they had been enrolled there. When they visited Rossini in Paris, neither of them was yet known as an operatic composer. Boito (1842–1918) did not see his first opera, *Mefistofele,* produced until 1868. Faccio's *I Profughi fiamminghi* (libretto by Emilio Praga) was put on for five nights at La Scala beginning on November 11, 1863; his *Amleto,* to Boito's first Shakespearean libretto, was staged at the Teatro Carlo Felice, Genoa, on May 30, 1865. After the fiasco of a single singing of *Amleto* at La Scala in 1871, Faccio gave up operatic composition and devoted himself to conducting symphony concerts and opera.

p. 316, l. 3 "in 1867" Giulio Ricordi's account of meeting Rossini in Paris was published as "*Conosco Gioachino Rossini,*" in *LGMM, Supplemento straordinario dedicato a Gioacchino Rossini,* 2/29/1892 (the centenary of Rossini's birth), 19.

p. 316, l. 23 "he published" First in the *Rivista romana di scienze e lettere,* then as a pamphlet entitled *Gioacchino Rossini: Appunti di viaggio,* and finally in his *Memorie: Studi dal vero.*

p. 317, l. 26 "and 'Memento'" No. 7 of the *Album des enfants dégourdis* and, almost certainly, "*Memente homo,*" No. 3 of the same album.

p. 320, l. 38 "the Exhibition" Rossini's letter to Castellani is in the

Raccolta Piancastelli, Forlì. The "marches" referred to included one by Auber. It was upon hearing that Auber, as representing France, would supply the Exhibition with a march that Verdi, who was to represent Italy, decided to compose a cantata instead.

p. 321, l. 4 "May 24, 1862)" Verdi's *Inno delle nazioni*, the tenor part designed for Enrico Tamberlik, had been intended for Covent Garden, then under the joint managership of Costa and Frederick Gye. Owing to disagreement between Verdi and the commisioners of the Exhibition, however, its performance was tranferred to Her Majesty's Theatre and the tenor role was transposed for singing by the soprano Thérèse Tietjens. With Luigi Arditi conducting, the peculiar work was sung six times in about three weeks.

p. 321, l. 9 "years old" Rossini's letter to Ivanoff of November 11, 1862, is in the Raccolta Piancastelli at Forlì. It again shows the bitterness with which, fourteen years later, Rossini looked back upon the events of 1848 in Bologna.

p. 322, l. 2 "a tam-tam" Number 12 of the *Album français*, the "*Choeur de chasseurs*," has been published in QR VII, 35. The anonymous text begins: "*En chasse, amis, en chasse;/du cerf suivons la trace;/d'un temps heureux qui passe/chasseur profite encor . . .*"

Notes to Chapter XVIII

p. 325, l. 21 "full score" The orchestrated version of the *Petite Messe solennelle* omits the "*Prélude Religieux*" for piano or harmonium of the original version, in which it is played during the Offertory preceding the *Sanctus*. The full score, of which only an organ part is not in Rossini's own hand, is in Pesaro; it is extremely legible and includes metronome indications.

p. 325, l. 23 "he lived;" A performance of the *Petite Messe solennelle* announced for the Birmingham Festival of 1867 did not take place.

p. 325, l. 30 "huband's memory" Verdi, writing to Conte Opprandino Arrivabene after hearing the orchestrated *Petite Messe solennelle*, referred to statements by several critics that it showed a great advance in Rossini's techniques: "Rossini made progress and studied during that last period? Auf! For me, I should have advised him to forget music and write another *Barbiere*." Thus Verdi echoed Beethoven.

p. 325, l. 38 "he said" *Souvenirs d'un impresario*, Paris, 1887, p. 73.

p. 326, l. 7 "Sydney, Australia" The first performance in Italy of the *Petite Messe solennelle* occurred at the Teatro Communale, Bologna, on March 23, 1869. Emanuele Muzio conducted; the soloists were Sofia Vera-Lorini, Erminia Spizert, Maria Waldmann, Carlo Vincentelli, Giovanni Valle, and Tommaso Costa. Although the Mass was repeated twice, its reception was much less enthusiastic than in northern countries. In Turin, it seems to have been disliked. It received its only singing at La Scala, Milan (as *Messa Solenne postuma*), on April 23, 1869. Nowhere, either in Italy or abroad, has its popularity ever equaled that of the *Stabat Mater*.

p. 326, l. 9 "to Verdi:" Escudier's letters are quoted from the Verdi *Coppialettere.*

p. 326, l. 30 "of ritornello'" Rossini later sent this *"Ritournelle pour l'Adagio du Trio d'Attila"* to Verdi, who presented it to Boito. Alessandro Luzio reproduced it in facsimile at the end of the pamphlet publication of his speech (Mantua, February 24, 1901) entitled *"Il Pensiero artistico e politico di Giuseppe Verdi nelle sue lettere inedite al Conte Opprandino Arrivabene."* At the bottom of the *"ritournelle"* can be seen, in Rossini's script: *"Sans la permission de Verdi/Rossini 1865."*

p. 327, ll. 4-5 "to write" One such letter of introduction, dated December 15, 1857, addressed from Paris to Felice Romani, is of peculiar interest. It reads: "Signor Bizet, 1st prize in composition at the Conservatoire Impérial de Paris, will bring you this letter. He is traveling to complete his practical musical education; he has done very well in his studies, he has had great success with an operetta performed here [*Le Docteur Miracle*, Bouffes-Parisiens, April 9, 1857]. He is a good pianist. He is an excellent fellow who deserves your and my solicitude. I recommend him to you and beg you to recommend him to the Ronzi brothers, for which I cordially thank you. Keep your warm friendship for me and believe me your affectionate friend." When Rossini wrote this letter, Bizet was just nineteen.

p. 327, l. 6 "musical writing" The present writer owns one such album leaf. On light cardboard measuring 12½" x 9¾" and decoratively outlined in gold printing, it is an eleven-measure *andante molto* for voice and piano on the usual Metastasian words ("*Mi lagnerò tacendo . . .*"). The inscription reads: *"a Mad^lle Palmyre Wertheimber/G. Rossini/Passi* [sic] *ce 29 Juin 1860."* On the obverse, Ernest Reyer wrote out twenty-four measures (for piano and voice) of his 1854 opera *Maître Wolfram.* Reyer's inscription reads: *"A Mademoiselle Palmyre Wertheimber, Artiste* [thrice underlined] *de l'Opéra"*; at the bottom of the page, he wrote: *"Son ami/28 mars 1864/E. Reyer."*

p. 327, l. 17 "ten-day illness" *L'Africaine* was given its *première* at the Opéra on April 28, 1865.

p. 327, ll. 22-3 *"muse sublime"* No. 1 of the *Morceaux réservés*, this *Choeur (Chant funèbre)* was published in QR VII, 84; it has been recorded.

p. 327, l. 26 "G. Rossini" The *Revue et Gazette musicale* reported that Rossini improvised this music at the piano, wrote it out, and then had it handed to Pacini with the request that he adapt appropriate words to it.

p. 328, ll. 8-9 "(Félix Tournachon)" Rossini's letter of June 6, 1864, to Fabi is in the Raccolta Piancastelli at Forlì. Later in the letter, after apologizing for not having written sooner and more often, Rossini added: "May my Old Likeness that I send you be more loquacious with my words!"

p. 328, l. 15 "of Memory" The sections quoted begin on pp. 56 and 59.

p. 328, l. 21 "von] Metternich" Prince Richard von Metternich

(1829–95), son of the longtime Austrian Minister of Foreign Affairs, was Austrian ambassador at Paris from 1859 to 1870. With his wife (*née* Countess Sándor), he was an important figure in the political and social life of the Second Empire.

p. 329, l. 1 "to mass" This appears to be the only reference to the mature Rossini's going to Mass.

p. 329, l. 10 "Auber" Auber, who had met Rossini at Carafa's home, wrote as follows of hearing Rossini accompany himself there while singing the "*Largo al factotum*" from *Il Barbiere di Siviglia*: "I shall never forget the impression I received from that dazzling performance. Rossini had a most beautiful baritone voice and sang his own music with a spirit and a brio that, in it, raised him above Pellegrini, Galli, and Lablache. Further, as to his art as an accompanist, it was marvelous: his hands appeared to gallop not over a piano, but over an orchestra. When he had finished, I mechanically looked at the ivory keys: I thought that I saw them smoking!" Auber shared the opinion of Verdi and many other musicians that *Il Barbiere* was Rossini's masterpiece, saying: "A sovereign perhaps could succeed in forcing Rossini to compose another *Guillaume Tell*, but not another *Barbiere di Siviglia*."

p. 329, ll. 15–16 "of 'Tannhäuser'" Rossini seems not to have attended any performance of *Tannhäuser*. Also, Mme de Hegermann-Lindencrone was writing of a period three years later than the performances of that opera in Paris (1861); *Tannhäuser* was not revived in Paris until May 13, 1895.

p. 329, l. 39 "Patricio] Garcia" Madame Moulton had studied singing with Manuel Patricio Garcia, son of the composer-tenor and brother of Malibran and Viardot-Garcia.

p. 330, l. 16 "One paper" Translated from the quotation in Italian by Radiciotti (*RAD* II, 457), which does not specify the now unrecoverable source.

p. 330, l. 25 "Lemmens-Sharrigton [*sic*]" Helen Sherrington, who had married the Belgian organist Nicolas-Jacques Lemmens.

p. 332, l. 24 "station there" The Rossini statue, mounted on a marble base, stood in the station *piazza* for some time before being installed in the courtyard of the Liceo Musicale, where it remains.

p. 332, l. 34 "Rossinian melodies" Both this hymn and the one by Pacini sung the next day were to texts supplied by Luigi Mercantini, who in 1858 had been asked by Garibaldi to write what (as set to music by Alessio Olivieri) became known as the *Inno dei Cacciatori delle Alpi* or *Inno di Garibaldi*.

p. 333, l. 1 "*Guglielmo Tell*" Several other towns and cities honored Rossini in 1864. Tiny Lugo sent him a patent of local nobility. Arezzo made him honorary president of an artistic commission to honor Guido d'Arezzo. A theater was named after him in Berlin. At Rome, the Accademia dei Quiriti mock-solemnly commemorated the eighteenth anniversary of his birth, there having been only eighteen February 29ths since 1792.

p. 333, l. 7 "main *piazza*" Also on Rossini's name-day in 1864, a commemorative incised stone was placed near the entrance to the Liceo Musicale in Bologna and that city changed the name of the contiguous *piazza* from San Giacomo to Rossini. The accompanying music had to be furnished by a military band because the renowned Bologna Municipal Band, accompanied by the *sindaco* of the city, had gone to Pesaro to take part in the festivities there. Radiciotti stated (*RAD* II, 452) that the first of the *Tell* performances in Pesaro occurred on August 14. In that chapter of his book, however, dates clearly became jumbled: he repeatedly places the Pesaro celebrations in May, though he himself etablished in other places that beyond doubt they took place in August.

p. 333, l. 8 "these celebrations" *Delle Feste fatte in Pesaro il 21 agosto 1864 in onore di G. Rossini.*

p. 333, l. 18 "by you)" Sometimes attributed to Conte Carlo Pepoli, then *sindaco* of Bologna and a senator, the inscription on this stone reads: "Here entered as a student who left here prince of the musical sciences, Gioachino Rossini, and Bologna, as a perennial document in honor of its adopted son named the surrounding *piazza* with his name and placed this here on August 21,1864."

p. 333, l. 21 "of Pesaro" Publishing this letter ("*Una Lettera inedita di Rossini*"), Claudio Sartori commented that in it Rossini "seems to want to justify abandoning the city by artistic motives," an interpretation that nothing in the letter supports. Sartori also wrote: "This new interpretation would explain his rancor's having remained so tenacious as to induce him in 1864 to sign 'Rossini from Pesaro,' thus to deny any rapport whatever with Bologna."

p. 334, l. 6 "architect Doussault" Doussault's account of this conversation was published in the *Revue de Paris*, March 1, 1856.

p. 334, l. 16 "quoted from" See p. 148.

p. 334, l. 31 "old men!" In 1855, Rossini had told Hiller, who had remarked that Weber's overtures remained very popular in Germany: "And with good reason, though I cannot condone the introduction of the most beautiful motives into the overture, if for no other reason than that on their later appearances in the opera, they will have lost the charm of novelty. And, in any case, no one can be aware of their interrelationships in advance. But Weber had charming ideas! In his *Conzertstück*, the introduction of the march by the deep clarinets is just enchanting [here Rossini sang the first part of it]. I always have loved hearing that piece."

p. 336, l. 12 "January 3, 1865:" Rossini's letter of January 3, 1865, to Costa is in the Raccolta Piancastelli, Forlì.

p. 337, l. 7 "answer was:" Louis Engel: *From Mozart to Mario: Reminiscences of Half a Century*, London, 1886, Vol. II, 52.

p. 337, l. 23 "years later:" In an interview by Ivan Lavretsky entitled "Madame Teresa Carreño," in *The Bellman*, June 26, 1915. Kindly called to my attention by Vincent de Sola, who had been given it by Carreño's last husband, Arturo Tagliapietra.

p. 338, l. 2 "Moreau] Gottschalk" Both of Rossini's letters introducing Carreño (the one to Arditi in facsimile) appear in Marta Milinowski: *Teresa Carreño*, New Haven, 1940.

p. 339, l. 16   *"vi credo'* "   These words initiate a quartet in Act I, Scene 9 of *Il Turco in Italia*.

p. 339, l. 37   *"ognor rammento'* "   Arsace's aria from Act I, Scene 5 of *Semiramide*.

p. 340, l. 32   "June 21, 1867"   Letter quoted in an article entitled "*Di giorno in giorno*," in *La Nazione*, Florence, 4/12/1893; reprinted in *Of*, p. 111.

p. 340, l. 37   "religious music!!!"   Rossini was almost ninety years ahead of the times: in 1955, the encyclical *Musicæ sacræ disciplinæ* finally permitted stringed instruments to be added to the organ in liturgical services —and women to sing in churches.

p. 341, ll. 5–6   "British orthography!)"   Translated from the catalogue description of a letter offered for sale at Sotheby's, London, in 1959.

NOTES TO CHAPTER XIX

p. 342, l. 5   "later wrote:"   In "*Conosco Gioachino Rossini*."

p. 345, l. 25   "later wrote:"   *Italienische Tondichter*. The quotation is translated from the 1883 Berlin edition, IV, 541.

p. 346, l. 8   "friends here"   Here Rossini referred to instruments recently invented and demonstrated by Adolphe Sax, the Belgian inventor of the saxhorn, saxophone, saxtromba, saxtuba, and related instruments; he had been awarded a Grand Prix for them at the Paris Exposition of 1867.

p. 347, l. 34   "von Schwind"   Schwind (1804–71) was a leading late German romantic painter.

p. 348, l. 4   "admit you"   Hanslick had believed the canard spread by some of Beethoven's friends and early biographers (including Schindler in 1840) that Beethoven had shut his door brusquely in Rossini's face. After hearing the facts from Rossini, he wrote: "I confess that this assurance, given me by Rossini himself, the truth of which was corroborated by many special circumstances, pleases me as much as an unexpected gift. I had always been irritated by that discourteous passage in the Beethoven biography, though I had seen in it a vicious move by the Jacobin musical party, which extols a German celebrity to the skies for the brutal act of having closed the door in the face of a man like Rossini. Fortunately, then, there is not a word of truth in the entire story." The story nonetheless was repeated by Wilhelm Joseph von Wasielewski in his biography of Beethoven (1888).

p. 348, l. 22   "belated accomplishment"   In actuality, Rossini's accomplishments at the piano had been noted from his young manhood on.

p. 348, l. 37   "Marlborough song"   This was probably the *allegretto tenero* section of "*L'Amour à Pekin*," a harmonization of "*Malbrouck s'en va-t-en guerre*."

p. 350, l. 7   "during 1867"   A third Rossini piece, composed in 1861, was heard in public for the first time in 1867 when "*Il Fanciullo smarrito*," which Rossini had presented to the author of its text, Antonio Castellani, in 1861, was sung by Italo Gardoni at the Théâtre-Italien, Paris.

p. 350, l. 20 "de l'Industrie" The Palais de l'Industrie was torn down and its site used (1900) for the Grand Palais and Petit Palais.

p. 350, ll. 33–4 "couldn't refuse" The *Hymne à Napoléon III* was announced for publication in one of four new *QR* to be issued at Pesaro in 1968 for the centenary of Rossini's death.

p. 351, l. 37 "future centuries" Olympe's letter is translated from Radiciotti's Italian version of it (*RAD* II, 479), the original being unavailable. Radiciotti thanked the "List and Franke bookshop of Leipzig" for permission to consult it.

p. 352, l. 9 "February 10, 1868" The actual five-hundredth performance of *Guillaume Tell* at the Opéra appears not to have occurred until May 22, 1868.

p. 353, l. 16 "less illustrious" Manzoni was eighty-three in 1868; he died in 1873. *I Promessi Sposi* (1825–6) was more than forty years old at the time of Broglio's letter.

p. 353, l. 31 "Meyerbeer and . . ." To speak only of Italian composers, Broglio thus airily disposed of Donizetti and the late Bellini—and of Verdi through *Don Carlos*. Boito said: "The dots that follow this profound observation are worth a Peru." Then he added: "Would you want to tell me, Your Excellency, what in your brain these four operas are? Not, of course, *Robert*, not *Le Prophète*, not *Les Huguenots*, not *L'Africaine*, seeing that they belong to that devilish class of the 'exterminating operas' (as you add farther down) 'that last five hours'; they belong to that race (as you say so charmingly), to that race of 'musical mastodons that have become a calamitous habit with the public.' "

p. 354, l. 1 "Mephistophelean presumptions . . ." The unsuccessful first performance of Boito's *Mefistofele* had taken place at La Scala, Milan, exactly twenty-four days before Broglio dated his letter to Rossini.

p. 356, l. 31 "*Trovatore* trial" In 1855, Verdi had sued Torribio Calzado, then impresario of the Théâtre-Italien, Paris, to prevent the staging of unauthorized versions of three of his operas, including *Il Trovatore*. As this was an action with which Rossini certainly would have sympathized, it is difficult to imagine what could have been in the now lost letter referred to by Verdi.

p. 357, l. 1 "Public Instruction" This renowned "Letter" was reprinted in full in Raffaello de Rensis, ed.: *Critiche e cronache musicali di Arrigo Boito*, p. 52, and in Franco Abbiati: *Giuseppe Verdi* III, 203. It is in four sections, the first three of which each contain several paragraphs. The fourth section is introduced at the end of the third with the suggestion that Broglio "meditate somewhat (for the good of the country, which needs it so much) on the profound significance of the following paragraph." That "fourth paragraph" consists entirely of the Italian alphabet: "*ABCDEFGHI-LMNOPQRSTUVZ*."

p. 357, l. 7 "*maestri* say" Here Boito makes an untranslatable pun on meanings of the verb *combinare* and refers obliquely both to Broglio's earlier correspondence with Manzoni about the purity and national desirability of Tuscan Italian and to a familiar distych by Carducci: "*Passai per San Fiorenza, intesi un raglio:/era un sospiro del ministro Broglio*" ("I passed through San Fiorenza, heard a braying; it was a sigh of Minister Broglio").

p. 357, l. 38   "of misunderstandings"   Untranslatable is Boito's clever pun, implied in the word *imbrogli* [im-Brogli(o)], the plural of *imbroglio*.

p. 360, l. 9   "he possesses . . ."   Fragment of a letter quoted in *RAD* II, 486–7, the present whereabouts of which cannot be determined.

p. 360, l. 29   "affectionate ROSSINI"   Letter in the Theatre Collection of the Harvard College Library, Cambridge. It was reproduced in facsimile in "Autograph Letters of Musicians at Harvard," by Hans Nathan (*Notes*, Washington, D. C., 9/1948, Second Series, V, 4, 475, misnumbered 575). Rossini misused the word "Quondam": Patti did not marry the Marquis Henri de Caux until July 29, 1868, two months after the date of this letter.

p. 360, l. 35   "G. Rossini"   An undated edition of this fanfare was published in Rome. The autograph manuscript went to G. Ricordi, Milan; a manuscript copy survived in the Conservatorio G. Rossini, Pesaro.

p. 361, l. 10   "the rights!! . . ."   From a letter quoted in *RAD* II, 488, footnote 2; its present whereabouts are unknown. The instruments called for by Rossini in *La Corona d'Italia* include three sizes of saxophones.

NOTES TO CHAPTER XX

p. 362, l. 14   "low spirits"   Bonato's report on Rossini's final illness was published in *Traslazione delle ceneri* [*di*] *Gioacchino Rossini da Parigi a Firenze*, Pesaro, 1887, p. 21.

p. 362, l. 20   "and admirers"   The group around Olympe during Rossini's final days included Dr. Giacomo D'Ancona, Gustave Doré and his brother Ernest, a Dr. Fortina, Nicholas Ivanoff, Domenico Liverani, a Maestro Lucantonio, Edmond Michotte, Andrea Peruzzi, Antonio Tamburini, and Auguste-Emmanuel Vaucorbeil.

p. 362, l. 22   "on November 3"   Nélaton (1807–73), Napoleon III's physician, had invented a porcelain-tipped probe for locating bullets in the body. It had been used first on Garibaldi at the battle of Aspromonte. He also developed the rubber catheter that long was known by his name.

p. 363, l. 35   "the patient"   This guestbook, now in the Library of the Royal Conservatory of Music at Brussels, shows—in addition to the names already mentioned—the signatures of Marietta Alboni, Ambroise Thomas, Émilien Pacini, Alexis-Jacob Azevedo, Italo Gardoni, Marie Battu, and Antoine Berryer (who was two years Rossini's senior and would outlive him by only seventeen days).

p. 364, l. 18   "this scene:"   *Le Figaro*, Paris, February 27, 1892.

p. 365, l. 7   "it now!"   Camille Du Locle wrote to Verdi (November 12, 1868) to say that Rossini had "sent away the Passy priest and the papal nuncio in person" because he wanted to die in peace.

p. 365, l. 28 "with difficulty"   Rossini's death certificate in the records of the sixteenth Paris *arrondissement* reads: "The year 1868, November 14 at two in the afternoon, there appeared before us, Henri Pierre Edouard Baron de BONNEMAINS, Officer of the Légion d'honneur, Mayor of the Sixteenth Arrondissement of Paris, Office of the État civil, Jean Frédéric POSSOZ, aged seventy-one, Officer of the Légion d'Honneur, former Mayor of Passy, member of the Municipal Council of the City of Paris, living in Paris, 8, chaussée de la Muette, and Luigi Francesco CERRUTI, aged forty-eight, Consul General of Italy in Paris, Officer of the Légion d'Honneur and of the Order of Sts. Maurice and Lazarus, living in Paris, rue Boissy d'Anglas, 45, who have declared to us that on the thirteenth of this month, at eleven o'clock in the evening, there died in his Paris domicile, avenue Ingres, 2, Gioacchino Antonio ROSSINI, aged seventy-six years, composer of music, member of the Institut, Grand Officer of the Légion d'honneur and Grand Cross of the Order of Sts. Maurice and Lazarus, Grand Cross of the Crown of Italy, (etc.), born at Pesaro (Italy), widower of his first marriage with Isabelle COLBRAN, and married for the second time to Olympe DESCUILLIERS, sixty-seven years, a woman of property [*rentière*], residing with him, son of Guiseppe [*sic*] ROSSINI and of GUIDERINI [*sic*], his wife, both deceased, without other information. After having been assured of the decease, WE have drawn up the present act, which the declarants have signed with US, after its having been read." (Translated from copy in *BdCRdS*, 1956, 2, p. 26.)

p. 365, l. 39 *"Due Orsi"*   Teatro San Radegonda, Milan, February 4, 1867.

p. 366, l. 30 "into oblivion"   Dall'Argine had had one earlier taste of notoriety. When Boito's *Mefistofele*, mostly a failure at its *première* at La Scala on March 5, 1868, had been repeated as divided between two nights—March 7 and 8—each section of it had been followed by a repetition of Dall'Argine's new ballet *Brahma* (*première*, La Scala, February 25, 1868), which the conservative, anti-Boito faction at once had taken up as a stick with which to belabor Boito's "music of the future." Dall'Argine died in 1877, when only thirty-four.

NOTES TO EPILOGUE

p. 367, l. 27 "his will"   The complete text of Rossini's will is given in Appendix C, p. 382.

p. 368, l. 3 "Théâtre-Italien"   Listed as among the members of the chorus were Marietta Alboni, Gilbert-Louis Duprez, Jean-Baptiste Faure, Italo Gardoni, Gabrielle Krauss, Nicholas-Prosper Levasseur, Mlle Méric, Nicolini, Christine Nilsson, Adelina Patti, Hippolyte Roger, and Antonio Tamburini.

p. 368, l. 22 "[Eleanora] Grossi"   At Cairo, on December 24, 1871, Grossi would create the role of Amneris in *Aida*.

p. 369, l. 14 "to Michelangelo"   A wreath placed on Rossini's coffin had been made from leaves cut from two trees that François-Joseph Méry had planted in 1859 in the garden of the Passy villa. One of them was a cutting from a tree at the "tomb of Vergil" in Naples; the other was a cutting from a tree at Tasso's tomb in the Giardino di San Onofrio in Rome. The coffin was placed temporarily in the family tomb of the Pepolis. On November 10, 1869, it was moved to the marble tomb that still stands in Père-Lachaise, but which now contains only the remains of Olympe. Over its entrance appears just the word ROSSINI.

p. 369, l. 34 "in London"   In a concert at the Crystal Palace attended by 18,500 people, 3,000 instrumentalists and singers took part; 700 performers joined in a concert at the Sacred Harmonic Society directed by Rossini's "beloved son," Sir Michael Costa.

p. 370, l. 5 "fourth string"   On November 17, 1868, the Consiglio Comunale of Florence had approved unanimously a motion to ask for the ashes of Rossini and to initiate a subscription for a monument to be erected to him in Santa Croce, a plan that it was to take nearly nineteen years to put into action.

p. 370, l. 7 "Tito Ricordi:"   Verdi's letter was reproduced in facsimile in the *LGMM Supplemento straordinario* of 2/29/1892, pp. 22–3, and was quoted in full in Alessandro Luzio, ed.: *Carteggi verdiani* II, 220, footnote 3.

p. 370, l. 10 "few measures)"   The seventy-three-year-old Mercadante had been totally blind since 1862.

p. 370, l. 39 "proposed Requiem"   The composers and the sections assigned to them were: Antonio Bazzini—*Dies irae,* C minor, *allegro maestoso,* chorus; Raimond Boucheron—*Confutatis,* D major, *allegro sostenuto,* bass solo; Antonio Buzzola—*Requiem aeternam,* G minor, *lento,* chorus; Antonio Cagnoni—*Quid sum miser,* A-flat major, *larghetto,* duet for soprano and contralto; Carlo Coccia (who was eighty-seven in 1869)—*Lacrymosa,* G major, *andante,* four solo voices, and *Amen,* C minor, fugue, *allegro*; Gaetano Gaspari—*Domine Jesu,* C major, *moderato,* chorus and solo voices; Teodulo Mabellini—*Lux aeterna,* A-flat major, *moderato,* chorus and solo soprano; Alessandro Nini—*Ingemisco,* A minor, *largo,* tenor solo; Carlo Pedrotti—*Tuba mirum,* E-flat major, *maestoso,* baritone solo with chorus; Errico Petrella—*Agnus Dei,* F major, *andante,* contralto solo; Pietro Platania —*Sanctus,* D-flat major, *maestoso,* chorus; Federico Ricci—*Recordare,* F major, *andantino,* quartet; and Verdi—*Libera me,* C minor, chorus with soprano solo, and fugue. Mercadante's blindness had prevented him from accepting the commission's invitation to contribute to the Mass. Angelo Mariani, though irritated over not having been asked to compose a section of it, had agreed to conduct it. But, as Alessandro Luzio wrote: ". . . his cold attitude and the rise of other difficulties, as well as the refusal of the impresario Scalaberni to cede singers and orchestra and the disinterest of the Community [Bologna], assured the shipwreck of the project." Verdi later adapted his *Libera me* for use in the "Manzoni" Requiem.

p. 371, ll. 4–5 "to cooperate"   The Comunale had opened, on October 1, 1869, a season during which Angelo Mariani was to conduct *Le Prophète, Les Huguenots,* Rossini's *Otello,* and *Un Ballo in maschera.* Five days later,

Scalaberni published in the *Monitore di Bologna* his reasons for refusing to collaborate with the commission. That revelatory document reads:

"First. I never assumed the obligation to cede my contracted artists for the Mass for Rossini.

"Second. I marvel at a private person's having been expected to bear the expenses for a national solemnity from which (it pleases me to note *en passant*) such young *maestri* as Boito, Dall'Argine, Faccio, Marchetti, etc., were excluded.

"Third. To say that the rehearsals for the performance of the Mass would not have upset the progress of the performances is a pleasantry that smells of the ridiculous.

"Fourth. My agreements with the City of Bologna consist of a contract agreed to three years ago, in which the death of Rossini was not foreseen.

"Fifth. If the committee for the Mass, instead of looking for a Maecenas of art in me, had turned to a businessman who does not have six children and is rich, that would have corresponded better to its program and, it cannot be doubted, they would have come to an understanding. Scalaberni."

p. 372, l. 24 "November 5, 1882" In 1892, the Liceo was removed to the reconstructed Palazzo Macchirelli. It is now the Conservatorio Gioacchino Rossini. Since 1923, when the endowment by Rossini no longer sufficed to support it, the school has received official subsidy.

p. 373, l. 5 "January 1889" At the ceremonies inaugurating the Maison de Retraite, Vio Bonato, a physician who had attended Rossini from 1865 to his death was present. Marietta Alboni, aged sixty-six, arrived on crutches—and sang.

p. 373, l. 7 "des Saints-Perrins" When I visited the Fondation Rossini in the late spring of 1964, it had long been unable to exist entirely on returns from Olympe's legacy, but was being maintained for its original purpose and still preserved a few mementos of Rossini, including the ceramic medallion illustrated in this book. Radiciotti had noted that of the thirty-seven women and twenty-six men housed in the retreat in January 1922, only one was an Italian—the regulations having specified that the pensioners must be either French men and women or Italians who had sung in France.

p. 373, ll. 12–13 "Santa Croce" When Verdi learned about the condition that Olympe wanted to impose, he wrote to Giulio Ricordi: "Have you read in the *Opinione* Mad.me Rossini's words to the Italian deputation? What beautiful things! What touching words! Now Mad.me finds (prodigy of prodigies) a word for *la bella Italia*!!! Oh, you'll see that Mad.me (our ministers are capable of this too) will end up having a monument among Dante, Michelangelo, etc., etc. If that happens, I'm going to turn Turk."

p. 373, l. 26 "Rossini's remains" Verdi was invited to preside over this committee in the role of honorary president. On June 16, 1878, he wrote from Sant'Agata to its president, asking to be excused. He pointed out the effort that he had put into the aborted collaborative Requiem Mass. "I too admire Rossini as much as anyone else," he wrote—and remained adamant. His attitude toward Rossini dead was as divided as it had been toward

Rossini living. In 1871, when his friend Conte Opprandino Arrivabene sent him some verses in praise of Rossini, asking him to set them to music, Verdi's answer was: "Your verses are extremely graceful, but I am no good (you know this well) at making fugitive pieces, separate pieces, etc. And then do you think that when I should have made some trill, some ascending scale, thinking to imitate the nightingale, I should have made a melody? I'll say even more: melodies are not made either with scales or with trills or with clusters of notes. . . . Notice what melodies are, for example, the *Coro dei Bardi*, the prayer in *Mosè*, etc., and what melodies are not, the cavatinas in the *Barbiere*, in *La Gazza ladra*, in *Semiramide*, etc., etc. What are they, will you say? . . . Whatever you wish, but certainly not melodies; and not even good music; don't fly into a rage if I mistreat Rossini to you a little, but Rossini is not afraid of being mistreated, and the art will gain a great deal when the critics will be be able to say, and will have the courage to say, the entire truth about him."

p. 374, l. 5   "500 voices"   Rossini certainly would have been entertained to know that the huge four-part chorus included numerous *contesse* and *marchese*, at least one *duchessa*—and the orchestra four *marchesi*.

p. 374, l. 11   "Romano Nannetti"   The compositions performed were: "*La Serenata*," a setting of words by Conte Carlo Pepoli which is No. 11 of the *Soirées musicales*; the "*Petite Polka chinoise*," No. 3 of the *Album de chaumière*; the "*Prélude convulsif*," No. 9 of the *Album pour les enfants adolescents*; "*L'Esule*," a setting of words by G. Torre which is No. 2 of the *Morceaux réservés* and was published in *QR* IV, 25; the "*Tarentelle pur sang (avec traversée de la Procession)*"; "*La promessa*," No. 1 of the *Soirées musicales*; and "*La Pastorella delle Alpi*," No. 6 of the *Soirées musicales*.

p. 374, l. 14   "of May 9"   Those taking part in this concert included Gottardo Aldighieri (who created the role of Barnaba in Ponchielli's *La Gioconda* and wrote the verse of Luigi Arditi's once endemic song "*Il Bacio*"), Mabellini, Barbara Marchisio, Jefté Sbolci, Camillo Sivori, and Enrico Tamberlik. The very long program consisted of the overture to *L'Italiana in Algeri*; Figaro's cavitina from *Il Barbiere di Siviglia*; a trio from *Guglielmo Tell*; a duet from *Mathilde di Shabran*; the overture to *La Gazza ladra*; Arsace's aria from *Semiramide*; a duet from *Otello*; Paganini's variations for one violin string on the prayer from *Mosè in Egitto*; the overture to *Guglielmo Tell*; a cavatina from *Semiramide*; Liszt's transcription of the *Cujus animam* from the *Stabat Mater*; and the concluding rondo from *La Cenerentola*. This concert followed by three days the solemn unveiling, in the presence of King Umberto and Queen Margherita, of the new façade of Santa Maria del Fiore, the Florence Cathedral.

p. 374, ll. 23–24   "resulting monument"   Romain Rolland ("*Rossini*," in *La Revue musicale*, Paris, 1902, II, 375) well said: "The style of the Rossini monument recalls both Canova and the nearby monument to Leonardo Bruni by Rossellino."

NOTE TO APPENDIX A

p. 378, l. 17   "Luigi Zamboni"   These quarters were in the Palazzo Pagliarini on the Vicolo de' Leutari, near the Piazza Navona. In 1872, the Roman municipal authorities placed on its façade an epigraph reading:

> Living in this house
> Gioacchino Rossini
> found the ever-new harmonies
> of *Il Barbiere di Siviglia.*
> S.P.Q.R.
> 1872.

NOTE TO APPENDIX C

p. 385, l. 43   "and punished!"   How or when the autograph score of *Otello* was recovered is not known. It is now in the collection of the Conservatorio Gioacchino Rossini at Pesaro.

THE MUSIC

The Music

This list of Rossini's compositions is divided into four sections, as follows:

A. The Operas—a chronological list by date of composition, with data on first productions and original casts.

B. Vocal Music—an alphabetical list of all nonoperatic vocal music.

C. Instrumental Music—an alphabetical list of all nonoperatic instrumental music.

D. *Péchés de vieillesse*—a catalogue of the fourteen collections of miscellaneous music grouped under this title.

For an explanation of the bibliographical abbreviations used, see page 391. In this section, *Péchés de vieillesse* has been abbreviated as *Pdv*, *Soirées musicales* as *Sm*.

Note for the Second Printing

Since the present book was completed, Dr. Philip Gossett has published some preliminary results of his research looking toward a systematic listing and thematic catalogue of Rossini's compositions. For this second printing, it has not proved possible to revise all of pp. 490–531 in view of Dr. Gossett's publications and intensely appreciated personal advice. Passages in the text and the following Section A, dealing with Rossini's operas, have been amended in view of some of that new information, but for detailed, extensive, and accurate data on the nonoperatic music, students should consult:

Gossett, Philip: "*Gli Autografi rossiniani al Museo Teatrale alla Scala di Milano*," in *BdCRdS*, 1967, 3, pp. 4854, and 4, pp. 65–68

"Rossini in Naples: Some Major Works Recovered," in *The Musical Quarterly*, New York, July 1968, pp. 316–340

"*Catalogo delle opere*," in Luigi Rognoni: *Gioacchino Rossini*, Turin, 1968, pp. 440–480

"*Le Fonti autografe delle opere teatrali di Rossini*," in (*Nuova*) *Rivista musicale italiana*, Turin, September–October 1968, pp. 936–960

New York, 1970   Herbert Weinstock

A. The Operas

1808

1. *Demetrio e Polibio*: opera seria, 2 acts; libretto by Vincenza Viganò Mombelli, after Metastasio's *Demetrio*; composed (completed in?) 1808. *Première*: Teatro Valle, Rome, May 18, 1812. Cast: Ester Mombelli (Lisinga), Marianna Mombelli (Siveno), Domenico Mombelli (Eumenio-Demetrio), and Lodovico Olivieri (Polibio). For more than twenty-five years, *Demetrio e Polibio* was staged intermittently throughout Italy; by 1820, it had also been heard in at least Vienna, Dresden, and Munich.

1810

2. *La Cambiale di matrimonio*: farsa, 1 act; libretto by Gaetano Rossi, after the play (1790) by the same name by Camillo Federici (pseudonym of Giovan Battista Viassolo); composed 1810. *Première*: Teatro San Moisè, Venice, November 3, 1810. Cast: Rosa Morandi (Fanny, spelled "Fanni" in the first printed libretto), Clementina Lanari (Clarina), Tommaso Ricci (Edoardo Milfort), Luigi Raffanelli (Sir Tobia Mill), Nicola De Grecis (Slook), and Domenico Remolini (Norton). Sung at least twelve times at the San Moisè between November 3 and December

1, 1810, *La Cambiale di matrimonio* was staged the next year in Trieste and Padua; during the 1814–15 season, it was sung in Cremona. Its extra-Italian history apparently began in Barcelona in 1816. It was sung in Vienna as *Der Bräutigam von Canada* in 1834 and in Italian in 1837; it was revived at the Teatro La Fenice, Venice, in 1910, its centenary year, since when it has been repeated intermittently throughout Italy. New York heard it in Italian on November 8, 1937; twenty years later, it was sung in the homeland of its Canadian character, Slook, by a student group at the University of British Colombia. It has been recorded more than once.

1811

3. *L'Equivoco stravagante*: opera buffa, 2 acts; libretto by Gaetano Gasparri; composed 1811. *Première*: Teatro del Corso, Bologna, October 26 (not 29), 1811. Cast: Marietta (Maria) Marcolini (Ernestina), Angiola (Angela) Chies (Rosalia), Domenico Vaccani (Gamberotto, spelled "Gambarotto" in the first printed libretto), Paolo (Pablo) Rosich (Buralicchio, spelled "Buralecchio" in the first printed libretto), Tommaso Berti (Ermanno), and Giuseppe Spirito (Frontino). *L'Equivoco*

stravagante has had fewer performances than any other of Rossini's operas, possibly excepting *Adina* and *Ermione*. It was revived at the twenty-second Settimana Musicale Senese, Siena (Teatro Comunale dei Rinnuovati), on September 7, 1965, in the "modern edition of the Accademia Musicale Chigiana, edited by V. Frazzi."

4. *L'Inganno felice: farsa*, 1 act; libretto by Giuseppe Foppa, after Giuseppe Palomba's libretto for Paisiello's opera of the same name (1798); composed 1811. *Première*: Teatro San Moisè, Venice, January 8, 1812. Cast: Teresa Giorgi-Belloc (Isabella), Raffaele Monelli (Bertrando), Filippo Galli (Batone), Luigi Raffanelli (Tarabotto), Vincenzo Venturi (Ormondo), and possibly Dorinda Caranti. *L'Inganno* went on to continuous popularity in other Italian opera houses. It became the second Rossini opera heard in Paris (Théâtre-Italien, May 13, 1819), possibly the first to be heard in Vienna (Kärnthnertortheater, 1816). It held the stages of Italy and the German-speaking countries for half a century. It was staged at the King's Theatre, London, on July 1, 1819, and in New Orleans on January 1, 1837, but seems never to have been performed in New York (though it was sung in Vera Cruz, Mexico, as early as 1831).

1812

5. *Ciro in Babilonia, ossia La Caduta di Balassare: dramma con cori* or *oratorio*, 2 acts: libretto by Conte Francesco Aventi; composed 1812. *Première*: Teatro Municipale

(Communale), Ferrara, March (March 14?), 1812. Cast: Marietta (Maria) Marcolini (Ciro), Elisabetta Manfredini (Amira), Anna Savinelli (Argene), Eliodoro Bianchi (Baldassare), Giovanni Layner (Zambri), Francesco Savinelli (Arbace), and Giovanni Fraschi (Daniele). *Ciro* was performed throughout Italy for about fifteen years. It was staged in Munich (1816), in Vienna (1817), in Weimar, and in Dresden (1822), but seems to have had few other performances outside Italy.

6. *La Scala di seta: farsa*, 1 act; libretto by Giuseppe Foppa, after the play *L'Échelle de soie*, by François-Antoine-Eugène de Planard and possibly a libretto made from it for Pierre Gaveaux (1808); composed 1812. *Première*: Teatro San Moisè, Venice, May 9, 1812. Cast: probably Maria Cantarelli (Giulia), Carolina Nagher (Lucilla), Raffaele Monelli (Dorvil), Gaetano Del Monte (Dormont), Nicola De Grecis (Blansac), and Nicola Tacci (Germano) *La Scala di seta* has had very few stagings in Italy; outside Italy, up to 1825 it had been staged in Barcelona and Lisbon. In England it has been seen only (1954) as produced by a company from Rome; it has not been staged in France, the German-speaking countries, or the United States. At the Piccola Scala, Milan, it was heard on February 6, 1961, with Graziella Sciutti, Luigi Alva, Franco Calabrese, and Sesto Bruscantini.

7. *La Pietra del paragone: melodrammo giocoso* or *opera buffa*, 2 acts; libretto by Luigi Romanelli; composed 1812. *Première*: Teatro

alla Scala, Milan, September 26, 1812. Cast: Marietta (Maria) Marcolini (La Marchesa Clarice), Carolina Zerbini (La Baronessa Aspasia), Orsola Fei (Donna Fulvia), Filippo Galli (Asdrubale), Claudio Bonoldi (Giocondo), Antonio Parlamagni (Il Conte Macrobio), Pietro Vasoli (Pacuvio), and Paolo Rossignoli (Fabrizio). *La Pietra del paragone* was very widely played in Italy for about twenty years. It began its foreign career at Munich in July 1817; during the next nineteen years, it was staged in Oporto, Paris, Vienna, Lisbon, Barcelona, Graz, Berlin, and Mexico City. It has had numerous more recent revivals, notably at the Maggio Musicale Fiorentino of 1952 and at the Piccola Scala, Milan, on May 29, 1959, when the cast included Fiorenza Cossotto (Clarice), Silvana Zanolli (Aspasia), Eugenia Ratti (Fulvia), Ivo Vinco (Asdrubale), Alvinio Misciano (Giocondo), Renato Capecchi (Macrobio), Giulio Fioravanti (Pacuvio), and Franco Calabrese (Fabrizio). A distorted German version (by Paul Friedrich and Günther Rennert) of *La Pietra del paragone* unfortunately has had some currency since 1963 and even has been translated into Italian for performance in Italy.

8. *L'Occasione fa il ladro, ossia Il Cambio della valigia: burletta per musica*, 1 act; libretto by Luigi Prividali; composed 1812. *Première*: Teatro San Moisè, Venice, November 24, 1812. Cast: Giacinta Canonici (Berenice), Carolina Nagher (Ernestina), Gaetano Del Monte (Don Eusebio), Tommaso Berti (Conte Alberto), Luigi Pacini (Don Parmenione), and Filippo Spada (Martino). Not a success at the San Moisè, *L'Occasione fa il ladro* won only a few performances in Italy subsequently (but was revived at Pesaro both in 1892, at the celebration of the centenary of Rossini's birth, and in 1916, at that of the centenary of *Il Barbiere di Siviglia*). It was produced in Barcelona in 1822, St. Petersburg in 1830, Vienna in 1834, but seems never to have been staged professionally in England, France, Germany, or the United States.

9. *Il Signor Bruschino, ossia Il Figlio per azzardo: farsa giocosa*, 1 act; libretto by Giuseppe Foppa, after a French comedy by Alisan (André-René-Polydore) de Chazet and E.-T. Maurice Ourry; composed 1812. *Première*: Teatro San Moisè, Venice, late January 1813. Cast: Teodolinda Pontiggia (Sofia), Carolina Nagher (Marianna), Luigi Raffanelli (Bruschino *padre*), Gaetano Del Monte (Bruschino *figlio* and Un Delegato di polizia), Nicola De Grecis (Gaudenzio), Tommaso Berti (Florville), and Nicola Tacci (Filiberto). *Il Signor Bruschino* has had several recent revivals: in Catania in 1955; at both the Festival of Two Worlds, Spoleto, and the Teatro San Carlo, Naples, in 1963; and at the Festival du Marais, Paris, on July 5, 1965. The Metropolitan Opera, New York, staged *Il Signor Bruschino* as a curtain-raiser for Strauss's *Elektra* on December 9, 1932, in a severely edited version that simplified the vocal lines. The cast consisted of Giuseppe DeLuca (Bruschino *padre*), Editha Fleischer

(Sofia), Elda Vittori (Marianna), Armand Tokatyan (Florville), Ezio Pinza (Gaudenzio), Louis D'Angelo (Commissar of Police), Marek Windheim (Bruschino *figlio*), and Alfred Gandolfi (Filiberto). With that season's fourth performance (January 12, 1933), *Il Signor Bruschino* left the Metropolitan.

1812-1813

10. *Tancredi*: *opera seria* or *melodramma eroico*, 2 acts, libretto by Gaetano Rossi, after Tasso's *Gerusalemme liberata* and Voltaire's *Tancrède*; composed 1812–13. *Première*: Teatro La Fenice, Venice, February 6, 1813. Cast: Adelaide Malanotte-Montresor (sometimes Melanotte-Montresor) (Tancredi), Elisabetta Manfredini-Guarmani (Amenaide), Teresa Marchesi (Isaura), Carolina Sivelli (Roggiero), Pietro Todràn (Argirio), and Luciano Bianchi (Orbazzano). From 1815 on, the popularity of *Tancredi* in Italy became enormous. Besides innumerable stagings there, it was heard in Munich on July 4, 1816; in Vienna, in Italian, on December 7 or 17, 1816 (probably the second Rossini opera there, following *L'Inganno felice* quickly); in Dresden in 1817, with the *castrato* Filippo Sassaroli in the title role; in Berlin, in German, in 1818; at the King's Theatre, London, on May 4, 1820; in Paris, in Italian, in 1822; and in New York, in Italian, on December 31, 1825. The only recent performances seem to have been during the Maggio Musicale Fiorentino of 1952 (with Giulietta Simionato

and Teresa Stich-Randall) and (in concert form, with two-piano accompaniment) at Wigmore Hall, London, on April 25, 1959.

1813

11. *L'Italiana in Algeri*: *melodramma giocoso*, 2 acts; libretto by Angelo Anelli, originally set, under the same title, by Luigi Mosca (1808); composed 1813. *Première*: Teatro San Benedetto, Venice, May 22, 1813. Cast: Marietta (Maria) Marcolini (Isabella), Luttgard Annibaldi (Elvira), Annunziata Berni Chelli (Zulma), Filippo Galli (Mustafà), Serafino Gentili (Lindoro), and Paolo Rosich (Taddeo). The popularity of *L'Italiana* became very great in Italy. On February 1, 1817, it became the first Rossini opera to be heard in Paris (Théâtre-Italien); it also was the first staged in Germany (Munich, June 18, 1816). It reached the Kärnthnertortheater, Vienna, in Italian, in 1817; His Majesty's Theatre, London, also in Italian, on January 26, 1819, with Teresa Giorgi-Belloc and Manuel Garcia; and New York, still in Italian, on November 5, 1832. The Metropolitan Opera, New York, got round to the first of its only four performances of *L'Italiana* on December 5, 1919. The cast, conducted by Gennaro Papi and displayed against lavish settings by Willy Pogany, consisted of Gabriella Besanzoni (Isabella), Marie Sundelius (Elvira), Kathleen Howard (Zulma), Charles Hackett (Lindoro), Adamo Didur (Mustafà), Giuseppe DeLuca (Taddeo), and Millo Picco (Haly). The

most important modern revival of *L'Italiana* began at the Teatro di Torino, Turin, on November 26, 1925, when Conchita Supervia's Isabella established a standard that later singers have had to accept. Vittorio Gui, who conducted, wrote Radiciotti that after a 1927 repetition of the opera in Turin, "Richard Strauss, who did not know this opera, seemed mad with enthusiasm after becoming acquainted with it here in Turin." Four performances of *L'Italiana* in which Supervia sang at the Théâtre des Champs-Elysées, Paris, in May 1929 occupy a special position in operatic lore. The opera has had many restagings since then, has been recorded, and has all but become a staple of the European opera-house repertoire.

12. *Aureliano in Palmira*: *opera seria* or *dramma serio*, 2 acts; libretto by Gian Francesco Roman(ell?)i; composed 1813. *Première*: Teatro alla Scala, Milan, December 26, 1813. Cast: Lorenza Correa (Zenobia), Luigia Sorrentini (Publia), Giambattista Velluti (Arsace), Luigi Mari (Aureliano), Gaetano Pozzi (Oraspe), Pietro Vasoli (Licinio), and Vincenzo Botticelli (Gran Sacerdote d'Iside). Although *Aureliano* never became one of Rossini's most popular operas, it had considerable diffusion throughout Italy. During its first decade, it was staged in about thirty opera houses; it was still being sung in 1832. Its extra-Italian history was less busy: it was performed in Barcelona in 1822; Lisbon in 1824; Corfu in 1825; London—with Velluti—on June 22, 1826; Graz, in German, in 1827;

and Buenos Aires in 1829. It seems never to have reached Paris or the United States.

1814

13. *Il Turco in Italia*: *opera buffa* or *dramma buffo*, 2 acts; libretto by Felice Romani; composed 1814. *Première*: Teatro alla Scala, Milan, August 14, 1814. Cast: Francesca Maffei-Festa (Fiorilla), Adelaide Carpano (Zaida), Giovanni David (Narciso), Filippo Galli (Selim), Luigi Pacini (Geronio), Pietro Vasoli (Prosdocimo), and Gaetano Pozzi (Albazar). Staged at the Teatro della Pergola, Florence, in 1814–15, *Il Turco* next was heard at the Teatro Valle, Rome, where Rossini supervised the production; presented at the Valle on November 7, 1815, it was sung there throughout that month. It then traveled the round of Italian and foreign opera houses (the latter beginning at Dresden in 1816) until about 1850. Its reviving career in the twentieth century was given impulse by a staging at Rome in 1950, with a cast headed by Maria Meneghini Callas, Cesare Valletti, Mariano Stabile, and Sesto Bruscantini. *Il Turco in Italia* was also revived at the Piccola Scala, Milan, on April 11, 1958. Gianandrea Gavazzeni conducted; the cast consisted of Eugenia Ratti (Fiorilla), Fiorenza Cossotto (Zaida), Luigi Alva (Narciso), Sesto Bruscantini (Selim), Franco Calabrese (Geronio), Giulio Fioravanti (Prosdocimo), and Angelo Mercuriali (Albazar).

14. *Sigismondo*: *opera seria* or *dramma*, 2 acts; libretto by Giuseppe Foppa; composed 1814.

Première: Teatro La Fenice, Venice, December 26, 1814. Cast: Marietta (Maria) Marcolini (Sigismondo, re di Polonia), Elisabetta Manfredini-Guarmani (Aldimira), Marianna Rossi (Anagilda), Claudio Bonoldi (Ladislao), Luciano Bianchi (Ulderico, re di Boemia, and Zenovito), and Domenico Bartoli (Radoski). Stendhal, who intensely admired Marcolini, said of her *"tour de force"* in singing the final aria in Sigismondo: "Where find a *prima donna* with lungs sufficiently robust to sing a grand *air à roulade* at the end of so wearying a work?" *Sigismondo*, which had some stagings in Italy up to 1827, seems not to have been performed elsewhere.

1815

15. *Elisabetta, regina d'Inghilterra*: *dramma*, 2 acts; libretto by Giovanni Federico Schmidt after a play by Carlo Federici based upon Sophia Lee's *The Recess*; composed 1815. *Première*: Teatro San Carlo, Naples, October 4, 1815. Cast: Isabella Colbran (Elisabetta), Girolama Dardanelli (Matilde), Maria(?) Manzi (Enrico), Andrea Nozzari (Leicester), Manuel Garcia (Norfolc), and Gaetano Chizzola (Guglielmo). That Maria Manzi created the travesty role of Enrico is not certain: at least six female Manzis singing in Naples in or about 1815 appear in the index to Florimo: *La Scuola musicale di Napoli*, vol. IV. The first printed libretto and the De Filippis-Arnese *Cronache del Teatro di San Carlo* call her simply "Manzi." *Elisabetta* was put on again in Naples (Teatro del

Fondo) in May 1816; thereafter, it was sung with some frequency throughout Italy until about 1840. Its first extra-Italian stagings occurred in Barcelona in August 1817 and in Dresden in January 1818 (it was repeated in Dresden in April and November and again in March 1819). It was a failure in Vienna in 1818, and was also heard at the King's Theatre, London, on April 30 of that year. It reached St. Petersburg, in Russian, in 1820; Paris, in Italian, in 1822; Berlin in 1824; Odessa in 1830; and Mexico City in 1834. It seems never to have been staged in New York.

16. *Torvaldo e Dorliska*: *dramma semiserio*, 2 acts; libretto by Cesare Sterbini; composed 1815. *Première*: Teatro Valle, Rome, December 26, 1815. Cast: Adelaide Sala (Dorliska), Agnese Loyselet (spelled "Loiselet" in the printed libretto, Carlotta), Domenico Donzelli (Torvaldo), Raniero Remorini (Giorgio), Filippo Galli (Il Duca d'Ordow), and Cristoforo Bastianelli (Ormondo). Agnese Loyselet should not be confused with Elisabetta Loyselet, the first Berta in *Il Barbiere di Siviglia*. After being staged at the Teatro San Moisè, Venice, during 1817–18, *Torvaldo e Dorliska* was produced throughout Italy until about 1840. Heard in Barcelona in May 1818, Munich and Lisbon in 1820, it thereafter won numerous foreign stagings. Paris first heard it in 1820 (November 21, Théâtre-Italien), Vienna in 1821, Prague (in German) in 1823, Madrid in 1824, Berlin (in German) in 1829. It apparently was never staged in London or New York.

1816

17. *Il Barbiere di Siviglia* (originally *Almaviva, ossia L'Inutile Precauzione*): *opera buffa* or *commedia*; 2 acts; libretto by Cesare Sterbini, after Beaumarchais's *Le Barbier de Séville* and Giuseppe Petrosellini's libretto for Paisiello's *Il Barbiere di Siviglia* (1782); composed 1816. *Première*: Teatro Argentina, Rome, February 20, 1816. Cast: Geltrude Righetti-Giorgi (Rosina), Elisabetta Loyselet (Berta), Manuel Garcia (Almaviva), Luigi Zamboni (Figaro), Bartolomeo Botticelli (Bartolo), Zenobio Vitarelli (Basilio), and Paolo Biagelli (Fiorello). Soon becoming one of the most popular of all operas both in Italy and abroad, *Il Barbiere* reached London (King's Theater), in Italian, on March 10, 1818 (twenty-two performances in two months), and was sung there in English, at Covent Garden, on October 13 of that year, with the music "arranged" by Henry Rowley Bishop. New York first heard it, in English, on May 3, 1819; on November 29, 1825, as the opening attraction of a season by the Garcia family troupe (which included Manuel Garcia, the future Maria Malibran, her mother, and her brother Manuel Patricio) at the Park Theater, it became the first opera ever sung in New York in Italian. Vienna heard it first in German on September 28, 1819; Paris in Italian on October 26, 1819; Berlin in German on June 18, 1822; St. Petersburg in Russian on December 9, 1822—and in German five days later, when the role of Figaro was sung by a woman, the Basilio was a tenor, and the Bartolo was a *"basse noble"*; Buenos Aires, where it was the first opera sung in Italian, on October 3, 1825. The Metropolitan Opera, New York, presented *Il Barbiere di Siviglia* during its first season, on November 23, 1883. Augusto Vianesi conducted, and the cast included Marcella Sembrich (Rosina), Emily (Emilia) Lablache (Berta), Roberto Stagno (Almaviva), Giuseppe Del Puente (Figaro), Baldassare Corsini (Bartolo), Giovanni Mirabella (Basilio), and Ludovico Contini (Fiorello).

18. *La Gazzetta, ossia Il Matrimonio per concorso* (subtitle not in first printed libretto): *dramma* [*sic*], really *opera buffa*, 2 acts; libretto a revision by Andrea Leone Tottola of a libretto by Giuseppe Palomba based on Goldoni's *Il Matrimonio per concorso*; composed 1816. *Première*: Teatro dei Fiorentini, Naples, September 26, 1816. Cast: Margherita Chabrand (spelled "Chambrand" in the first printed libretto; Lisetta), Francesca Cardini (Doralice), Maria(?) Manzi (Madama La Rosa), Alberico Curioni (Alberto), Carlo Casaccia (Pomponio), Felice Pellegrini (Filippo), Giovanni Pace (Anselmo), and Francesco Sparano (Monsù Traversen). After a few evenings at the Fiorentini, *La Gazzetta* lapsed into oblivion. A studio performance of it was broadcast by RAI (Italian radio network) on September 29, 1960.

19. *Otello, ossia il Moro di Venezia*: *opera seria* or *dramma*, 3 acts; libretto by Francesco Berio di Salsa, after Shakespeare's *Othello*; com-

posed 1816. *Première*: Teatro del Fondo, Naples, December 4, 1816. Cast: Isabella Colbran (Desdemona), Maria (?) Manzi (Emilia), Andrea Nozzari (Otello), Michele Benedetti (Elmiro Barberigo), Giovanni David (Rodrigo), and Giuseppe Ciccimarra (Jago), Gaetano Chizzola (Doge), Mollo (Lucio). The first libretto shows Ciccimarra as Jago, but its creation often is credited to Manuel Garcia. An undated Ricordi edition of *Otello* in the present writer's possession (plate no. 43971) assigns Jago to Garcia, "*Un Gondoliere*" to Ciccimarra (perhaps reflecting the 1817 San Carlo cast), and lists no singers for Emilia, the Doge, and Lucio. *Otello* soon became standard both in Italy and abroad. Its first extra-Italian staging occurred in Munich, in Italian, on September 13, 1818. Vienna heard it first in German, on January 19, 1819; Frankfurt-am-Main on April 9, 1820, with (for perhaps the first time) a soprano as Otello; Lisbon, in Italian, in 1820; Berlin, in German, on January 16, 1821; Paris, in Italian, on June 5, 1821; London, in Italian, on May 16, 1822; New York, at the Park Theater, in Italian, as sung by the Garcia troupe, on February 7, 1826; St. Petersburg, in Italian, in February 1829 (and in German in 1835, Russian in 1860). It was being played in German in Prague and Berlin as late as 1889. Among concert performances given more recently, one was presented at Town Hall, New York, on November 23, 1954, by the American Opera Society. Arnold U. Gamson conducted; leading roles were sung by Jennie Tourel (Desdemona), Carol Brice (Emilia), Thomas Hayward (Otello), Albert Da Costa (Rodrigo), and Thomas Lo Monaco (Iago). *Otello* was revived at the Teatro dell'Opera, Rome, on March 31, 1964, when Carlo Franci conducted; costumes and scenery were by Giorgio De Chirico; and the cast was made up of Virginia Zeani (Desdemona), Luisa Ribacchi (Emilia), Agostino Lazzari (Otello), Franco Ventriglia (Elmiro Barbarigo), Pietro Bottazzo (Rodrigo), Gastone Limarilli (Jago), Tommaso Frascati (Il Doge and Un Gondoliere), and Fernando Jacopucci (Lucio); the production was taken over into the 1964-5 season.

1816-1817

20. *La Cenerentola, ossia La Bontà in trionfo: dramma giocoso*, 2 acts; libretto by Jacopo Ferretti, after Charles Perrault's *Cendrillon, ou La Petite Pantoufle* (1697) and probably both Charles-Guillaume Étienne's libretto for Niccolò Isouard's *Cendrillon* (1810) and Felice Romani's libretto for Stefano Pavesi's *Agatina, o La Virtù premiata* (1814); composed 1816-17. *Première*: Teatro Valle, Rome, January 25, 1817. Cast: Geltrude Righetti-Giorgi (Angiolina-Cenerentola), Caterina Rossi (Clorinda), Teresa Mariani (Tisbe), Giacomo Guglielmi (Don Ramiro), Andrea Verni (Don Magnifico), Giuseppe De Begnis (Dandini), and Zenobio Vitarelli (Alidoro). Enormously popular in Italy, *La Cenerentola* soon was heard in many European countries

and in both Americas. On February 12, 1844, in English, it became the first opera to be staged in Australia. It was first played in London, in Italian, at the King's Theatre, on January 8, 1820, nearly two years after its first extra-Italian performance had taken place in Barcelona (April 15, 1818). The first Vienna production, in German, was heard on August 29, 1820—and Rossini himself conducted it there in German on March 30, 1822. It was sung in Paris, in Italian, on June 8, 1822. The earliest Berlin performance, in German, took place on October 29, 1825. It was sung in Moscow, in Italian, on November 5, 1825, and in that language in Buenos Aires on May 4, 1826. New York heard it on June 27, 1826, at the Park Theater, given by the Garcia troupe. Since World War II, *La Cenerentola* has had numerous revivals on stage and has been sung in concert performances. It was staged stylishly by the New York City Opera Company at the New York City Center of Music and Drama in 1953, when Joseph Rosenstock conducted and the cast consisted of Frances Bible (Angelina-Cenerentola), Laurel Hurley (Clorinda), Edith Evans (Tisbe), Riccardo Manning (Prince Ramiro), George Gaynes (Dandini), Richard Wentworth (Don Magnifico), and Arthur Newman (Alidoro). The American Opera Society presented a concert performance of *La Cenerentola* at Carnegie Hall, New York, on April 10, 1962, when Nicola Rescigno conducted; the cast was made up of Teresa Berganza (her New York debut; Cenerentola), Elizabeth Carron (Clorinda), Edith Evans (Tisbe), Charles Anthony (Don Ramiro) Ezio Flagello (Dandini), René Miville (Alidoro), and Fernando Corena (Don Magnifico). The Metropolitan Opera National Company made the mistake of presenting, during its inaugural (1965–1966) season a "new version" of *La Cenerentola* (as *Cinderella*) in English translation; the handsome sets and costumes by Beni Montresor could not redeem a pointless distortion of both Ferretti's libretto and Rossini's music.

1817

21. *La Gazza ladra: melodramma* or *opera semiseria*, 2 acts; libretto by Giovanni Gherardini, after *La Pie voleuse* (1815), by Jean-Marie-Théodore Baudoin d'Aubigny and Louis-Charles Caigniez. *Première*: Teatro alla Scala, Milan, May 31, 1817. Cast: Teresa Giorgi-Belloc (Ninetta), Teresa Gallianis (Pippo), Marietta Castiglioni (Lucia), Savino Monelli (Giannetto), Vincenzo Botticelli (Fabrizio Vingradito), Filippo Galli (Fernando Villabella), Antonio Ambrosi (Gottardo, the *podestà*), Francesco Biscottini (Isacco), Paolo Rossignoli (Giorgio), and Alessandro De Angeli (Ernesto). In addition to its very great popularity in Italy, *La Gazza ladra* quickly won numerous stagings abroad. It was staged in Munich, in Italian, in November 1817; in Vienna, in German, on May 3, 1819; in St. Petersburg, in Russian, on February 7, 1821; in Lon-

don, in Italian, on March 10, 1821, and in English—as *Ninetta, or The Maid of Palaiseau*, the music "adapted by Henry Rowley Bishop"—at Covent Garden on February 4, 1830; in Paris at the Théâtre-Italien, in Italian, on September 18, 1821, and at the Odéon, in French, on August 2, 1824; in Berlin (after an earlier concert performance) on December 31, 1824, in German; in Warsaw, in Polish, on February 22, 1825; in Philadelphia, in French, in October 1827; and in New York, in French, on August 28, 1830 (and in Italian on November 18, 1833, and in English on January 14, 1839). *La Gazza ladra* has had numerous recent productions, including one in Eire (the Wexford Music Festival of 1959) and one at the Teatro Comunale, Florence (the Maggio Musicale Fiorentino, May 11, 1965). On March 10, 1954, the American Chamber Opera Society (which later dropped "Chamber" from its name) presented *La Gazza ladra* in concert form at Town Hall, New York; the most notable members of the cast were Laurel Hurley (Ninetta), Charles Anthony (Gianetto), Salvatore Baccaloni (Podestà), and Thomas Lo Monaco (Giorgio).

22. *Armida*: opera seria or *dramma*, 3 acts; libretto by Giovanni Federico Schmidt, after Tasso's *Gerusalemme liberata*; composed 1817. *Première*: Teatro San Carlo, Naples, November 11, 1817. Cast: Isabella Colbran (Armida), Andrea Nozzari (Rinaldo), Giuseppe Ciccimarra (Goffredo and Carlo), Michele Benedetti (Idraste—"Idraote" in the printed libretto),

Claudio Bonoldi (Gernando and Ubaldo), and Gaetano Chizzola (Eustasio and Astarotte). *Armida* received some later performances in Italian and foreign opera houses, but seems never to have been staged in London, New York, or Paris. It was revived at the Maggio Musicale Fiorentino in 1952, with Tullio Serafin conducting a cast that included Maria Meneghini Callas as Armida.

23. *Adelaide di Borgogna, ossia Ottone, re d'Italia*: *dramma*, 2 acts; libretto by Giovanni Federico Schmidt; composed 1817. *Première*: Teatro Argentina, Rome, December 27, 1817. Cast: Elisabetta Manfredini-Guarmani (Adelaide), Elisabetta Pinotti (Ottone), Anna Maria Muratori (Eurice), Luisa Bottesi (Iroldo), Savino Monelli (Adalberto), Antonio Ambrosi (Berengario), and Giovanni Puglieschi (Ernesto). The libretto issued for the first performance of *Adelaide* lists Gioacchino Sciarpelletti as singing the role of Berengario. On December 27, 1817, however, Prince Chigi-Albani noted in his diary: "The theaters opened this evening. Argentina: the *dramma* is *Adelaide di Borgogna*, music by Rossini. . . . Everything turned out rather badly except a third, added [singer, a] *buffo* named Ambrogi [Ambrosi], who found favor as a replacement." Evidently Ambrosi substituted for Sciarpelletti at a late hour. Of Elisabetta Pinotti in *Adelaide*, Alberto Cametti wrote: "The role of Ottone, by one of those strange customs of the time, was sustained by a woman; it was the part of the contralto, also

called that of the *primo musico*, a denomination that explains itself when one thinks that the contralto *donna* had taken the place of the elephant songbirds [*castrati*] of the seventeen hundreds . . . The part that Rossini wrote for her rises from a deep B to the high F, and a few times pushes from the deep G to the high B-flat." *Adelaide di Borgogna* had a few later stagings in Italy, but appears not to have been heard abroad.

1818

24. *Mosè in Egitto: azione tragico-sacra* or *oratorio*, 3 acts; libretto by Andrea Leone Tottola, after Padre Francesco Ringhieri's *Sara in Egitto* (1747); composed 1818. *Première*: Teatro San Carlo, Naples, March 5, 1818. Cast: Isabella Colbran (Elcia), Friderike Funk (Amaltea), Maria(?) Manzi (Amenofi), Michele Benedetti (Mosè), Andrea Nozzari (Osiride), Giuseppe Ciccimarra (Aronne), Raniero Remorini (Faraone), and Gaetano Chizzola (Mambre). The 1819 libretto shows the 1818 cast except for the Amenofi (Raffaela De Bernardis), the Amaltea (Maria[?] Manzi), and the Faraone (Matteo Porto). Before Rossini's 1827 revision of *Mosè* as a French opera (for which see *Moïse*, under 1827), the Italian original had won considerable distribution in Italy. It had also been staged in German in Budapest (1820), Vienna (1821), and Frankfurt-am-Main (1822) and in Italian in Paris (Théâtre-Italien) in 1822. *Mosè in Egitto* was heard in London for the first time as a concert

oratorio at Covent Garden on January 30, 1822. In *The Financial Times* (London) of May 24, 1965, Andrew Porter wrote that "though described as a 'selection from the most approved Pieces,'" this singing "included most of the opera, dropping only (with one exception [the tenor-baritone duet that Rossini later transferred to *Moïse*]) those numbers which Rossini was later to drop when fashioning *Moïse*. The roles were not consistently assigned. The cast included Ronzi de Begnis and her husband De Begnis . . ." Later in the 1822 season, Biblical subjects being banned from the stage in England, the opera became, at the King's Theatre, *Pietro l'eremita*, with a cast including Violante Camporese (Agia), Giuseppina Ronzi De Begnis (Fatima), and Carlo Zucchelli (Noraddin). Later, *Mosè* was heard in Italian in Lisbon and Dresden (1823), in Prague in German in that year, and in Barcelona in Italian in 1825. After 1830, it is often impossible to determine what version of Rossini's Moses opera was being sung. On November 6, 1852, Joseph Méry wrote to Rossini (letter in the Moldenhauer Archive) to describe a splendid revival of *Moïse* at the Opéra (Paris); the cast had included Louis-Henry Obin as Moïse (November 4, 1852). The first Italian version was heard in New York on March 2, 1835. During the fall of 1957, RAI (Radio Italiana) broadcast a much-admired studio performance of the opera, conducted by Tullio Serafin; the cast included Anita Cerquetti, Rosanna Carteri, Gianni

Iaia, Giuseppe Taddei, and Nicola Rossi-Lemeni. On December 2, 1958, at Carnegie Hall, New York, the American Opera Society presented a concert performance of a mixed version in Italian. Arnold U. Gamson conducted; the principal roles were sung by Gloria Davy (Anaïde), Jennie Tourel (Sinaïde), Jon Crain (Amenophi), and (his New York debut) Boris Christoff (Mosè). When the Society repeated this version at Carnegie Hall on October 28, 1966, Lamberto Gardelli conducted, and the roles were in the hands of Rita Orlandi Malaspina (Anaïde), Ruza Pospinov (Sinaïde), Luigi Ottolini (Amenophi), and Nicolai Ghiaurov (Mosè).

25. *Adina, o Il Califfo di Bagdad*: *farsa*, 1 act; libretto by the Marchese Gherardo Bevilacqua-Aldobrandini, derived from Felice Romani's two-act libretto *Il Califfo e la schiava*, which was set by Francesco Basilj (La Scala, Milan, 1819), and possibly from Andrea Leone Tottola's version (for Manuel Garcia's *Il Califfo di Bagdad*) of Claude Godard d'Aucour de Saint-Just's libretto for Boieldieu's *Le Calife de Bagdad* (1800); composed 1818. *Première*: Teatro São Carlos, Lisbon, June 22, 1826. Cast: Luigia Valesi (Adina), Luigi Ravaglia (Selimo), Giovanni Orazio Cartagenova (Califfo), Gaspare Martinelli (Alì), and Filippo Spada (Mustafà). It shared a triple bill with Act II of *Semiramide* and a ballet. (*RAD* III, 228, gives an incorrect list of the singers at the *première*, omitting Valesi and mistaking Ravaglia for a female singer. *ROG* repeats these errors, 376.)

No other production of *Adina* has been traced until September 1963, when it shared a double bill with Donizetti's *Le Convenienze ed inconvenienze teatrali* at the Teatro dei Rinnuovati, Siena; Bruno Rigacci conducted a cast including Mariella Adani (Adina), Giorgio Tadeo (Il Califfo), Mario Spina (Selimo), Paolo Pedani (Mustafà), and Florindo Andreolli (sometimes Andreoli; Alì).

26. *Ricciardo e Zoraide*: *dramma* or *opera seria* or *opera semiseria*, 2 acts; libretto by the Marchese Francesco Berio di Salsa, after Niccolò Forteguerri's *Ricciardetto*; composed 1818. *Première*: Teatro San Carlo, Naples, December 3, 1818. Cast: Isabella Colbran (Zoraide), Benedetta Rosmunda Pisaroni-Carrara (Zomira), Maria(?) Manzi (Fatima), Raffaela De Bernardis (Elmira), Giovanni David (Ricciardo), Andrea Nozzari (Agorante), Michele Benedetti (Ircano), and Giuseppe Ciccimarra (Ernesto). The *première* had been announced for November 28, but Colbran had injured herself in a fall; the audience on December 3 was handed a notice stating that she had not recovered entirely, but would carry out her duty as well as she could. *Ricciardo e Zoraide* was staged in German in Vienna on October 3, 1819, and had later performances in that language in Stuttgart and Budapest (1820), Munich (1821), Graz (1823), and elsewhere. It was staged with some frequency in Italy until a revival at La Scala, Milan, on October 13, 1846, after which it seems to have vanished from Italian theaters. *Ricciardo*

was staged in Italian in Paris (Théâtre-Italien) in 1824; at the King's Theatre in London, with Violante Camporese, Manuel del Popolo Vicente Garcia, Lucia Elizabeth Vestris, Alberico Curioni, Domenico Reina, and Matteo Porto in 1823 (it was also heard there, in a one-act version, in 1829, with Rosmunda Pisaroni, Virginia De Blasis, Curioni, and Domenico Donzelli). It appears not to have been staged in the United States.

1819

27. *Ermione*: *azione tragica*, 2 acts; libretto by Andrea Leone Tottola, after Racine's *Andromaque*; composed 1819. *Première*: Teatro San Carlo, Naples, March 27, 1819. Cast: Isabella Colbran (Ermione), Rosmunda Pisaroni (Andromaca), Maria(?) Manzi (Cleone), De Bernardis *minore* (Cefisa), Andrea Nozzari (Pirro), Giovanni David (Oreste), Michele Benedetti (Fenicio), Giuseppe Ciccimarra (Pilade), Gaetano Chizzola (Attalo), and "A pupil of the Royal School of Dance" (Astianatte). No later performances of *Ermione* have been traced.

28. *Eduardo e Cristina*: *dramma*, 2 acts; libretto a refashioning by Andrea Leone Tottola and the Marchese Gherardo Bevilacqua-Aldobrandini of Giovanni Federico Schmidt's libretto for Stefano Pavesi's *Odoardo e Cristina* (1810); composed 1819. *Première*: Teatro San Benedetto, Venice, April 24, 1819. Cast: Rosa Morandi (Cristina), Carolina Cortesi (Eduardo), Eliodoro Bianchi (Carlo, re di Svezia), Luciano Bianchi (Gia-

como, principe di Scozia), and Vincenzo Fracalini (sometimes Fracabini, Fraccalini; Atlei). *Edoardo e Cristina*, now so spelled, was transferred to La Fenice in 1820, during which it also was staged in many cities in Italy and elsewhere. For obvious reasons, it was not staged in Naples, but it reached La Scala, Milan (with Caroline Unger as Edoardo), on January 26, 1828. It was staged in German in Budapest on October 25, 1820, in Vienna on October 16, 1821, in Bucharest in November 1830, and in Graz on September 21, 1833. Meanwhile, it had been heard in Italian in Munich (January 26, 1821), Vienna (May 4, 1824), St. Petersburg (1831), and New York (November 25, 1834). It seems not to have been staged in London.

29. *La Donna del lago*: *melodramma* or *opera seria*, 2 acts; libretto by Andrea Leone Tottola, after Scott's *The Lady of the Lake*; composed 1819. *Première*: Teatro San Carlo, Naples, September 24, 1819. Cast: Isabella Colbran (Elena), Rosmunda Pisaroni (Malcolm Groeme—*sic* in the first printed libretto, though often "Graeme" elsewhere), Maria (?) Manzi (Albina), Giovanni David (Giacomo V, re di Scozia, alias Cavaliere Uberto), Andrea Nozzari (Rodrigo di Dhu), Michele Benedetti (Douglas d'Angus), Gaetano Chizzola (Serano), and Massimo Orlandini (Bertram). *La Donna del lago* at once became popular. After repetitions at the San Carlo in 1820 and 1821, it spread throughout Italy. In 1821, in Italian, it was sung in Dresden and Munich; in

1822 it was sung in Lisbon and (in German) in Vienna. London first heard it in Italian on February 18, 1823; St. Petersburg, in German, in 1824; Paris (Théâtre-Italien), in Italian, on September 7, 1824 (and in French in 1825); New York, in French, on August 25, 1829 (and in Italian in 1833); and Berlin, in German, in 1831. *La Donna del lago* has been revived intermittently in the twentieth century. One notable staging of it occurred at the Maggio Musicale Fiorentino of 1958, when Tullio Serafin conducted, Rosanna Carteri was the Elena, and others in the cast were Irene Companeez (Malcolm Graeme), Cesare Valletti (Giacomo V, re di Scozia), Eddy Ruhl (Rodrigo di Dhu), and Paolo Washington (Douglas d'Angus).

30. *Bianca e Falliero, ossia Il Consiglio dei tre*: opera seria, 2 acts; libretto by Felice Romani, after Manzoni's *Il Conte di Carmagnola*; composed 1819. *Première*: Teatro alla Scala, Milan, December 26, 1819. Cast: Violante Camporesi (Bianca), Carolina Bassi (Falliero), Adelaide Chinzani (or Ghinzani; Costanza), Claudio Bonoldi (Contareno), Alessandro De Angeli (Priuli, doge di Venezia), Giuseppe Fioravanti (Capellio), and Francesco Biscottini (Un Concellerie—*sic* in the first printed libretto, which lists no singer for the role of Loredano). Never one of the most widely staged of Rossini's operas, *Bianca e Falliero* nonetheless traveled. It was staged in Lisbon in 1824, Vienna in 1825, and Barcelona in 1830. One of its last stagings occurred in Cagliari, Sardinia, in the autumn of 1856.

It was never staged in London, Paris, or New York.

1820

31. *Maometto II*: dramma or opera seria, 2 acts; libretto by Cesare della Valle, duca di Ventignano, after Voltaire's *Mahomet, ou Le Fanatisme*; composed 1820. *Première*: Teatro San Carlo, Naples, December 3, 1820. Cast: Isabella Colbran (Anna), Adelaide Comelli (Calbo), Andrea Nozzari (Paolo Erisso), Filippo Galli (Maometto II), Giuseppe Ciccimarra (Condulmiero), and Gaetano Chizzola (Selimo). Adelaide Comelli (born Adele Chaumel), recently had married Giovanni Battista Rubini (she later was billed as Comelli-Rubini). Never one of Rossini's great successes, *Maometto II* nevertheless was staged in Venice in 1823 and at La Scala, Milan, in 1824; Vienna heard it in German in 1823, Lisbon in Italian in 1826. After the triumphs of Rossini's recasting of this opera as *Le Siège de Corinthe* (see under 1826), *Maometto II* seems to have slid from the repertoire.

1820–1821

32. *Matilde Shabran* (later *Matilde di Shabran*), *ossia Bellezza e Cuor di Ferro*: melodramma giocoso (really *opera semiseria*), 2 acts; libretto by Jacopo Ferretti, after François Benoît Hofmann's libretto for Méhul's *Euphrosine, ou Le Tyran corrigé* (1790); composed 1820–1. *Première*: Teatro Apollo, Rome, February 24, 1821. Cast: Caterina Lipparini (Matilde),

Annetta Parlamagni (Edoardo), Luigia Cruciati (Contessa d'Arco), Giuseppe Fusconi (Corradino), Giuseppe Fioravanti (Aliprando), Antonio Parlamagni (Isidoro), Antonio Ambrosi (Ginardo), Gaetano Rambaldi (Egoldo and Rodrigo), and Carlo Moncada (Raimondo). In the first printed libretto, Ambrosi is spelled "Ambrogi." Although Carlo Moncada is listed in that libretto as the Raimondo, Luigi Rognoni (*ROG*) gives the tenor Gioacchino Moncada as creating this role, perhaps repeating an error made by Radiciotti (*RAD* I, 271). As *Bellezza e Cuor di Ferro*, *Matilde Shabran* was heard in 1821 at the Teatro del Fondo Naples. Thereafter, increasingly billed as *Matilde di Shabran*, it rapidly visited other Italian and foreign opera houses. It was staged in Milan (as *Corradino*) in 1821; in London in 1823, and at the Théâtre-Italien, Paris, in 1829. New York first heard it on February 10, 1834, Philadelphia little more than two months later (April 28).

1821(?)-1822

33. *Zelmira*: *dramma* or *opera seria*, 2 acts; libretto by Andrea Leone Tottola, after the *Zelmire* (1762) of Dormont de Belloy (Buyrette); composed 1821(?)-2. *Première*: Teatro San Carlo, Naples, February 16, 1822. Cast: Isabella Colbran (Zelmira), Anna Maria Cecconi (Emma), Antonio Ambrosi (Polidoro), Giovanni David (Ilo), Andrea Nozzari (Antenore), Michele Benedetti (Leucippo), Gaetano Chizzola (Eacide), and Massimo

Orlandini (Gran Sacerdote). The *Cronache del Teatro di S. Carlo* of F. De Filippis and R. Arnese, lists Giacinta Canonici in the first cast of *Zelmira* and omits Colbran. But as that book also gives the date of the *première* incorrectly as February 24, the authors may have referred to a later performance, in which, Colbran having left Naples, Canonici replaced her. *Zelmira* achieved the first of the Viennese performances for which it had been intended on April 13, 1822. During that year, too, it began its extensive career in other cities, both in Italy and elsewhere. In 1824, it was staged in London, Barcelona, Dresden, and Prague; in 1825, in Moscow, Graz, Budapest, Stuttgart, and Amsterdam; in 1826 in Madrid and Paris —where Rossini himself supervised its staging at the Théâtre-Italien. On April 10, 1965, *Zelmira* was revived poorly at its first home, the San Carlo in Naples. The title role was sung by Virginia Zeani. Carlo Franci's conducting was admired, but Margherita Wallman's staging was not. *Zelmira* seems never to have been staged in the United States after a production in New Orleans about 1835.

1822-1823

34. *Semiramide*: *melodramma tragico* or *opera seria*, 2 acts; libretto by Gaetano Rossi, after Voltaire's *Sémiramis*; composed 1822-3. *Première*: Teatro La Fenice, Venice, February 3, 1823. Cast: Isabella Colbran (Semiramide), Rosa Mariani (Arsace), Matilde Spagna (Azema), Filippo Galli (Assur),

John Sinclair (Idreno), and Luciano Mariani (Oroe). Within a few years, *Semiramide* became one of the most popular of all operas. Its extra-Venetian career seems to have begun during 1823 at Naples and Vienna. In 1824, it was heard two separate times at the San Carlo, Naples, and three at La Scala, Milan; it was also staged in Padua, Munich, London —where Rossini conducted it at the King's Theatre—and Berlin, where Pauline Anna Milder-Haputmann, who had created the title role in Beethoven's *Fidelio*, was the Semiramide and the role of Arsace was sung by a tenor. *Semiramide* was heard in New York in shortened form on May 29, 1835, complete on January 1, 1845. The first Russian-language staging occurred at St. Petersburg in 1836; the first in English at Covent Garden, London, on October 1, 1842, when Sir Julius Benedict conducted, Adelaide Kemble was the Semiramis, and the Arsaces was Mrs. Alfred Shaw. The first singing in French occurred in Lyon in 1844, the first in Czech in Prague in 1864. The Metropolitan Opera, New York, staged *Semiramide* on January 12, 1894; Luigi Mancinelli conducted, and the cast was made up of Nellie Melba (Semiramide), Sofia Scalchi (Arsace), Édouard de Reszke (Assur), Pedro Guetary (Idreno), Armand Castelmary (Oroe), and Antonio de Vaschetti (Spettro di Nino). In 1940, *Semiramide* opened the sixth Maggio Musicale Fiorentino. It was restaged at La Scala, Milan, on December 17, 1962, when the cast included Joan Suth-

erland (Semiramide), Giulietta Simionato (Arsace), Gianni Raimondi (Idreno), and Wladimiro Ganzarolli (Assur). The American Opera Society presented a concert version of *Semiramide* at Carnegie Hall, New York, on February 18, 1964; Richard Bonynge conducted, and the cast was made up of Joan Sutherland (Semiramide), Marilyn Horne (Arsace), Richard Cross (Assur), Walter Carringer (Idreno), Spiro Malas (Oroe), and Louis Sgarro (Ghost of Ninus).

1825

35. *Il Viaggio a Reims, ossia L'Albergo del Giglio d'Oro: cantata scenica*, 2 parts; libretto by Luigi Balocchi; composed 1825. *Première*: Salle Louvois (Théâtre-Italien), Paris, June 19, 1825. Cast: Giuditta Pasta (Corinna), Laure Cinti-Damoreau (La Contessa di Folleville), Ester Mombelli (Madama Cortese), Adelaide Schiassetti (La Marchesa Melibea), Domenico Donzelli (Il Cavalier Belfiore), Marco Bordogni (Il Conte di Libenskof), Carlo Zucchelli (Lord Sidney), Felice Pellegrini (Don Profondo), Francesco Graziani (Il Barone di Trombonok), Nicholas-Prosper Levasseur (Don Alvaro), Pierre Scudo (Don Luigino), Trevaux (Gelsomino), Amigo (Delia), Rossi (Maddalena), Dotty (Modestina), Giovanola (Zefirino), Auletta (Antonio), and Amigo, Dotty, Giovanola, and Scudo (Quattro Virtuosi ambulanti). After another performance or two, Rossini withdrew the score, reusing much of it in *Le Comte Ory*. A scene for soprano

and bass has been published (*QR X*, 62).

1826

36. *Le Siège de Corinthe*: grand *opéra*, 3 acts; libretto by Luigi Balocchi and Alexandre Soumet, a refashioning of the Duca di Ventignano's two-act libretto for *Maometto II*; composed 1826. *Première*: Salle Le Peletier (Opéra), Paris, October 9, 1826. Cast: Laure Cinti-Damoreau (Pamyre), Mlle Frémont (Ismène), Louis Nourrit (Cléomène), Adolphe Nourrit (Néoclès), Henri-Étienne Dérivis (Mahomet II), Ferdinand Prévost (Omar), Alex Prévost (Hiéros), and M. Bonel (sometimes Bonnel; Adraste). During 1827, the opera was heard in Frankfurt-am-Main (in German), in Brussels and Mainz, and in concert form in Rome. The first staged performance of the Italian translation (*L'Assedio di Corinto*) was heard in Parma on January 26, 1828; thereafter it was staged throughout Italy until about 1870. The Italian version was heard in Paris (Théâtre-Italien) on February 4, 1829. Vienna heard the opera first in July 1831, New York in 1833. It was heard at Her Majesty's Theatre, London, in 1834(?), with Giulia Grisi, Rubini, and Tamburini. It was one of the first operas performed at the Teatro Carlo Felice, Genoa (1828). Donizetti, present for the *première* of his *Alina, regina di Golconda*, composed a cabaletta for insertion into the Act II Pamira-Maometto duet in *L'Assedio*; his "*Pietosa all'amor mio*" was sung by Adelaide Tosi and Antonio Tamburini, arousing the Genoese audience to wild applause. The cabaletta became an all but integral part of *L'Assedio* thereafter, particularly after it stirred up similar enthusiasm at the Teatro Apollo, Rome, in 1830. *L'Assedio di Corinto* was revived at the 1949 Maggio Musicale Fiorentino, when Renata Tebaldi was the Pamira, a role that she also sang in Rome in 1951.

1827

37. *Moïse et Pharaon, ou Le Passage de la Mer Rouge*: grand *opéra*, 4 acts; libretto by Luigi Balocchi and Étienne de Jouy (Victor-Joseph-Étienne Jouy), a refashioning of Andrea Leone Tottola's three-act libretto for *Mosè in Egitto* (listed under 1818); composed 1827. *Première*: Salle Le Peletier (Opéra), Paris, March 26, 1827. Cast: Laure Cinti-Damoreau (Anaï), Mlle Mori (Marie), Louise-Zulme Dabadie (Sinaïde), Adolphe Nourrit (Aménophis), Alexis (Pierre-Auguste) Dupont (Eliézer), Ferdinand-Prevôt (Ophide), Nicholas-Prosper Levasseur (Moïse), Henry-Bernard Dabadie (Pharaon), and M. Bonel (sometimes Bonnel; Osiride). The libretto of *Moïse* was quickly translated into Italian; in Italy, the revised opera became known as *Il Mosè nuovo*. Because some performances of the original *Mosè in Egitto* continued to be staged in Italy, it often is impossible to determine whether a specific post-1827 staging in Italy was of it, of the translated *Moïse*, or of some

amalgam of the two. The first performance of the translated *Moïse* was given in concert form by the Accademia Filarmonica, Rome, in 1827; the first staged production of it in Italy took place in Perugia on February 4, 1829. In a variety of versions and languages, Rossini's Moses opera continues to be heard.

1828

38. *Le Comte Ory; opéra-comique*, 2 acts; libretto an expansion of a one-act *comédie* (1817) by Augustin-Eugène Scribe and Charles-Gaspard Delestre-Poirson, after "an old Picard legend" narrated (1785) by Pierre-Antoine de La Place; composed 1828, but making large use of numbers from *Il Viaggio a Reims* (1825). *Première:* Salle Le Peletier (Opéra), Paris, August 20, 1828, with François-Antoine Habeneck conducting. Cast: Laure Cinti-Damoreau (Comtesse de Fourmoutiers), Constance Jawureck (Isolier), Mlle Mori (Ragonde), Adolphe Nourrit (Comte Ory), Henry-Bernard Dabadie (Raimbaut, also called Robert), and Nicholas-Prosper Levasseur (Le Gouverneur). The original French version of *Le Comte Ory* was sung in Liège, Antwerp, and Brussels in 1829; in New York on August 22, 1831; at St. James's Theatre, London, on June 20, 1849; and in Baden-Baden in 1863. In Italian translation, as *Il Conte Ory*, it was presented first at His Majesty's Theatre, London, on February 28, 1829, probably to honor Rossini's thirty-seventh birthday; it was also staged that spring at the Teatro San Benedetto, Venice, and later in Mexico City (1833), Odessa (1839), St. Petersburg (1849), Malta (1870), and Lisbon (1879). In one of several German translations, probably that of Ferdinand Leopold Karl von Biedenfeld, it was produced at Berlin, Budapest, and Vienna in 1829 and at Bucharest in 1843. Two not very successful performances of *Le Comte Ory*, notable chiefly for their cast, were offered at Covent Garden, London, in 1854; the singers, with Costa conducting, included Angiolino Bosio, Constance Nantier-Didiée, and Joseph-Dieudonné Tagliafico. The opera was sung in various cities in German, Polish, and Russian. The French original was performed thirty-six times in four years (1954–8) by the Glyndebourne Festival Opera; that version was recorded in drastically compressed form, and in the succeeding years interest in Rossini's only French comic opera has increased slowly. As *Il Conte Ory*, it never has been popular in Italy. When it was staged in Milan in May 1830, *La Gazzetta di Milano* commented: "The poetry was inspired by Midas rather than by Apollo." *Il Conte Ory* was revived at the 1952 Maggio Musicale Fiorentino; and on January 17, 1958, at the Piccola Scala, Milan, with this cast: Graziella Sciutti (Contessa Adele), Teresa Berganza (Isoliero), Fiorenza Cossotto (Ragonda), Juan Oncina (Conte Ory), Rolando Panerai (Roberto), and Franco Calabrese (L'Ajo), with Nino Sanzogno conducting.

1828-1829

39. *Guillaume Tell*: *grand opéra*, 4 acts; libretto by Étienne de Jouy (Victor - Joseph - Étienne Jouy), Hippolyte-Louis-Florent Bis, and Armand Marrast, after Schiller's *Wilhelm Tell*; composed 1828–9. *Première*: Salle Le Peletier (Opéra), Paris, August 3, 1829. Cast: Laure Cinti-Damoreau (Mathilde), Louise-Zulme Dabadie (Jemmy), Mlle Mori (Hedwige), Henry-Bernard Dabadie (Guillaume Tell), Adolphe Nourrit (Arnold), Nicholas-Prosper Levasseur (Walter Fürst), Bonel (sometimes Bonnel; Melcthal), Alex (?) Prévost (Gessler), Alexis Dupont (Ruodi), Ferdinand-Prevôt (Leuthold), Jean-Étienne Massol (Rodolphe), Pouilley (Chasseur); and Trevaux and Didier in unspecified roles. The *affiche* issued to announce the *première* of *Tell* reads: "M^rs Ad.-Nourrit, Dabadie, Levasseur, Bonel, Prévost, Alex [*sic*], Ferdinand-Prevôt, Massol, Pouilley, Trevaux; Mmes Cinti-Damoreau, Dabadie, Mori, Didier." One of the dancers was Marie Taglioni, who had been at the Opéra since 1827. On February 10, 1868, *Guillaume Tell* reached its official 500th singing at the Opéra (*Guglielmo Tell* also had been sung at the Théâtre-Italien from December 26, 1838, on). It was heard at the Palais Garnier for the 911th and last time to date on June 4, 1932. At some Opéra performances of *Tell* in its centenary year (1929), the Arnold was James Joyce's protégé John (O') Sullivan. In 1929, Joyce noted: "I have been through the score of *Guillaume Tell*, and I dis-cover that Sullivan sings 456 G's, 93 A-flats, 54 B-flats, 15 B's, 19 C's, and 2 C-sharps. Nobody else can do it." (Quoted by Herbert Gorman: *James Joyce*, New York, 1939.)

The first performance of *Guglielmo Tell* in Italy had occurred at the Teatro del Giglio, Lucca, on September 17, 1831; it omitted "*Selva opaca*" ("*Sombre forêt*"). The Arnold was Duprez, thus being introduced in what was to become his characteristic role. In one version or another—complete, abridged, translated, disguised by change of title to placate nervous censors—*Tell* has been sung throughout the world. The first extra-Parisian performance occurred in Brussels on March 18, 1830; six days later, it was heard in German in Frankfurt-am-Main. On March 27, its first two acts were heard in German in Budapest, to be followed by the final two acts on April 3. The first London performance—an adaptation of the text by James Robinson Planché, librettist of Weber's *Oberon*, and with the music adapted by Henry Rowley Bishop—was entitled *Hofer, or The Tell of the Tyrol*; it was sung at Drury Lane Theatre on May 1, 1830. *Tell* was also staged in London in Italian (July 11, 1839) before a Belgian troupe took it to Covent Garden in French (June 6, 1845). Vienna heard a much-truncated version in German on June 24, 1830, and a nearly complete version, still in German, on June 26, 1848. *Tell* was staged in New York in an English version on September 19, 1831; in the French original on June 16, 1845; in Italian on April 9, 1855; and in German on April 18, 1866. St. Petersburg first heard *Tell* in Russian, as *Charles the Bold*, on November 11, 1836. The opera was staged in French in New Orleans on December 13, 1842.

The Metropolitan Opera, New York, presented the first of its twenty-three singings to date of *Tell* on November 28, 1884; it was *Wilhelm Tell*, with Walter Damrosch conducting this cast: Adolf Robinson (Tell), Josef Kögel (Walter Fürst), Josef Miller (Melchthal), Anton (Antal) Udvardy (Arnold), Ludwig Wolf (Leuthold), Emil Tiffero (Fisher-man), Josef Staudigl, Jr. (Gessler), Otto Kemlitz (Rudolf), Marie Schröder-Hanfstängl (Mathilde), Marianne Brandt (Hedwig), and Anna Slach (Jemmy). The last Metropolitan singing, in Italian, occurred on April 4, 1931, with Tullio Serafin conducting and a cast made up of Giuseppe Danise (Tell), Giacomo Lauri-Volpi (Arnold), Léon Rothier (Walter Fürst), Louis D'Angelo (Melchthal), Alfio Tedesco (Fisherman), George Cehanovsky (Leuthold), Alfredo Gandolfi (Gessler), Angelo Bada (Rudolph), Editha Fleischer (Mathilde), Faina Petrova (Hedwig), and Aida Doninelli (Jemmy).

Pastiches (*pasticci* or *centoni*) sometimes listed as operas by Rossini

1. *Andremo a Parigi?*: *opera comica*, 2 acts; libretto by Luigi Balocchi and Henri Dupin, a free revision of Balocchi's text for *Il Viaggio a Reims*, from which the music was adapted. *Première*: Théâtre-Italien, Paris, October 26, 1848. The cast included Fanny Tacchinardi-Persiani, Jeanne-Anaïs Castellan, Angiolina Bosio, Sara Clari-Bellini, Giorgio Ronconi (then co-director of the Italien), Filippo Morelli, Paolo Bordas, and Arnoux (bass). A failure.

2. *Cinderella, or The Fairy and the Little Glass Slipper*: comic opera, 2 acts; libretto an adaptation by Michael Rophino Lacy of Jacopo Ferretti's text for *La Cenerentola*, music a mélange of pieces from that opera, *Armida*, *Maometto II*, and *Guillaume Tell*. *Première*: Covent Garden, London, April 13, 1830. Cast: Mary Ann Paton (Cinderella), Miss H. Cawse (Clorinda), Miss Hughes (Tisbe), Joseph Wood (Felix, Prince of Salerno), and G. Penson (Baron Pumpolino). *Cinderella* remained in the Covent Garden repertoire intermittently for about fifteen years and also became popular in New York, Washington, and elsewhere in the United States.

3. *Un Curioso Accidente*: *opera buffa*, 2 acts; libretto by G. Berettoni, music borrowed from *Aureliano in Palmira*, *La Cambiale di*

matrimonio, *L'Occasione fa il ladro*, and *La Pietra del paragone*. *Première*: Théâtre-Italien, Paris, November 27, 1859. Cast included Marietta Alboni, Signora Cambardi, Cesare Badiali, Giovanni Zucchini, Giuseppe Lucchesi, and Domenico Patriossi. Given only once.

4. *La Fausse Agnès*: *opéra-bouffon*, 3 acts, libretto by Castil-Blaze after a one-act play by Destouches (Philippe Néricault), music a mélange of pieces by Cimarosa, Meyerbeer, Rossini, and others. *Première*: Théâtre de Madame, Paris, date unknown; revived at the Théâtre de l'Odéon, Paris, June 13, 1826, when the cast included M. Bellemont, Mme Mondonville, Alexandrine Duperron-Duprez, and Gilbert-Louis Duprez.

5. *Ivanhoé*: *opera seria*, 3 acts; libretto by Emile Deschamps and Gabriel-Gustave de Wailly, after Scott's *Ivanhoe*, music adapted by Antonio Pacini from *La Cenerentola*, *La Gazza ladra*, *Mosè*, *Semiramide*, *Tancredi*, *Zelmira*, and possibly other Rossini operas. *Première*: Théâtre de l'Odéon, Paris, September 15, 1826. Cast: Mme Lemoule, Gilbert-Louis Duprez, and M. Lecomte. Successful (Porel and Monval, *L'Odéon* II, 87, called it a "*succès d'argent*"). Also staged in Strasbourg in 1826, Coburg in 1833.

6. *M. de Pourceaugnac*: *opéra-bouffon*, 3 acts; libretto by Castil-Blaze (?), after Molière, music arranged from operas by Rossini and Weber. *Première*: Théâtre de l'Odéon, Paris, February 24, 1827. Cast unknown. A success.

7. *Le Neveu de Monseigneur*: *opera-bouffe*, 2 acts. libretto by Jean-François-Alfred Bayard, Romieu, and Thomas-Marie François Sauvage, music adapted by Luc Guénée from operas by Morlacchi, Pacini, Fioravanti, and Rossini. *Première*: Théâtre de l'Odéon, Paris, August 7, 1826. Cast included Mme Meyssin, Léon Bizot, and Gilbert-Louis Duprez.

8. *Robert Bruce*: *opéra*, 3 acts; libretto by Alphonse Royer and "Gustave Vaëz" (Jean-Nicolas-Gustave van Nieuwenhuysen), music adapted by Abraham-Louis Niedermeyer from *Armida*, *Bianca e Falliero*, *La Donna del lago*, *Moïse*, *Torvaldo e Dorliska*, and *Zelmira*. *Première*: Opéra, Paris, December 30, 1846. Cast: Rosine Stoltz (Maria), Marie Nau (Nelly), Moisson (Un Page), Paul Barroilhet (Robert Bruce), Louis Paulin (Édouard II), Raffaele Anconi (Douglas-le-Noir), Geremia Bettini (Arthur), Rommy (Morton), and Bessin (Dickson). Mildly successful; staged in Brussels and The Hague in 1847; revived at the Opéra, Paris, in 1848.

9. *Le Testament*: *opéra*, 2 acts; libretto by Joseph-Henri de Saur and Léonce de Saint-Géniès, music adapted from Rossini scores by Jean-Frédéric-Auguste Lemierre (Lemière) de Corvey. *Première*: Théâtre de l'Odéon, Paris, January 22, 1827. Cast undetermined except that it included Gilbert-Louis Duprez. A complete failure.

Edoardo e Cristina, in effect a *pasticcio*, includes music that Rossini composed for it, and is therefore listed among the operas.

B. Vocal Music

(See also *Péchés de vieillesse*, page 523)

All pieces are with piano accompaniment unless otherwise specified.

À Grenade, ariette espagnole: French text by Émilien Pacini, Italian by Achille de Lauzières; n.d., pub. Escudier, Paris, w. *La Veuve andalouse*, as *Deux Chansons espagnoles*; pub. *QR* V, 90.

À Ma Belle Mère (Requiem): see *Pdv* XI, 4.

Absence, L': *romance*; n.d.

Addio ai viennesi: aria; text by Rossini (?); 1822.

Addio di Rossini ai parigini: *cavatina*; 8/5/1829; pub. Pacini, Paris, 9/-1829.

Adieu à l'Italie: see *Deux Nocturnes*.

Adieux à la vie, Les (élégie sur une seule note): see *Pdv* II, 9.

Adieux à Rome, Les: aria; composed for Adolphe Nourrit, who sang it at Rouen in 1829 at dedication of a statue of Corneille.

Agli italiani: see *Inno dell'indipendenza*.

Ahi! qual destin: aria (tenor, chorus); 1824; MS. in British Museum, London.

Album français: see *Pdv* II.

Album per canto italiano: see *Pdv* I.

Alle voci della gloria: *scena* and aria (?); see *GR* VII, 255, col. 2.

Allegrezza e malanconia: see *Pdv* II, 10.

Amants de Séville, Les (tirana pour deux voix): c, t; see *Pdv* III, 3.

Amour à Pekin, L': see *Pdv* III, 5.

Amour sans espoir (tiranne à l'espagnole rossinisée): see *Pdv* XI, 3; see also *Pdv* I, 3.

Animali parlanti del giorno: perpetual canon for 4 s; composed 10/1855 for album of Louis-James-Alfred Lefébure-Wély; pub. Sonzogno in *Musica popolare* IV (1885); facsimile in front matter of *AZ* and in *ROG*, opposite 257.

"*Anzoletta avanti la regata*," "*Anzoletta co passa la regata*," "*Anzoletta dopo la regata*": see *La Regata veneziana (Pdv* I, 8-10).

Aragonese, L': s; see *Pdv* XI, 6.

Argene e Melania: incomplete cantata; see *Pdv* XIV, 16.

Aria di Filippuccio (sopra una sola nota, il la): w. orch. acc.; pub. 1892; see *RAD* III, 250.

Arietta: 1833; pub. Lomax, London ("Composed expressly for the Bazaar for the Foreigners in Distress . . . ").

Arietta all'antica (dedotta dal "O salutaris Hostia"): s; see *Pdv* XI, 7.

Ariette à l'ancienne (text beginning "*Que le jour me dure!*"): ms.; see *Pdv* III, 11.

Ariette villageoise: ms.; see *Pdv* XI, 1.

Armonica Cetra del nume, L': see *Quartettino*.

Au Chevet d'un mourant: *élégie*; s; see *Pdv* III, 8.

Augurio felice, L': cantata (soloists,

chor., orch.); 1822.

Aurora: cantata; pub. *Sovietskaya Muzika*, Moscow, 1955 (see *BdCRdS* 1955, 4, 78; 1956, 3, 51).

Ave Maria: s; see *Pdv* III, 4.

Ave Maria: s, c, t, bs, organ; pub. *QR* XI, 43 (same as *Ave Maria a 4 voci*, pub. Hutchings Romer, London).

Ave Maria: 3/20/1850; see *Preghiera alla Vergine*.

Ave Maria (setting only "*Ave Maria, gratia plena*"): see *Pdv* XIV, 9.

Ave Maria (*su due note*, G and A flat): 1861 (?); see *Pdv* I, 7.

Bardo, Il: cantata (soloists, chor., orch. [?]); said to have been composed for the Congress of Verona (1822).

Bell'alme generose a questo sen venite: *romanza*; pub. *The Carcanet*, "a new Musical Album—1842—Edited and Arranged by Joseph [Giuseppe] de Begnis—New York—published by Joseph de Begnis, 341 Broadway."

Beppa la napolitaine: *mélodie*; pub. Schlesinger, Paris, 1840.

Bolero on Metastasio's "*Mi lagnerò tacendo*": see *RAD* III, 250; see also "*Mi lagnerò tacendo*."

Bolero: s, c; 1861 or 1863; comp. for Barbara and Carlotta Marchisio.

Brindisi (*corifeo e coro*), *cianciafruscola musicale offerta al M.o Busca pel suo onomastico del giugno 1862*: see *Pdv* XIV, 11.

Candore in fuga, Il: 2s, c, t, bs; see *Pdv* XI, 8.

Canone antisavant a 3 voci: see *Pdv* XIV, 1.

Canone perpetuo per quattro soprani indicante i modi vocali usitati dai Cantori della Pontificia Cappella Sistina: annotations in Rossini's script include: "*Or che s'oscura il ciel, il canto strano udiam de' castrati.*" See Hirt: "*Di Alcuni autografi di G. Rossini.*"

Cantata ("*Tu che il verde prato*"): according to *RAD* III, 251, performed at Turin, 1898.

Cantata a tre voci con cori: text by Giulio Genoino, 1819. Printed text reads: "*Cantata da eseguirsi La sera del dì 9 Maggio 1819 in occasione che sua Maestà Cesarea Reale ed Apostolica Francesco I Imperatore di Austria ec. ec. ec. onora la prima volta di Sua Augusta Presenza Il Real Teatro S. Carlo Napoli. Dalla Tipografia Flautina 1819. Corifea—Colbran; Corifeo—Gio. David; Araldo—Gio. Battista Rubini.*"

Cantata ad Onore del Sommo Pontefice Pio IX: text by Conte Giovanni Marchetti, 1846; music from Rossini operas. *Première*: Accademia Filarmonica, Bologna, 8/-16/1846; also performed in the Campidoglio, Rome, 1/1/1847.

Cantata con cori (referred to as *Corifea* and as both *Partenope* and *Igea*): solo cantata w. chor.; text by Antonio Niccolini; performed Teatro San Carlo, Naples, 2/20/-1819. Printed text reads: "*Omaggio Umiliato a Sua Maestà Dagli Artisti del Real Teatro S. Carlo In occasione di essere per la prima volta la M. S. intervenuta in detto Real Teatro dopo la sua felicissima guarigione La sera del dì 20 Febbrajo 1819. La Musica e del Signor Maestro Gioacchino Rossini. Corifea—Signora Isabella Colbran; Coro di Cantori—Tutti li Cantanti addetti ai RR. Teatri.*" In 1959, a 26-page autograph of a cantata was found in the Bibliothèque du Conservatoire, Paris (see *BdCRdS*

1960, 4, 77); it is headed: "*Cantata in occasione della ricuperata salute di S. Maestà Ferdinando 1° Re delle Due Sicilie . . . nel 1818.*"

Cantata per il battesimo del figlio del banchiere Aguado: sung by Rosmunda Pisaroni, Paris, 7/16/-1827.

Cantemus Domino: eight real voices; see *Pdv* III, 10.

Canzonetta ("Mi lagnerò tacendo"): 1850; MS. in British Museum, London. See also "*Mi lagnerò tacendo.*"

Canzonetta ("Mi lagnerò tacendo"): for album of the Baucardé-Albertini couple, 4/5/1852. See also "*Mi lagnerò tacendo.*"

Cara, voi siete quella: aria ded. to Antonio Chies; ms. formerly possession of the Malerbi family, Lugo.

Carnevale di Venezia, Il: chor., 4 voices; pub. Ricordi, Milan, n.d.

Cavatina: Dolci aurette che spirate: t; 1809 or 1810 (?).

Chanson de Zora: ms.; see *Pdv* II, 5.

Chanson du bébé, La: ms; see *Pdv* XI, 2.

Chant de Requiem: c; dated Passy, 8/19/1864; MS. in Bibliothèque du Conservatoire Royal de Musique, Brussels.

Chant des Titans, Le: 4 bs in unison; acc. harmonium or piano and bassoon; see *Pdv* III, 6.

Chant funèbre à Meyerbeer: chor.; composed with piano acc., but adapted to drum acc.; see *Pdv* III, 1.

Choeur de chasseurs démocrates: t,t,b,bs; see *Pdv* II, 12.

Cipresso e la rosa, Il: see *Pdv* II, 10.

Compositions diverses et esquisses: see *Pdv* XIV.

Corifea: see *Cantata con cori*.

Coro: text by Conte Giovanni Marchetti; music adapted from the "*Coro dei Bardi*" in *La Donna del lago*; performed at Turin, 3/10 (11?)/1844.

Coro dedicato alla guardia civica di Bologna ("Inno nazionale"): text by Filippo Martinelli; scored for band by Domenico Liverani, performed under Liverani's direction, Bologna, 6/21/1848; repeated at Florence, 6/29/1848; the Liverani arrangement having been lost, reinstrumentated by Ottino Ranalli and performed at Bologna, 9/26/-1915.

Dalle quete e pallid'ombre: cantata (s, bs); MS. in the Museo Teatrale alla Scala; see Philip Gossett: "*Gli Autografi rossiniani al Museo teatrale alla Scala di Milano,*" *BdCRdS*, 1967, 4, pp. 66–68.

Dall'Oriente l'astro del giorno: quartet; 1823; MS. in British Museum, London.

Danza (tarantella napoletana): see *Sm* 8.

Départ, Le: see *Pdv* III, 12; see also *Deux Nocturnes*.

Deux Chansons espagnoles: see *À Grenade* and *La Veuve andalouse*.

Deux Nocturnes: 1. Adieu à l'Italie, 2. Le Départ: pub. Schott, Mainz, 1836.

Didone abbandonata: misnomer for *La Morte di Didone* (q.v.).

Dodo des enfants, Le: see *Pdv* II, 7.

Dolci aurette che spirate: see *Cavatina: Dolci aurette che spirate*.

Due "Riens" (su versi del Metastasio): b; see *Pdv* XIV, 10.

Duetto: see *O giorno sereno*.

Duetto buffo di due gatti: text consisting of repetitions of "*Miau*"; pub. *QR* IV, 1. See Gossett: "*Catalogo delle opere,*" in Rognoni: *Gioacchino Rossini* (1968),

p. 464, for its partial derivation from an aria in *Otello* and for its very dubious authenticity.

Edipo a Colono: incidental music for Gian Battista Giusti's Italian translation of Sophocles' *Œdipus at Colonos*; 1813–16(?). See note for page 232 for description of the score, taken from Natale Gallini's "*La Musica di Scena dell'Edipo a Colono di Sofocle Ritrovata nella sua Integrità*," *La Scala: Rivista dell' Opera* 31, Milan, 5/15/1952; see also *Foi, L'Espérance, La Charité, La,* and *Oedipe.*

Egle ed Irene: cantata (2 voices); 1814.

Esule, L': t; see *Pdv* III, 2.

Fanciullo smarrito, Il: t; see *Pdv* I, 11.

Fede, La Speranza, La Carità, La: see *Foi, L'Espérance, La Charite, La.*

Fioraia fiorentina, La: s; see *Pdv* I, 5.

Foi, L'Espérance, La Charité, La: chorus, 3 female voices. The first two were revisions of numbers from the incidental music to *Edipo a Colono* (*q.v.*), supplied with French texts by, respectively, Prosper Goubaux and Hippolyte Lucas; the third, composed 1844 to an Italian doggerel hymn to the Virgin, was given a French text by Louise Colet. Pub. Troupenas, Paris, 1844. First performed Paris, 11/20/1844. First performance as translated into Italian by Geremia Vitali as *La Fede, La Speranza, La Carità*, Bologna, 3/14/1845; pub. Ricordi, Milan. Liszt transcribed *La Charité* for voice and organ (pub., with transcription by him of the *Cujus animam* from the *Stabat Mater*, Schott, Mainz, and Brandus, Paris, 1848).

(*Francesca da Rimini*): rhythmic recitative on verses from Dante ("*Farò come colui che piange e dice . . .* "); composed 1848 for inclusion in the edition of the *Inferno* published by Lord Vernon in 1865 (which includes facsimile of the MS., which was also reproduced in F. Mariotti: *Dante e la statistica delle lingue,* Florence, 1880, page 121); pub. Ricordi, Milan, n.d., as *Racconto di Francesca da Rimini nella Divina Commedia.*

Genio del Cristianesimo, Il: sketches for a cantata?; see *Pdv* XIV, 14.

Giovanna d'Arco: cantata or grande scena; see *Pdv* XI, 10.

Gitane, Le: s, c; see *Pdv* I, 6.

Gondolieri, I: quartet; see *Pdv* I, 1.

Gorgheggi e Solfeggi per soprano (Vocalizzi e solfeggi per rendere la voce agile ed apprendere a cantare secondo il gusto moderno): vocal exercises; 1822–7(?); pub. Pacini, Paris, 1827; repub. with 12 new exercises for ms or b, as *Praktische Schule des modernen Gesanges,* Schlesinger, Berlin.

Graduale a tre voci concertato: 3 male voices w. acc. of small orch. 1. Allegro, D major. 2. *Ave Maria,* t, B-flat major, obbligato oboe. 3. *Alleluja,* D major; 1808; facsimile in front matter of *SIL.*

Grande Coquette, La (Ariette Pompadour): ms; see *Pdv* II, 3.

Grande Scena "Giovanna d'Arco" or *Grande Scène Jeanne d'Arc*: see *Pdv* XI, 10.

Grido di Esultazione Riconoscente al Sommo Pontefice Pio IX (alternatively *Grido di esultazione riconoscente alla paterna clemenza di PIO*): male chorus; text attributed to a Canon Golfieri, 1846; a refashioning of the *"Coro dei Bardi"* in *La Donna del Lago*; first sung at Bologna, 7/23/1846.

Hymne à Napoléon III et à son vaillant peuple: cantata for soloists, chor., piano (later orch. and band); text by Émilien Pacini; first performed at Paris, 8/18/-1867; announced (1967) for publication with original piano acc. in one of the four new *QR* to be issued at Pesaro in 1968 for the centenary of Rossini's death.

Igea: see *Cantata con cori.*

In giorno si bello (alternatively *In si bel giorno*): nocturne (3 voices); MS. in British Museum, London.

Inno alla pace: text a translation from Bacchilides by Giuseppe Arcangeli; composed 1851 for vocal soloists and chor., with piano acc.; instrumentated by Giovanni Pacini; announced (1967) for publication in original form in one of four new *QR* to be issued at Pesaro in 1968 for the centenary of Rossini's death.

Inno dell'indipendenza (*"Agli italiani"*): text by Giovanni Battista Giusti; first performed at Bologna 4/15/1815.

Inno nazionale: see *Coro dedicato alla guardia civica di Bologna.*

Kyrie and *Qui tollis*: 1808; see first and second examples of *Messa*, below.

Larme, Une: bs; see *Pdv* XIV, 2.

Laudamus: orch. acc.; very early.

Laus Deo: scherzo (ms); it consists of introduction; seven measures in which *"Laus Deo"* is repeated twice; three measures of close; pub., with date *"Passy, 1861,"* in *Il Piovano Arlotto*, 1861.

Lazzarone, Le: b; see *Pdv* II, 8.

Lontananza, La: t; see *Pdv* I, 2.

Marina(r)i, I (alternatively *Li*): see *Sm* 12.

Mass: see *Messa.*

Messa: male voices, chor., orch., organ; composed 1808, first performed Ravenna, 1808; three sections of it were used in the next composition below.

Messa (only *Graduale*, *Kyrie*, and *Qui tollis* by Rossini): 1808; sung at Bologna, 1808.

Messa solenne: collaboration with Pietro Raimondi, 1820; performed Naples, 3/19/1820.

"Mi lagnerò tacendo": opening line of a speech in Metastasio's *Siroe*, Act I, Scene 1:

Mi lagnerò tacendo
Del mio destino amaro;
Ma ch'io non t'ami, o caro,
Non sperar da me.
      Crudele! in che t'offendo,
Se resta a questo petto
Il misero diletto
Di sospirar per te?

Rossini made hundreds of distinct settings of these lines in autograph albums, in the six songs of *Musique anodine* (see *Pdv* XIII), and elsewhere. The present writer owns one such album setting. It is an *andantino mosso* for voice and piano ded. *"à Mad*lle *Palmyre Wertheimber/ G. Rossini/ Passi [sic] ce 29 Juin 1860"*: its obverse contains a passage from Ernest Reyer's opera *Maître Wolfram*, also inscribed to Palmyre Wertheimber and signed *"Son ami E. Reyer/ 29 mars 1864."*

Miscellanée de musique vocale: see *Pdv* XI.

Morceaux réservés: see *Pdv* III.

Morte di Didone, La: solo cantata;

1811; first sung by Ester Mombelli at Venice, 5/2/1818. Two numbers from it—"*Se dal Ciel pietà non trovo*" and "*Per tutto l'orror*"— pub. Ricordi, Milan, as from Rossini's "opera" *Didone abbandonata*.

Mottetto: quartet; see *Pdv* XI, 9.

Musique anodine: see *Pdv* XIII.

National Hymn: b and chor., to English text beginning: "Oh! Lord most High!"; first performed at Birmingham, England, 1867.

Nizza: song pub. Chabal, Paris, 5/1840.

Non posso, o Dio, resistere: see *GR* VII, 255.

Notturno: see *In giorno si bello*.

Nozze di Teti e di Peleo, Le: cantata (six solo voices and chorus); text by Angelo Maria Ricci; first performed Naples, 4/24/1816.

Nuit de Noël, La (*La Notte del Santo Natale*): bs and 4-voice chor.; see *Pdv* II, 6.

O giorno sereno: duet (t, bs) with chor.; MS. in British Museum, London.

O quanti son grati: duet (?); see *GR* VII, 255.

O salutaris . . . de champagne: c; see *Pdv* XI, 5.

O salutaris Hostia: s,c,t,bs; pub. in facsimile in *La Maîtrise*, Paris, 1851, no. 1, and in *AZ*. The MS. bears the inscription: "*Petit souvenir offert à mon ami I. D'Ortigue.—G. Rossini.—Paris, ce 29 Nov. 1857.*"

Oedipe: aria (bs); from incidental music for *Edipo a Colono* (*q.v.*); pub. Troupenas, Paris, and Breitkopf & Härtel, 1850; see also *Foi, L'Espérance, La Charité, La*.

Omaggio pastorale, cantata (3 voices); composed for inauguration of bust of Antonio Canova;

first performed at Treviso, 4/1/-1823.

Orpheline du Tyrol, L' (*ballade-élégie*): s; see *Pdv* II, 11.

Partenope: see *Cantata con cori*.

Passeggiata, La: *quartettino*; see *Pdv* I, 12.

Pastori, I: alternative title for *Il Serto votivo* (*q.v.*).

Péchés de vieillesse: see separate section, page 523.

Petitie Bohémienne, La: see *Pdv* II, 5.

Petite Messe solennelle: composed 1863-4. First (semiprivate) performance, Paris, 3/14/1864; soloists: Barbara and Carlotta Marchisio, Italo Gardoni, and Agnesi (Louis Agniez); acc. played on two pianos (George Mathias, Andrea Peruzzi) and a harmonium (Albert Lavignac). First performance of orchestrated version, Paris, 2/24/1869. Soloists: Gabrielle Kraus, Marietta Alboni, Nicolini (Ernest Nicolas), and Agnesi (Louis Agniez).

Pezzi caratteristici: catch-all substitute title for many of the *Pdv*.

Pianto d'Armonia sulla morte d'Orfeo, Il: cantata (t and chor.); text by Girolamo Ruggia, 1808; first performance, Bologna, 8/11/1808.

Pianto delle muse in morte di lord Byron, Il: cantata (solo voice, chor., orch.); composed 1824; incorporates music from *Maometto II*; first performance at London, 6/9/1824, with Rossini as vocal soloist; MS. in British Museum, London; pub. T. Boosey, London, for Rossini, 1824(?).

Preghiera ("*Tu che di verde il prato*"): see *Pdv* III, 7.

Preghiera alla Vergine ("*Salve, o Vergine Maria*"): s,c,t,ba; MS. bears the inscription: "*Al diletis-*

*simo mio amico Abbate Gordini.
—Gioacchino Rossini.—Firenze, li
20 marzo 1850"*; in facsimile in
RAD III, after p. 252; pub. *QR*
VI, 77.

Prière, La: 8 male voices; see *Pdv*
III, 7.

Quartetti da camera: see *Tre Quartetti da camera*.

*Quartettino: L'Armonica Cetra del
nume ("scritto espressamente per
la sera del 2 aprile 1830, giorno del
nome del suo amico Zampieri
[sic]. G. Rossini")*: MS. was in
the Stadtbibliothek, Berlin (*RAD*
III, 252).

Qui tollis and *Qui sedes*: solo voice
w. obbligato horn; before 1808(?).

Quoniam: bs. w. orch. acc.; 1832.

*Racconto di Francesca da Rimini
nella Divina Commedia*: see (*Francesca da Rimini*).

Recitativo ritmato su versi di Dante:
see (*Francesca da Rimini*).

Regata veneziana, La: 3 songs; see
Pdv I, 8–10; duet (s,t), see *Sm* 9.

Requiem (À Ma Belle Mère): see
Pdv XI, 4.

Riconoscenza, La: cantata (4 solo
voices); text by Giulio Genoino;
1821; first performance at Naples
12/27/1821; for later performance
in revised form, see *Serto votivo, Il*.

Rien, Un (Ave Maria): see *Pdv*
XIV, 9.

Ritorno, Il: 1823; see *GR* VII, 255.

Ritorno d'Astrea, Il: supposed name
given by Rossini to the *Inno dell'-
indipendenza* (*q.v.*) as recomposed
to please Austrian authorities; actually a cantata, to a text by Vincenzo Monti, music by Joseph
Weigl, first performed at Milan
1/6/1816.

Romanza: otherwise unidentified
song composed for and dedicated

to Adelaide Borghi-Mamo, who
sang it at the Opéra, Paris, 1/22/
1859.

Roméo: see *Pdv* II, 2.

Salve Maria: see *Preghiera alla Vergine*.

Santa Alleanza, La: cantata (solo
voices, chor., orch.); text by Gaetano Rossi; first performance at
Verona, 11/24/1822.

Saul: oratorio (but misattribution?);
see *GR* VII, 255.

Se il vuol la marinara: arietta buffa;
1806(?); to a text by an unknown
writer; pub. Ricordi, Milan, in
Biblioteca di musica moderna II
as Rossini's first published composition; quoted, perhaps unintentionally, in introduction to Ruggero's "*Torni alfin ridente e bella*"
in *Tancredi*.

Separazione, La: ms; pub. Breitkopf
& Härtel, Leipzig.

Serenata, La: duet (s,t); text by
Conte Carlo Pepoli; see *BdCRdS*
1956, 2, 38.

Serto votivo, Il (or *I Pastori*): alternative title for *La Riconoscenza*
(*q.v.*) in revision; sung under this
title at Bologna, 1829; a copy in
the Bibliothèque Nationale, Paris,
states that it was composed for "D.
Nicola Pegnalverd"; pub. Ricordi,
Milan, with ded. "*a Madimigella
Lewis, esimia dilettante di canto.*"

Soirées musicales: 8 ariettas and 4
duets, 1830–5; pub. Troupenas,
Paris, with Italian texts, 1835; pub.
Ricordi, Milan, with Italian and
French texts (tr. by Louis-Ernest
Crevel de Charlemagne); other
edns. by Girard, Naples, and
Brandus, Paris. As issued by Troupenas, the *Soirées musicales* are:
1. "*La Promessa*" (*canzonetta, s*);
2. "*Il Rimprovero*" (*canzonetta,*

c); 3. "*La Partenza*" (*canzonetta*, ms); 4. "*L'Orgia*" (arietta, ms); 5. "*L'Invito*" (bolero, ms); 6. "*La Pastorella delle Alpi*" (Tyrolienne, ms); 7. "*La Gita in gondola*" (barcarole, ms); 8. "*La Danza (tarantella napoletana*, ms); 9. "*La Regata veneziana*" (duet, s,t); 10. "*La Pesca*" (duet, s,c); 11. "*La Serenata*" (duet, s,t); 12. "*I Marinai*" (duet, t,bs). "*I Marina(r)i*" incorporates musical matter from the backstage chorus "*Il tuo pianto, i tuoi sospiri*" in *Ricciardo e Zoraide*, Act II, Scene 10—which in turn reflected the gondolier's song "*Nessun maggior dolore*" in *Otello*, Act III, Scene 1. Franz Liszt published as his Opus 8 a two-part fantasia based on (part 1) "*La Serenata e L'Orgia*" and (part 2) "*La Pastorella dell'Alpi e Li Marinari.*" Liszt made new versions of these four numbers when making a complete transcription (not in the published order) of the *Soirées musicales.* Wagner orchestrated "*I Marinai*" and conducted it at Riga, 3/1838.

Sou, Un (*complainte à deux voix*): t,b; see *Pdv* II, 4.

Soupir et sourire (*élégie*): duet (s,t); see *Pdv* II, 10.

Stabat Mater, a setting of the 13th-century Latin hymn attributed to Jacopone da Todi; composed 1831(?)–2; completed 1841. First (partial) performances at Madrid, Holy Saturday 1833; Paris, 10/-

1841. First complete public performance, Paris, 1/7/1842.

Sylvain, Le: ms; see *Pdv* III, 9.

Tantum ergo: 2t, bs; 1847; performed "on the occasion of the solemn restoration to the Catholic Cult of the Church of San Francesco dei Minori Conventuali . . . November 28, 1847 . . . performed by the *signori* Donzelli, Gamberini and Badiali"; pub. G. Ricordi & C., Milan; for a sketch for a *Tantum ergo,* see *Pdv* XIV, 12.

Teodora e Riccardino: sketch for a cantata scene (?); see *Pdv* XIV, 13.

Tirana alla spagnola rossinizzata: s; see *Pdv* I, 3; see also *Pdv* XI, 3.

Toast pour le nouvel an: ottettino (2 each, s,c,t,bs); see *Pdv* II, 1.

Tre Quartetti da camera, 1826–7; pub. Pacini, Paris, and Ricordi; No. 2 ded. to Aguado, No. 3 to Mme Carmen Aguado.

Trois Choeurs: see *Foi, L'Espérance, La Charité, La.*

Tyrolienne sentimentale: 2s, 2c; see *Pdv* III, 12.

Ultimo Ricordo, L': t; see *Pdv* I, 4.

Vero Omaggio, Il: cantata (solo voices, chor., orch.); said to have been composed for and performed at the Congress of Verona, 1822.

Veuve andalouse, La: pub. Escudier, Paris, w. *À Grenade,* as *Deux Chansons espagnoles.*

Voto filiale: misnomer for *Il Serto votivo?* See *GR* VII, 255.

Zora: ms; see *Pdv* II, 5.

C. Instrumental Music

(See also *Péchés de vieillesse*, page 523)

All pieces are for solo piano unless otherwise specified.

À mon ami Panseron: see Pdv XII, 3.

Album de château: see Pdv VIII.

Album de chaumière: see Pdv V.

Album des enfants dégourdis: see Pdv VII.

Album pour les enfants adolescents: see Pdv VI.

Album pour piano, violon, violoncelle, harmonium et cor: see Pdv IX.

Allegro agitato: cello; see *Larme, Une*.

Amandes, Les: see Pdv IV–B2.

Âme du Purgatoire, L': pub. Schlésinger, Paris, 1832.

Anchois, Les: see Pdv IV–A2.

Andante con variazioni per violino e arpa ("*Composte espressamente e dedicate alla Signora Carolina Barbaja da Gioacchino Rossini, Napoli*"): pub. Girard, Naples, and QR VI, 1; includes quotation of "*Di tanti palpiti*" from *Tancredi*, Act I, Scene 5.

Assez de memento: dansons: see Pdv VII, 4.

Bagatelle, Une: see Pdv X, 4.

Bagatelle, Une (In nomine patris, mélodie italienne): see Pdv X, 5.

Barcarolle: see Pdv VII, 8.

Beurre, Le: see Pdv IV–A4.

Boléro tartare: see Pdv VIII, 4.

Caresse à ma femme, Une: see Pdv VII, 7.

Cauchemar, Un: see Pdv V, 9.

Chansonette: see Pdv IX, 3.

Congresso di Verona, Il: 4 hands; 1823.

Cornichons, Les: see Pdv IV–A3.

Corona d'Italia, La: military band ("*Fanfara per musica militare offerta a S. M. Vittorio Emanuele II dal riconoscente G. Rossini*"); 1868.

Danse sibérienne: MS. in the Bibliothèque Nationale, Paris ("*Passy—1864 G. Rossini*"); see also Pdv XII, 12; rep. on p. 331 of present book.

Des Tritons, s'il vous plait: see Pdv X, 2.

Dodici Valzer: two flutes; 1827.

Doublebass, pieces for: see GR VII, 255, "Pieces for double bass (1808)."

Douce Reminiscences: see Pdv XII, 16.

Duets, 2 horns: 1806; one melody became that of *Rendez-vous de chasse* (*q.v.*).

Échantillon de blague mélodique sur les noires: see Pdv IX, 11.

Échantillon du Chant de Noël à l'italienne: see Pdv IX, 6.

Encore un peu de blague: see Pdv XIV, 7.

Enterrement en carnaval, Un: see Pdv VII, 12.

Étude asthmatique: see Pdv VII, 11.

Fanfare for 4 trumpets: see *Rendez-vous de chasse*.

Fausse Couche de polka-mazurka: see *Pdv* VII, 10.

Figues sèches, Les: see *Pdv* IV–B1.

Grande Fanfare: 4 trumpets; see *Rendez-vous de chasse*.

Gymnastique d'écartement: see *Pdv* V, 1.

Hachis romantique: see *Pdv* VI, 12.

Hors d'oeuvres, Les: see *Pdv* IV–A.

Huile de ricin, L': see *Pdv* V, 6.

Impromptu: violin, piano; 1853; ded. to Adelaide Borghi-Mamo; pub. in facsimile in *L'Album du grand monde*, Paris.

Impromptu anodin: see *Pdv* VI, 6.

Impromptu tarentellisé: see *Pdv* IX, 5.

Innocence italienne, L'—La Candeur française: see *Pdv* VI, 7.

Lagune de Venise à l'expiration de l'année 1861 ! ! ! ! , La: see *Pdv* VI, 9.

Larme, Une (Thème et variations): cello; pub. (as *Allegro agitato per violoncello*) in *QR* VI, 9; incorporates the song *Une Larme* (q.v.).

March: 4 hands; probably one of the *Trois Marches militaires*, below; Louis Diémer mentioned (quoted *RAD* II, 368, footnote) playing it with Rossini.

Marche: see *Pdv* V, 12.

Marche et réminiscences pour mon dernier voyage: see *Pdv* IX, 7.

Marches, three miiltary: band; see *Mariage de S.A.R. le duc d'Orléans, Le*.

Marcia militare: band; 1851 (1852?— as in *GR* VII, 255); ded. to Sultan Abdul-Medjid of Turkey; exists in arrangements for piano, 2 hands, and piano, 4 hands, both pub. Brandus, Paris.

Mariage de S.A.R. le duc d'Orléans, Le: band; 1837; performed at Fontainebleau, 5/30/1837; pub. for band and for piano, 2 hands, and piano, 4 hands, Breitkopf & Härtel, Leipzig.

Mélodie candide: see *Pdv* IX, 1.

Memento Homo: see *Pdv* VII, 3.

Miscellanée pour piano: see *Pdv* X.

Moderato: undated autograph signed "*G. Rossini*"; see Schlitzer, Franco: *Rossini a Siena*, 11.

Mon Prélude hygiénique du matin, see *Pdv* VII, 1.

Mot à Paganini, Un (élégie pour violon): see *Pdv* IX, 4.

Noisettes, Les: see *Pdv* IV–B3.

Ouf! les petits pois: see *Pdv* VI, 10.

Overture, D major: 1808; see *GR* V, 255.

Passo doppio: band; 1822; later revised as *allegro vivace* finale of the overture to *Guillaume Tell*.

Pensée à Florence, Une: see *Pdv* V, 11.

Pésarèse, La: see *Pdv* VII, 5.

Petit Caprice (style Offenbach): see *Pdv* X, 6.

Petit Train de plaisir, Un—Comique imitatif: see *Pdv* VII, 9.

Petite Fanfare à quatre mains: 4 hands; see *Pdv* IX, 12.

Petite Galette allemande: see *Pdv* XII, 15.

Petite Pensée, Une: see *Pdv* X, 3.

Petite Polka chinoise: see *Pdv* V, 3.

Petite Promenade de Passy à Courbevoie: see *Pdv* XIV, 4.

Petite Valse: L'Huile de ricin: see *Pdv* V, 6.

Peu de tout, Un: subtitle covering volumes V, VI, VII, and VIII of *Pdv*.

Piano solo, untitled: six-page score dedicated to the Baronne Charlotte Nathaniel de Rothschild; in the Bibliothèque Nationale, Paris.

Plein-chant chinois: see *Pdv* V, 8.

Prélude baroque: see *Pdv* VII, 2.

Prélude blagueur de bon train-train: see *Pdv* X, 1.

Prélude convulsif: see *Pdv* VI, 8.

Prélude fugassé: see *Pdv* V, 2.

Prélude inoffensif: see *Pdv* V, 5.

Prélude italien: see *Pdv* IX, 9.

Prélude moresque: see *Pdv* VI, 4.

Prélude pétulant-rococo: see *Pdv* VIII, 2.

Prélude prétentieux: see *Pdv* VIII, 5.

Prélude semi-pastoral: see *Pdv* VIII, 8.

Prélude soi-disant dramatique: see *Pdv* VIII, 11.

Prélude, thème et variations pour cor: piano acc.; see *Pdv* IX, 8.

Première Comunion: see *Pdv* VI, 1.

Profond Sommeil, Un—Un Reveil en sursaut: see *Pdv* V, 7.

Quartets for flute, *clarino*, horn, oboe: six juvenilia, 1808–9; pub. Schott, Paris; No. 1 (F major) also pub. Breitkopf & Härtel, Leipzig.

Quartets for flute, violin, viola, cello: four (G, A, B-flat, D), pub. Schott, Paris, are transcriptions of quartets for strings (*q.v.*), which in turn are revisions of *sonate a quattro* (*q.v.*).

Quartets for strings (2 violins, viola, cello): 1806–8; five (G, A, B-flat, E-flat, D), pub. Schott, Paris, and Ricordi, Milan, are revisions of the six *sonate a quattro* (*q.v.*), but omitting No. 3, and with the cello part recast for viola, the double-bass part for cello.

Quatre Hors d'oeuvres et quatre mendiants pour piano: see *Pdv* IV.

Quatre Mendiants, Les: see *Pdv* IV-B.

Quelques Riens pour album: see *Pdv* XII; an album entitled *Quelques Riens pour piano* (8 pieces) was pub. Suivini-Zerboni, Milan, 1951 (ed. Luigi Rognoni).

Raisins, Les: see *Pdv* IV-B4.

Reggia di Nettuno, La: 4 hands, 1823.

Réjouissance, Une: see *Pdv* XIV, 5.

Rendez-vous de chasse: 4 cors de chasse or trumpets; also known as *Grande Fanfare*; 1828; ded. to Schickler; derived from 1806 duets for 2 horns; pub. Breitkopf & Härtel, Leipzig, and *QR* IX, 45.

Rêve, Un: see *Pdv* VIII, 10.

Rien sur le mode enharmonique, Un: see *Pdv* XII, 24.

Ritournelle gothique: see *Pdv* XIV, 6.

Ritournelle pour L'Adagio du Trio d'Atilla: 2/10/1865; pub. in facsimile in Luzio: "*Il Pensiero artistico e politico di Giuseppe Verdi* . . . "

Rondeau fantastique: horn and piano; 1856; composed for Eugène-Léon Vivier.

Saltarello à l'italienne: see *Pdv* VI, 3.

Sauté, Un: see *Pdv* VI, 11.

Savoie amante, La: see *Pdv* IX, 2.

Scherzo: pub. Carisch e Jänichen, Milan, 1908, from MS. in the Biblioteca Estense, Modena.

Sei Quartetti per flauto: *see* quartets for flute, *clarino*, horn, oboe.

Sei Sonate: see *sonate a quattro*.

Sérénade: see *Serenata per piccolo complesso*.

Serenata per piccolo complesso: E-flat major; violins, viola, flute, oboe, English horn, cello; 1823; composed expressly for Vincenzo(?) Bianchi; pub. *QR* VI, 31.

Sinfonia ("Bologna"): D major; flute, 2 oboes, 2 C clarinets, bassoon, 2 D horns, 2 D trumpets, strings, timpani; 1808; pub. *QR* VIII, 1.

Sinfonia: 1809; later used as overture to *La Cambiale di matrimonio*; MS. in Bibliothèque du Conservatoire Royal de Musique, Brussels.

Sinfonia ("Odense"): A major; flutes, oboes, A clarinets, bassoons,

A horns, E horns, D trumpets, trombones, strings, timpani; found at Odense, Denmark, by Povl Ingerslev-Jensen; pub. *QR* VIII, 17.

Solo per violoncello: untitled; see *Pdv* XIV, 15.

sonate a quattro: 2 violins, cello, doublebass; six *sonate* (1. G major; 2. A major; 3. C. Major; 4. B-flat major; 5. E-flat major; 6. D major); MS. copy in Library of Congress, Washington, D. C.; title page reads: "*Opera di sei sonate Composta Dal Sig.r Giovacchino Rossini in età di anni XII in Ravenna, l'Anno 1804.*" The first page of the violin part contains this inscription by Olympe Rossini: "*Offert à mon excellent ami, en souvenir d'amitié O. V.ve Rossini ce 22 Mars 1873 à Monsieur Mazzoni*"; the next page contains this gloss by Rossini: "*Parti di Violino Primo, Violino Secondo, Violoncello Contrabasso, e questi*[?] *di Sei Sonate* orrende *da me composte alla villeggiatura (presso Ravenna) del mio amico mecenate, Agostino Triossi alla età la più infantile non avendo preso neppure una Lezione di accompagnamento, il Tutto composto e copiato in Tre Giorni ed eseguite cagnescamente dal Triossi Contrabasso, Morri*[?] *(di Lui Cugino) Primo Violino, il fratello di questo il Violoncello, ed il Secondo Violino da me stesso, che ero per dio non il meno cane. G. Rossini.*" Pub. *QR* I; the third of the *sonate* pub., as edited by Alfredo Casella, by Carisch, Milan, 1951; *see also* quartets for strings.

Spécimen de l'ancien régime: see *Pdv* VIII, 1.

Spécimen de l'avenir: see *Pdv* VIII, 12.

Spécimen de mon temps: see *Pdv* VIII, 6.

string quartets: *see* quartets for strings.

Tarentelle pur sang (avec traversée de la Procession): see *Pdv* VIII, 9.

Tema con variazioni per quattro strumenti a fiato: F major; flute, C clarinet, F horn, bassoon; 1812; pub. *QR* VI, 18.

Thème et variations sur le mode majeur: see *Pdv* XII, 23.

Thème et variations sur le mode mineur: *Pdv* XII, 22.

Thème naïf et variations: see *Pdv* VI, 2.

Tourniquet sur la gamme chromatique ascendante et descendante: see *Pdv* XIV, 8.

Trois Marches militaire: 4 hands, 1823.

Valse antidansante: see *Pdv* VIII, 7.

Valse boîteuse: see *Pdv* V, 10.

Valse lugubre: see *Pdv* VI, 5.

Valse torturée: see *Pdv* VII, 6.

Valser: E-flat; composed at Venice, 1823, for Signora Francesca Barbaja.

Variazioni in do maggiore per clarinetto obbligato con accompagnamento di orchestra: flute, C clarinet, bassoon, 2 C horns, strings, solo C clarinet; 1810; pub. Breitkopf & Härtel, Leipzig, and *QR* VI, 57.

Variazioni in fa maggiore per più strumenti obbligati con accompagnamento d'orchestra: flute, 2 C clarinets, bassoon, 2 F horns, strings, *concertante* B-flat clarinet; 1809; pub. *QR* IX, 1.

Vénitienne, La: see *Pdv* XIV, 3.

waltzes: see *Dodici Valser*; *Valse*; *Valser*.

D. *Péchés de vieillesse*

Rossini appears to have given the title *Sins of Old Age* only to the volumes listed below as V, VI, VII, VIII, and IX. I have thought it easiest for reference, however, to extend that title (as was done originally by *RAD* III, 256–63, and, using a somewhat different system, by *ROG*, 383–90) to fourteen collections of miscellaneous compositions for voices, chorus, piano, instrumental ensembles, and orchestra belonging to Rossini's later years and left to the Liceo Musicale, Pesaro, by Olympe Rossini. The lack of systematic control—and often the refusal or inability to cooperate—by the Fondazione Rossini at Pesaro continues to make impossible definitive cataloguing of the thousands of pages of Rossini manuscript in its keeping. New Rossini manuscripts (and particularly album leaves) materialize constantly in many parts of the world; any list of his small compositions is unavoidably tentative.

All vocal pieces have solo-piano accompaniment unless otherwise specified.

Volume I—*Album per canto italiano*

1. *I Gondolieri*: s,c,t,bs; pub. *QR* VII, 1.
2. *La Lontananza*: t; text by Giuseppe Torre; pub. *QR* IV, 12.
3. *Tirana alla spagnola rossinizatta*: s; pub. *QR* IV, 30 (translation into Italian of *Amour sans espoir, Pdv.* XI, 3?).
4. *L'Ultimo Ricordo*: t; ded. to Olympe; text by Rossini ending "*Quest'appassito fiore ti lascio, Olimpia, in don*"; pub. *QR* IV, 19.
5. *La Fioraia fiorentina*: s; pub. *QR* IV, 5.
6. *Le Gitane*: s,c; composed originally to the Metastasian lines beginning "*Mi lagnerò tacendo,*" later adapted to lines beginning "*Il suon, le danze, il canto son nostro sol tesoro.*"
7. *Ave Maria (sopra due note* [G and A flat]): c; text beginning "*A te, che benedetta fra tutte sei, Maria*"; composed 1861(?); pub. *QR* IV, 51.
8–10. *La Regata veneziana*: three songs; s; texts by Conte Carlo Pepoli(?): 1. "*Anzoletta avanti la regata*"; 2. "*Anzoletta co passa la regata*"; 3. "*Anzoletta dopo la regata.*" Published several times.
11. *Il Fanciullo smarrito*: t; text by Antonio Castellani, 1861; MS. inscribed "*Al carissimo mio A. Cas-*

tellani *per uso suo esclusivamente personale, G. Rossini.—Parigi, 10 marzo 1861.*" The autograph score carries notes for "*campanello,*" indicating *campanelli levati,* bells added to pianos before the mid-19th century to vary and increase the volume of sound; placed in the piano's tail, they were removable at will and were operated by foot, one or two extra pedals being supplied.

12. *La Paseggiata* [*sic*]: s,c,t,bs; pub. QR VII, 16.

Volume II—*Album français*

1. *Toast pour le nouvel an*: 2 each s,c,t,bs; pub. QR VII, 50.
2. *Roméo*: t.
3. *La Grande Coquette (Ariette Pompadour)*: ms; text by Émilien Pacini.
4. *Un Sou (complainte à deux voix)*: t,b; pub. QR V, 58.
5. *Zora* (two parts: "*La Chanson de Zora,*" "*La Petite Bohémienne*"): ms; text by Émile Deschamps; pub. (partial?) QR V, 49.
6. *La Nuit de Noël (La Notte del Santo Natale)*: *pastorale* for Un Vecchio (bs) and chor. of 2 each s,c,t,b; 1864(?); pub., with bilingual text, QR VII, 62; see also *Échantillon du chant de Noël à l'italienne*, Pdv IX, 6.
7. *Le Dodo des enfants*: text by Émilien Pacini; pub. QR V, 9.
8. *Le Lazzarone, chansonette de cab-*aret: b; text by Émilien Pacini; this parody of gluttony was marked by Rossini "*Parlé en se lechant les lèvres.*"
9. *Les Adieux à la vie (élégie sur une seule note)*: ms; pub. QR V, 75.
10. *Soupir et sourire (élégie)*: duet (s,t); text by Émilien Pacini; versions exist in Italian (*Il Cipresso e la rosa* and *Allegrezza e malanconia,* the latter with text by Giuseppe Torre).
11. *L'Orpheline du Tyrol (L'Orfana del Tirolo) (ballade-élegie)*: s; text by Émilien Pacini; pub. QR V, 31.
12. *Choeur des chasseurs démocrates*: t 1, t 2, b, bs, with acc. of tamtam, 2 bass drums; 1862; composed for the Baronne Rothschild, sung at the Château de Ferrières, 12/1862; pub. QR VII, 35.

Volume III—*Morceaux réservés*

1. *Chant funèbre à Meyerbeer*: t 1, t 2, b, bs, with drum-roll acc.; text by Émilien Pacini, 1864; inscription on MS. reads: "*Quelques mésures de chant funèbre à mon pauvre ami Meyerbeer. 8 heures du matin. Paris, 6 mai 1864. Paroles de Émilien Pacini*"; pub. QR VII, 84.
2. *L'Esule*: t, text by Giuseppe Torre; pub. QR IV, 25.
3. *Les Amants de Séville (tirana pour*

deux voix): c,t; pub. *QR* V, 37.

4. *Ave Maria*: s, with organ acc.

5. *L'Amour à Pekin (petite mélodie sur la Gamme chinoise*—a whole-tone scale); c; text by Émilien Pacini; composed for Marietta Alboni. As pub. in *QR* V, 81, it consists of *Montée* (piano), *Descente* (piano), *Montée* (piano), *Descente* (piano), *Montante et Descendante: I Gamme chinoise* (piano), *Montante et Descendante: II Gamme chinoise* (piano), *Petite Mélodie sur la Gamme chinoise* (c, piano acc., text beginning "*Mon coeur blessé gémit tout bas*").

6. *Le Chant des Titans*: 4 bs in unison, with acc. of harmonium or piano (and bassoon?); text by Émilien Pacini; composed 1861 for Conte Pompeo Belgiojoso; pub. Hutchings and Romer, London. *See* Bonaccorsi: "*Prefazione*" to *QR* VIII for discussion of the doubtful statement by *RAD* II, 431, that the original version of *Le Chant des Titans* was for solo bs to lines in Italian beginning (like the Conte-Susanna duet in Act III of *Le Nozze di Figaro*) "*Crudel, perchè finora . . .*" Orchestrated by Rossini, 1861 (piccolo, 2 flutes, 2 oboes, 2 B-flat clarinets, 2 bassoons—bassoons III and IV *ad*

libitum—2 F horns, 2 C horns, 2 C trumpets, 3 trombones, ophicleide, 24 first violins, 24 second violins, 6 violas, 6 cellos, 6 double-basses, timpani, tam-tam); first performed at the Opéra, Paris, 12/22/61; this version pub. *QR* VIII, 66.

7. *Preghiera* ("*Tu che di verde il prato*"): t 1, t 2, b 1, b 2, bs 1, bs 2; pub. *QR* VII, 89.

8. *Au Chevet d'un mourant (élégie)*: s; text by Émilien Pacini; the autograph ded. reads: "*Dédié à Madame de Lafitte née Pacini par son ami G. Rossini—Paroles d'Émilien Pacini*"; pub. *QR* V, 17.

9. *Le Sylvain*: ms; text by Émilien Pacini; pub. *QR* V, 1.

10. *Cantemus Domino*: 8 real voices; at end of autograph manuscript, Rossini wrote "*Voilà du temps perdu!*"; pub. *QR* XI, 53.

11. *Ariette à l'ancienne*: ms; text by Jean-Jacques Rousseau; pub. *QR* V, 69 (same text set as *Ariette villageoise*, *Pdv* XI, 1, the two settings being related).

12. *Le Départ (tyrolienne sentimentale)*: s 1, s 2, c 1, c 2; text by Émilien Pacini; subtitled "*Le départ des promis—Quatuor—Tyrolesienne* [sic] *sentimentale pour 4 voix. Paroles d'Émilien Pacini.*"

Volume IV—*Quatre Hors d'oeuvres et quatre mendiants pour piano*

The cover of the collection made up of Vols. IV–VIII (all for solo piano) has this inscription: "*UN PEU DE TOUT. Recueil de 56 morceaux sémicomiques pour le piano, savoir*

Quatre mendiants, Quatre hors d'œuvres, Quatre Album [sic] *de douze numéros chaque un. Je dédie ces péchés de vieillesse aux pianistes de la quatrième classe à la quelle j'ai l'honneur d'appartenir. G. Rossini, Passy—Mes autographes."*

A. *Les Hors d'œuvres*
  1. *Les Radis*
  2. *Les Anchois (thème et variations)*
  3. *Les Cornichons (introduction—thème et varations)*
  4. *Le Beurre (thème et variations)*

B. *Les Quatres Mendiants*
  1. *Les Figues sèches*: has the valedictory inscription *"Me voilà—Bonjour, Madame."*
  2. *Les Amandes*: with the subtitle *"Minuit sonne—bon soir, Ma-*

dame."
  3. *Les Noisettes*: with the subtitle *"A ma chère Nini—Pensée d'amour à ma chienne."*
  4. *Les Raisins*: with the inscription *"À ma petite perruche—Foutre, foutre. Bonjour, Rossini! Bonjour, farceur!—Oh c'te tête—Oh c'te tête—Portez l'arme. Presentez l'arme.—En joue—feu!—rataplan, rataplan, plan, plan, tu n'en auras—Quand je bois du vin clairet, tout tourne au cabaret."*

Volume V—*Album de chaumière*

1. *Gymnastique d'écartement*
2. *Prélude fugassé*
3. *Petite Polka chinoise*
4. *Petite Valse de boudoir*
5. *Prélude inoffensif*: pub. QR II, 8.
6. *Petite Valse: L'Huile de ricin*
7. *Un Profond Sommeil—Un Reveil*
en sursaut
8. *Plein-chant chinois (scherzo)*
9. *Un Cauchemar*
10. *Valse boîteuse*
11. *Une Pensée à Florence*
12. *Marche*

Volume VI—*Album pour les enfants adolescents*

1. *Première comunion (andantino religioso)*: with the inscription *"Passage de l'Ostie—Recréation."*
2. *Thème naïf et variations*
3. *Saltarello à l'italienne*
4. *Prélude moresque*
5. *Valse lugubre*
6. *Impromptu anodin*
7. *L'Innocence italienne suite de la candeur française*: pub. QR II, 19.
8. *Prélude convulsif*
9. *La Lagune de Venise à l'expiration de l'année 1861!!!!*: with the opening instruction *"pppppppp"* and the inscription *"L'Ombre de Radetzky!!!—Arrivée de S. M.!!!—La lagune baissante d'une tièrce."*
10. *Ouf! Les Petits Pois*: pub. QR II, 30.
11. *Un Sauté*
12. *Hachis romantique*

Volume VII—*Album des enfants dégourdis*

1. *Mon Prélude hygiénique du matin*: pub. *QR X*, 28.
2. *Prélude baroque*
3. *Memento Homo*: pub. *QR X*, 87.
4. *Assez de memento; dansons*: pub. *QR X*, 94.
5. *La Pésarèse*: pub. *QR X*, 60.
6. *Valse torturée*
7. *Une Caresse à ma femme*: marked "*semplice . . . affetuoso . . . litigioso . . . lusingando . . . affetuoso . . . semplice*"; pub. *QR II*, 37.
8. *Barcarolle*
9. *Un Petit Train de plaisir* (*Comique-imitatif*): with the indications "*Allº.—Cloche d'appel—Montée en Wagon—En avant la machine—Sifflet satanique—Douce mélodie du Frein—Arrivée à la Gare—Andante—Les Lions Parisiens offrant la main aux Biches pour descendre du Wagon—Primo tempo—(Suite du voyage)—Terrible Déraillement du convoi—Premier Blessé—Second Blessé—Premier mort en Paradis—Second mort en Enfer—Largo—Chant funébre—Amen—On ne m'y attrapera pas G. R.—Douleur aiguë des héritiers—Tout ce ci est plus que naïf mais c'est vrai. G. Rossini*"; pub. *QR II*, 42.
10. *Fausse Couche de polka-mazurka*
11. *Étude asthmatique*
12. *Un Enterrement en carneval*: pub. *QR X*, 68.

Volume VIII—*Album de château*

1. *Spécimen de l'ancien régime*
2. *Prélude pétulant-rococo*
3. *Un Regret, un espoir*
4. *Boléro tartare*
5. *Prélude prétentieux* (first called *Prélude orgueilleux*): pub. *QR X*, 1.
6. *Spécimen de mon temps* (first called *Prélude prétentieux*): pub. *QR X*, 38.
7. *Valse antidansante*
8. *Prélude semi-pastoral*
9. *Tarentelle pur sang* (*avec traversée de la Procession*): with the gloss "*Choeur, harmonium, clochette à la fin et ad libitum—Traversée de la Procession—Retour de la Procession*"; pub. *QR II*, 83.
10. *Un Rêve*: pub. *QR X*, 11.
11. *Prélude soi-distant dramatique*
12. *Spécimen de l'avenir* (first called *Prélude de l'avenir*): pub. *QR X*, 104.

Volume IX—*Album pour piano, violon, violoncelle, harmonium et cor*

1. *Mélodie candide*: piano.
2. *La Savoie amante* (first called *L'Arrivée des zouaves*): piano.
3. *Chansonette*: piano.
4. *Un Mot à Paganini* (*élégie pour violon*)
5. *Impromptu tarentellisé*: piano.
6. *Échantillon du Chant de Noël à l'italienne*: piano; subtitled *Album pour les enfants emmaillottes*; pub. *QR* II, 102; see also *La Nuit de Noël*, of which this is a transcription, *Pdv* II, 6.
7. *Marche et réminiscences pour mon dernier voyage*: piano; with the gloss "*Frappons ff—Tancredi—Cenerentola—Donna del lago—Semiramide—Conte Ory—G. Tell —Otello—Barbiere—Mon portrait —allons—on ouvre—j'y suis—Requiem*"; passages from the operas named are quoted; pub. *QR* II, 108.
8. *Prélude, thème et variations pour*
cor: piano acc.; included is a "*Variante pour les paresseux!!*"; inscribed "*À l'aimable Vivier, petit souvenir d'amitié de G. Rossini, Paris, ce 11 Mai 1857*"; pub. *QR* III, 1.
9. *Prélude italien*: piano.
10. *Une Larme* (*thème et variations pour violoncello*): quotes song of the same name, *Pdv* XIV, 2; pub. *QR* VI, 9.
11. *Échantillon de blague mélodique* (*sur les noirs de la main droite*): piano; first called *Petite Plaisanterie*, it has the gloss "*Chante, cochon . . .* "
12. *Petite Fanfare à quatre mains*: piano, 4 hands; with the gloss "*La droite à Mademoiselle. La gauche à Monsieur*"; at the end, it has the note "*Je prie mes interprètes de vouloir executer avec amour (des mains et des genoux) ma petite fanfare.*"

Volume X—*Miscellanée pour piano*

1. *Prélude blagueur de bon train-train*
2. *Des Tritons, s'il vous plait* (*montée-descente*)
3. *Une Petite Pensée*
4. *Une Bagatelle*
5. *Une Bagatelle* (*In Nomine Patris —mélodie italienne*)
6. *Petite Caprice* (*style Offenbach*), *allegretto grotesco*: perhaps Rossini's amused reply to the *Guillaume Tell* trio parody in Offenbach's *La Belle Hélène*; exists for 2 hands, 4 hands; pub. (2 hands) *QR* II, 1.

Volume XI—*Miscellanée de musique vocale*

1. *Ariette villageoise*: ms; text by Jean-Jacques Rousseau; also used in *Ariette à l'ancienne*, pub. *QR* V, 69.—the two settings are related.
2. *Chanson du bébé*: ms; text by Émilien Pacini; pub. *QR* V, 25.
3. *Amour sans espoir (tiranne à l'espagnole rossinisée)*: s (a translation into French by Emilien Pacini of *Tirana alla spagnola rossinizatta*, *Pdv* I, 3?).
4. *Requiem (à ma belle mère)*: c; "*belle mère*" rather than "*belle-mère*" is almost certainly correct; pub. *QR* XI, 58.
5. *O salutaris . . . de champagne*: c. According to Hirt: "*Di Alcuni autografi di G. Rossini*," "At the Madeleine in Paris, Halévy had brought out a sublime Offertory for tenor; one of the leading artists of the Opéra had sung it deliciously, and Rossini, the old and unrepentant burlesquer, composed his '*O salutaris . . . de cham-*

pagne.'"
6. *Aragonese, L'*: s; a setting of the Metastasian "*Mi lagnerò tacendo*"; pub. *QR* IV, 44.
7. *Arietta all'antica*: s; a setting of the Metastasian "*Mi lagnerò tacendo*," the music derived from *Pdv* XI, 5; pub. *QR* IV, 60.
8. *Il Candore in fuga*: fugued quintet for s 1, s 2, c,t,bs.
9. *Mottetto*: vocal quartet; ded. "*A Maria Santissima Annunziata.*"
10. *Grande Scena*: "*Giovanna d' Arco*": s; autograph manuscript has the inscription "*Cantata a voce sola con accompagnamento di piano, espressamente composta per Madamigella Olimpia Pélissier da Rossini. Parigi 1832*"; revised text (by Luigi Crisostomo Ferrucci?), with string acc. (2 violins, viola, doublebass), 1852 or 1853; original version pub. *QR* X, 1; fragment of revised version pub. *QR* XI, 30.

Volume XII—*Quelques Riens pour album*

These are brief pieces that Rossini composed in autograph albums, a small part of the vast number of such album leaves in existence. 1. Allegretto; 2. Allegretto moderato; 3. Allegretto moderato ("*À mon ami Panseron, Passy*"); 4. Andante sostenuto; 5. Allegretto moderato; 6. Andante maestoso; 7. Andante mosso; 8. Andante sostenuto; 9. Allegretto moderato; 10. Andantino mosso; 11. Andantino mosso; 12. *Danse sibérienne* (see also under Instrumental Music); 13. Allegretto brillante; 14. Allegro vivace; 15. *Petite*

Galette allemande; 16. *Douce réminiscences: "Offerte à mon ami Carafa pour le nouvel an 1866; 'Oh Fricaine!' "* (Meyerbeer's *L' Africaine* had had its première in 1865; "*fricain*" could be an adjective manufactured from "*fric*," a slang word for money); 17. Andantino mosso quasi allegretto; 18.

Andantino mosso; 19. Allegretto moderato; 20. Allegretto brillante; 21. Andantino sostenuto (with the gloss "*In tempo à l'Offen.* . . . "); 22. *Thème et variations sur le mode mineur*; 23. *Thème et variations sur le mode majeur*; 24. *Un Rien sur le mode enharmonique.*

Volume XIII—*Musique anodine*

Prélude pour le piano suivi de six petites mélodies composées sur les mêmes paroles ["*Mi lagnerò tacendo*"] *dont deux pour soprano, une pour mezzo-soprano, une pour contralto et deux pour baryton, avec accompagnement de piano.* With this dedication: "*J'offre ces modestes mélodies à ma chère femme Olimpia comme simple témoignage de reconnaissance pour les soins affectueux, intelligents qu'elle me prodigua dans ma trop longue et terrible maladie (opprobre de la faculté). Gioacchino Rossini. Paris, ce 14 avril 1857*"; pub. QR IV, 62.

I. Andantino, c
II. Andantino mosso, b
III. Andantino moderato, s
IIII. Allegretto moderato, s
IIIII. Andantino moderato, ms
IIIIII. Allegretto moderato, b

Volume XIV—*Compositions diverses et esquisses*

1. *Canone antisavant*: 3 voices; "*Dédié au* [sic] *Turcos par le Singe de Pesaro. Paroles et Musique du Singe, Passy*"; the text reads "*Vive l'Empereur, de France la splendeur. Vive! Vive! Vive! Vive!*"; at the end appears the instruction "*Da capo sine fine dicentibus.*"
2. *Une Larme*: bs; see also *Pdv* IX 10.
3. *La Vénitienne: canzonetta* (piano).

4. *Petite Promenade de Passy à Courbevoie*—"*La percourant (homéopathiquement et à la pésarèse) dans tous les tons de la gamme chromatique)*"; near the close is the gloss "*Mi gran-dièze, pardon de t'avoir oublié!! Rassure-toi, je suis encore en mésure de te fourrer dans ma petite promenade. Suive et tu verras . . .* "
5. *Une Réjouissance*: piano.
6. *Ritournelle gothique*: piano.

7. *Encore un peu de blague*: piano.
8. *Tourniquet sur la gamme chromatique ascendante et descendante*: piano; *ROG* 390, footnote 4, says: "The whole piece is made up of lines of three measures, each one of which is performed alternately, one in tempo and the other ritenuto."
9. *Un Rien: Ave Maria*: voice and piano; the text consists entirely of "*Ave Maria, gratia plena*"; pub. *QR* XI, 60.
10. *Due "Riens"*: b; on lines by Metastasio ("*Mi lagnerò tacendo*"?).
11. *Brindisi*: coryphée and chor.
12. *Tantum ergo*: sketch.
13. *Teodora e Riccardino*: sketch (for a cantata scene?).
14. *Il Genio del Cristianesimo*: sketches for a cantata?
15. *Solo per violoncello*: untitled.
16. *Argene e Melania*: cantata (incomplete?) for 2 solo voices, with acc. including clarinets and trombones; announced (1967) for publication in one of four new *QR* to be issued at Pesaro for the 1968 centenary of Rossini's death.

BIBLIOGRAPHY

Bibliography

For an explanation of the abbreviations used, see page 391.

Abbiati, Franco: *Giuseppe Verdi*, 4 vols., Milan, 1959.
—— "*Rossini inedito*," La Scala, Milan, 12/15/1949.
Adam, Adolphe: *Derniers Souvenirs d'un musicien*, Paris, 1859.
Adami, Giuseppe: *Giulio Ricordi*, Milan, 1945.
Alaleona, D.: "*Variazioni rossiniane e donizettiane*," Il Mondo 3, 2/1922.
Albarelli, Padre Giuseppe: "*L'Infanzia di Gioacchino Rossini (Da documenti inediti dell'Archivio storico del Comune di Pesaro)*," BdCRdS 1958, 6, 101; 1958, 1, 6; 1958, 2, 28.
Albertini, Luciano: "*Rossini oggi, nella testimonianza di un giovane*," BdCRdS 1956, 2, 27; 1957, 3, 45.
Albini, Eugenia: "*Rossiniana*," RMI XLIV, 3–4, 1940.
Albini, Giuseppe: "*Il Centenario di domani*," FdD XIV, 9, 2/28/1892.
—— "*Di un articolo sul Rossini*," FdD, 3/6/1892.
"*Alcune parole sullo 'Stabat Mater' di Rossini eseguito nella grande aula dell'Archiginnasio di Bologna le sere del 18, 19 e 20 marzo*," Teatri, arti e letteratura XX, 57, Bologna, 3/24/1842.
Allmaÿer, Alessandro: *Undici Lettere di Gioachino Rossini pubblicate per la prima volta . . .*, Siena, 1892.
Arcozzi, Masino: *Parole dette dal Vice-Presidente del Liceo musicale di Torino Comm. Arcozzi Masino in occasione del Saggio in onore di Rossini*, Turin, 1892.
Armani, Franco, and Bascapé, Giacomo: *La Scala: Breve Biografia (1778–1950)*, Milan, n.d.
Arnese, R.: *see* De Filippis, F.
Ashbrook, William: *Donizetti*, London, 1965.
Aulagnier, Antoine: *G. Rossini: Sa Vie et ses œuvres*, Paris, 1864.
—— *Quelques Observations sur la publication du "Stabat Mater" de Rossini*, Paris, 1842.
Azevedo, Alexis-Jacob: *G. Rossini: Sa Vie et ses œuvres*, Paris, 1864.
—— "*Rossini chez lui*," La Cronique musicale, Paris, 7/1873.
Azzuri, Francesco: *Rossini scultore*, Pesaro, 1896.

Bacchelli, Riccardo: *"Come ho studiato Rossini senza sapere la musica,"* LRM 1947, 3.

———— *Rossini e Esperienze rossiniane* (definitive edn.), Milan, 1959.

———— *"Rossini patetico e lirico,"* XVM 1952.

"Bach": *"Rossini nelle memorie di 'Rosina,'"* GdI 2/21/1916.

Baldacchini, Michele: *A Gioacchino Rossini: Iscrizioni e discorso*, Naples, 1869.

Baldassini, Alessandro: *A Giovacchino Rossini rinnovatore delle musicali armonie . . .*, Bologna, 1830.

Barbèri, Pio: *"Ferretti,"* Giornale di Roma 75, Rome, 4/2/1852.

Barberio, Francesco: *"La Regina d'Etruria e Rossini,"* RMI LV, 1, 63, 1–3/1953.

Barbiera, Raffaele: *Vite ardenti nel Teatro (1700–1900) . . .*, Milan, 1931.

Barblan, Guglielmo: *"Il Rossiniano farsesco ne 'La Scala di seta,'"* XVM.

Barini, G.: *"Il Nuovo Teatro Quirino e il 'Mosè' del Rossini,"* NA 5/16/1915.

Bascapé, Giacomo: see Armani, Franco.

Battaglia, G.: *"Milano—Teatro Carcano—Seconda Produzione del Barbiere di Siviglia,"* BdS 8/16/1834 (see also, L'Eco).

———— (?, signed *"L'Estensore"*): *"Polemica: Risposta dell'estensore di questo giornale alla lettera inserita nel num. 100 dell' 'Eco,'"* BdS 8/23/1834.

Becherini, Bianca: *"A Proposito di un segno particolare in Rossini,"* BdCRdS 1956, 5, 90.

Becker, Heinz, ed.: *Giacomo Meyerbeer: Briefwechsel und Tagebücher*, Vol. I (to 1824), Berlin, 1960; Vol. II, Berlin, 1967(?).

Bell, Georges: *"Rossini,"* Les Grands et les petits personages du jour, par un des plus petits, Paris, n.d.

Bellaigue, Camille: *Portraits et silhouettes des musiciens*, Paris, 1896.

Benadduci, Giovanni: *Una Lettera inedita di Gioachino Rossini*, Tolentino, 1890.

Berkel, Cor van: *Gioacchino Rossini* (Dutch), Harlem, 1950.

Berlioz, Hector: *"Guillaume Tell,"* La Gazette musicale, Paris, 10–11/1834.

Berton, Henri-Montan: *De la Musique mécanique et de la musique philosophique*, Paris, 1821.

———— *Épître à un célèbre compositeur français . . .*, Paris, 1829.

Berton, Pierre: *Souvenirs de la vie de théâtre*, Paris, n.d.

Bertù, Berto: *Lo Spirito di Rossini (Aneddoti)*, Pesaro, 1927.

Betti, Salvatore: *Decreto latino fatto dall'Accademia pesarese di scienze, belle lettere ed arti in onore del celebre Gioacchino Rossini di Pesaro* (handbill), Pesaro, n.d., but 1819.

Bettoni, Nicolò: often cited as author of Zanolini's life of Rossini, of which he was actually the first publisher (in his periodical *L'Ape italiana*, Paris).

Beulé, Charles-Ernest: *Éloge de Rossini . . . 18 décembre 1869* (Institut Impérial de France, Académie des Beaux-Arts), Paris, 1869.

Bevilacqua-Aldobrandini, Marchese Gherardo: *"G. Rossini,"* Omnibus, Naples, 10/5/1839.

Biaggi, G. Alessandro: *"Gioacchino Rossini nel centenario della sua nascita,"* NA 3/16/1892.

―――― *"Memoria letta nell'adunanza solenne del dì 2 febbraio 1869 . . . Della vita e delle opere di Gioacchino Rossini,"* Atti, Regio Instituto Musicale, Florence, 1869, 15; also NA 12/1868–3-4/1869.

―――― *"La Musica religiosa e la 'Petite Messe,' "* NA 7/1870.

―――― *"Lo 'Stabat Mater' di Rossini,"* La Gazzetta dei teatri, Milan, 1888.

Biagi, Guido: *"Undici lettere inedite di G. Rossini,"* Of (q.v.).

Biamonti, G.: *"Il Barbiere di Siviglia" di Gioacchino Rossini*, Rome, 1929.

―――― *Guglielmo Tell*, Rome, 1929.

Bianchi, Nerino: *"Il Barbiere di Siviglia" e il sentimento patrio di Gioacchino Rossini*, Rome, 1916.

―――― *"Rossini e il suo carattere,"* La Scena illustrata 7, 4/1/1892.

Bianchini, Giuseppe Nicolò: *Lettere di Gioacchino Rossini a Giuseppe Ancillo, Speziale veneziano*, Venice, 1892.

Bisogni, Fabio: *"Rossini e Schubert,"* in (Nuova) Rivista musicale italiana, Turin, September–October 1968, pp. 920–935.

Blaze de Bury (Henri Blaze, Baron de Bury): *"Rossini,"* Revue des deux mondes, Paris, 12/1869 (reprinted in *Musiciens du passé, du présent et de l'avenir*, Paris, 1880).

―――― *"Rossini: Sa Vie et ses œuvres,"* Revue des deux mondes, Paris, 5-6/1854.

―――― *"Le 'Stabat' de Rossini,"* Revue des deux mondes, Paris, 2/1842 (reprinted in *Musiciens contemporains*, Paris, 1856).

Boggio, Camillo, and others: *La Cantante Teresa Belloc*, Milan, 1895.

Bollettino del Centro Rossiniano di Studi, Pesaro (30 issues), 1955–60. In addition to the important articles listed herein under authors' names, BdCRdS published the following unsigned items of value: *"La Critica musicale rossiniana nella prima metà dell'Ottocento,"* 1956, 2, 32; 1957, 3, 47; 1957, 4, 69; *"Goethiana,"* 1958, 4, 73; 1958, 5, 93, 1958, 6, 114; *"Opere di Rossini a Bologna,"* 1957, 2, 37; 1958, 3, 55; 1958, 4, 74; 1958, 5, 96; 1958, 6, 115; 1958, 1, 13; 1958, 2, 37; 1959, 3, 53; *"Rossini nel giudizio della stampa inglese,"* 1956, 2, 34; 1957, 3, 49; 1957, 4, 72. The chronological sequence (scholastic year, September–September) was: 1955, 1, 2; 1956, 3, 4, 5, 6, 1, 2; 1957, 3, 4, 5, 6, 1, 2; 1958, 3, 4, 5, 6, 1, 2; 1959, 3, 4, 5, 6, 1; 1960, 2, 3, 4, 5, 6; 1967, 1, 2, 3, 4, 5, 6; 1968, 1, 2, 3, 4-5-6; 1969, 1. To be issued three times per year beginning in 1970.

Bollettino del Primo Centenario Rossiniano, Pubblicato dal Comitato Ordinatore (18 issues), Pesaro, 2/29–9/15/1892.

Bonaccorsi, Alfredo: *"Abbellimenti e coloratura,"* BdCRdS 1957, 5, 81.

―――― *"Arie classiche dell'Ottocento,"* BdCRdS 1958, 3, 41.

―――― *"L'Arsi come inciso melodico iniziatore,"* BdCRdS 1959, 6, 101.

―――― *"Come componeva Rossini?"* BdCRdS 1955, 1, 1.

―――― *"Un Crescendo di qualità,"* BdCRdS 1960, 6, 110.

―――― *"Edipo a Colono,"* BdCRdS 1957, 1, 41.

———— *Giacomo Puccini e i suoi antenati musicali*, Milan, n.d., but 1950.

———— ed.: *Gioacchino Rossini: Symposium—Collana di saggi musicali diretta da Guido M. Gatti* (mostly reprints), Florence, 1968(?).

————"*Hum-ta-ta Musik*," BdCRdS 1957, 1, 1.

———— "*Inno di Bacchilide alla Pace*," BdCRdS 1960, 4, 61; 1960, 5, 83.

———— "*Invenzione e invenzioni*," BdCRdS 1959, 4, 61.

———— "*Il Leitmotiv*," BdCRdS 1958, 1, 1.

———— "*Paragone per una marcia funebre (fra Rossini e Wagner)*," BdCRdS 1955, 2, 21.

———— "*I Punti colorati nell'Ottocento*," BdCRdS 1957, 2, 21.

———— ed.: *Quaderni Rossiniani*, Pesaro, 1954–65; see *Quaderni Rossiniani*.

———— "*Qualche Sviluppo*," BdCRdS 1958, 2, 21.

———— "*42° Bisestile*," BdCRdS 1960, 4, 77.

———— "*Schede per Rossini: scheda uno*," BdCRdS 1960, 2, 21.

———— "*La Sinfonia del 'Barbiere' prima del 'Barbiere*,'" LRM 7–9/1954, 210.

———— "*Una Sinfonia ciclica*," BdCRdS 1956, 6, 101.

———— "*Il Silenzio come espressione drammatica*," BdCRdS 1959, 3, 41.

———— "*Spunti popolari*," BdCRdS 1956, 1, 1.

———— "*Temporali dell'Ottocento*," BdCRdS 1958, 5, 81.

———— "*Terminologia*," BdCRdS 1956, 4, 1.

———— "*29 Febbraio 1792/29 febbraio 1956*," BdCRdS 1956, 4, 70.

———— "*Una 'Via crucis' e una 'Bonamorte' rossiniane*," LRM 7–9/1954, 270

————, ed.: *Gioacchino Rossini*, Florence, 1968 (largely reprints of articles by Massimo Mila, Riccardo Bacchelli, Ada Melica, Bonaccorsi, Luigi Magnani, André Schaeffner, Ildebrando Pizzetti, Andrea Della Corte, Guido Pannain, and Roman Vlad); genealogical tables.

Bonafé, Félix: "*Une Amie di Rossini*," BdCRdS 1955, 2, 23.

———— *Rossini e son œuvre*, Le-Puy-en-Velay, 1955.

Bonaventura, Arnaldo: *Rossini*, Florence, 1934.

———— "*Rossini e una satira di Giuseppe Barbieri*," LCM 1896, 9.

Bonavia, Michael: "Rossini in London," *Monthly Musical Record*, London, 1930, 297.

Bonetti, Gaetano: "*A Rossini per l'esecuzione solenne della sua musica sullo 'Stabat Mater' . . .*," Bologna, 1842.

Bonfiglioli, Gianni: "*La 'Piccola Messe solenne*,'" ROS (q.v.).

Bontempelli, Ettore: "*Introduzione biografica e critica*" (to libretto of *Il Barbiere di Siviglia*), Milan, 1932.

Bosdari, F.: *La Vita musicale a Bologna nel periodo napoleonico*, Bologna, 1914.

Bourgault-Ducoudray, Louis-Albert: "*L'Opéra italien: Rossini*," *Annales de Paris*, 1909 (reprinted in LCM 1909, 12).

Bouvet, Charles: *Cornélie Falcon*, Paris, 1927.

———— *Spontini*, Paris, 1930.

Branca, Emilia: *Felice Romani ed i più riputati maestri di musica del*

suo tempo, cenni biografici ed aneddotici raccolti e pubblicati da sua moglie,
Turin, etc., n.d., but 1892.

    Brevi Cenni sull'ex R. Teatro Rossini, ecc., Florence(?), 1889.

    Brigante Colonna, Gustavo: *Vita di Rossini, Florence,* 1947.

    Brighenti, Pietro: *Della Musica rossiniana e del suo autore,* Bologna, 1830.

    Brisson, Adolfo: "*Gli Amori di Rossini,*" BdPCR 13, 7/20/1892, 97.

    Caffi, F.: *Analisi delle opinione pubblicate nelle gazzette intorno allo* "*Stabat*" *del Cav. Maestro Rossini,* Venice, 1847.

    Caldarella, Antonio: "*Il Primo Incontro di Bellini con Rossini,*" LRM 1/1949, 46.

    Camaiti, V.: *Gioachino Rossini: Notizie biografiche, artistiche e aneddotiche,* Florence, 1887.

    Cambi, Luisa: *Bellini* [*La Vita*], Milan, 1938.

    —— *Vincenzo Bellini: Epistolario,* Milan, 1943.

    Cambiasi, Pompeo: *La Scala 1778–1906—note storiche e statistiche . . . 5 ed. completamente rifusa, accresciuta e corretta,* Milan, etc., 1906.

    Cametti, Alberto, ed.: *Una Conferenza inedita di Jacopo Ferretti sulla storia della poesia melodrammatica romana,* Pesaro, 1896.

    —— "*Il 'Guglielmo Tell' e le sue rappresentazioni in Italia,*" RMI 1899, 1, 580, and LCM 1899, 3.

    —— *La Musica teatrale a Roma cento anni fa, Annuario della Regia Accademia di Santa Cecilia,* Rome, 1915–30.

    —— *Un Poeta melodrammatico romano: Appunti e notizie in gran parte inedite sopra Jacopo Ferretti e i musicisti del suo tempo, con ritratti e fac-simili,* Milan, etc., n.d., but 1898.

    —— *Il Teatro di Tordinona poi Apollo,* 2 vols., Tivoli, 1928.

    Cantarini, A.: "*La Scoperta di un manoscritto*" (Wagner's transcription of "*I Marinai*"), *Musica,* Rome, 6/1912.

    Capri, Antonio: "*Rossini e l'estetica teatrale della vocalità,*" RMI 1942, 353.

    —— "*Il Silenzio di Rossini,*" *Bollettino mensile di vita e cultura musicale,* Milan, 12/1936.

    Caputo Montalto, Francesco: see *Lettere inedite di Gioachino Rossini a Filippo Santocanale.*

    Carletti, Domenico: *A Gioacchino Rossini nell'apertura del teatro in Pesaro dopo le funebri pompe . . .* (2 flyers: "*La Mesta Mia Scordata Cetra appesa*" and "*O fulgid'Astro assiso fra le sfere*"), Pesaro, 1869.

    —— *Nel Dì trigesimo di lutto universale . . .* (flyer, second edition, containing two sonnets from above flyers and a third sonnet, "*Chi e mai costei che (solo) in bruno ammanto*"), Pesaro, 1868.

    Carpani, Giuseppe: *Lettera del Professore Giuseppe Carpani sulla musica di Gioacchino Rossini . . . ,* Rome, 1826.

    —— *Le Rossiniane, ossia Lettere musicò-teatrali,* Padua, 1824.

    Casamorata, L. F.: "*G. Rossini,*" LGMF 1853.

    —— "*Lo 'Stabat' di Rossini,*" LGMM 4/5/1842.

Casella, Alfredo: *"Di un 'Si naturale' e di qualche altra cosa,"* *MdO* 7/1931.

———— *"Una Ignota 'Sonata' per archi di G. Rossini,"* *ROS* (*q.v.*).

Casini, Tommaso: *"Rappresentazioni di opere rossiniane in Pesaro,"* *BdPCR* 10, 77.

———— *"Rossini e Pio IX,"* *BdPCR* 7, 53; *BdPCR* 8, 62.

———— *"Rossini in patria,"* *NA* 3/1/1892, 109.

Castil-Blaze (François-Henri-Joseph Blaze): *L'Académie imperiale de musique de 1655 à 1855,* 2 vols., Paris, 1855.

———— *L'Opéra-Comique de 1753 à 1856,* MS. in the Bibliothèque Nationale, Paris.

———— *L'Opéra-Italien de 1548 à 1856,* Paris, 1856.

Catalogo del Museo Teatrale alla Scala . . . compilato da Stefano Vittadini, prefazione di Renato Simoni, Milan, 1940.

Cavazzocca Mazzanti, Vittorio: *Rossini a Verona durante il Congresso del 1822,* Verona, 1922.

Celani, F.: *"Musica e musicisti in Roma (1750–1850), con documenti su la prima rappresentazione del 'Barbiere di Siviglia,'"* *RMI* 1925, 2.

Celebrazione marchigiane, 16 agosto–16 settembre 1934 (with monographs by Franco Alfano, G. Mulè, M. Puccini), Urbino, 1935.

Celletti, Rodolfo: *"Origini e sviluppi della coloratura rossiniana,"* in *(Nuova) Rivista musicale italiana,* September–October 1968, pp. 872–919.

Checchi, Eugenio: *"Il Centenario di Rossini,"* *FdD* 12/31/1892.

———— *"Le Lettere di G. Rossini"* (review of the Mazzatinti-Manis collection), *FdD* 12/8/1901.

———— *Rossini,* Florence, 1898.

———— *"Rossini,"* *FdD* 2/21/1892.

Chilesotti, Oscar: *I Nostri Maestri del passato,* Milan, 1882(?).

Cicconnetti, Filippo: *Nella Morte di Gioacchino Rossini . . . ,* Rome, 1869.

Cinelli, Carlo: *Carolina di Brunswick principessa di Galles,* Pesaro, 1890.

———— *Memorie cronistoriche del Teatro di Pesaro dall'anno 1637 al 1807,* Pesaro, 1898.

Cinque, Vincenzo: *"Istituzione poco nota: La 'Fondation Rossini' di Parigi,* *BdCRdS* 1960, 2, 27.

Cipollone, Ernesto: *"Rossini interpretato da Papini,"* *BdCRdS* 1958, 1, 10.

———— *"Rossini secondo Pascoli,"* *BdCRdS* 1958, 2, 31.

Clément, Félix: *Musiciens célèbres depuis le XVIᵉ siècle jusqu'à nos jours,* Paris, 1868; 4th edn., 1887.

Colombani, Alfredo: *L'Opera italiana nel secolo XIX,* Milan, 1900.

Commetant, Oscar: *"Relics of Rossini,"* *Monthly Musical Record,* London, 1875, p. 33.

Confalonieri, Giulio: *" 'Il Conte Ory,' "* *XVM.*

Conti, Augusto: *"Religiosità, bontà, malinconia del Rossini,"* *Of* (*q.v.*).

Cooke, James Francis: *Rossini: A Short Biography,* Philadelphia, 1929.

Cordara, C.: *"Rossini nell'intimità,"* *Marzocco,* Florence, 1902, 15.

Cottrau, Guglielmo: *Lettres d'un mélomane pour servir de document à l'histoire musicale de Naples de 1829 à 1847* (preface by F. Verdinois), Naples, 1885.

Cowen, Sir Frederick Hymen: *Rossini*, London and New York, 1912.

Crémieux, Adolphe: *Collection d'autographes*, Paris, 1885.

Cristal, M.: *"Rossini," Le Correspondant*, Paris, 12/25/1868.

Cronaca musicale, La, Pesaro: *Numero rossiniano*, 1916, 1, 2.

Cucchetti, Gino: *"La 'Vie de Rossini' de Stendhal," ROS* (q.v.).

Cugino, Giovanni: *In Morte di Giovacchino Rossini, canzone*, Palermo, 1872.

Damerini, Adelmo: *"Il Coro 'La Carità,' " LRM* 7–9/1954.

———*"La Prima Ripresa moderna di un'opera giovanile di Rossini: 'L'Equivoco stravagante' (1811)," Chigiana* XXII, Florence, 1965.

———*"Il Rossini vero," MdO* 5/1942.

———*"Signore del canto," La Scala*, Milan, 1950.

D'Amico, Lele (Fedele): *Rossini*, Turin, 1939.

D'Ancona, Alessandro: *"Il 'Gran Rifiuto' di Rossini," Of* (q.v.).

D'Angeli, A.: *"Autografi musicali di G. R.," LCM* 1908, no. 2.

———*"G. R., la sua scuola, la sua opera," LCM* 1908, no. 3.

———*"Gli 'Stabat Mater' di Pergolesi e quello di G. R.," LCM* 1912, nos. 1–2.

———*"Lettere inedite di Giuseppe e Gioacchino Rossini," LCM* 1908, no. 21.

———*" ' L'Occasione fa il ladro' di G. R.," LCM* 1916, nos. 7–8.

———*"Il Padre di Rossini, poeta," LCM* 1898, no. 3.

———*"Rossini e Liszt," LCM* 1911, nos. 8–9.

———*"Rossiniana," LCM* 1912, no. 12.

Da Prato, Cesare: *Genova: Teatro Carlo Felice, relazione storico-esplicativa*, Genoa, n.d.

D'Arcais, F.: articles on Rossini in *L'Opinione*, Florence, during 1869 (5/10, 5/18, 8/2, 8/23, 8/24, 11/17, 11/18).

———*"L'Eredità in R.," NA*, 10/16/1879.

———*"Rossini in Santa Croce," NA* 5/1/1887.

D'Arienzo, N.: *Pel Centenario di G. R.*, Naples, 1892.

Dal Fabbro, Beniamino: *"Crome e biscrome (dal Diario)," XVM*.

Dauriac, Lionel: *La Psychologie dans l'opéra français: Auber, Rossini, Meyerbeer*, Paris, 1920.

———*Les Musiciens célèbres*, Paris, 1907(?).

D'Azeglio, Massimo (Massimo Taparelli, Marchese d'Azeglio): *I Miei Ricordi*.

De Angelis, Alberto: *"Il Conte Gioacchino Antonio Rossini," Scenario*, 9/1933 (reprinted as pamphlet, Milan, n.d.).

———*La Musica a Roma nel secolo XIX*, Rome, 1935.

De Boigne, Charles: *Petits Mémoires de l'Opéra*, Paris, 1857.

De Curzon, Henri: *Rossini*, Paris, 1930.

———*"Rossini et la musique d'église," Le Ménestrel*, Paris, 5/5/1922.

——— *"Un Souvenir de Rossini à propos de voix,"* Le Guide musicale, Brussels, 1911, no. 9.

De Eisner-Eisenhof, Baron Angelo: *Lettere inedite di Gaetano Donizetti a diversi e lettere di Rossini, Scribe, Dumas, Spontini, Adam, Verdi a Gaetano Donizetti*, Bergamo, 1897.

De Filippis, F., and Arnese, R.: *Cronache del Teatro di S. Carlo 1737–1960)*, 2 vols, Naples, 1961.

De Gubernatis, Angelo: *Le Feste rossiniane a Pesaro, Museo di famiglia*, 8/28/1864, 544.

——— *"Gioacchino Rossini,"* Natura ed arte, 3/1892.

——— *"Un Giudizio sul Rossini,"* BdPCR 12, 89.

De Hegermann-Lindencrone, L.: *In the Courts of Memory, 1858–1875, from Contemporary Letters*, New York and London, 1912.

De La-Fage, I. A. (Juste-Adrien Lenoir de Lafage): *Memoria intorno la vita e le opere di Stanislao Mattei, P. Minorità bolognese*, Bologna, 1840.

De Loménie, Louis: *M. Rossini, par un homme de rien*, Paris, 1842.

De Mirecourt, Eugène (pseudonym of Ch.-J.-B Jacquot): *Rossini*, Paris, 1855.

De Morginis, L.: *"Rossini d'après sa correspondance,"* Le Correspondant, Paris, 1/10/1902.

De Rensis, Raffaello, ed.: *Critiche e cronache musicale di Arrigo Boito (1862–1870)*, Milan, 1931.

——— *"Rossini intimo: Lettere all'amico Santocanale,"* MdO 8–9/1931.

De Sanctis, Guglielmo: *Gioacchino Rossini: Appunti di viaggio* (reprinted from *Rivista romana di scienze e lettere* I, 3, 4), Rome, 1878.

——— *Memorie: Studie dal vero*, Rome, n.d.

De Zerbi, Rocco: *Rossini e la musica nuova*, Florence, 1892.

Del Lungo, Isidoro: *"Dello Stile rossiniano,"* Of (q.v.).

(Delaire, J.-A.): *Observations d'un amateur non dilettante au sujet du "Stabat" de M. Rossini* . . . , Paris, 1842.

Délécluze, Étienne-Jean: *Le "Stabat" de Rossini*, Paris, n.d.

Della Corte, Andrea: *"La 'Cenerentola' di G. R.,"* Arti e vita, II.

——— *"La Drammaturgia nella 'Semiramide' di G. R.,"* LRM 1938, 1.

——— *"Fra Gorgheggi e melodie di Rossini,"* Musica I, Florence, 1942.

——— *Paisiello (con una tavola tematica); L'Estetica musicale di P. Metastasio*, Turin, 1922.

——— *"Su 'Guglielmo Tell,'"* XVM.

——— with Guido Pannain: *Vincenzo Bellini: Il Carattere morale, i caratteri artistici*, Turin, etc., n.d.

Delle Feste fatte in Pesaro in onore di G. R. nel suo dì onomastico 21 agosto, 1864, Pesaro, 1864.

Derwent, George Harcourt Johnstone, Baron: *Rossini and Some Forgotten Nightingales*, London, 1934.

Desnoyers, Luigi (Louis): *De l'Opéra en 1847*, Paris, 1847.

Di Marzo, Gioacchino: *"Del Genio di Gioacchino Rossini,"* see *Omaggio a Gioacchino Rossini.*

Diddi, Stefano: *"La Corona d'Italia," BdCRdS* 1960, 4, 71.
—— *"Rossini strumentatore per banda," BdCRdS* 1959, 1, 9.
D'Indy, Vincent: *"La Messe solennelle de Rossini," Le Correspondant,* Paris, 3/25/1869.
Donati, Francesco: *In Lode di Giovacchino Rossini,* Urbino, 1869.
Donna e l'artista, La: Musicisti inamorati, Rome, 1927.
D'Ortigue, Joseph-Louis: *De la guerre des dilettanti, ou De la Révolution opérée par Rossini dans l'opéra français, et des rapports qui existent entre la musique, la littérature et les arts,* Paris, 1830.
—— *Le "Stabat" de Rossini,* Paris, 1841.
Du Bled, Victor: *"Le Salon de Rossini," La Revue musicale,* Paris, 1921, 143.
Dupré, Giovanni: *Ricordi autobiografici,* Florence, 1895; 2nd edn., as *Pensieri sull'arte e ricordi autobiografici,* Florence, 1898.
Duprez, Gilbert-Louis: *Souvenirs d'un chanteur,* Paris, 1880.
Ebers, John: *Seven Years of the King's Theatre,* London, 1828.
Eco, L', Milan, 1834, 100: *"Carteggio"* (letter attacking G. Battaglia).
Edwards, Henry Sutherland: *Famous First Representations,* London, 1886.
—— *Rossini's Life,* London, 1869; reissued in condensed form as *Rossini and His School,* London, 1881.
Enciclopedia dello spettacolo, 9 vols., Rome, 1952–62; *Aggiornamento 1955–1965* (vol. 10), Rome, 1966.
Enciclopedia italiana, Rome, 1936.
Engel, Louis: *From Mozart to Mario: Reminiscences of Half a Century,* 2 vols., London, 1886.
Eredità Rossini: *Relazione della Commissione al Consiglio comunale,* Pesaro, 1879.
Ernouf, Baron: *"Rossini, sa vie et son œuvre," Revue contemporaine,* Paris, 12/15/1868.
Escudier, Léon: *Mes Souvenirs,* Paris, 1863.
Escudier, Les Frères (Léon and M.): *Rossini: Sa Vie et ses œuvres* (introduction by M. Méry), Paris, 1854.
Fabri-Scarpellini, E.: *Della Cantata eseguita nel Campidoglio la sera del 1.° gennaio 1847 in onore del clementissimo pontefice PIO NONO,* Rome, 1846.
Fara, Giulio: *Genio e ingegno musicale: Gioachino Rossini,* Turin, 1915.
—— *"G. R. nel 150° anniversario della sua nascita," Rassegna dorica,* Rome, 3/1942.
Faustini, L.: *Di Rosmunda Pisaroni: Cenni biografici e aneddotici,* Piacenza, 1884.
Favre, Georges: *Boieldieu: Sa Vie—son œuvre,* 2 vols., Paris, 1944–5.
Ferrato, Pietro, ed.: *Poesie musicali inedite ed anonime del secolo XIV,* Padua, 1870.
Ferrer, "Le Chevalier de," tr.: *Essai de littérature concernant l'origine, les progrès et les revolutions de la musique italienne, avec des rémarques*

critiques . . . sur le nouveau style de Rossini, traduit de l'italienne . . . , Nare-brouk, n.d.

———— tr.: *Rossini e Bellini*; see San Jacinto, Stefano Mira e Sirignano, Marchese di.

Ferrucci, Luigi Crisostomo: *A Gioachino Rossini nel LXXVI anniversario della sua nascita (29 febbrajo 1792)*, Imola, 1868.

———— "*Accademia: Esecuzione dello 'Stabat Mater' del maestro Rossini nelle private sale del Palazzo Hercolani*," *Teatri, arti e letteratura*, Bologna, 3/31/1853.

———— "*Al Sig. Cav. Giuseppe Spada*," *L'Album*, Rome, 3/23/1861.

———— *Giudizio perentorio sulla verità della patria di Gioachino Rossini impugnata dal Prof. Giuliano Vanzolini* (a reply to Vanzolini: *Della Vera Patria di Gioacchino Rossini*), Florence, 1874.

———— "*Sulla Patria di Rossini*," *La Gazzetta del popolo*, Florence, 1868, 315, 329, 339; also in *Il Romagnolo*, Ravenna, 8/28/1869.

Fétis, François-Joseph: *Biographie universelle des musiciens et bibliographie générale de la musique*, 2nd edn., 9 vols., Paris, 1873; *Supplément et complément publiés sous la direction de M. Arthur Pougin*, 2 vols., Paris, 1878.

Filippi, Filippo: *Musica e musicisti: Critiche, biografie ed escursioni (Haydn-Beethoven-Weber-Meyerbeer-Rossini-Schumann-Wagner-Verdi)*, Milan, 1876.

Fiorentino, Vincenzo: *Musica, lavoro storico, filosofico, sociale: Storia, scienze ed arte, teatro e società*, 1886.

Florimo, Francesco: *Bellini: Memorie e lettere*, Florence, 1892.

———— *Cenno storico sulla scuola musicale di Napoli*, 2 vols., Naples, 1869–71.

———— *La Scuola musicale di Napoli: I suoi conservatorii con uno sguardo sulla storia della musica in Italia*, 4 vols., Naples, 1881.

Fracassi, Ferruccio: "*Appunti da Oriani*" (criticism of Alfredo Oriani's "*L'Arciero*," *Fuochi di bivacco*), *BdCRdS* 1957, 4, 66.

———— "*Rileggendo il 'Rossini' di Bacchelli*," *BdCRdS* 1958, 6, 108.

———— "*Tamburi, caisse roulante, tam-tam, ecc.*," *BdCRdS* 1958, 1, 9.

———— "*Uno del pubblico*," *BdCRdS* 1956, 4, 67.

Fraccaroli, Arnaldo: *Rossini*, Milan, 1941.

Fradeletto, A.: "*Commemorazione rossiniana*," *LCM* 1904, 12.

———— "*G. R.: I. L'Artista, II. L'Uomo*," *La Lettura*, Milan, 10–11/1925.

Fragapane, Paolo: *Spontini*, Bologna, 1954.

Francavilla, Luigi Maria Majorca Mortillaro, Conte de: *Il Real Teatro S. Cecilia e le sue vicende MDCXVII–MCMVIII*, Palermo, 1909.

"Gaianus": "*Centocinquant'anni dopo: Rossini e la sua festa bolognese*," *ROS* (*q.v.*).

Galeati, P.: see *Lettere inedite di G. Rossini e G. Donizetti*.

Gallesi, Sidney: "*Rossini e l'oboe*," *BdCRdS* 1959, 5, 92.

Gallet, Abbé: account of Rossini's last confession and extreme unction, *Le Figaro*, Paris, 2/27/1892.

Galli, Philippe (Filippo): "*L'Inno nazionale di G. R.*," *La Scala: Rivista dell'Opera* 39, Milan, 2/1953.

Gallini, Natale: *"Importante inedito rossiniano: La Musica di scena dell'* 'Edipo a Colono' di Sofocle ritrovata nella sua integrità," *La Scala: Rivista dell'Opera* 31, Milan, 1952.

Gallo, F. Alberto: *"Ironia romantica di Rossini,"* BdCRdS 1960, 5, 81.

Gandolfi, Riccardo Cristoforo Daniele Diomede: *Gioacchino Rossini*, Florence, 1887.

────── ed.: see *Of*.

Gara, Eugenio: *"(Rossini) I suoi cantanti,"* XVM.

Garibaldi, A., ed.: *Giuseppe Verdi nelle lettere di Emanuele Muzio ad Antonio Barezzi*, Milan, 1931.

Gasparoni, F. & B.: *Arti e lettere, scritti raccolti*, 2 or more vols., Rome, 1865.

Gatti, Carlo: *Il Teatro alla Scala nella storia e nell'arte (1778–1963)*, 2 vols., Milan, 1964 (with *"Cronologia completa degli spettacoli e dei concerti a cura di Giampiero Tintori"*).

Gatti, Guido M.: *Le "Barbier de Séville" de Rossini*, Paris, 1926.

────── see Bonaccorsi, Alfredo: *Gioacchino Rossini*.

Gavazzeni, Gianandrea: *"Così lo vide Stendhal,"* *La Scala: Rivista dell'-Opera* 5, Milan, 1950.

Gazzetta musicale di Milano, La: Supplemento straordinario dedicato a Gioachino Rossini, 29 febbraio, 1892, Milan, 1892.

────── Supplemento straordinaro: 'Commemorazione rossiniana," Milan, 4/8/1892.

Gherardi, Pompeo: *"Letteratura—Giovacchino Rossini,"* *Rivista urbinate*, Urbino, 1868.

Giazotto, Remo: *"Alcune Ignote Vicende riguardante la stampa e la diffusione della 'Semiramide,' "* in *(Nuova) Rivista musicale italiana*, September–October 1968, pp. 961–970.

Giorgi-Righetti, Geltrude: *Cenni di una donna già cantante sopra il maestro Rossini*, Bologna, 1823.

Giraldi, R.: *"Rossini,"* *Il Musicista*, Rome, 6/1942.

Giulini, Maria Ferranti Nob.: *Giuditta Pasta e i suoi tempi: Memorie e lettere*, Milan, 1935.

Gossett, Philip: for his important preliminary publications leading toward a definitive *catalogue raisonné* of Rossini's works, see p. 489.

Gozzano, Umberto: *Rossini: Il Romanzo dell'opera*, Turin, 1955.

Grosso, Emma: *"Rossini attraverso alcune notizie di un giornale torinese del suo tempo,"* RMI 1943, 381.

Guerrazzi, Francesco Domenico: *Manzoni, Verdi e l'albo rossiniano*, Milan, 1874.

Guerrini, P.: *"Lo 'Stabat' di Rossini,"* Turin, 1905.

Guglielmo Tell: Melodramma tragico in 4 atti tradotto dal francese da Calisto Bassi, musica di Gioacchino Rossini, da rappresentarsi in Pesaro nell'-agosto del 1864 per l'inaugurazione della statua dell'immortale maestro (with program of the celebrations), Milan, 1864.

Gui, Vittorio: *" 'Si naturale' o 'La naturale,' a proposito del Guglielmo Tell,"* MdO 5/1931.

Guidicini, Ferdinando: *Albo rossiniano: Voto musicale di Gioachino*

Rossini, commentato ed illustrato da un epistolario di celebri contemporanei . . . , Bologna, 1880.

⸻ *Parere musicale del celebre cav. maestro Gioacchino Rossini dato il 12 maggio 1851*, Bologna, 1867.

Hanslick, Eduard: *Aus dem Concert-Saal: Kritiken und Schilderungen aus 20 Jahren des Wiener Musiklebens 1848–1868*, Vienna, Leipzig, 1897; 1st edn., 1870.

⸻ *Die moderne Opera*, 2 vols., Berlin, 1892.

⸻ *Musikalisches Skizzenbuch*, Berlin, 1888.

Heine, Heinrich: *Französische Maler: über die französische Bühne*, Hamburg.

⸻ "*Rossini und Mendelssohn,*" *Werke* X, 331 (Italian tr. as "Lo 'Stabat Mater' del Rossini giudicato da Enrico Heine," *FdD* 5/8/1887).

Hiller, Ferdinand: *Plaudereien mit Rossini*, Vol. II of *Aus dem Tonleben unserer Zeit*, 2 vols., Leipzig, 1868.

Hirt, Giulio C. (pseudonym of L. Torchi): "*Di Alcuni autografi di G. Rossini,*" *RMI* 1895, 1, 23.

Hoefer, F.: *Nouvelle biographie générale*, Paris, 1863 (article on Rossini, 42, 667).

Hughes, Spike: "Introduction to Rossini's 'Cenerentola,' " *Opera*, London, 1952.

Hullah, John: *The History of Modern Music*, London, 1862.

Huyard, Étienne: "*Rossini,*" *Actes de l'Académie Nationale des Sciences. Belles-Lettres et Arts de Bordeaux*, series 4, 7, 155–76.

Iconografia musicale, ovvero Ritratti e biografie di varj del più celebrati maestri, professoi e cantanti moderni, Turin, 1838.

"*Il 'Barbiere' dopo cent'anni,*" *GdI* 3/24/1916.

Imbert de Laphalèque, G.: "*G. Tell de Rossini,*" *Revue de Paris*, Paris, 1829 (reprinted in *De la Musique en France*, Brussels, n.d.).

Ingerslev-Jessen, Povl: "An Unknown Rossini Overture: Report of a Discovery in Odense," *Music Review*, Cambridge, 2/1950, 19.

⸻ *Rossini* (Danish), Cophenhagen, 1959.

Istel, Edgar: "*Rossiniana: 1. In Rossini's Heimat,*" *Die Musik* X, Berlin, Leipzig, 1910–11, 19.

Jarro (pseudonym of Giulio Piccini): *Attori, cantanti, concertisti, acrobati: Ritratti, macchiette, aneddoti, memorie umoristiche*, 2nd edn., Florence, 1897.

⸻ *Giovacchino Rossini e la sua famiglia: Notizie aneddotiche tolte da documenti inediti*, Florence, 1902.

⸻ "*Lettere di G. R. a L. G. Ferucci,*" *La Nazione*, Florence, 8/12/1893.

⸻ *Memorie di un impresario fiorentino*, Florence, 1892.

⸻ *Storia aneddotica dei teatri fiorentini: 1. Il Teatro della Pergola (da documenti inediti)*, Florence, n.d., but 1912(?).

Jullien, Adolphe: *Airs variés: Histoire, critique, biographie musicales et dramatiques*, Paris, 1877.

K. M.: *"Wagner et Rossini,"* Le Guide musicale, Brussels XIV, 46.

Kienzl, Wilhelm: *Aus Kunst und Leben, Berlin,* 1904.

Kirby, P. R.: "The Overture to Rossini's *Guillaume Tell,"* Music and *Letters,* London, 4/1962.

Klefisch, Walter: *"Rossini als Ausdrucksmusiker,"* BdCRdS 1956, 1, 12.

────── *"Rossini im heutigen Deutschland,"* BdCRdS 1956, 3, 47.

────── *"Rossini und Schopenhauer,"* BdCRdS 1958, 4, 69.

Kolodin, Irving: *The Metropolitan Opera . . . 1883–1966,* New York, 1966.

Kuhe, Wilhelm: *My Musical Recollections,* London, 1896.

Labroca, Mario: *"Modo di rappresentare Rossini,"* Musica I, Florence, 1942, 67.

Laget, Auguste: *Le Chant et les chanteurs,* Paris, Toulouse, 1874.

Lancellotti, Arturo: *Gioacchino Rossini, 1772 [sic]–1868,* Rome, 1942.

Lapiccirella, Leonardo: *Autografi di musicisti* (catalogue), Florence, 1956.

Lauzières de Thémines, Achille de: *"L'Asilo Rossini,"* La Gazzetta musicale di Milano: Supplemento straordinario, Milan, 2/29/1892, 25.

────── *"Funerali di Rossini,"* La Gazzetta musicale di Milano: Supplemento straordinario, 2/29/1892, 23.

────── *"Memorie di un giornalista,"* Capitan Fracassa, Rome, 9/1885.

Lavignac, Albert: *La Musique et les musiciens,* Paris, n.d.

Lejeune, André, and Wolff, Stéphane: *Les Quinze Salles de l'Opéra de Paris, 1669–1955,* Paris, n.d.

"Lettera di Rossini all'avvocato Filippo Santocanale sul 'Puritani' di Bellini," Omnibus, Naples, 1835, 5.

Lettere di G. Meyerbeer, G. Rossini, ecc., Cremona, 1882.

Lettere di G. R. e Gaetano Donizzeti ad Alessandro Lanari, Florence, 1891.

Lettere di Gioacchino Rossini a Giuseppe Ancillo: see Bianchini, Giuseppe Nicolò.

Lettere inedite di Gioachino Rossini a Filippo Santocanale, avvocato palermitano, ora per la prima volta pubblicata da Francesco Caputo Montalto, Palermo, 1898.

Lettere inedite di G. Rossini e G. Donizetti, ed. P. Galeati, Imola, 1889.

"Lettere inedite di Olimpia Pélissier-Rossini," LCM 1916, 9–12.

Lianovosani, Luigi (pseudonym of Giovanni Salvioli): *La Fenice: Gran Teatro di Venezia (Serie degli spettacoli dalla primavera 1792 a tutto il Carnovale 1876),* Milan, n.d., but 1877(?).

Lippmann, Friedrich: *"Rossini,"* in Vol X of Die Musik in Geschichte und *Gegenwart,* Kassel, 1966(?).

──────*"Per un esegesi dello stile rossiniano,"* in (Nuova) Rivista musicale *italiana,* Turin, September–October 1968, pp. 813–856.

Lumbroso, Alberto: *"Stendhaliana: Da Enrico Beyle a Gioacchino . . . con una inedita lettera rossiniana,"* Rivista storica italiana 19 (reprinted as pamphlet, Pinerolo, 1902).

Lupo, B.: *"Romanze, notturni, ariette nel primo Ottocento,"* LRM 4/ 1941.

Luzio, Alessandro: *Carteggi verdiani,* 4 vols., Rome, 1947.

———— *"Il Pensiero artistico e politico di Giuseppe Verdi nelle sue lettere inedite al conte Opprandino Arrivabene,"* Lettura, Milan, 3–4/1901, 295.

Macarini-Carmignani, G.: *"La Musica per pianoforte di Rossini negli autografi pesaresi,"* LRM 1954, 3, 229.

Maffei, Andrea: *Rossini,* Florence, 1898.

Magnanini, Mariano: *Discorso letto nell'Accademia tenuto in onore di G. R. dai soci del 'Convegno dei buoni amici,'* Pesaro, 1893.

Magnico, Carlo: *Rossini e Wagner, o La Musica italiana e la musica tedesca,* Genoa, 1875; also Turin, 1877.

Malerbi, Giuseppe: *Pagine secrete,* Bologna, 1921.

Malherbe, Charles: *Auber,* Paris, n.d.

Mancini, D.: *"'L'Italiana in Algeri' di Rossini,"* Rivista nazionale di musica, Rome, 1/1936.

Manferrari, Umberto: *Dizionario universale delle opere melodrammatiche,* Florence, 1955.

Manis, F. and G.: *see* Mazzatinti, Giuseppe.

Mantovani, Tancredi: *"Il Centenario del 'Barbiere di Siviglia,'"* La Lettura, Milan, 3/1916.

———— *Gioacchino Rossini a Lugo e il cembalo del suo maestro Malerbi,* Pesaro, 1902.

———— *"G. R. direttore del Liceo di Bologna,"* LCM 1916, 5, 6 (also Musica, Rome, 5/10/1916).

———— *"Le 'Lettere' di G. R.,"* LCM 1901, 8, 9.

———— *"Il Museo rossiniano di Pesaro,"* Musica e musicisti, Milan, 3/1904.

———— *"Rossini maestro di canto,"* Musica, Rome, 2/23/1922.

Mapleson, James Henry: *The Mapleson Memoirs, 1848–1888,* 2 vols., London, New York, 1888 (an edition in 1 vol., ed. and annotated by Harold Rosenthal, London and New York, 1966).

Marchesi, S. de Castrone: *"Souvenirs de Rossini,"* Le Ménestrel, Paris, 2/10/1889.

Marinelli, Carlo: *"Discografia rossiniana,"* LRM 7–9/1954.

Martini, Ferdinando: *Confessioni e ricordi,* Florence, 1922.

———— *Di Palo in frasca,* Modena, n.d.

———— *Firenze granducale,* Florence, 1902.

———— *"Gioacchino Rossini e Ferdinando Martini,"* BdPCR 14, 7/31/ 1892.

———— *"Rimembranze giovanili,"* Of (q.v.).

Masi, Ernesto: *"Spigolature epistolari rossiniane,"* Of (q.v.).

Massi, F. P.: *"Parliamo dunque di Rossini,"* L'Ordine, Ancona, 2/24–25/1892 et seq.

Mastrigli, Leopoldo: *Gli Uomini illustri nella musica . . . ,* Turin, 1883 (article on Rossini, 265).

Mauri, Alfredo: *"Il Dialetto di Rossini,"* BdCRdS 1957, 1, 15.

Mazzatinti, Giuseppe: *Lettere inedite di Gioacchino Rossini*, Imola, 1890.

────── *Lettere inedite e rare di G. Rossini*, Imola, 1892.

────── *"Per la Storia dell'Otello rossiniano,"* BdPCR 11, 6/12/1892, 84.

────── and Manis, F. and G.: *Lettere di G. Rossini*, Florence, 1902.

Mazzini, Giuseppe: *Scritti letterari di un italiano vivente (Filosofia della musica)*, Lugano, 1847.

Mazzoni, Guido: "*G. Rossini classico e romantico*," Of.

Melica, Ada: "*L'Aria in rondò de 'La Donna del lago,'*" BdCRdS 1958, 6, 101.

────── "*L'Armonia,*" BdCRdS 1957, 6, 102.

────── "*Auto-citazioni o rielaborazioni?*" BdCRdS 1956, 5, 88.

────── "*La Casa di Rossini, oggi,*" BdCRdS 1955, 1, 4.

────── "*Catalogo ragionato della Raccolta Rossini del Conservatorio di Pesaro,*" BdCRdS 1960, 2, 31; 1960, 3, 53; 1960, 5, 90.

────── "*Ciò che si può vedere di Rossini nel Conservatorio pesarese,*" BdCRdS 1955, 2, 25.

────── "*Il Concertato,*" BdCRdS 1958, 1, 4.

────── "*Il Conservatorio 'G. Rossini,'*" BdCRdS 1957, 1, 6.

────── "*Contemporanei di Rossini,*" BdCRdS 1956, 1, 4.

────── "*Il Contrappunto: 1. Musica teatrale, 2. Musica religiosa,*" BdCRdS 1957, 2, 25; 1958, 3, 44.

────── "*Il Crescendo,*" BdCRdS 1957, 5, 84.

────── "*Le Critiche,*" BdCRdS 1959, 4, 63; 1959, 5, 86; 1959, 6, 108; 1959, 1, 10; 1960, 2, 29; 1960, 4, 74.

────── "*Del Recitativo sinfonico,*" BdCRdS 1956, 2, 21.

────── "*Di Padre in figlio: il corno,*" BdCRdS 1957, 3, 42.

────── "*'La Donna del lago' nella revisione di Frazzi,*" BdCRdS 1959, 3, 43.

────── "*Forma delle sinfonie,*" BdCRdS 1956, 6, 102.

────── "*Forme e spirito dell'aria,*" BdCRdS 1957, 4, 61.

────── "*'La Gazza ladra' nella revisione di Zandonai,*" BdCRdS 1956, 3, 48.

────── "*I Libretti,*" BdCRdS 1958, 2, 24.

────── "*Pezzi dedicati a Rossini,*" BdCRdS 1960, 4, 73.

────── "*Quadreria rossiniana,*" BdCRdS 1956, 4, 70.

────── "*'Ricordo Bòdoira,'*" BdCRdS 1959, 1, 8.

────── "*Ritmo, periodo e metro,*" BdCRdS 1958, 5, 84.

────── "*Rossini nella musica degli altri,*" BdCRdS 1956, 3, 56; 1956, 4, 76; 1956, 5, 98; 1956, 6, 118; 1956, 1, 15; 1956, 2, 17; 1957, 3, 57; 1957, 4, 77; 1957, 5, 96; 1957, 6, 117; 1957, 1, 17; 1957, 2, 38; 1958, 3, 58; 1958, 4, 77; 1958, 5, 97; 1958, 6, 119; 1958, 1, 17.

────── "*La Strumentazione,*" BdCRdS 1958, 4, 66.

Mereaux, A.: "*Anecdotes sur la bonté de Rossini en ses relations avec Meyerbeer,*" *Le Moniteur universel*, Paris, 11/22/1868.

────── *Variétés littéraires et musicales*, Paris, 1878 (includes "*Rossini l'homme et l'artiste*").

Merle, Jean-Toussaint: *Lettre à un compositeur français*, Paris, 1827.

Méry, M.: *see* Escudier, Les Frères.

Michelant, L.: *Notice sur Rossini*, 2nd edn., Paris, 1842.

Michotte, Edmond: *"Rossini e sua madre: Ricordi della sua infanzia,"* in *LCM 1913*, 5.

———— *Souvenirs: Une Soirée chez Rossini à Beau-Sejour (Passy) 1858; Exposé par le maestro des principes du "bel canto,"* Brussels, n.d. but after 1893 (Italian translation, as *"Autobiografia rossiniana,"* *FdM* 5/29 and 7/24/1887). English tr., by Herbert Weinstock, Chicago, 1968.

———— *Souvenirs: La Visite de R. Wagner à Rossini (Paris 1860): Détails inédits et commentaires*, Paris, 1906. English tr., by Herbert Weinstock, Chicago, 1968.

Mila, Massimo: *"Le Idee di Rossini,"* in *Rassegna musicale Curci*, 1968, No. 5.

———— *"Rossini, tutto musica,"* *NA* 9/16/1934 (also in *Cent'Anni di musica moderna*, Milan, 1944).

———— *" 'Selva opaca,' "* in *La Scala: Rivista dell'Opera* 1, Milan, 1949.

———— *" 'Il Turco in Italia,' manifesto di dolce vita,"* in *(Nuova) Rivista musicale italiana*, Turin, September–October 1968, pp. 857–871.

Monaldi, Gino: *Cantanti celebri del secolo XIX*, Rome, n.d.

———— *Impresari celebri del secolo XIX*, Rocca San Casciano, 1918.

———— *I Teatri di Roma negli ultimi tre secoli*, Naples, 1929.

Monaldi, Guido: *Gli Uomini illustri: Gioacchino Rossini nell'arte, nella vita, negli aneddoti*, Milan, n.d.

Montanelli, Archimede: *Gioachino Rossini e il melodramma in Italia*, Carrara, 1892.

Montazio, Enrico: *Giovacchino Rossini (I Contemporanei italiani: Galleria nazionale del secolo XIX, 39)*, Turin, 1862.

Montefiore, T.: article including letter from Rossini to Pietro Groggia, *Gdl* 2/20/1916.

———— *"Paisiello, Rossini, il 'Barbiere,' "* *Gdl* 2/16/1916.

Montegut, E.: *"Du Génie de Rossini,"* *Le Moniteur universel*, Paris, 12/1/1862.

Montrond, Clément Fourcheux de: *Rossini: Étude biographique*, Lille, 1870.

Monvel, Georges: *see* Porel, Paul.

Morand, Félix: *L'Année anecdotique: Petits Mémoires du temps*, Paris, 1860 (p. 143 and Ch. xxiii).

Mordani, Filippo: *Della Vita privata di Giovacchino Rossini: Memorie inedite*, Imola, 1871.

Morgan, Sydney (Lady Morgan): *Italy* ("A New Edition in Three Volumes"), London, 1821.

Morini, Nestore: *La Casa di Rossini in Bologna*, Bologna, 1916.

———— *Mobili ed arredi di Rossini*, Bologna, 1919.

———— *"Rossini al teatro del Corso,"* *Il Pensiero musicale* 5, 1925.

Morini, U.: *La Reale Accademia degli Immobili ed il suo Teatro "La Pergola" (1649–1925)*, Pisa, 1926.

(Moscheles, Ignaz): *Life of Moscheles, with Selections from His Diaries and Correspondence, by His Wife*, adapted from the German by A. D. Coleridge, 2 vols., London, 1873 (*Aus Moscheles Leben*, Leipzig, 1872).

Moutoz, A.: *Littérature musicale: Rossini et son Guillaume Tell*, Paris, etc., 1872.

Mozzoni, Eugenio: "*Gioachino Rossini: Lettere inedite*," LRM 7–8/1902.

Mussumerci, Conte Liborio: *Parallelo fra i due maestri Rossini e Bellini*, Palermo, 1832.

Nardi, Piero: *Vita di Arrigo Boito*, Milan, 1942.

Nascimbeni, Giovanni: "*L'Altro Rossini*," *Marzocco*, Florence, 2/25/1919.

——— "*Le Case e le donne di Rossini a Bologna*," *Emporium*, Bergamo, 2/1920.

Nauman, Emil: *Italienische Tondichter, von Palestrina bis auf die Gegenwart*, 1876.

Nel XVIII Bisestile Anniversario di Gioacchino Rossini, sole della musica nel secolo XIX . . . 29 febbraio 1864, Florence, 1864.

Nelle Nozze Odetti Santini-Giustiniani (includes letter of Rossini to the Marchesa Maria Martellini, 12/26/1850), n.d.

Neretti, L.: *I Due Inni patriottici di G. R.*, Florence, 1918.

Neri, A.: "*Aneddoti rossiniani*," FdD 11/23/1902.

Neumann, Wilhelm: *Die Komponisten der neuen Zeit*, Cassel, 1855–8.

Newman, Ernest (pseudonym of William Roberts): *The Life of Richard Wagner*, 4 vols., London and New York, 1933–46.

Nordio, Cesare: "*Preludio*," ROS.

Notarnicola, Biagio: *Saverio Mercadante nel III cinquantennio dalla nascita: Biografia critica*, Rome, 1945.

(Novello, Clara): *Clara Novello's Reminiscences Compiled by Her Daughter Contessa Valeria Gigliucci, with a Memoir by Arthur D. Coleridge*, London, 1910.

Nozze Donzelli-Ferroni (Rossini letters), 2/1886.

Occelli, Celso: "*Discoteca*," BdCRdS 1957, 3, 54; 1957, 4, 74; 1957, 5, 93; 1957, 6, 112; 1957, 2, 31; 1958, 4, 69; 1959, 6, 115.

——— "*Fondo Biaggi*," BdCRdS 1957, 6, 106; 1957, 1, 8; 1957, 2, 31; 1958, 4, 69.

——— "*Libretti a Pesaro*," BdCRdS 1959, 4, 72.

——— "*Musica all'aria aperta*," BdCRdS 1960, 5, 93.

Oettinger, Eduard Maria: *Rossini, komischer Roman*, Leipzig, 1845 (many trs.; in French, as *Rossini: L'Homme et l'artiste*, Brussels, etc., 1858; Italian tr., Venice, 1867).

Omaggio a Gioacchino Rossini celebrato dagli artisti di musica di Palermo . . . 28 aprile 1869, Palermo, 1869.

Onoranze fiorentine a Gioachino Rossini inaugurandosi in Santa Croce il monumento al grande maestro (XXIII giugno MCMII): Memorie pubblicate da Riccardo Gandolfi, Florence, 1902.

L'Opera italiana in musica (*Festschrift* for Eugenio Gara), Milan, 1965.

L'Opera italiana nel secolo XIX, Milan, 1900.

Ortigue, Joseph-Louis d': *see* D'Ortigue, Joseph-Louis.

Pacini, Giovanni: *Agli Onorevoli componenti la Giunta artistica della Società rossiniana pesarese*, Pescia, n.d.

—— *Le Mie Memorie artistiche (edite ed inedite): Autobiografia del maestro cav. Giovanni Pacini riscontrata sugli autografi e pubblicata da Ferdinando Magnani*, Florence, 1865 (another version, prepared by Filippo Cicconnetti, Rome, 1872).

Paglia, Gioachino: *Sulla Musica rossiniana: Pensieri*, Bologna, 1875.

Pagliara, Rocco E.: "*Rossini e i maccheroni*," *Capitan Fracassa*, Rome, 9/2/1883 (also included in *Intermezzi musicali*, Naples, 1896).

—— "*Rossiniana*," *FdD* 5/15/1887 (also included in *Intermezzi musicali*, Naples, 1896); English tr., *The Athenaeum*, London, 2/27/1892, 4/2/1892.

Pancaldi, Carlo: *Dello Stabat Mater del celebre cavaliere Gioachino Rossini: Lettere storico-critiche d'un lombardo*, Bologna, 1842.

—— *Vita di Lorenzo Gibelli celebre contrappuntista e cantore*, Bologna 1830.

Pannain, Guido: "*Gioacchino Rossini*," *Il Mattino*, Naples, 9/7/1934.

—— "*L'Opera italiana dell'Ottocento*," *Il Pianoforte* 5-6, Turin, 1927.

—— "*Personalità di Rossini*," *Musica* I, Florence, 1942 (also included in *Ottocento musicale italiano: Saggi e note*, Milan, 1952).

—— "*Rossini nel' 'Guglielmo Tell,'* " *RMI* 1924, 4.

—— with Andrea Della Corte: *Vincenzo Bellini*; *see* Della Corte, Andrea.

Panzacchi, Enrico: *Nel Centenario di Rossini . . .* , Bologna, 1892 (reprinted, *BdPCR* 3/25/1892, 25; 4/6/1892, 33; 4/15/1892, 41).

—— *Nel Mondo della musica*, Turin, etc., n.d.

Paoli, Rodolfo: "*Le 'Melodie francesi,'* " *BdCRdS* 1958, 3, 47.

Parigi, Luigi: "*Rossini e le arti figurative*," *LRM* 7-9/1954.

Parisotti, Alessandro: "*I Collaboratori di Rossini*," *FdD* 3/13/1892.

Pasolini-Zanelli, G.: *Il Teatro di Faenza dal 1788 al 1888*, Faenza, 1888.

Pastura, Francesco: *Bellini secondo la storia*, Parma, 1959.

—— *Le Lettere di Bellini*, Catania, 1935.

Pavan: "*Catalogo cronologico degli spettacoli del T. San Benedetto*," *Ateneo veneto*, Venice, 1916 (and as book, Venice, 1916).

Per le Nozze dell Dott. Lino Sighinolfi con la gentile signorina Prof.a Ginevra Baruzzi (letters), Bologna, 1909.

Per l'Inaugurazione del busto di Gioachino Rossini scolpito in marmo da Cincinnato Baruzzi per L'I. R. Stabilimento musicale di Giovanni Ricordi (includes Felice Romani's "*Inno a Gioachino Rossini*" set to music by Placido Mandanici), Milan, 1846.

Perotti, G. A.: "*Lo Stabat di Rossini*," *LGMM* 3/15/1842, 3/20/1842.

Pesci, Ugo: "*Nel Primo Centenario del Liceo Musicale Rossini in Bologna*," *Musica e musicisti*, Milan, 12/1904.

Pestalozza, Luigi, ed.: *La Rassegna musicale: Antologia*, Milan, 1966.

Petrocchi, Giorgio: *"Avvenimenti dell'uomo Rossini,"* ROS.

Pettinelli, Diego: *"Guardando un disegno,"* BdCRdS 1957, 5, 87.

Peyser, Herbert F.: "The 'Cenerentola' of Rossini," *Musical America*, New York, 6/1929.

Pfister, Kurt: *Das Leben Rossinis: Gesetz und Triumph der Oper*, Vienna, Berlin, 1948.

Pizzetti, Ildebrando: *"Colloquio con Rossini,"* Musica, Rome, 4/30/1947.

———*"L'Immortalità del Barbiere di Siviglia,"* Marzocco, Florence (included in *Intermezzi critici*, Florence, 1921).

——— *La Musica italiana dell'Ottocento*, Turin, 1947.

Pizzoli, Gaetano: *Cenni filosofici sopra il cavaliere Gioacchino Rossini, dedicati . . . a madama Olimpia Pelisiè [sic] Rossini*, Bologna, 1847.

Planté, Francis: *"Souvenirs de Rossini,"* Le Courrier musicale, Paris, 5/1/1928.

Ploner, Luigi: *Le Statue di Perticari e di Rossini a Pesaro . . .*, Bologna, n.d., but 1854 (?).

Podestà, B.: *"Alcune Lettere di Giuseppe Rossini scritte da Bologna al figliuolo GIOACHINO a Parigi dal 1827 al 1834*, Of.

Poesie musicale ed anonime del secolo XIV, Padua, 1870.

Porel, Paul, and Monvel, Georges: *L'Odéon: Histoire administrative, anecdotique et littéraire du second Théâtre français*, 2 vols., Paris, 1876, 1882.

Porresini, G.: *Lo "Stabat" di Rossini a Faenza*, Faenza, 1933.

Porter, Andrew: "A Lost Opera by Rossini," *Music and Letters*, London, 1/1964; reprinted in *Opera 66*, ed. Charles Osborne, London, n.d. (but 1966).

Pougin, Arthur: *"Les Deux Mariages de Rossini,"* Le Ménestrel, Paris, 1892, 387–8, 395–6, 404–5.

——— *Hérold: Biographie critique*, Paris, n.d.

——— *Marie Malibran*, Paris, 1911.

——— *Marietta Alboni*, 3rd edn., Paris, 1912.

——— *Musiciens du XIX siècle*, Paris, 1911.

——— *Rossini: Notes, impressions, souvenirs, commentaires*, Paris, 1871.

——— *Supplément et complément* (to Fétis: *Biographie universelle*); see Fétis, François-Joseph.

Pratella, Francesco Balilla: *"Rossini a Lugo,"* Vedetta, 7/31/1902.

Prato, Cesare da: *see* Da Prato, Cesare.

Programma dell'Accademia di musica per l'inaugurazione del busto di G. Rossini . . ., Milan, 1846.

Prose e rime in onore di Gioacchino Rossini . . . 29 febbraio 1864 . . ., Pesaro, 1864.

Prunières, Henri: *"Stendhal et l'opéra buffa de Rossini,"* L'Opéra-comique, Paris, 4/1929.

Pugliese, Giuseppe: *"Scoprire Rossini?"* XVM, Florence, 1952.

——— *"Stendhal et Rossini,"* La Revue critique des idées et des livres, Paris, 1920, 29, 35–47, 162–75 (English tr., *The Musical Quarterly*, New York, 1921, 7, 133–55).

Quaderni Rossiniani, 11 volumes of music by Rossini, with introductions by Alfredo Bonaccorsi, Pesaro, 1954–65 (index to Vols. I-VI, *BdCRdS* 1958, 1, 16; contents of later volumes as follows: VIII: *Sinfonia [di Bologna]*, *Sinfonia [di Odense]*, *Le Chant des Titans*; IX: *Variazioni a più strumenti obbligati*, *Grande Fanfare par Rossini*, *Scena da "Il Viaggio a Reims"*; X. *Second Scelta di pezzi per pianoforte (Prélude prétentieux, Un Rêve, Mon prélude hygiénique du matin, Spécimen de mon temps, La Pésarèse, Un Enterrement en carnaval, Memento Homo, Assez de memento: dansons, Spécimen de l'avenir)*; XI: *Giovanna d'Arco per una voce e pianoforte: idem, recitativi con archi, Ave Maria, Cantemus, "À Ma Belle Mère," Un Rien: Ave Maria*; XII: *Inno alla pace, Inno a Napoleone III*; XIII: *"Argene e Melania"*; XIV: *Composizioni per pianoforte*. Not all of the scores issued are musicologically reliable.

Radiciotti, Giuseppe: *"Aggiunte e correzioni ai dizionari biografici di musicisti,"* La Critica musicale, 1922, 138.

——— *Aneddoti rossiniani autentici*, Rome, 1929.

——— *"Il Barbaia nella leggenda e nella storia,"* L'Arte pianistica, Naples, 1920, 3.

——— *Il Barbiere di Siviglia: Guida attraverso la commedia e la musica*, Milan, 1923.

——— *"Due Lettere inedite di G. Rossini e la sua definitiva partenza da Bologna,"* RMI 1925, 2.

——— *"La Famosa Lettera a Cicognara non fu scritta dal Rossini,"* RMI 1923, 3.

——— *Gioacchino Rossini (Profili 37)*, Genoa, 1914.

——— *"Gioacchino Rossini e il 'leitmotiv,' "* MdO 3/1925.

——— *"Gioacchino Rossini et son école,"* Encyclopédie de la musique et Dictionnaire du Conservatoire, Paris, 1931.

——— *Gioacchino Rossini: Vita documentata, opere ed influenza su l'arte*, 3 vols., Tivoli, 1927–9.

——— *G. B. Pergolesi: Vita, opere ed influenza su l'arte*, Rome, 1910.

——— *" 'L'Italiana in Algeri' di Gioacchino Rossini,"* Il Pianoforte, Turin, 11/1925.

——— *Lettere inedite di celebri musicisti annotate e precedute dalle biografie di Pietro, Giovanni e Rosa Morandi a cui sono dirette*, Milan, 1890.

——— *"I Primi Anni e studi di Gioacchino Rossini,"* RMI, Turin, 1917, 24, Nos. 2, 3, 4.

——— *"Rossini à Londres,"* La Revue musicale, Paris, 2/1/1924 (English tr., The Sackbut, London, 4/1924).

——— "Rossini Misunderstood" (Hungarian), Crescendo, Budapest, 10/1927.

——— *"Rossini pianista è compositore per piano,"* Il Pianista, Turin, 8/1908.

——— *" 'Il Signor Bruschino' ed il 'Tancredi,' "* RMI 1920, 2.

——— *"Stendhal e Rossini,"* Il Pianoforte, Turin, 12/1923.

——— *Teatro e musica in Roma nel secondo quarto del secolo XIX*, Rome, 1905.

———— *"Un Opéra fantastique [Armida] de Rossini,"* La Revue musicale, Paris, 1921, 3.

Radius, Emilio: *"Rossini nella vita d'oggi,"* XVM.

Raffaelli, P.: *Il Melodramma in Italia,* Florence, 1881.

Raggi, Alessandro and Luigi: *Il Teatro Communale di Cesena: Memorie cronologiche (1500–1905),* Cesena, 1906.

La Rassegna musicale (special issue containing articles on Rossini and his works), Rome, etc., 7–9/1954.

R. Accademia dei Rozzi di Siena: A. G. Rossini nel 1 centenario della sua nascita, Siena, 1892.

Reggiani, Vincenzo: *Lettere al marchese Torquato Antaldi e a Giuseppe Vaccai,* Pesaro, 1886.

———— *Tre Lettere di G. Rossini . . . ,* Pesaro, 1886.

Regli, Francesco: *Dizionario biografico dei più celebri poeti ed artisti melodrammatici, tragici e comici, maestri, concertisti, coreografi, mimi, ballerini, scenografi, giornalisti, impresari, ecc., ecc., che fiorirono in Italia dal 1800 al 1860,* Turin, 1860.

———— *Elogio di Gioachino Rossini . . . 21 agosto 1864 . . . ,* Turin, 1864.

Résumé des opinions de la presse sur le "Stabat" de Rossini exécuté pour la première fois en public, au Théâtre-Italien le 7 janvier 1842, Paris, 1842.

Riboli, Bruno: *"Malattia di Gioacchino Rossini secondo una relazione medica del 1842,"* Note e riviste di psichiatria, 7/1955, 12/1955 (republished as pamphlet, Pesaro, 1956).

———— *"Profilo medico psicologico di G. Rossini,"* LRM 7–9/1954, 291.

Ricci, Corrado: *Figure e figuri del mondo teatrale,* Milan, 1920.

———— *"Pel Centenario di Gioachino Rossini,"* L'Illustrazione italiana, 1892, 131.

———— *Rossini: Le Sue Case e le sue donne,* Milan, 1889 (also included in *Figure e figuri del mondo teatrale*).

Ricordi, Giovanni, ed.: *I Nostri Maestri del passato,* Milan, n.d.

Ricordi, Giulio: *"Conosco Gioachino Rossini,"* La Gazzetta musicale di Milano: Supplemento straordinario, 2/20/1892, 18.

Righetti-Giorgi, Geltrude: see Giorgi-Righetti, Geltrude.

Rinaldi, Mario: *Felice Romani: Dal Melodramma classico al melodramma romantico,* Rome, 1965.

Rognoni, Luigi: *Rossini, con un'appendice comprendente lettere, documenti, testimonianze,* Parma, 1956.

———— *Gioacchino Rossini,* Turin, 1968. Important for analyses of Rossini's musical methods and for its *"Appendice II,"* which includes an extensive bibliography edited by Maria Ajani, a catalogue of Rossini's music by Philip Gossett, and a discography by Edward D. R. Neill.

Rolandi, Ulderico: *"Alcune Deformazioni del 'Barbiere di Siviglia,'"* Le Maschere, Rome, 9/1920.

———— *"Librettistica rossiniana,"* Musica I, Florence, 1942.

———— *Il Libretto per musica attraverso i tempi,* Rome, 1951.

Rolland, Romain: *"Rossini,"* La Revue musicale, Paris, 9/1902, 374.

Romagnoli, G.: *"Gioacchino Rossini, Giulio Perticari e la 'Gazza ladra,' "* *La Vita italiana,* 7/1/1897, 106.

Romani, Luigi: *Teatro alla Scala: Cronologia di tutti gli spettacoli, ecc.,* Milan, n.d.

Roncaglia, Gino: *"I Centoventicinque Anni del 'Barbiere di Siviglia,' "* *Rivista nazionale di musica,* Rome, 1941, 393.

——— *" 'La Pietra del paragone,' "* *XVM.*

——— *Rossini l'olimpico,* Milan, 1946 (2nd edn., 1953).

Ronga, Luigi: *"Vicende del gusto rossiniano nell'Ottocento,"* *Musica* I, Florence, 1942; *"Svolgimento del gusto rossiniano fino al Novecento,"* *Musica* II, Florence, 1943. As *"Breve Storia del gusto rossiniano,"* in *Arte e gusto nella musica,* Milan-Naples, 1956.

Roqueplan, Nestor: *"Rossini"* (obituary), *Le Constitutionnel,* Paris, 1869.

Rosadi, Giovanni: *"Per il Centenario del 'Barbiere di Siviglia,' "* *Conferenze e prolusioni,* Rome, 1916.

——— *"Rossini a Firenze nella casa che fu sua,"* *Il Marzocco,* Florence, 2/13/1916.

Rosenthal, Harold: *Two Centuries of Opera at Covent Garden,* London, 1958.

Rossi-Scotti, G. B.: *Del M.o Morlacchi: Ricordo storico con due lettere inedite de C. M. Weber al Morlacchi e una di Gioacchino Rossini all'autore,* Perugia, 1872.

Rossini e la musica, ossia Amena Biografia musicale, Milan, 1827.

Rossini e la sua musica (attributed by Niccolò Bettoni to Fétis; said to have been translated into French as *Rossini et la musique,* 1836; its existence denied by *ZAN,* but that of the French version affirmed by Pougin), Milan, 1824(?).

"Rossini, ses ouvrages et son influence sur la musique actuelle," *Revue nationale de Belgique,* Brussels, 1841, 5.

Rossiniana (*"a cura del R. Conservatorio 'G. B. Martini' di Bologna"*), Bologna, 1942.

Rovani, Giuseppe: *La Mente di Gioachino Rossini,* Florence, 1871.

——— *Le Tre Arti considerate in alcuni illustri italiani contemporanei,* Milan, 1874.

Royer, Alphonse: *Histoire de l'Opéra,* Paris, 1875.

——— *Histoire universelle du théâtre—Histoire du théâtre contemporain en France et à l'étranger,* Paris, 1878.

Rudakova, E.: *"A Cantata Discovered in Russia"* (Russian), *Sovietskaya Muzika,* Moscow, 1955, supplement to no. 8 (Italian tr., *BdCRdS,* 1956, 3, 49).

Ruggeri, Augusto: *Alla Memoria di Gioacchino Rossini,* Fano, 1869.

Sainsbury, John H., compiler: *A Dictionary of Musicians,* London, 1824.

Saint-Saëns, Charles-Camille: *École buissonière,* Paris, 1913.

San Jacinto, Stefano Mira e Sirignano, Marchese di: *Osservazioni sul merito musicale dei maestri Rossini e Bellini . . . ,* Palermo, 1834; Bologna, 1836 (French tr. by Ferrer, *q.v.,* as *Rossini et Bellini,* Paris, 1836; translated back into Italian as *Rossini e Bellini*).

Sandelewski, Wiaroslaw: *"Influssi rossiniani nell'opera di Chopin,"* *BdCRdS* 1959, 3, 45; 1959, 4, 69.

Sartori, Claudio: *"Dagli Archivi del Liceo musicale: 1. Il Consulente perpetuo in funzione; 2. I Concerti del consulente,"* *ROS* (*q.v.*).

—— *"Il Riso dell'uomo buono,"* *XVM*.

—— *"Rossini 1808,"* *ROS* (*q.v.*).

—— *"Soirées musicales,"* *ROS* (*q.v.*).

—— *"Una Lettera inedita di Rossini,"* *RMI* XLVI, 4 (reprinted as pamphlet, Milan, 1942).

Scala Theatre Museum, The: Illustrated Guide, Milan, 1966.

Schaeffner, A. R.: *"L'Italiana in Algeri,'"* *LRM* 1929, 7.

Schlitzer, Franco: *"Accenni a Rossini nelle lettere degli altri,"* *BdCRdS* 1956, 1, 13; 1956, 2, 31; 1957, 4, 67; 1957, 5, 88; 1957, 6, 107.

—— *"Ancora del Teatro 'Rossini' di Firenze,"* *BdCRdS* 1956, 6, 113.

—— *Gli Auguri di Rossini con zamponi, cotechini e panettoni*, Florence, 1959.

—— *"Contributi all'epistolario rossiniano"* (for which *see also* Titus), *BdCRdS* 1956, 3, 43; 1956, 4, 63; 1956, 5, 83; 1956, 6, 109.

—— *"Il Fondo francese dell'Archivio rossiniano di Pesaro: Confidenze di Olimpia Pélissier,"* *LRM* 7–9/1954.

—— *Mobili e immobili di Rossini a Firenze: Lettere inedite a un avvocato* (Leopoldo Pini), Florence, 1957.

—— *Mondo teatrale dell'Ottocento: Episodi, testimonianze, musiche e lettere inedite*, Naples, 1954.

—— *Un Piccolo Carteggio inedito di Rossini con un impresario italiano a Vienna*, Florence, 1959.

—— *Rossini a Siena e altri scritti rossiniani (con lettere inedite)*, Quaderni dell'Accademia chigiana XXXIX, Siena, 1958.

—— *Rossiniana: Contributo all'epistolario di G. Rossini*, Quaderni dell'Accademia chigiana XXXV, Siena, 1956.

—— *"Il Teatro 'Rossini' di Firenze,"* *BdCRdS* 1956, 5, 94.

—— *"Una Lettere di G. B. Rubini per la dedica del 'Robert Bruce,'"* *BdCRdS* 1956, 5, 93.

—— *"Una Lettera inedita di Verdi per la progettata Messa in memoria di Rossini,"* *BdCRdS* 1956, 4, 72.

Schloesser, Louis: "Retrospects of Rossini and the Italian Opera Season in Vienna During the Year 1822," *Monthly Musical Record*, London, 1910, 40, nos. 476, 477.

Scipioni, G. S.: *"Giovacchino Rossini,"* Biblioteca della provincia di Pesaro e Urbino 1, Pesaro, 1884.

Scudo, Pierre (Pietro): *L'Art ancien et l'art moderne: Nouveaux Mélanges de critique et de littérature musicales*, Paris, 1854.

—— *Critique et littérature musicale* I, Paris, 1850; II, Paris, 1859.

Servières, G.: *"La Première Représentation de 'Guillaume Tell' à Paris en 1829,"* *RMI* 1929, 2.

Silvestri, Lodovico Settimo: *Della Vita e delle opere di Gioachino Rossini: Notizie biografico-artistco-aneddotico-critiche compilate su tutte le biografie di questo celebre italiano e sui giudizi della stampa italiana e straniera intorno alle sue opere*, Milan, 1874.

Simoni, Renato: see *Catalogo del Museo Teatrale alla Scala*.

Sittard, Josef: *Gioachimo Antonio Rossini*, Leipzig, 1882.

Smith, William C.: *The Italian Opera and Contemporary Ballet in London 1789–1820: A Record of Performances and Players with Reports from the Journals of the Time*, London, 1953.

Solustri, Ubaldo M.: *Alcune Lettere inedite di Rossini e Pacini*, Monte Cassino, 1870.

Soubies, Albert: *Le Théâtre-Italien de 1801 à 1913*, Paris, 1913.

Spada, Luigi: "*Rossini e la cantata per Pio IX*," *Giornale d'Italia*, Rome, 3/21/1916.

Spadoni, Domenico: *Bologna e Pellegrino Rossi per l'independenza d'Italia nel 1815*, Città di Castello, 1916.

Lo Stabat del celeberrimo cavaliere Gioacchino Rossini eseguito in Pesaro sua patria le sere 16 e 17 febbraio 1843, Pesaro, 1843.

Lo "Stabat" del celeberrimo Gioacchino Rossini eseguito in Pesaro sua patria le sere 22 e 23 agosto 1869, Pesaro, 1869.

"*Lo 'Stabat' fatto eseguire dalla principessa Donna Maria Hercolani nel suo palazzo nel marzo 1853 sotto la direzione del prof. Domenico Liverani*," *Teatri, arti e letteratura*, Bologna, 3/31/1853.

Stacchiotti, E.: *Commemorazioni di Giuseppe Verdi e Gioacchino Rossini* (preface by Giuseppe Baldassarri), Milan, 1942.

Stendhal (Henri Beyle): *Rome, Naples et Florence en 1817* (1817), *suivi de L'Italie en 1818*, edited and annotated by Henri Martineau, Paris, 1956 (English tr. of *Rome, Naples et Florence en 1817*, as *Rome, Naples and Florence*, tr. and annotated by Richard N. Coe, London and New York, 1959).

―――― *Vie de Rossini* (1824), ed. and annotated by Henri Martineau, 2 vols., Paris, 1929 (English tr., as *Life of Rossini*, tr. and annotated by Richard N. Coe, London and New York, 1957).

Struth, A.: *Rossini, sein Leben, sein Werke und Charakterzüge*, Leipzig, n.d.

Sull'Istituto da erigersi in Pesaro, Pesaro, 1880.

Taccone Gallucci, Barone Niccola: *Gioacchino Rossini e la musica italiana nel secolo XIX*, Naples, 1869.

Tebaldini, G.: "*Da Rossini a Verdi*," *Aversa a Domenico Cimarosa*, Naples, 1901.

―――― "*Rossini*," *RMI* 1929, 1.

Testoni, Alfredo: *Gioachini Rossini: Quattro Episodi della sua vita . . .* (dramatizations), Bologna, 1909.

Tiersot, Julien: "*Une Lettre inédite de Rossini et l'interruption de sa carrière*," *Le Ménestrel*, Paris, 1908, 25.

Tintori, Giampiero: see Gatti, Carlo.

"Titus": "*Condoglianze*," BdCRdS 1959, 6, 110.

——— "*Conti di cassa*," BdCRdS 1959, 3, 49.

——— "*Contributi all'epistolario rossiniano*" (for which *see also* Schlitzer, Franco): BdCRdS 1957, 1, 10; 1958, 3, 49; 1958, 4, 70; 1958, 5, 89; 1958, 6, 111; 1958, 1, 12; 1958, 2, 33.

——— "*Malumore di Rossini*," BdCRdS 1959, 5, 94.

Tommaseo, N.: "*Gioacchino Rossini*," *Rivista urbinate di scienze, lettere ed arti*, Urbino, 1868.

Toni, Alceo: "*Nuovo Contributo allo studio della psiche rossiniana*," *RMI* 1909, 2.

——— with Serafin, Tullio: *Stile, tradizioni e convenzioni del melodramma italiano del Settecento e dell'Ottocento*, Milan, 1958.

Torrefranca, Fausto: "*Il Momento dell' 'Armida,' *" *XVM*.

——— "*Parere musicale del 1851*," BdCRdS 1956, 3, 41.

Toye, Francis: *Rossini: A Study in Tragi-Comedy*, London and New York, 1934 (paperbound edn., with new preface, New York, 1963).

Traslazione delle cenere [di] Gioacchino Rossini da Parigi a Firenze (XXX aprile–III maggio MDCCCLXXXVII), Pesaro, 1887.

Trebbi, Oreste: *Le Grandi Esecuzioni musicali a Bologna: Lo "Stabat" di Rossini*, Bologna, 1918.

——— *Il Teatro Contavalli (1814–1914)*, Bologna, 1914.

Valeri, Antonio (pseudonym: Carletta): "*La Prima della Cenerentola*," *La Tribuna*, Rome, 10/7/1894.

(Van Damme, Jean): *Vie de G. Rossini . . .*, Antwerp, 1830.

Vander Straeten, Edmond: *La Mélodie populaire dans l'opéra Guillaume Tell de Rossini*, Paris, 1879.

Vanzolini, Giuliano: *Della Vera Patria di Gioacchino Rossini*, Pesaro, 1873.

——— *Delle Feste fatte in Pesaro il 21 agosto 1864 in onore di G. Rossini*, Pesaro, 1864.

——— *Relazione delle pompe funebri fatte in Pesaro in onore di G. Rossini . . . 21 di agosto 1869 . . .*, Pesaro, 1869.

Vatielli, Francesco: *La Biblioteca del Liceo musicale di Bologna*, Bologna, 1916–17.

——— "*Bologna e Rossini*," ROS (*q.v.*).

——— "*Il Liceo musicale e l'Accademia filarmonica*," *Vita cittadina*, Bologna, 1918.

——— *Rossini a Bologna*, Bologna, 1918.

Vauthier: "*Le Jury de lecture de l'Opéra . . . d'après les papiers de la Maison du roi*," *La Revue musicale*, Paris, 1910, 1–3.

Verdinois, F.: *see* Cottrau, Guglielmo.

"*Il Vero Libretto del 'Barbiere,' *" GdI 3/22/1916.

Vianello, Carlo Antonio: *Teatri, spettacoli, muische a Milano nei secoli scorsi*, Milan, 1941.

Viannini-Simoni, Carla: "*Rossini e Pacini*," BdCRdS 1956, 6, 106.

La Vie amoureuse et anecdotique de G. Rossini (documents inédits), Paris, n.d.

Vittadini, Stefano: see *Catalogo del Museo Teatrale alla Scala*.

Viviani, Vittorio, ed.: *I Libretti di Rossini*, Milan, 1965.

Vlad, Roman: "*Rossini e i compositori moderni*," LRM 1954, 3, 251.

Wagner, Richard: "*Eine Errinerung an Rossini*," *Allgemeine Zeitung*, Augsburg, 12/17/1868; reprinted in *Gesammelte Schrifte* VIII.

────── *Gesammelte schrifte*, ed. Julius Kapp, Leipzig, 1914.

────── *Mein Leben*, 2 vols. (written 1865–70; parts 1–3 printed at Basel, 1870–5, part 4 at Bayreuth, 1881), Munich, 1911.

────── "*Rossini's 'Stabat Mater,'*" *Neue Zeitschrift für Musik*, Leipzig, 12/28/1841; reprinted in *Gesammelte Schrifte* I.

Walker, Frank: "*Lettere disperse e inedite di Vincenzo Bellini*," *Rivista del Comune di Catania*, Catania 10–12/1960.

────── "*Rossiniana in the Piancastelli Collection*," *Monthly Musical Record*, London, 7–8/1960, 138; 11–12/1960, 203 (Italian tr., as "*Rossiniana nella Raccolta Piancastelli*," BdCRdS 1960, 3, 41; 1960, 4, 62).

Weber, Max Maria von: "*Ein Name, besser als eine Hausnummer: Erinnerungen an K. M. von Weber und Rossini*," *Deutsche Rundschau*, 1875, 5, 257.

Weinstock, Herbert: *Donizetti and the World of Opera in Italy, Paris, and Vienna in the First Half of the Nineteenth Century*, New York and London, 1963.

Wendt, Amadeus: *Rossini's Leben und Treiben*, Leipzig, 1824.

Winternitz, Emanuel: *Musical Autographs: Monteverdi to Hindesmith*, Princeton, 1955.

Wolff, Stéphane: *see* Lejeune, André.

Woollet, H.: "*L'Art théâtrale de Mozart à Rossini*," *Le Monde musical*, Paris, 1910, 1.

Zanetti, Emilia: "*Il Conte Ory*," ROS (*q.v.*).

────── "*Motivi della vocalità rossiniana*," LRM 11/1942.

Zanolini, Antonio: *Biografia di Gioachino Rossini*, Paris, 1836 (several later editions, most importantly Siena, 1841, and Bologna, 1875, the latter including *Nuovi Ricordi* and *Una Passeggiata in compagnia di Rossini*).

────── "*Rossini e la sua musica: Una Passeggiata con Rossini, estratti dal Ricoglitore Fiorentino*," Florence, 1841.

Zavadini, Guido: *Donizetti: Vita, musiche, epistolario*, Bergamo, 1948.

Zolfanelli, Cesare: *Lettere apuane: Nuovi Studii sulla regione*, 2nd edn., Florence, 1877.

INDEXES

General Index

of Text, Notes, and List of Operas

(A separate index of Rossini's compositions begins on p. xli)

Abbiati, Franco, 479
Abdul-Aziz, Sultan of Turkey, 350
Abdul-Medjid, Sultan of Turkey, 253, 465, 469
Académie des Beaux-Arts (Paris), 134, 369, 383
Académie Philharmonique (Brussels), 192
Académie Royale (later Impériale) de Musique (Paris): *see* Opéra
Académie Royale des sciences, lettres, et beaux-arts (Brussels), 236–7
Accademia (Pesaro), 95, 99
Accademia dei Concordi (Bologna), 20, 24, 395
Accademia dei Quiriti (Rome), 476
Accademia del Real Istituto di Musica (later Conservatorio Luigi Cherubini [Florence], *q.v.*), 373
Accademia di Santa Cecilia (Rome), 395, 421
Accademia Filarmonica (Bologna), 13–14, 15, 241, 393, 395, 396, 455
Accademia Filarmonica (Rome), 507
Accademia Filarmonica (Turin), 231
Accademia Musicale Chigiana (Siena), 491
Accademia Polimniaca (Bologna), 15, 19, 395
Accademia Pontificale di Bologna, 208
Accursi (violinist, Paris), 304
Achilli, Luigi, 83

Adam, Adolphe: quoted, 160; 215; quoted, 233
Adani, Mariella, 501
Adelaide di Borgogna (libretto, Schmidt), 82, 499
Adelaide di Guesclino (ballet, Clerico), 129
Adelina (Generali), 21, 399, 424–5
Adelson e Salvini (Fioravanti), 21, 416
Adina (libretto, Bevilacqua-Aldobrandini), 89, 128, 501
Aeneid (Vergil): quoted, 86, 433
Africaine, L' (Meyerbeer), 156, 327, 472, 475, 479
Agatina (Pavesi), 72, 497
Agatina (libretto, Romani), 72, 497
Agnese di Fitz-Henry (Paër), 436
Agnesi, Luigi (Louis Agniez), 307, 324, 325, 368, 369, 467
Agniez, Louis: *see* Agnesi, Luigi
Agolini, Luca, 71, 420–1
Agoult, Marie de Flavigny, Comtesse d', 202–3
Aguado, Alexandre-Marie (Alejandro María), Marqués de las Marismas, 158, 160, 161, 177, 179, 181, 203–4, 212, 226–7, 291, 292, 442, 446, 450, 459
Aguado, Carmen, Marquesa de las Marismas, 181
Aida (Verdi), 481
Ajo nell'imbarazzo, L' (Donizetti), 402, 412, 423

Francis I, King of the Two Sicilies, 50, 64, 450
Französische Maler: über die französische Bühne (Heine), 456
Frapolli Suini, Antonietta, 406
Frascati, Tommaso, 497
Fraschi, Giovanni, 401, 491
Frazzi, Vito, 400, 491
Freischütz, Der (Weber), 114, 144, 440, 443
Frémol (male dancer, Paris), 447
Frémont, Mlle (singer, Paris), 443, 506
French Academy (Rome), 182
Freudenberg, Theophilus, 118
Frezzolini, Erminia, 229, 273, 467
Friedrich, Paul, 492
Friedrich Wilhelm III, King of Prussia, 102
Friedrich Wilhelm IV, King of Prussia, 227
From Mozart to Mario (Engel), 426, 469, 477
"*Frühlingslied*" (Moscheles), 309
Funk, Frederike, 424, 500
Furioso all'isola di San Domingo, Il (Donizetti), 442
Fusco, Cecilia, 402
Fusconi, Giuseppe, 430, 504
Fyson & Beck (solicitors, London), 141

"G. Rossini" (Bevilacqua-Aldobrandini), 435
G. Rossini: Sa vie et ses oeuvres (Azevedo), 396, 397, 404, 405; quoted, 407–8; 415, 427; quoted, 467
Gabriella di Vergy (Carafa), 416, 423
Gabrielli, Annibale: quoted, 223
Gabrielli, Conte Nicolò, 278–9
Gabussi, Vincenzo, 208, 231–2
Gaetano Donizetti (Gabrielli), 456
Gafforini, Elisabetta, 414
Galleria teatrale (Rome), 74
Gallet, Abbé: quoted, 364–5
Galli, Filippo: 31, 59; quoted, 103; 128, 129, 146, 151, 190, 401, 403, 404, 406, 408, 412, 421, 422, 429, 434, 435, 476, 491, 492, 493, 494, 495, 498, 503, 504
Gallianis, Teresa, 422, 498
Gallini, Natale, 452, 460
Gallo, Conte Cesare: quoted, 414

Galoppe d'Onquaire, 273, 304
Galvani, Giacomo, 307
Galzerani, Giovanni, 125
Gamba Papers (Ravenna), 426
Gambaro (orchestra leader, Paris), 132
Gamson, Arnold U., 497, 501
Gandolfi, Alfredo, 493, 509
Ganzarolli, Wladimiro, 505
Garcia, Manuel del Popolo Vicente, 53, 55, 56, 57, 59, 60, 62, 131, 132, 135, 137, 411, 415, 417, 418, 425, 436, 437, 476, 493, 495, 496, 497, 502
Garcia, Manuel Patricio, 329, 330, 411, 437, 476, 496
Garcia family, 496, 497, 498
Gardelli, Lamberto, 501
Gardoni, Italo, 236, 305, 306, 307, 324, 326, 345, 352, 467, 479, 480, 481
Garibaldi, A. (editor), 451
Garibaldi, Giuseppe, 301, 302, 476, 480
Garrick, David, 28
Gaspar(r)i, Gaetano (musician-bibliophile, Bologna), 229, 250, 332, 399, 482
Gasparri (sometimes Gasbarri), Gaetano (librettist, Bologna), 24, 399, 490
Gavazzeni, Gianandrea, 494
Gaveaux, Pierre, 402, 491
Gaynes, George, 498
Gazette de France, La (Paris), 132
Gazette musicale, La (Paris), 455
Gazza ladra, La (libretto, Gherardini), 75, 498
Gazzetta, La (libretto, Palomba), 65, 424, 496
Gazzetta di Milano, 116; quoted, 507
Gazzetta di Pesaro: quoted, 7
Gazzetta musicale, La (Florence), 255
Gazzetta musicale, La (Milan), 274, 402; quoted, 430; 433, 473, 482
Gazzetta musicale, La (Naples), 465
Gazzetta privilegiata di Bologna, La, 221; quoted, 244
Gazzetta privilegiata di Milano, La, 224
Gazzetta privilegiata di Venezia, La: quoted, 86, 93
Gemma di Vergy (Donizetti), 185
Genari, Francesco: quoted, 8
Generali, Pietro, 21, 31, 40, 265, 359, 424–5

Valet de chambre, Le (Carafa), 278
Valle, Giovanni, 474
Valletti, Cesare, 494, 503
Vambianchi, Arturo, 372
Vandyke, Sir Anthony, 191
Vanotti (friend of Rossini, Milan), 187
Vanzolini, Giuliano: quoted, 88; 333, 394
Varela, Manuel Fernández: *see* Fernández Varela, Manuel
Variations for one violin string on the prayer from *Mosè in Egitto* (Paganini), 484
Vaschetti, Antonio de, 505
Vasoli, Pietro, 403, 407, 408, 492, 494
Vasselli, Antonio, 223, 224, 226, 458
Vaucorbeil, Auguste-Emmanuel, 480
Vauthier (writer, Paris), 447
Vauthrot, François-Eugène, 330
Vecchi, Luigi, 372
"Vecchio Teatrofilo, Un": quoted, 9–10
Veggetti, Serafino, 222
Velluti, Giambattista (Giovanni Battista), 14, 19, 40, 102, 125, 407, 408, 434, 494
Vendetta di Nino, La (Prati), 434
Ventaglio, Il (Goldoni), 72
Ventignano, Cesare della Valle, duca di, 66, 102, 150, 317, 428, 503, 506
Ventriglia, Franco, 497
Venturi, Vincenzo, 401, 491
Vêpres siciliennes, Les (Verdi), 260, 447, 449, 465, 470
Vera-Lorini, Sofia, 474
Verconsin (writer, Paris), 330
Verdi, G., 7
Verdi, Giuseppe, xv, xvii, 15; quoted, 55–6; 67, 69, 81, 131, 160, 167, 223; quoted, 227; 229, 231, 233–4, 246, 252, 254, 255, 260; quoted, 274, 275, 280, 281, 303, 305, 307, 320–1, 326; quoted, 327; 337, 342, 344, 345, 353; quoted, 356; 358; quoted, 370, 371; 372, 373, 403, 408, 413, 417; quoted, 418; 422, 437, 443, 447; quoted, 448–9; 449, 456, 464; quoted, 465; 468, 470, 472, 473; quoted, 474; 475, 476, 479, 480, 482; quoted, 483; 483–4; quoted, 484
Verdi, Giuseppina (Strepponi): quoted, 254, 303; 326
Vergil (Publius Vergilius Maro): quoted, 86; 420, 482

Vernet, Horace, 132, 182, 451
Verni, Andrea, 72, 421, 497
Vernoy, Jules-Henri, Marquis de Saint-Georges; *see* Saint-Georges, Jules-Henri Vernoy, Marquis de
Véron, Louis-Désiré, 180
Vestale, La (Spontini), 57, 80, 99, 396
Vestri, Luigi, 104, 429
Vestris, Auguste, 437
Vestris, Auguste-Armand, 437
Vestris, Lucia Elisabeth, 135, 136–7, 437, 502
Viaggio a Reims, Il (libretto, Balocchi), 144, 247, 505, 509
Vianesi, Augusto, 326, 496
Viardot, Louis, 20
Viardot-Garcia, Pauline, 201, 215, 345, 411, 437, 476
Vicar of Wakefield, The (Goldsmith), 38
Victoria, Queen of the United Kingdom of Great Britain and Ireland, 138
Vie de Lord Byron en Italie, La (Guiccioli), 426
Vie de Rossini (Stendhal), xvii, 62, 406, 426
Vies de Haydn, Mozart et Métastase (Stendhal), 406
Viganò, Elena, 234, 461
Viganò, Salvatore, 49, 125, 234, 396
Viganò, Vincenz(in)a: *see* Mombelli, Vincenz(in)a (Viganò)
Villa Casalecchio (Bologna), 170, 172
Villa Cornetti (Bologna), 210, 232, 433
Villa Loretino (Florence), 249
Villa Normanby (Florence), 250
Villa Pellegrino (Florence), 250
Villa Rossini (Passy), 267–8, 277–8, 300, 308, 311, 316–17, 321, 323, 335, 362, 384, 466, 482
Villaret (singer, Paris), 330, 352, 471
Villet d'Epagny, Jean-Baptiste, 441
Vincentelli, Carlo, 474
Vincenzo (Rossini servant), 250
Vinci, Leonardo, 434
Vinco, Ivo, 492
Viotti, Giovanni Battista, 445
Virtuosi ambulanti, I (Fioravanti), 416, 440
Virtuosi ambulanti, I (libretto, Balocchi), 440

Index

of Rossini Compositions Mentioned in the Text, Notes, and List of Operas

A Note About the Author

HERBERT WEINSTOCK is the author of such biographical studies of composers as *Tchaikovsky* (1943), *Chopin: The Man and His Music* (1949), *Donizetti* (1963), and *Vincenzo Bellini* (1971). He is also the author (in collaboration with Wallace Brockway) of *Men of Music* and *The World of Opera*. A well-known historian and critic of the musical scene, Mr. Weinstock was, until his death in 1971, a frequent contributor to musical publications and was the New York correspondent for *Opera* (London).

A Note on the Type

The text of this book was set on the Linotype in Janson, a recutting made direct from type cast from matrices long thought to have been made by the Dutchman Anton Janson, who was a practicing type founder in Leipzig during the years 1668–87. However, it has been conclusively demonstrated that these types are actually the work of Nicholas Kis (1650–1702), a Hungarian, who most probably learned his trade from the master Dutch type founder Kirk Voskens. The type is an excellent example of the influential and sturdy Dutch types that prevailed in England up to the time William Caslon developed his own incomparable designs from these Dutch faces.

Typography by Anthea Lingeman, adapted from original design by Herbert H. Johnson.

Binding design by Anthea Lingeman